# Textbook for Midwives

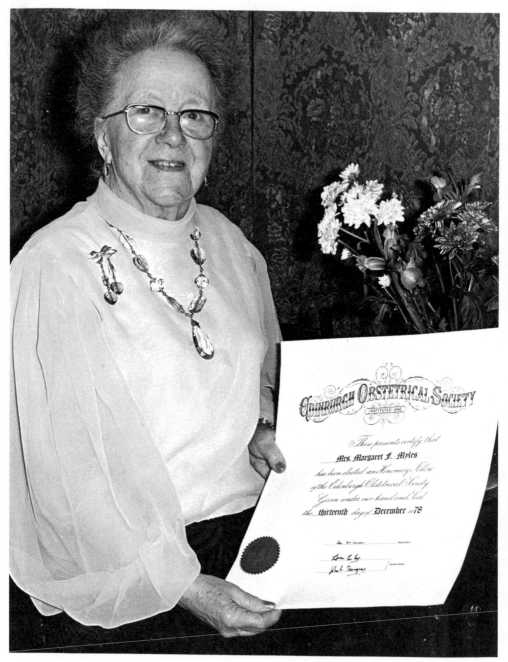

Margaret F. Myles elected an Honorary Fellow of the Edinburgh Obstetrical Society
December 1978

# Textbook for Midwives

## with modern concepts of Obstetric and Neonatal care

## Margaret F. Myles

S.R.N., S.C.M., H.V.CERT., SISTER TUTOR CERT., M.T.D.

*Formerly Examiner to Central Midwives Board, Scotland: Principal Midwife Tutor, Simpson Memorial Maternity Pavilion, Edinburgh: Director of Education, Woman's Hospital, Detroit, U.S.A.: Examiner to The Council for Midwives, Northern Ireland: Tutor, Midwife Teachers Diploma (Scot.) Course*

### *NINTH EDITION*

## CHURCHILL LIVINGSTONE

EDINBURGH LONDON MELBOURNE AND NEW YORK
1981

CHURCHILL LIVINGSTONE
Medical Division of Longman Group Limited

Distributed in the United States of America by Churchill
Livingstone Inc., 19 West 44th Street, New York, N.Y. 10036,
and by associated companies, branches and representatives
throughout the world.

| | |
|---|---|
| *First Edition* | 1953 |
| *Reprinted* | 1955 |
| *Second Edition* | 1956 |
| *Reprinted* | 1956 |
| *Third Edition* | 1958 |
| *Reprinted* | 1959 |
| *Fourth Edition* | 1961 |
| *Reprinted* | 1962 |
| *Fifth Edition* | 1964 |
| *Reprinted* | 1966 |
| *Sixth Edition* | 1968 |
| *Reprinted* | 1969 |
| *Seventh Edition* | 1971 |
| *Reprinted* | 1972 |
| *Eighth Edition* | 1975 |
| *Reprinted* | 1977 |
| *Reprinted* | 1978 |
| *Reprinted* | 1979 |
| *Ninth Edition* | 1981 |
| *ELBS Edition of Sixth* | |
| *Edition first published* | 1968 |
| *ELBS Reprinted* | 1968 |
| *ELBS Reprinted* | 1969 |
| *ELBS Edition of Seventh Edition* | 1971 |
| *ELBS Reprinted* | 1972 |
| *ELBS Reprinted* | 1974 |
| *ELBS Edition of Eighth Edition* | 1975 |
| *ELBS Reprinted* | 1976 |
| *ELBS Reprinted* | 1978 |
| *ELBS Reprinted* | 1979 |
| *ELBS Edition of Ninth Edition* | 1981 |

ISBN 0 443 02011 6 (cased)
ISBN 0 443 02010 8 (limp)

**British Library Cataloguing in Publication Data**
Myles, Margaret Fraser
  Textbook for midwives. – 9th ed.
  1. Obstetrics
  I. Title
  618.2    RG524    80–40700

Printed in Hong Kong by
C & C Joint Printing Co., (H. K.) Ltd.

# Preface to the Ninth Edition

**Massive extension of the text has been undertaken to** accommodate subject matter selected from the recent upsurge of obstetric and neonatal knowledge and the increased utilisation of ultrasonic screening devices and electronic monitors. The whole text has been updated, much of it rewritten, with alterations or additions on almost every page. Three new chapters, 124 photographs and 132 line drawings have been introduced.

**Further expansion of the midwife's role** has necessitated definitive widening of horizons and deepening of her insights. These, combined with subjects that impinge on the midwife's role, such as family centred maternity care; principles, psychology and methods of teaching; counselling, ethical problems, bonding, sex education and bereavement, have been included in the 9th edition. The modern midwife must identify personally with her extended role. This entails the cultivation of a progressive, flexible, attitude of mind: being receptive to new ideas and scientific procedures. She should manifest willingness to adopt modern concepts, such as team membership, specialisation of function and shared responsibility.

### The midwife, a team member

As a member of the obstetric team, the midwife is given more and even greater responsibility than the individual practitioner: this sanction being intellectually challenging and emotionally fulfilling. Job satisfaction is intensified by contributing to the benefits and safety that the team effort confers on mother and child.

**Throughout the text the midwife's professional heritage and traditional role as a caring, competent practitioner, have been staunchly upheld.** This does not preclude the expansion of her role to that of an obstetric team member, nor does it negate her participation in the use of modern screening, diagnostic and monitoring devices.

**Inexorably the midwife practising in the eighties must adapt to the requirements of a scientific and technological age.** To enable her to collaborate intelligently with the obstetrician, illustrations have been introduced to depict the use of up-to-date equipment. Information supplied will provide a reference source for her comprehension of monitor signals and interpretation of deviations from normal as in fetal heart rate patterns.

**As a member of the neonatal team,** the midwife requires knowledge, skill and manual dexterity to achieve proficiency in giving special and intensive care to high risk and seriously ill babies. Enhanced perception of the biochemistry and biophysics of the neonate in association with screening and diagnostic tests, intubation and pulmonary ventilation, electronic monitoring and intravenous therapy, have helped to reduce the perinatal mortality rate and improved the quality of infant life.

### Practising Midwives

**Bringing the text up-to-date will assist practising midwives in pursuing their ongoing obstetric education** and in maintaining the high level of technological competence so essential in obstetric care today. Not only must the midwife be familiar with new drugs, tests and procedures; she must also be aware of modern trends and pay attention to the reaction of expectant parents to the obstetric service provided by midwives.

**Critical appraisal of patient-midwife-relationships** and current means of communication, indicate the need to explore fresh avenues of approach. Midwives are now expected to make a more dynamic contribution to the motivation and education of expectant mothers: this has been dealt with in a new chapter on the principles and psychology of education.

**The Student Midwife**

Her educational needs during the proposed extended period of training, have been given due consideration: the wider aspects of obstetric practice having been included. Anatomical details and physiological processes are presented when such information provides a foundation on which sound obstetric practice can be established. Principles are co-related to, and integrated with, clinical practice. The new chapter containing over 1500 test-questions, will enable the student to revise and assess her knowledge and clinical competence.

To compensate for the newly qualified midwife's limited experience in coping with the understandable, but sometimes unwarranted statements, demands and objections, made by a minority of expectant mothers, suggestions are given for dealing with certain controversial subjects. Decisions on professional management should be the prerogative of the qualified person who is ultimately responsible for obstetric care as would occur in other medical disciplines. Reasoned judgment transcends emotional bias as a basis for obstetric decisions and care.

**Midwives returning to hospital practice**

After some years absence, the midwife may feel insecure and apprehensive at the prospect of participating in procedures that have recently been updated, e.g. (a) dealing with complications of pregnancy: (b) management of normal labour: (c) motivating, counselling and screening patients: (d) new tests: (e) application of metric and SI units: (f) administration of vaginal prostaglandin$_E$, topping up epidural analgesics, supervising automated i.v. drip induction: (g) intensive neo-natal care.

**This new edition provides information, explanation and illustrations that will help to extend the returning midwife's knowledge** and revive her expertise and confidence as a proficient obstetric practitioner and team member.

## SUBJECT MATTER ADDED OR AMPLIFIED

**Prenatal.** Screening for fetal growth and wellbeing: Counselling procedure; genetic and abortion, unsupported mother. Menstrual regulation. Real-time ultrasonic scanning. Kick count chart. New ideas on management of pre-eclampsia, diabetes, cardiac disease, anaemia, placental abruption, blood coagulation disorders.

**Intranatal.** Causes of onset of labour. Oxytocin challenge test. Bishop's pre induction cervical score. Induction by prostaglandin$_E$, electronic induction systems and dosage. Use of the cervicograph and partogram, foam rubber wedges. Monitoring F.H. rate pattern. Epidural management. Malpresentation. Caesarean section. Bonding.

**Neonatal.** Intubation. Pulmonary ventilation: CPAP—CNP—PEEP. Modern views on breast and bottle feeding. Neurological responses and tests. Screening. Management of low birth weight babies. Metabolic disorders. Acid base status.

**Postnatal.** 'The blues'. Psychiatric disorders. Deep vein thrombosis. Family planning. Billing's cervical mucus test.

**Miscellaneous.** Ethical problems: Family centred maternity care: Social problems and pressures: Bereavement: Sex education.

## CONTENT OF THREE NEW CHAPTERS

**Chapter 44. The Use of Medicines by Midwives.** Legislation; Regulations: CMB directives: pethidine: Addition of drugs to i.v. fluids: 'Topping up' epidural analgesics: teratogenic drugs: storage of controlled drugs: SI units.

**Chapter 47. Principles and Psychology of Education.** The learning process; arousing interest; promoting understanding; motivation, making contact; methods of learning; methods of teaching: drawing, teaching aids: discussion: demonstration: television broadcasting.

**Chapter 49. Questions for Revision and Assessment of Knowledge.** Twenty seven tests are set out, each having 40 to 70 practical questions: 'when', 'where', 'why', 'how'. Reasons why: Advice: differentiate: How 'could', 'would', 'should' you act: Method preferred: Time in minutes, hours, days, weeks. Medicines (a) condition for which prescribed, (b) pharmacological and pharmaceutical names: appliances and why used.

14 Ashley Park South           MARGARET F. MYLES
Aberdeen AB1 6RP.

# Acknowledgements

**My indebtedness to British obstetricians,** neonatologists and other medical specialists, increases with each subsequent edition. Without the benefit of their authoritative knowledge, clinical expertise, and mature judgment it would be impossible to write a balanced textbook for midwives and give an accurate account of current obstetric practice. I gladly express my thanks to those who, with exceeding courtesy, have shared the fruits of their experience and interpreted to one no longer in practice, some of the more abstruse aspects of their speciality.

**Updating the text** involves extensive perusal of contemporary obstetric and paediatric literature as well as the selection of subject matter suitable for midwives, from the vast amount of new available information. Findings are discussed with midwife colleagues who are actively engaged in the subject under consideration: when necessary the critical appraisal of a medical authority is sought prior to submission for publication.

## Visits to Maternity Hospitals

**To maintain the practical and clinical bias of the text** and to enhance its value as a source of reference on new obstetric and paediatric equipment and techniques, a number of hospitals are visited every year. This furthers my comprehension of modern obstetric concepts, procedures and mechanical devices.

**Nursing officers and ward sisters** have been most co-operative in 'setting up' for photographic demonstrations of modern procedures and the use of electronic monitoring and ultrasonic diagnostic equipment. Tutors and senior nursing officers generously discussed modern trends in patient care as well as the widening education of student midwives and the extended role of the practising midwife. To them I accord my gratitude.

**Mr K. D. Bagshawe,** F.R.C.P., Director of Medical Oncology, Charing Cross Hospital (Fulham), London, scrutinised with precision the section on Choriocarcinoma and gave advice re cytotoxic chemotherapy. For the procedure advocated by this world authority my gratefulness is profound.

**Miss Sarah Roch,** Senior Nursing Officer (Teaching), Maternity Section, Southampton General Hospital, has been resourceful and indefatigable in her response to requests for information and the verification of facts and figures. With exactitude she has translated mg to mmol throughout the text and has made an admirable contribution in presenting the English aspects of obstetric practice, the National Health Service and drug usage and legislation. Miss Roch has diligently scrutinised the page proofs and made some desirable recommendations, also participating in updating the index. For her interest, industry and collaboration I extend my appreciation and thanks.

**Professor Ian Macgillivray** generously allowed me to visit Aberdeen Maternity Hospital, observe new procedures and photograph modern equipment. It gives me pleasure to acknowledge this privilege.

**Professor A. G. M. Campbell** has given me every opportunity to update my knowledge of intensive neonatal care and permitted me to take photographs depicting some topical procedures carried out in his department in Aberdeen Maternity Hospital. For this courtesy I gratefully record my thanks.

**Professor Arnold Klopper,** Department of Endocrinology of Reproduction, is an eminent authority on this subject. For his explanation of the hormonal treatment of anovular infertility, the feto-placental unit and other aspects of obstetric endocrinology, I have much pleasure in expressing my appreciation.

**Professor J. M. Stowers,** Diabetic Department, Aberdeen Royal Infirmary, cordially afforded me the benefit of his erudite knowledge and specialised clinical acumen in revising the section on diabetes in pregnancy. With exceeding courtesy he read and amended the final proofs. For his patience in lucidly amplifying many enigmatic points and for applying biochemical principles to practical procedures I gratefully record my indebtedness.

**Dr M. E. Tunstall,** the obstetric anaesthetist, Aberdeen, who initiated Entonox, has had extensive experience in his speciality. He read the script with assiduous care and gave me wise counsel on the various forms of obstetric analgesia, including epidural. I record with thanks his excellent advice on the prevention of Mendelson's syndrome and on the preparation of the patient for anaesthesia. It is a pleasure to express my gratitude for his courteous professional guidance and help.

**Dr Vijay Jandial,** Consultant Obstetrician, Aberdeen is a reliable source of theoretical and clinical obstetric knowledge. His courteous response to requests for elucidation of obscure problems and the practical application of academic information deserves commendation. I acknowledge with thanks his professional advice.

**Dr D. J. Lloyd,** Consultant Paediatrician, Aberdeen, gave helpful counsel and constructive criticism on the section devoted to intensive care of the neonate. He made a number of up-to-date recommendations regarding the treatment of serious disorders and by his lucidity of exposition, several complicated conditions and scientific procedures were illuminated and clarified. For his competent professional advice I record my appreciation.

**Dr H. W. Rutherford,** Physician-in-Charge, Department of Sexually Transmitted Diseases, Royal Infirmary, Aberdeen, read with precise care the section on his speciality concerning the pregnant woman and neonate. For bringing treatment in line with modern concepts and making other pertinent recommendations, I tender my thanks.

**Dr J. K. Finlayson,** Consultant Cardiologist, Aberdeen scrutinised the script with cognitive vigilance and made a number of beneficial amendments: e.g. that the four grades of functional capacity are no longer relied on as a prognostic criterion or a guide to management. His recommendations for care of the woman with cardiac impairment throughout pregnancy, labour and the puerperium include much wise guidance and prudent counsel. For Dr Finlayson's exceeding courtesy in sharing some of his expert knowledge and experience, I express my appreciation and thanks.

**Dr John R. C. Logie,** when Senior Registrar in the Department of Vascular Surgery at Aberdeen Royal Infirmary, scanned the section on Venous Thrombosis and made a number of valid recommendations for improvement. These involved a more modern approach to diagnostic techniques and to the essential features of management; including that of thrombo-pulmonary embolism. For his assistance, I record my gratitude.

**Miss M. Turner,** Divisional Nursing Officer (Midwifery) cordially welcomed me to the Aberdeen Maternity Hospital. With gracious competence she arranged for the setting up of photographs to be taken in various departments depicting contemporary obstetric and neonatal practice. Her observations on the wider aspects of the education and role of the modern midwife were perceptive: her timely suggestions on patient care were commendable and enlightened. With appreciation, I record my indebtedness to her.

**Miss M. MacKay,** Senior Nursing Officer (Teaching), and her colleagues Miss D. Reid and Miss M. Watt, read some of the proofs and made a number of relevant recommendations. For their interest and discerning advice, I express my appreciation.

**Miss Ruth Allan,** Nursing Officer, Abderdeen Neonatal Intensive Care Unit, magnanimously shared with me some of the expertise she has acquired during her extensive clinical experience, based on scientific knowledge, of low birth weight and 'high risk' babies. In her unit the concept of 'tender loving care' (T.L.C.) is personalised: babies who are receiving mechanical aids to respiration, nutrition, or being monitored electronically, are given almost constant devoted nursing care. I gladly register my thanks to Miss Allan.

**Dr John Horn,** Chest Physician, City Hospital, Edinburgh, gave from his expert knowledge and extensive experience, professional advice to bring the section on Pulmonary Tuberculosis in line with modern thought and practice. For his prudent counsel given with lucidity and benevolence, I record my thanks.

**Dr. John L. Cox,** Senior Lecturer, University Department of Psychiatry (Royal Edinburgh Hospital), read the script on psychiatric disorders with skill and discernment. From his knowledge and experience of psychiatric illness in childbearing women and his intense interest in the mentally disturbed postnatal woman, he advised some radical amendments to the section on depressive illness in the puerperium. For his expert guidance and counsel and the elucidation of some concepts relating to organic psychoses, I express my appreciation and thanks.

**Miss A. S. Grant,** Education Officer, Central Midwives Board (Scotland), has read the text and amended sections on which she has expert knowledge and professional experience, i.e. The Central Midwives Board (Scot.) directives and code of practice, The Education of the Student Midwife, The National Health Service (Scot.), Social Aspects of Obstetrics. Miss Grant read and corrected the page proofs with her customary diligence and meticulous care and has made a number of invaluable recommendations. For her continued assistance and co-operation, I gratefully express my thanks.

**Miss Elizabeth Venters,** Labour Ward Sister, Simpson Memorial Maternity Pavilion, Edinburgh, has made a worth while contribution to the section of the book devoted to operative obstetrics. She has verified and when necessary corrected lists of instruments and other equipment. Her instructions on induction of labour by i.v. infusion of Syntocinon is an example of her painstaking work. While Labour Ward Sister recently in Aberdeen, she assisted in the setting up of photographic demonstrations of obstetric procedures. I am most appreciative of her expert assistance and collaboration in updating the aspects of operative procedures that are of interest to midwives.

**Miss M. E. Herbertson,** Nursing Officer, renal dialysis unit, Royal Infirmary, Edinburgh, read and revised the section on acute renal failure. For her excellent counsel based on extensive clinical experience, I express my appreciation.

**Miss M. M. Grieve,** Divisional Nursing Officer (midwifery) Forth Park Maternity Hospital, Kirkcaldy, gave me every opportunity to observe some modern clinical obstetric procedures. Aided by the tutorial staff and ward sisters, she was indefatigable in demonstrating obstetric operative situations for illustrative purposes. My thanks are willingly expressed.

**Mrs B. B. Maclennan,** Principal Nursing Officer and **Miss E. Creighton,** Senior Nursing Officer (Teaching), Royal Maternity Hospital, Rottenrow, Glasgow, were cordial and most cooperative in setting up photographic demonstrations in the neonatal intensive care unit and other departments. I am deeply grateful for their timely suggestions and comments on current obstetrical techniques and educational trends.

**Professor Forrester Cockburn** Queen Mother's Hospital Glasgow has been a source of enlightenment on the specialised care of low birth weight babies and other neonates at 'high risk'. I acknowledge my obligation for his elucidation of various biochemical haematological and other investigations and express my thanks for his courtesy.

**Dr N. P. Robinson,** when in charge of the Department of Diagnostic Ultrasonics, Queen Mother's Hospital, courteously explained some of the rudiments of ultrasonography to me, including the use of the portable real-time scanner. For his kindness in supplying a series of ultrasound illustrations for the text, I am deeply grateful. To Dr Robinson, who is now in Melbourne, Australia, I tender my thanks.

**Miss M. E. Marr,** Divisional Nursing Officer (Midwifery), was most helpful in arranging visits to the various departments of the Queen Mother's Hospital. With courtesy and proficiency her staff set up procedures for photography. Miss Marr's competence, and resourcefulness enhanced the illustrative and educational value of the subject being documented. Her progressive approach to the midwife's education and role was manifest at all levels. I record my indebtedness with gratitude.

**Miss S. P. O. Bramley,** Divisional Nursing Officer (Midwifery), Bellshill Maternity Hospital, Larnarkshire, with her customary enthusiasm and ingenuity, did her utmost to ensure the successful presentation for photography of practical obstetrical and neonatal techniques, as well as demonstrations of health teaching and education for parenthood. I extend my sincere thanks to Miss Bramley, the tutorial staff and sisters who so ably assisted in coping with the various projects.

**Miss P. M. Forrest,** Divisional Nursing Officer, Forth Valley Maternity Hospital, Stirling, with intuitive skill combined with resolute industriousness, organised the setting up of various teaching situations and elicited the participation of a number of expectant parents. **Miss Forbes Walker** and other members of the tutorial staff collaborated in providing the educational aids. To them I express my sincere thanks.

### Illustrations and Production

**Mr T. McFetters,** Photographer, Department of Obstetrics, University of Edinburgh, produced over 100 photographs taken at various hospitals in Scotland. His technical proficiency is manifest in the excellent photographs depicted throughout the text. The author's efforts were enhanced by his willing co-operation, calm assurance and admirable tolerance in the inexorable demands for exactitude with equipment and naturalness in situations involving midwives, expectant parents, and he deserves the high praise I am delighted to give.

**Mr R. A. Morton,** Director of Medical Illustrations, University of Aberdeen, is responsible for the photographs taken at Aberdeen Maternity Hospital and in the Department of Medical Illustration. For his co-operation and unremitting efforts to achieve the highest possible standard of clinical excellence I express my thanks.

**Mr Edward Smith,** when in the Department of Medical Illustration, University of Aberdeen, made a unique visual contribution to this the 9th edition of the text. His patient co-operation, intelligent approach, acute perception and meticulous draughtsmanship have been combined in the execution of over 130 illustrations. The serial delineations of certain of his ideas are effective and most commendable. I gratefully record my thanks for his artistic skill in the pictorial clarification of points verbally obscure.

**The publishers deserve great credit** for the masterly way in which this edition has been prepared for publication. Mr A. D. Lewis, Director of Production, deserves special mention for his unfailing good advice and forbearance throughout a long and arduous operation. I deeply appreciate the scope given to me as author. Mr Graham Birnie, Editor, has shown perceptive comprehension in dealing with the manuscript and proofs. To all members of Churchill Livingstone and the printers who have contributed to the preparation for publication of this the 9th edition, I have pleasure in expressing my grateful thanks.

M.F.M.

# CONTENTS

# 1
# Orientation to the British Midwife

*The midwife's role:* (a) *member of the obstetric team,* (b) *competent practitioner,* (c) *teacher. Evolution and education. Preventive concept of maternity care. Duties imposed by Statute. Some procedures and drugs sanctioned by the Central Midwives Boards. Specialised duties and responsibilities. Midwife versus obstetric nurse. Maintaining her identity. Need for professional midwives in developing and in affluent countries. International definition of a midwife. Family centred maternity care.*

The British midwife, a highly competent professional woman, is legally licensed as a practitioner of normal obstetrics. During pregnancy she supervises and teaches the expectant mother; throughout labour she makes observations, examinations and decisions on which maternal and fetal life and wellbeing depend; having delivered the baby she attends to mother and child during the postnatal period. Should a complication arise she gives emergency treatment pending the arrival of the doctor.

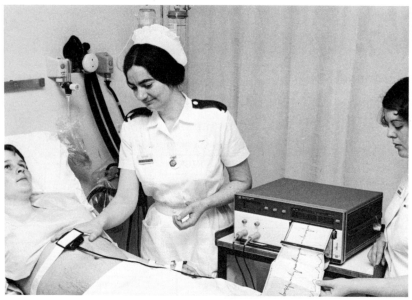

Fig. 1-1   Modern midwife palpating for uterine tonus. Uterine contractions monitored by an external pressure transducer on the abdomen. Fetal heart rate recorded via an ECG electrode on the fetal scalp.

*Hewlett Packard Cardiotocograph model 8030A*
*Aberdeen Maternity Hospital.*

In preparation for her onerous responsibilities the midwife receives a comprehensive, sound, professional education; deep knowledge of the physiological processes of human reproduction being an essential foundation for proficient obstetric practice. During her training, adequate clinical experience is provided to

1

enable her to acquire manual dexterity in carrying out the various examinations and skills associated with childbirth.

The modern midwife requires a degree of expertise in the use of the electronic monitoring equipment which has added a new dimension to the management of labour by improving the quality of fetal life and the safety of mother and child.

## THE ROLE OF THE MIDWIFE

The basic role of the British professional midwife was originally that of a 'delivery woman' who practised independently and gave rudimentary maternity care, proficient but minimal by modern standards. This role has been superseded. The midwife's knowledge has been greatly extended; fresh insights having enabled her to adapt her role in order to keep pace with the scientific advances in obstetrics and neonatology. To meet the needs of an enlightened community with improved socio-economic standards the midwife has adopted the wider concepts of obstetric care, i.e. social, educational and psychological. Her understanding of behavioural science is applied to patient and family.

Only when seconded to developing countries, where medical, technological and financial resources are not available to administer high-quality maternity care, would the midwife revert to the basic 'delivery woman' role. It would now be considered a retrograde step for a midwife to take sole charge of an expectant mother, thereby depriving her of the scientific expert care that only the obstetric team can provide. Delivery in hospital is strongly advocated and over 96 per cent of babies in England and 99·5 per cent in Scotland are born in hospital.

### The midwife, a member of the obstetric team

The modern role of the midwife is that of a team member, functioning within an obstetric unit,. The central team with whom she collaborates consists of an obstetrician, anaesthetist and paediatrician. Surrounding this central core is a group of authorities each member having expert knowledge of the obstetric or paediatric implications of his speciality. A supportive team of obstetric and neonatal

THE MIDWIFE

A MEMBER OF THE OBSTETRIC TEAM

paediatric nurses provides some of the basic nursing care. Health visitors maintain close liaison with the maternity hospital and assist with health education and in family planning programmes. The general practitioner and the community midwife are members of the primary health care team and co-operate in the provision of prenatal care and undertake the postnatal supervision of mothers and babies transferred from hospital 24-48 hours after delivery.

### The neonatal paediatric team

The midwife is an efficient member of the neonatal intensive care team: her knowledge of obstetric conditions that put the fetus at 'high risk' gives her added awareness of the significance of neonatal disorders. She assists the paediatrician in carrying out biochemical, haematological and neurological investigations, Rh replacement transfusion, monitoring respiratory disorders and caring for preterm babies.

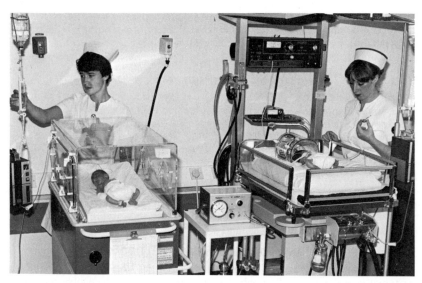

Fig. 1-2   Neonatal intensive care unit. On left, preterm baby with RDS in Vickers 79 servo incubator receiving i.v. laevulose 20 per cent monitored by Ivac 53. On right, baby RDS in Ohio intensive baby care centre receiving positive pressure from Vickers CPAP: perspex chamber over head. On table, Vickers continuous positive airway pressure alarm.

*Bellshill Maternity Hospital, Lanarkshire.*

### The midwife, a teacher of expectant mothers

This is one of the definitive and most exigent roles of the modern midwife, who by giving appropriate instruction can motivate and prepare prospective mothers to fulfil their reproductive and maternal roles successfully and happily. The Central Midwives Boards require that student midwives shall receive instruction on the principles and methods of education as well as practice in teaching mothers-to-be subjects such as health education, nutrition, preparation for childbirth, baby care and development. The midwife also gives counsel to parents of babies with a congenital handicap, and participates in family planning programmes by advising, motivating and encouraging.

**The midwife in a supportive role** provides professional companionship and demonstrates a 'caring' attitude as an integral part of good obstetric practice. Her presence is assuring and comforting to the woman in labour who is aware of the midwife's competence to deliver the baby in the doctor's absence. Physical safety engenders emotional security.

## THE MIDWIFE, A COMPETENT PRACTITIONER

One of the assets of the British midwife is her ability as a craftswoman; the tendency in some quarters to denigrate this fundamental faculty is to be deprecated. Her clinical expertise in anticipating as well as recognising an abnormal situation, appreciating the necessity for medical assistance and coping with an obstetric or neonatal emergency is one area in which her supremacy is irrefutable. The midwife's professional education provides a rich soil that germinates clinical acumen, proficiency in specialised skills, prudent judgment and behavioural insights. Technical facility in the manipulation and interpretation of electronic monitors and other diagnostic devices is an essential component of the midwife's clinical competence in this technological age. Mechanical equipment extends the midwife's powers of observation and thereby improves the physical and mental quality of fetal and neonatal life. Although childbirth is safer and has been made easier than at any previous time this can only be achieved by diligent supervision and vigilant perceptive observation.

### EVOLUTION OF THE BRITISH MIDWIFE 1902–1974

Since 1902 when the first Midwives Act was passed and the Central Midwives Board was set up as the statutory body governing the training, certification and practice of midwives in England, it has been illegal for any midwife to practise there unless qualified and State Certified.

During the first twenty years of this century the midwife was an economic necessity; practising in the homes of the socially less privileged groups who could not afford a doctor's fee. The midwife at that time, defiantly aware of her legal position as an independent practitioner, staunchly defended that right. During this period prenatal care was practically non-existent; other than delivering the baby the midwife's abilities were mainly directed to dealing with obstetric tragedies such as obstructed labour, haemorrhage and sepsis.

## EDUCATIONAL DEVELOPMENT OF THE MIDWIFE

Horizons in obstetric care widened as scientific, social, educational and psychological influences were applied to the management of childbearing. Midwives realised that they could no longer function effectively as independent practitioners. Only doctors could make the diagnostic tests and provide the therapeutic aids so beneficial to mother and child. Existing basic concepts were not sufficient: the midwife needed fresh insights to broaden her outlook.

**The Central Midwives Board** since 1902 has consistently increased the content of the student midwives' curriculum and lengthened the prescribed period of training in order that the standard of midwifery as practised by midwives would be maintained at a high level. The Central Midwives Boards also stipulate that every practising midwife shall attend a full-time refresher course lasting four days every five years: some elect to attend a two weeks hospital course.

**The Midwives Institute**, now the Royal College of Midwives, recognised the need for properly qualified midwife tutors, well informed in regard to expanding obstetric knowledge and therapeutic procedures. Teaching facilities also needed amplification and greater utilisation of modern educational methods. With admirable vision the Midwives Institute in 1926 introduced the Midwife Teachers Diploma for which a course of instruction was given jointly by the College of Nursing and the Institute. The Central Midwives Board took over responsibility for the examination in 1931. This Diploma, not lightly awarded, is obtained annually by approximately 80 candidates who must be experienced midwives from authorised training schools. A prescribed course of instruction, with University or other Educational Institution affiliation, must be attended prior to the examination.

**A critical period in the educational evolution of the British midwife ensued.** Fortunately a sense of perspective was maintained and although her role was expanded to provide a more positive scientific approach and to incorporate the preventive, social and supportive aspects as well as giving health education and providing family-centred, high-quality maternity care her basic function as an obstetric practitioner always remained dominant. The student midwives' curriculum was orientated primarily to comprehension of the sound principles and practice of obstetrics; to the inculcation of desirable supportive attitudes and to gaining manual dexterity in the essential skills. By steadfastly fostering clinical instruction and applying knowledge to diligent supervision the midwife has developed an enviable standard in the skill of perceptive observation. Her proficiency in practical obstetrics gives her job satisfaction as well as the desire and the fortitude to practise with confidence even in remote areas.

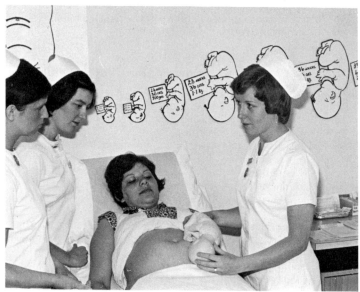

Fig. 1-3  Student midwives receiving clinical instruction on abdominal examination at the midwives prenatal clinic.

*Maternity Hospital, Stirling.*

## THE PREVENTIVE CONCEPT OF MATERNITY CARE

When socio-economic standards improved, the community became receptive to health education and more interested in maternity care and child welfare. Factors such as the introduction of the National Health Service, the obstetric team concept; more intensive supervision during pregnancy and the increased antenatal beds available for complications of pregnancy combined with improved nutrition and education for parenthood have helped to enhance the quality of maternity care. Active measures have reduced the maternal and perinatal mortality rates.

**The introduction of the National Health Service in 1948** made the provision of a doctor and a midwife for every pregnant woman in Britain compulsory. Although the midwife still retains her legal right to practise midwifery, her employing authority will require her to function in collaboration with the doctor who can and does delegate part of the maternity care to her, including delivery of the baby.

## DUTIES IMPOSED ON THE BRITISH MIDWIFE BY STATUTE

**By Act of Parliament.** Eng. 1902. Scot. 1915, the midwife is given legal sanction to practise. The Central Midwives Board Rules 1951 regulating, supervising and restricting the practice of midwives (within due limits) must be observed.

**Registration of Births and Deaths Act.** In default of the parents the midwife, in Britain, may have to register the baby's birth. In certain circumstances she may issue a certificate of stillbirth.

**Notification of Births Act.** The midwife notifies the birth or stillbirth to the Chief Administrative Medical Officer of the Area: Health Authority (Eng.), Health Board (Scot.) within 36 hours of birth.

**Certificate of expected confinement** and of confinement can be given by the midwife to enable the woman to claim the Maternity Allowance and the Maternity Grant from the Department of Health and Social Security.

**Population Statistics Act.** The midwife states the cause of stillbirth (if known).

**Misuse of Drugs Amendment Regulations 1974** permits community midwives to prescribe pethidine for the relief of pain in labour.

## Some Drugs and Procedures sanctioned by the Central Midwives Board(s)

**Inhalational analgesia.** The midwife must be competent to administer appropriate inhalational analgesics during labour, e.g. Entonox, Penthrane.

Administration of pethidine by community midwives. Pentazocine (Fortral), Trilene. In England promazine (Sparine).

To control postabortum and postpartum haemorrhage the midwife may administer ergometrine or Syntometrine intravenously.

The midwife is permitted to 'top up' epidural analgesic drugs if she has been suitably instructed, but must not administer the initial dose.

In Scotland the midwife may 'top up' prostaglandins being given by the extra amniotic route.

**Episiotomy** may be made by the midwife under local analgesia (lignocaine). Repair of episiotomy or perineal laceration may be performed by the midwife if she has received instruction and the doctor is satisfied that she is proficient. The doctor must take the responsibility.

**Intubating the asphyxiated baby** is permitted if the midwife has been properly trained to do so.

### SPECIALISED DUTIES OF THE MIDWIFE

#### (Compared with those of the obstetric nurse)

In order to compare the functions of the midwife with those of the obstetric nurse the following abridged account of some of the midwife's professional responsibilities and obligations is set out. The more simple routine skills are too numerous to mention: the wider aspects of her role have already been stated in this chapter.

**The obstetric nurse** gives nursing care under the jurisdiction of the doctor who makes all diagnoses and decisions. Her theoretical knowledge of the complex processes of reproduction and the brief period of clinical practice allotted during her training do not provide a sound foundation on which subsequent experience becomes perceptive and meaningful. The obstetric nurse is neither qualified nor competent to deliver the baby; neither is she capable of coping with an obstetric or neonatal emergency.

**The midwife** is more than a nurse; she is a practitioner of normal obstetrics qualified to make diagnoses and decisions that are based on knowledge, experience and judgment. She supervises normal pregnancy and labour and delivers the baby. The midwife also recognises an abnormal situation, appreciates the need for obtaining medical assistance and deals proficiently with complications; giving obstetric first aid treatment in an emergency until the doctor's arrival. It is obvious that her professional education and clinical skill must transcend that of the obstetric nurse.

### Some diagnoses the midwife makes

That the woman is pregnant and period of gestation. Screening for 'high risk' conditions, e.g. pre-eclampsia and diabetes that necessitate medical aid, abnormal presentation of the fetus, cephalo-pelvic disproportion, fetal growth, fetal death, twins. The midwife's expertise in performing abdominal and vaginal examinations is an admirable aid in diagnosis, e.g. to assess the onset and progress of labour, spontaneous, induced and accelerated.

**Some congenital abnormalities** and complications which the midwife must diagnose and deal with are asphyxia, intracranial injury, oesophageal and anal atresia, the light for date baby.

### Prevention and management of emergencies

Anticipation and early recognition of conditions that would give rise to emergencies constitute modern preventive practice, a concept which surpasses concentration on the active treatment of established complications, e.g. shoulder presentation, fetal distress, prolapse of cord, rupture of uterus. Some emergencies are so urgent that immediate action must be taken to support or save life, e.g. controlling postpartum haemorrhage, intubating the severely asphyxiated baby. Although plans are made to deliver twins and babies presenting by the breech in hospital, labour may be preterm, or the condition undiagnosed, so midwives must be competent to cope proficiently with such cases.

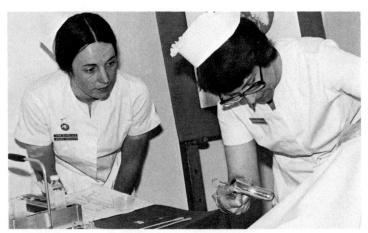

Fig. 1-4 Taking Papanicolaou smear at midwives prenatal clinic.
*Maternity Hospital, Stirling.*

### Conditions demanding specialised obstetric care

The following complications occur only in association with pregnancy, their skilful treatment therefore being appropriate to midwives: eclampsia, antepartum haemorrhage, hydatidiform mole.

Supervising a woman under epidural analgesia whose labour is being accelerated by oxytocin via an electronic infusion unit and monitored by cardiotocograph demands obstetric efficiency and technological expertise.

**Obstetric and paediatric investigations the midwife participates in** are abdominal amniocentesis for (*a*) genetic anomalies, (*b*) bilirubin, (*c*) lecithin sphingomyelin ratio. Serial oestriol assays. Neonatal neurological responses, blood chemistry, metabolic disorders, rubella antibodies, cervical cytology. Guthrie, Kleihauer, Dextrostix, and Uricult tests.

### MAINTAINING THE IDENTITY OF THE MIDWIFE

The midwife should be accorded the status and prestige of her own profession: submerging her in public health administration negates her role. This sometimes occurs when midwives seconded to developing countries are required to concern themselves with environmental health and the epidemiology of disease when the urgent need is to diminish the tragic sequelae of poor obstetric practice. That the midwife is the only available person with medical knowledge does not justify fragmenting or dissipating her professional talents: she should be allowed to function to her full potential as a midwife.

## THE NEED FOR PROFESSIONAL MIDWIVES IN DEVELOPING COUNTRIES

In underdeveloped and developing countries the need for qualified midwives is greatest. Approximately 80 million babies are born in the world every year and 50 million women receive no obstetric care from a doctor or professional midwife; the babies being delivered by neighbours or traditional birth attendants (T.B.A.). These attendants have had no midwifery training nor have they any conception of the need for cleanliness. Obstetric disasters are commonplace; medical help not usually being sought until labour has lasted for more than three days or the placenta not having been expelled within 12 hours. Obstructed labour, rupture of uterus, haemorrhage and sepsis cause extensive loss of maternal and infant life. These countries need help.

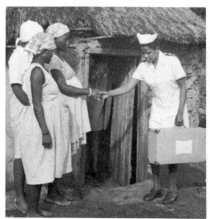 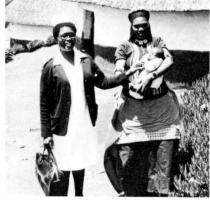

Fig. 1-5  Professional African midwife from Mosvold Mission Hospital, Ingwavuma, Natal, arrives to give prenatal care to Zulu women.

Fig. 1-6  Professional African midwife from Murchison Mission Hospital, Port Shepstone, Natal, visiting one of the babies she delivered.

**Midwives seconded to developing countries** should have received a professional education that equipped them to be capable practitioners; obstetric acumen and practical experience being of more value than erudition in ancillary subjects such as bio-statistics and social science. The midwives must be adaptable, resourceful and sufficiently imaginative to appreciate the influence of culture and tradition on the outlook of the people. Racial or tribal customs and religious scruples that dictate practices concerned with reproduction should be studied and respected, otherwise resentment is created. As many as 40 fast days are imposed by some tribes and meat and eggs are forbidden during pregnancy. Existing methods of practice should be subjected to critical appraisal and not condemned outright: it being prudent to build on the best as a foundation for future projects. The temptation to set up a replica of the regimen the midwife has been accustomed to must be strenuously resisted. She should not expect her ideas and methods to be accepted just because they are modern; they may not be practicable for various reasons, viz. financial, political, medical, cultural or climatic.

Midwives should be able and willing to function at basic level if required; teaching the traditional birth attendants in the homes during labour. Gaining the good will of the traditional birth attendants is absolutely essential for without their co-operation very little will be accomplished: care being taken not to undermine their prestige in the village community. Observing them at work will reveal undesirable practices such as using cow dung as an umbilical dressing. Advance should be made slowly with patience and tact: a pleasant manner surmounts many obstacles. Although the abolition of obstetric disasters will be high on the list of priorities, community health education should proceed concurrently. Extending the teaching of health into the homes will help to eradicate the causes of anaemia and the infectious diseases that undermine the health of child-bearing women and their babies. Progress should proceed from grass roots level upwards as well as from governmental administrative level downwards.

## THE NEED FOR PROFESSIONAL MIDWIVES IN AFFLUENT COUNTRIES

It is quite erroneous to believe that professional midwives are only needed in underdeveloped lands: in fact some opulent, highly developed countries have areas that are obstetrically underdeveloped, where non-professional midwives deliver

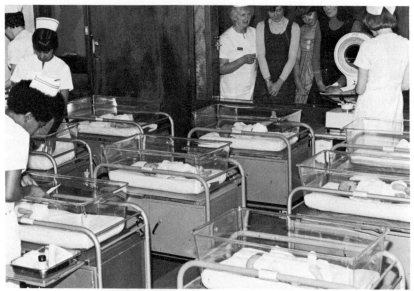

Fig. 1–7    Parenthood class having a preview of the nursery.
*Bellshill Maternity Hospital, Lanarkshire.*

thousands of babies every year. Other sophisticated countries have vast, isolated areas in which sheer distance precludes the doctor's attendance. In large cities immigrants tend to congregate and some of the expectant mothers neither seek nor receive the attention of a doctor: neighbours acting as midwives. It has been traditional in some well-developed countries where the ratio of doctors to population is high or the distance from specialised obstetric units prohibitive, for maternity care to be undertaken by a doctor with an obstetric nurse in attendance. Such an arrangement may have been acceptable when obstetric knowledge was limited and the team concept had not evolved, but the tremendous upsurge in obstetric and neonatal paediatric knowledge, to which has been applied advances in anaesthesiology, immunology, haematology, technology, genetics, bacteriology, ultrasonography, biochemistry and biophysics, has changed the pattern of administering maternity care. The collaboration of these medical and scientific experts who apply their specialised knowledge in saving and improving the quality of maternal, fetal and infant life demands concomitant obstetric nursing care of a high order. The midwife has proved to be an able member of such a team.

Educational concepts are now woven into the fabric of maternity care but many women in highly civilised countries do not receive adequate prenatal instruction on how to maintain fetal and maternal wellbeing during pregnancy, to enable them to cope successfully during labour and to fulfil their maternal role in caring for their baby's physical, mental and emotional development. Those in the upper income groups should not be deprived of the high-quality maternity care currently being provided for those in less well favoured circumstances.

## Groups who could be motivated to accept professional midwives

**The medical profession.** Doctors who have not been accustomed to the collaboration of professional midwives should reconsider the modern situation in which midwives are supplementary to and not substitutes for the doctor. They are an extension of his eyes, ears and hands, and helpful assistants in abnormal and operative obstetrics.

**The nursing profession.** Recent advances and radical changes in maternity care must surely create doubt as to whether existing patterns of obstetric nursing care are adequate. An exchange of innovative ideas on the provision of high-quality maternity care might reveal that the services of professional midwives would be beneficial to childbearing women.

**The community.** Prospective mothers have been enlightened regarding the need for, but not the quality of, maternity care. They ought to be given an authentic image of the modern professional midwife as a highly proficient obstetric team member. They should also be aware that the midwife's services are in addition to and not instead of the doctor's care. The outmoded idea that the midwife is second rate should be eradicated.

**For rich or poor, in every sphere, professional midwives are needed.**

### DEFINITION OF THE WORD MIDWIFE

The word 'midwife' is derived from the Anglo-Saxon words 'mid' = together with, and 'wif' = a woman. Literally it means a helping woman. The word 'obstetrics' includes midwifery: the Latin derivation being 'ob' = before and 'sto' = to stand. From usage the word 'obstetrics' has assumed a wider connotation than midwifery: being associated with the scientific and more advanced concepts of human reproduction.

### INTERNATIONAL DEFINITION OF A MIDWIFE

*The following definition was accepted by the Council of the International Confederation of Midwives (I.C.M.) at their 16th International Congress in November 1972 held in Washington U.S.A. It was also accepted by the 7th Ceneral Assembly of the International Federation of Gynaecology and Obstetrics (F.I.G.O.) which took place in August 1973, in Moscow.*

'A midwife is a person who, having been regularly admitted to a midwifery educational programme, duly recognised in the country in which it is located, has successfully completed the prescribed course of studies in midwifery and has acquired the requisite qualifications to be registered and/or legally licenced to

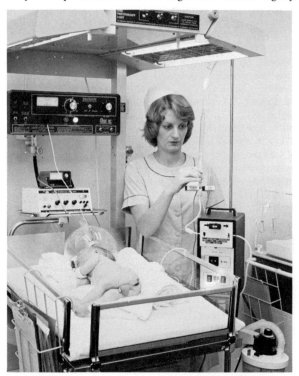

Fig. 1-8 Baby with intracranial injury in Ohio intensive care centre, glass oxygen head box. On top (a) Servo control, (b) apnoea alarm, (c) $O_2$ analyser. Lower right, Bennett humidifier. Midwife adjusting flow of milk.

*Aberdeen Maternity Hospital.*

practise midwifery. She must be able to give the necessary supervision, care and advice to women during pregnancy, labour and the post-partum period, to conduct deliveries on her own responsibility and to care for the new born and the infant. This care includes preventive measures, the detection of abnormal conditions in mother and child, the procurement of medical assistance and the execution of emergency measures in the absence of medical help. She has an important task in health counselling and education, not only for patients but also within the family and the community. The work should involve ante-natal education and preparation for parenthood and extend to certain areas of gynaecology, family planning and child care. She may practise in hospitals, clinics, health units, domiciliary conditions or in any other service.'

## FAMILY CENTRED MATERNITY CARE

**This modern concept extends the role of the midwife** beyond the provision of obstetric care *per se* and takes cognizance of the pregnant woman in the family and home situation; not just as a parturient individual.

Throughout the text promotive and therapeutic aspects of health and maternity care that concern the family, and are within the jurisdiction of the midwife, have been dealt with, e.g. health education, nutrition, keeping fit, the expectant and the new father, home confinement, baby care, breast feeding, immunisation, the toddler and the new baby, family planning, accidents in the home and the prevention of non-accidental injury.

### The midwife, a counsellor

**Midwives should be concerned with the wider features of family life** which incorporate the behavioural sciences, moral codes, and the enhancement of emotional as well as healthful living. Childbearing and child rearing are greatly influenced by human relationships within the family: both parents may need counsel regarding this.

At the present time, the stability of family life is being threatened, i.e. parental obligations are not always adequately fulfilled, marital infidelity, desertion and divorce being increasingly common. The midwife has such an intimate association with the pregnant woman that she should utilise the opportunity to counsel her re the establishment of a secure, happy home by giving sensible, practical advice on how to accomplish this.

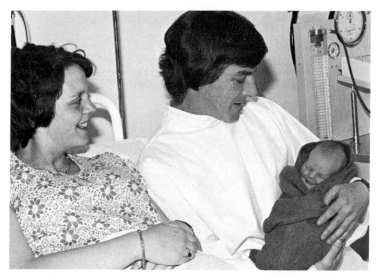

Fig. 1-9   Bonding process obviously successful: one hour after birth.
*Maternity Hospital, Stirling.*

### MARRIAGE

Society has proved that when people marry and set up a nuclear family, this is in the best interests of the children during their years of dependence and education. Having entered matrimony as a loving, trusting relationship, most women appreciate the durability of the commitment and the security of the emotional anchorage it provides. Marriage is a relationship with social, emotional, sexual, intellectual and spiritual aspects: good companionship and shared interests should be advocated as a basis for living together amicably.

**Harmonious human relationships** depend greatly on personal qualities such as kindliness, unselfishness and consideration. Approval or admiration should be freely expressed; carping criticism and nagging avoided.

**Qualities of character that enable husband and wife to be faithful to their marriage vows,** should be fostered and appreciated. Wives should be advised to create a pleasant, comfortable home and to endeavour to acquire some culinary expertise. Both should contribute in promoting a congenial marital environment and furthering the establishment of a home that is an admirable abode for child rearing and happy, stable family life. Immature, irresponsible parents need patient understanding and a great deal of support and advice.

### THE MIDWIFE AND THE FAMILY

To undertake her commitment as a teacher of family-centred parenthood, the midwife ought to be aware of the functions of the family.

**The nuclear family** is a home-based social structure; parents and their offspring living together permanently. In a well-established close-knit family, children can develop physically, intellectually and emotionally to their full potential. The young expectant mother may have little understanding of how to create such an environment: she needs guidance and midwives should act as counsellors.

**The extended family** is comprised of members of the families from which the parents are derived. Both husband and wife bring to their marriage the customs and beliefs of their extended families. These may be cultural, religious, political and along with food-habits and social behaviour may give rise to conflict. Some wives, because of temperament, immaturity or selfishness, are incapable of forming an amicable relationship with the extended family group. Any attempt to alienate the husband from his parents puts an intolerable strain on the marriage and deprives the children of what can be a meaningful and pleasant relationship with the grandparents. The mother plays a large part in fostering peaceable relationships within the extended family group; some need helpful advice.

Family life today is conditioned by the fact that wives are having to work outside the home to provide necessities as well as luxuries. Not all women have the stamina to cope with the physical and emotional stress such employment imposes. The husband, may be deprived of the companionship and domestic comfort that makes home a desirable place to return to. The children may not receive the sustenance, devotion and moral supervision they so urgently need today. Midwives can give some of the counsel and emotional support young mothers need.

### The mother's influence

**If the mother is a loving person, she derives pleasure in creating a kindly atmosphere;** making the home a haven to which the children gladly return even when they reach adulthood. In such a home, the husband finds contentment in the duties as well as the joys of family life. The midwife should motivate prospective parents to provide such a home for their children; her concern for the baby she delivers should extend beyond his physical welfare.

**Husbands need counsel** for their new role as expectant fathers; (a) in maintaining a caring partnership during pregnancy (b) in providing emotional support and companionship during labour (c) in observing his paternal duty in the home as a loving, helpful, dependable member of the family group.

Parents do not always realise that they are teachers by example as well as by word. The midwife should explain to them that young children are imprinted with patterns of speech and behaviour and that they tend to respond in the same manner as that in which they are approached. Gentleness begets gentleness.

### LIBERAL ATTITUDES TO SEXUALITY

Admittedly, attitudes to sexual behaviour are more lax than previously and midwives should be competent to refute the argument of permissive-minded individuals who question the need for marriage and the stable family group: such an irresponsible attitude being anti-social, selfish and immature.

**Many thoughtful persons are alarmed at the effect of liberal sexual codes on schoolgirls.** In the year 1975 in Britain, babies were born to one girl of 11 years, to three girls of 12 years, to thirty-seven girls of 13 years, to 230 girls of 14 years and to 1272 girls of 15 years.

**Equally disturbing is the large number of abortions** deemed necessary in this age group. Parents seem to be afraid they will alienate their children if they condemn pre-marital sex, but to ignore is to condone.

### The midwife a realist

In the pursuit of her profession, the midwife encounters the sequelae of lax sexual behaviour, e.g. abortion, sexually transmitted disease, unwanted, unloved children, broken marriages and misery. The increase among children of truancy, vandalism, dishonesty, and violence may be due to lack of discipline (which should be wise guidance) in the home.

**Parents need advice** regarding (a) imbuing their children with high ideals (b) encouraging good behaviour and (c) motivating them to recognise and pursue that which is honourable and worthwhile. Standards of behaviour learned in the home are reflected (a) at school (b) in the local community and (c) at national level.

**Family centred maternity care,** it is hoped will provide encouragement and support to parents, strengthen the family bond, improve standards of behaviour and increase the happiness of individuals.

# 2
# The Female Pelvis: The Generative Organs

*Pelvic bones, joints, measurement, types. Pelvic floor. Vulva. Vagina. Uterus. Fallopian tubes. Ovaries. Hormones, ovarian, pituitary, in pregnancy*

## THE BONY PELVIS

The pelvis forms a bony canal through which the fetus must pass during the process of birth, and if the canal is of average shape and dimensions the baby of normal size will negotiate it without difficulty. But pelves vary in size and shape, even within normal limits, so it is essential that the midwife should be competent to recognise a normal pelvis in the pregnant woman; she must also be able to detect deviations from normal. Gross deformities due to maldevelopment or disease are fortunately rare: their diagnosis presents little difficulty and the appropriate treatment, in such cases, is usually Caesarean section. Knowledge of pelvic anatomy is also needed in the conduct of labour, for the progress made is estimated by the relationship of the fetus to certain pelvic landmarks.

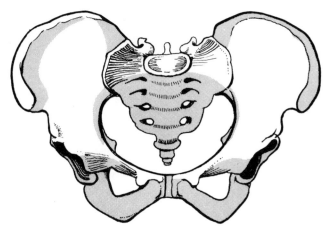

Fig. 2-1   Normal female pelvis. Pubic arch 90°.

### PELVIC BONES

**The pelvis is composed of four bones;** two innominate or hip bones, the sacrum and coccyx. The innominate bone consists of three parts: the **ilium, ischium** and **os pubis.**

**The ilium** is the large flared-out part, and the concave anterior surface is known as the iliac fossa. The upper curved border is called the iliac crest, the terminal points of which are known as the anterior superior and the posterior superior iliac spines.

**The ischium** is the lowest part of the innominate bone, and upon the large prominences, known as the *tuberosities* of the ischium, the body rests when in a sitting position. Posterior and superior to the tuberosity is a projection, the spine of the ischium, a useful landmark when making a vaginal examination during labour; the station (level) of the fetal head being assessed in centimetres above or below the ischial spines.

**The os pubis** consists of a body, a superior and an inferior ramus: the two inferior rami forming the pubic arch; at the symphysis pubis the two pubic bones meet.

**The sacrum** is a wedge-shaped bone composed of five sacral vertebrae: the centre of the upper surface of the first sacral vertebra being known as the **promontory of the sacrum.** Because it encroaches on the antero-posterior diameter of the pelvic inlet and in some cases may prevent the fetal head from entering the brim, it is an important landmark. The anterior surface of the sacrum is concave and is referred to as the *hollow of the sacrum.*

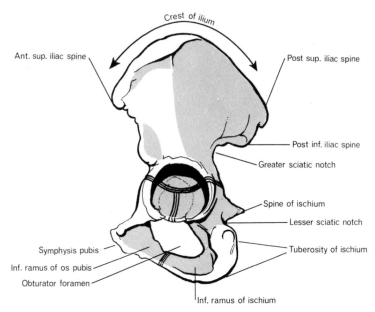

Fig. 2-2    Innominate bone, showing important landmarks.

**The coccyx** is a small bone consisting of four coccygeal vertebrae, tiny nodules of bone fused together.

### PELVIC JOINTS

**There are four pelvic joints:** two sacro-iliac, the symphysis pubis and the sacro-coccygeal. In the non-pregnant state there is very little movement in these joints, but during pregnancy a certain amount of softening and stretching of the ligaments takes place, probably due to endocrine activity, which results in slight separation of the joints. In cases where there is a minor degree of disproportion between the fetal head and maternal pelvis, the additional space provided by the 'give' of the joints may permit passage of the fetal head.

**The sacro-iliac joint** is formed at the articulation of the sacrum with the ilium, and allows for a limited backward and forward movement of the tip and promontory of the sacrum. During pregnancy there is a good deal of strain on these joints, and multiparous women frequently complain of backache at this time and in the weeks following childbirth.

**The symphysis pubis** is formed at the junction of the two pubic bones which are united by a pad of cartilage. This joint widens appreciably during the later months of pregnancy, and the degree of movement permitted may give rise to pain on walking.

**The sacro-coccygeal joint** is formed where the base of the coccyx articulates with the tip of the sacrum, and allows the coccyx to bend backwards during the actual birth of the head.

### PELVIC LIGAMENTS

The ligaments binding the sacrum and ilium at the sacro-iliac joint are the strongest in the whole body. The interpubic ligaments strengthen the symphysis

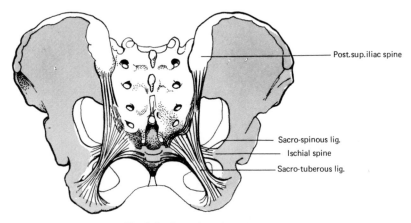

Fig. 2-3   Posterior view of the pelvis.

pubis. The sacro-tuberous ligament forms an attachment between the sacrum and the tuberosity of the ischium, the sacro-spinous ligament connects the sacrum with the spine of the ischium and both ligaments form the posterior wall of the pelvic outlet.

### THE FALSE PELVIS

The bony pelvis is divided into two parts, the false and the true. The false pelvis is that part above the brim and consists mainly of the flared-out iliac bones. It has little obstetrical importance.

### THE TRUE PELVIS

The true pelvis is the curved bony canal through which the fetus must pass during birth. It consists of a brim, cavity and outlet.

**The pelvic brim or inlet.** The pelvic brim is bounded posteriorly by the promontory and alae of the sacrum, and in front by the pubic bones. Where the superior ramus of the pubic bone meets the ilium a roughened area known as the iliopectineal eminence is formed. In the gynaecoid or female pelvis the brim is round, except where the promontory of the sacrum projects into it. Three diameters are measured.

1. **The antero-posterior diameter** is measured from the sacral promontory to a point 1·25 cm down, on the posterior surface of the symphysis pubis, and measures 11 cm. This measurement is known as the **obstetrical conjugate,** and differs from

the true or anatomical conjugate, 12 cm, which is measured to the summit of the symphysis pubis. The thickness of the pubic bone diminishes the space available for the passage of the fetal head, so the obstetrical conjugate is utilised not the wider anatomical conjugate. **The diagonal conjugate,** the distance from the lower border of the symphysis pubis to the promontory of the sacrum 12 to 13 cm, is measured per vaginam to assess the length of the antero-posterior diameter of the pelvic brim (see p. 127. Fig. 8–5).

2. **The oblique diameters** of the brim are measured from the sacro-iliac joints to the ilio-pectineal eminences on the opposite sides, and are named right and left, according to the sacro-iliac joint from which they are measured. Both are 12 cm in length, but the descending colon encroaches on the left oblique diameter and diminishes the available space.

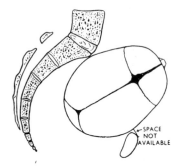

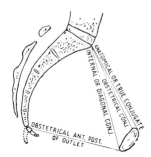

Fig. 2-4   Note the narrow obstetrical conjugate through which the head must pass. Because of the thickness of the pubic bone, the extra space provided by the anatomical or true conjugate is not available for the passage of the fetal head.

Fig. 2-5   Median section of the pelvis showing antero-posterior diameters.

3. **The transverse diameter** is the widest part of the brim, and extends from side to side, immediately behind the ilio-pectineal eminences. It measures 13 cm, but is encroached on by the psoas muscles. The fetal head commonly enters in the transverse diameter of the pelvic brim.

**The sacro-cotyloid** dimensions 9 cm, which lie between the promontory of the sacrum and the ilio-pectineal eminences are of practical importance. The bi-parietal eminences may become caught between the promontory of the sacrum and the ilio-pectineal eminence during vertex presentation posterior position and be held up during labour.

### The pelvic cavity

The cavity is the curved canal between the inlet and outlet. The anterior wall is 4 cm—the depth of the pubic bone. The posterior wall is 12 cm—the length of the sacrum and coccyx. The cavity is circular in shape and curves forwards. Its diameters cannot be accurately measured as the cavity is not entirely surrounded by bone, but all the diameters are considered to be 12 cm.

### The pelvic outlet

The upper border of the pelvic outlet is at the level of the ischial spines; the distance between these being known as the bispinous diameter 10 cm. This diameter has great obstetrical importance because it is the transverse measurement of the 'narrow pelvic plane.' The lower border of the pelvic outlet is diamond-shaped, and is bounded anteriorly by the pubic arch which, in the gynaecoid pelvis, forms an angle of 90°. Laterally it is bounded by the ischial tuberosities, and posteriorly by the coccyx and sacro-tuberous ligaments.

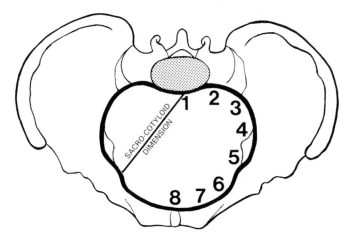

Fig. 2-6   Brim or inlet of female pelvis

1. Promontory of sacrum
2. Ala of sacrum
3. Sacro-iliac joint
4. Ilio-pectineal line
5. Ilio-pectineal eminence
6. Ramus of os pubis
7. Summit of symphysis pubis
8. Symphysis pubis

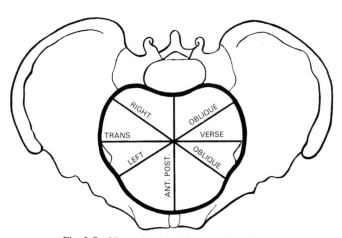

Fig. 2-7   View of pelvic inlet, showing diameters.

**The antero-posterior diameter** is measured from the apex of the pubic arch to the tip of the coccyx, but as the coccyx bends backwards during the birth of the head the diameter is increased by 1·25 cm. This larger diameter is known as the obstetrical antero-posterior diameter, and measures 13 cm.

**The oblique diameters** of the outlet having no fixed points are therefore not measured.

**The transverse (intertuberischial) diameter** is at the lower border of the outlet, extending from the inner borders of the ischial tuberosities and measures 11 cm.

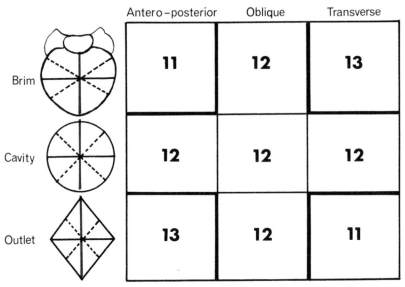

|  | Antero-posterior | Oblique | Transverse |
|---|---|---|---|
| Brim | 11 | 12 | 13 |
| Cavity | 12 | 12 | 12 |
| Outlet | 13 | 12 | 11 |

Fig. 2-8   Measurements of the pelvic canal in centimetres.

The above measurements of the pelvic canal, simplified for ease in learning, are within the minimal limit of normal range. They will, it is hoped, provide midwives with an impression of the average dimensions and shape of the pelvic inlet, cavity and outlet.

### Pelvic inclination

When a woman is standing in the upright position, her pelvis is not at right angles to her spine, as one might think: the inlet slopes at an angle of 60° with the floor; the tip of the sacrum will be on a level with the summit of the symphysis pubis. The inclination of the cavity is 30°, and at the outlet the inclination is only 11°, being nearly horizontal. In some negro women the inclination of the plane of the brim is nearer 90° and this causes delay in engagement of the head during labour.

### Pelvic planes

These are imaginary flat surfaces at various levels of the pelvic canal. The three commonly described are on a level with the brim, cavity and outlet. The fetus will enter at right angles to the plane of the brim, and the inclination of that plane, as already stated, is 60°. When trying to determine whether the fetal head is small enough to enter the pelvic inlet, the inclination of the plane of the brim should be kept in mind. This will be better understood if Fig. 2-10 is turned sideways to give the impression of a patient in the recumbent position.

Because the plane of the outlet is at an inclination of 11°, it will be necessary for the fetus to turn at an acute angle to enter it. This plane extends from the lower border of the symphysis pubis to the ischial spines and tip of the sacrum.

### Axis of the pelvic canal

A line drawn at right angles to the planes of the inlet, cavity and outlet would represent the anatomical axis of the pelvic canal, sometimes known as the curve of Carus. During the actual birth the midwife facilitates the natural upward curving movement of the baby's head and body as they emerge from the pelvic canal.

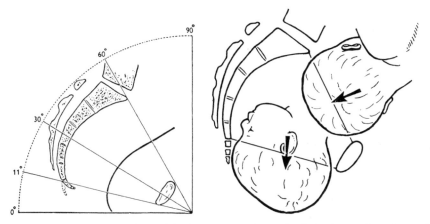

Fig. 2-9 Median section of the pelvis, showing the inclination of the planes and the axis of the pelvic canal.

Fig. 2-10 Fetal head entering plane of pelvic brim and leaving plane of pelvic outlet.

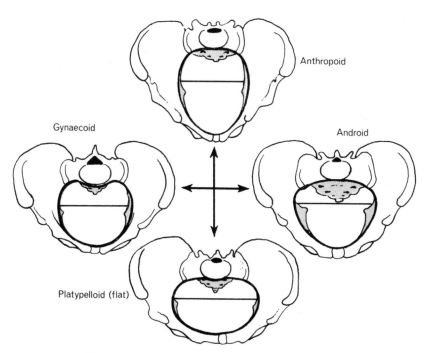

Fig. 2-11 Characteristic inlet of the four types of pelvis.

### THE FOUR BASIC TYPES OF PELVIS

Female pelves have been classified into four parent groups, according to the shape of the brim.

1. **The gynaecoid,** or true female pelvis, has a round brim (inlet).
2. **The android** has a heart-shaped brim.
3. **The anthropoid** has an oval brim, narrow in the transverse.
4. **The platypelloid,** or simple flat pelvis, has a kidney-shaped brim, narrow in the antero-posterior diameter.

**The gynaecoid pelvis,** is eminently suited for childbearing. The brim is round, except where it is encroached upon by the promontory of the sacrum. The cavity is shallow with a broad well-curved sacrum. The greater sciatic notch is wide, the pubic arch forms a right angle, the iliac crest is broad and well curved. This pelvis would be found in a woman of average build whose hips are broader than her shoulders—height over 1·5 metres, with shoes size 4 or larger, and in whom no deformity is present.

Pelves vary in size and shape as much as faces and feet, and women's shoes range from size 2 to 10, with nine widths in each of the average sizes.

### THE PELVIC FLOOR

Although it is desirable that the midwife should be acquainted with the general formation and functions of the pelvic floor, she need not have a detailed knowledge of its anatomy. It is made up mainly of muscular tissue, but skin, fat, fascia and connective tissue go to form this structure which fills in the irregular-shaped pelvic outlet.

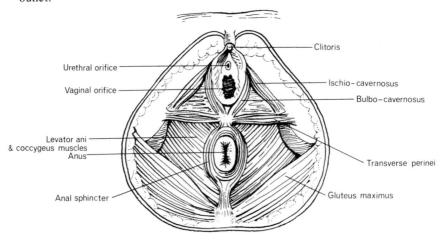

Fig. 2-12   The pelvic floor—superficial structures. Clitoris. Urethral orifice. Vaginal orifice. Levator ani and coccygeus muscles. Sphincter ani externus. Anus. Gluteus maximus. Transverse perinei. Bulbo-cavernosus. Ischio-cavernosus.

The levatores ani are the most substantial of the six pairs of muscles included in its construction, and by their mode of attachment to the pelvis they act like a sling or hammock. In front they are attached to the lateral part of the os pubis; behind, to the ischial spines and coccyx, and laterally, to the obturator fascia. The two levator ani muscles meet to form a gutter which slopes forwards and is perforated by three canals, the *urethra*, *vagina* and *rectum*. These canals are embraced by fascia which serves to augment the area where they pass through the pelvic floor.

The external aspect of the pelvic floor is mainly muscular; the transverse perinei which stretches from the perineum to the ischial tuberosity being the most superficial. The ischio-cavernosus runs from the ischial tuberosity to the region of the clitoris. The bulbo-cavernosus surrounds and strengthens the vaginal orifice and the sphincter ani externus guards the anal canal.

Internally the pelvic floor constitutes the base of the abdominal cavity; it is lined with peritoneum; and the cervix, upper vagina, bladder and rectum are securely anchored in it. These organs are surrounded by connective tissue and sustained by muscle and strong fascial attachments. The connective tissue surrounding the uterus is known as parametrium and it merges with the fascia of the transverse cervical ligaments and with the fibres of the levator ani muscles.

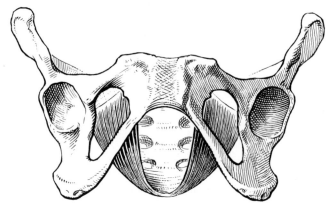

Fig. 2-13   Diagrammatic representation of the gutter shape of the pelvic floor.

**Injury to pelvic floor during labour**

During the last weeks of pregnancy the pelvic floor softens in preparation for labour. If, during the first stage of labour, the patient 'bears down'—when she will, of course, be advised to desist—the paracervical tissue and transverse cervical ligaments will be subjected to excessive strain. The uterus may then sag downwards and become retroverted. When, during the second stage, the fetal head distends the pelvic floor, the perineal body is flattened out until it is quite thin. The stress to which the pelvic floor is subjected may be very great, and should the second stage be unduly prolonged, the fascia supporting the bladder may become overstretched; subsequently the anterior vaginal wall prolapses and forms a sac containing bladder, known as a cystocele. When the head is on the perineum too long, the excessive strain to which this structure is subjected will give rise to a lax, sagging pelvic floor that will afford inadequate support to the pelvic organs.

## THE VULVA

The term 'vulva' is applied to the external genital organs, extending from the mons veneris to the perineum. The labia majora, or greater lips, are two elongated masses of areolar tissue and fat, covered with skin on their outer surfaces. They arise anteriorly in the mons veneris—a pad of fat lying over the pubic area: posteriorly they merge into the perineum; the round ligaments of the uterus are inserted into their anterior portion. The labia minora are two thin folds of skin, lying between the inner surfaces of the labia majora. Posteriorly they fuse and form a thin fold of skin known as the *fourchette*, or anterior edge of the perineum. In front, the labia minora unite and enclose the clitoris, one fold passing under that structure, the other passing over it like a hood to form the prepuce of the clitoris.

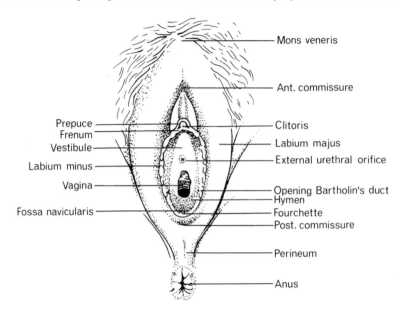

Fig. 2-14   Female external genital organs.

**The clitoris,** a rudimentary organ analogous to the penis in the male, is a sensitive, highly vascular structure, situated about 2·5 cm above the external urethral orifice. It serves as a useful landmark in locating this orifice for catheterisation if following childbirth, extensive vulval bruising and laceration are present.

**The external urethral orifice** is situated in the vestibule, a triangular-shaped area, bounded anteriorly by the clitoris, laterally by the labia minora and posteriorly by the fourchette. Skene's ducts which open just within the urethra are sometimes inflamed, due to infection which may be gonococcal.

**The introitus, or orifice of the vagina,** is partially closed by the hymen, a thin membrane which tears during the birth of the first child, if it has not previously been torn during coitus. The remaining tags of hymen are known as carunculae myrtiformes.

**Bartholin's glands** lie embedded in the posterior region of the labia majora, and their ducts open on either side of the vaginal orifice. They secrete a lubricating fluid. If infected, abscess formation may result, and this is frequently, but not invariably, due to the gonococcus. Repeated attacks of infection result in a cystic condition of the gland, which can be recognised on palpating it.

### THE PERINEUM

The perineum is the area extending from the fourchette to the anus, and forms the base of the perineal body—a triangular mass of connective tissue, muscle and fat, measuring 4 cm×4 cm. The perineal body fills the wedge-shaped area between the lower ends of the rectum and vagina, and forms a central attachment for the muscles and fascia of the pelvic floor. When, during the second stage of labour, the perineal body is flattened out by the descending fetal head, the perineum elongates and becomes so thin that it is liable to tear.

**First degree tear.** The fourchette only is torn.
**Second degree tear.** Beyond the fourchette and not involving rectum or anus.
**Third degree tear.** The anal sphincter is torn, the rectum occasionally.

## THE VAGINA

The vagina is a canal extending from the vestibule to the cervix. The posterior wall is 8 to 10 cm long and the anterior wall is 5 to 7·5 cm being 2·5 cm shorter because the cervix enters its upper third; the uterus therefore lies almost at right angles to the vagina. The upper end of the vagina is known as the vault and is divided into four arches or **fornices** by the cervix protruding down into it. The largest arch, known as the posterior fornix, is behind the cervix, the one in front is the anterior fornix, and on the right and left sides are the two lateral fornices.

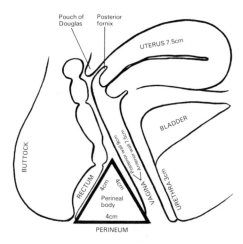

Fig. 2-15  Diagrammatic representation of vagina and uterus with their relation to bladder, urethra and rectum. (As an aid to learning the student midwife should first draw the perineal body to obtain correct measurements of adjoining structures.)

The vagina has four coats and is lined with stratified epithelium which is similar to skin, without the horny layer. This epithelium is thrown into ridges or rugae which tend to be obliterated with repeated childbearing. The outer connective tissue coat is richly supplied with blood vessels, mainly from the vaginal arteries and branches of the uterine arteries. The muscular layer is not well developed and the vagina is capable of great distension. There are no glands in the vagina; its secretion is a transudation of lymph and cast-off epithelial cells. During pregnancy the vaginal secretion is increased, but if it is profuse, red, purulent, frothy or irritating, this should be investigated. The acid medium of the vagina tends to inhibit the growth of organisms, and this acidity is maintained by the action of Doderlein's bacillus—a normal inhabitant of the vagina. Certain organisms are found fairly constantly in the vagina, e.g. aerobic and anaerobic streptococci, but not haemolytic streptococci which are always introduced from without. Gram-positive cocci and diphtheroids are also found.

### Anatomical relations of the vagina

The lower half of the anterior wall of the vagina is in close contact with the urethra which runs parallel to it; the upper half is in contact with the bladder. (When obtaining a urethral smear for gonococci the gloved finger is inserted into the vagina, and by stroking its anterior wall, secretion can be 'milked' from the urethra.) During labour, if difficulty is encountered in inserting a catheter, the gloved finger placed against the anterior wall of the vagina can be used as a guide to direct the catheter into the bladder and thus avoid injury to the urethra.

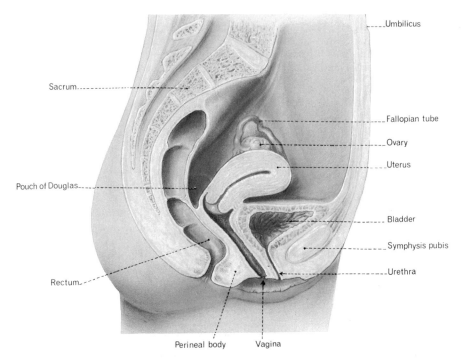

Fig. 2-16   A median section through the female pelvis, showing bladder, uterus, rectum, vagina and their anatomical relations.

The lower third of the posterior vaginal wall adjoins the perineal body; the middle part is in apposition with the rectum. The upper part is in contact with the peritoneum at the base of the pouch of Douglas. Laterally, the vagina is in relation to the levator ani muscles of the pelvic floor.

## THE UTERUS

The uterus, a hollow muscular organ shaped like a flattened pear, is situated in the cavity of the true pelvis, behind the bladder and in front of the rectum. In it the fertilised ovum embeds, is nourished and protected for 40 weeks until, during labour, the fetus is expelled by the powerful contractions of the uterine muscle.

The non-pregnant uterus weighs about 60 g and measures $7 \cdot 5 \times 5 \times 2 \cdot 5$ cm. The corpus or body is 5 cm long, the cervix 2.5 cm long: the upper part of the corpus is 5 cm broad, the lower part and cervix are $2 \cdot 5$ cm broad. The walls of the uterus are $1 \cdot 25$ cm thick, and as the anterior and posterior walls are in apposition the thickness of the uterus is $2 \cdot 5$ cm.

### THE CORPUS

The corpus or body forms the greater part of the uterus, and the rounded upper part of the corpus above the insertion of the Fallopian tubes is known as the **fundus**. The angle where the Fallopian tube is inserted is known as the *cornu* or horn. The body gradually tapers downwards and the constricted area immediately above the cervix is known as the **isthmus** which distends during pregnancy to form the lower uterine segment.

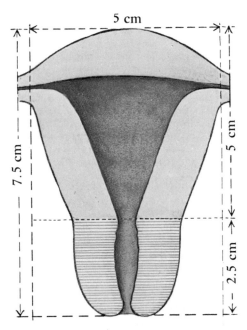

Fig. 2-17 Measurements of uterus.

**The endometrium** lines the body of the uterus and consists of columnar epithelium, glands, which produce an alkaline secretion, and stroma or connective tissue cells capable of the rapid regeneration necessary following menstruation. It is also a rich source of prostaglandins. The endometrium is richly supplied with blood and is about 1·5 mm thick. When embedding of the fertilised ovum occurs the endometrium is known as the **decidua**, because after labour it will be shed.

**The myometrium,** or muscle coat has very great expansile properties. It forms seven-eighths of the thickness of the uterine wall and consists of three layers, an inner circular layer of fibres, a thick intermediate layer, the fibres of which form an encircling figure of eight arrangement surrounding the blood vessels, and by constricting them act as living ligatures to control bleeding during the third stage of labour. The fibres of the outer muscle layer are arranged longitudinally and because they are four times more plentiful in the fundus the decreasing gradient plays a part in the expulsion of the fetus.

**The perimetrium** is a layer of peritoneum, which covers the uterus except at the sides, beyond which it extends to form the **broad ligaments.** The perimetrium is firmly attached to the uterine wall except at the lower anterior part where, at the level of the isthmus, the peritoneum is reflected on to the bladder.

## THE CERVIX

The cervix or neck is the lowest part of the uterus and the vaginal portion projects into the vault of the vagina. The cervical canal is 2·5 cm long, and the constricted area where the cervix and isthmus meet forms what is known as the internal os (mouth): the external os is a small round opening at the lowest point of the uterus, but after childbirth it is a tranverse slit. In structure the cervix differs from the body of the uterus, containing fewer muscle cells and more collagen fibres. Lining the canal is mucous membrane, with glands of the deep racemose type which secrete glairy alkaline mucus. The mucosa covering the outer surface of the cervix is similar to the stratified epithelium of the vagina.

### Position of uterus

The uterus lies in a position which is almost horizontal when the woman stands erect. It leans forwards, and this position is known as anteversion; it bends forwards on itself, producing anteflexion, with the fundus resting on the bladder. When this position of anteflexion and anteversion is maintained, prolapse is less likely to occur. When the uterus is backwardly displaced or retroverted, it lies in the same axis as the vagina and is more liable to prolapse. The uterus is maintained in position by four pairs of ligaments and indirectly by the **pelvic floor.** It is capable of a wide range of movement: a full bladder alters its position from horizontal to vertical: a distended colon pushes it downwards and forwards.

## THE LIGAMENTS (4 pairs)

**The broad ligament** is a double fold of peritoneum continuous with the perimetrium, extending outwards from the uterus and attached to the side wall of the pelvis. The lower border of the broad ligament is thickened and strengthened with fascia, fibrous tissue and muscle to form the most important uterine support, **the transverse cervical ligament,** which, if overstretched or damaged during labour, will cause the uterus to sag downwards.

**The round ligament** arises at the cornu of the uterus, in front of and below the insertion of the Fallopian tube, and runs between the folds of the broad ligament, passes through the inguinal canal and is inserted into the labium majus. It has little value as a support, but tends to hold the uterus forwards in the position of anteversion.

**The utero-sacral ligament** consists of folds of peritoneum containing muscular and fibrous tissue, extending backwards from the sides of the isthmus and attached to the sacrum. It forms the lateral border of the base of the pouch of Douglas, and by pulling the cervix backwards helps to maintain uterine anteversion.

## THE UTERINE BLOOD SUPPLY

The vessels supplying blood to the uterus are the two uterine and the two ovarian arteries. The uterine artery, a branch of the internal iliac, is ensheathed in the paracervical tissue forming the transverse cervical ligament, and joins the uterus at the level of the isthmus. It sends a branch to the upper part of the vagina, but the larger branch runs in a convoluted fashion up alongside the uterus between the folds of the broad ligament, giving off branches to the body of the uterus and eventually anastomosing with the ovarian artery. Uterine veins accompany the arteries.

The ovarian artery is a branch of the abdominal aorta and arises just below the renal artery. It enters the pelvis, passes between the folds of the broad ligament, supplies ovary and Fallopian tube, and enters the uterus at the fundus. The veins that drain the upper part of the uterus unite between the folds of the broad ligament to form the pampiniform plexus and from it on either side arise the two ovarian veins which fuse to form one vein: the left joining the left renal vein, the right joining the inferior vena cava. The uterine blood supply is increased during pregnancy and decreased during the puerperium. The fetus depends on a constant supply, via the maternal blood, of oxygen, nutrients and metabolites.

The lymphatic drainage from the uterus is abundant and accounts for the successful outcome of many uterine infections.

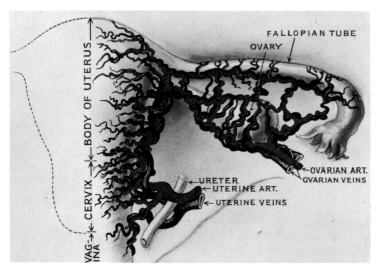

Fig. 2-18   Blood supply of the uterus and its appendages.

### THE UTERINE NERVE SUPPLY

The main nerve supply to the uterus is now considered to be from the pelvic autonomic system, sympathetic and parasympathetic. It is suggested that impulses transmitted by the sympathetic nerves may be stimulative or inhibitive to the uterus depending on whether they are influenced by chemical agents within the uterus, or by hormonal factors in the feto-placental unit.

Sympathetic nerve fibres from the hypogastric plexus pass to the pelvic (Frankenhauser's) plexus, in the base of the utero-sacral ligaments, from which are supplied the uterus, vagina, bladder and rectum. Sympathetic nerves from the pelvic plexus pass to the paracervical ganglia, which are sheaths of sympathetic nerve fibres situated close behind and on either side of the cervix. The contact or pressure on the cervix of a well-fitting presenting part results in the transmission of a stimulus through the paracervical ganglia from the nerve endings in the cervix. These stimulative impulses result in stronger contractions of the muscle fibres in the upper uterine segment.

## THE FALLOPIAN TUBES

The Fallopian tubes are two muscular canals, extending from the cornua of the uterus and opening into the peritoneal cavity near the ovaries. Each tube measures about 11 cm in length and is enveloped in the upper fold of the broad ligament. The ciliated mucous membrane, lining the tube, produces a current of lymph which, in conjunction with the rhythmic peristaltic action of the muscle coat furthers the passage of the ovum from the ovary along the tube to the uterus.

*Four parts of the tube are described, as follows:*

**The interstitial** passes through the 1·25 cm thickness of the uterine wall. Its lumen is about 1 mm in diameter (the size of a common pin).

**The isthmus** is the narrow part, immediately adjoining the uterus.

**The ampulla** is the wider portion in which fertilisation of the ovum usually occurs.

**The infundibulum** is the funnel-shaped extremity, the terminal margins of which are fimbriated (fringed); one of the longer fimbria being in contact with the ovary, the fimbria ovarica.

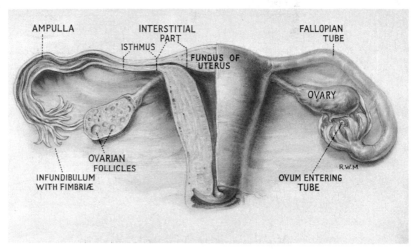

Fig. 2-19 Diagrammatic representation of Fallopian tube in section, demonstrating the narrow interstitial and isthmic portions. Note ovum entering the fimbriated end of the tube.

## THE OVARIES

The ovaries are two small organs (about the size of an unshelled almond), 4 cm long, 2 cm broad, and 1·25 cm thick. They are situated on the posterior surface of the broad ligaments to which they are attached by the mesovarium. Blood vessels and nerves enter the ovary at the hilum, a stalk-like structure, on its anterior edge. One end of the ovary is attached to the cornu of the uterus by the ovarian ligament which is about 2·5 cm long; the other end is connected to the pelvic wall by the suspensory or infundibulo-pelvic ligament. The ovary is brought into contact with the Fallopian tube by one of its longer fimbria.

The ovary consists of a medulla and a cortex. The medulla is a supporting framework of connective tissue, blood vessels and nerves, but the cortex (covering or bark) is the important functioning part and is composed of germinal epithelium, stroma cells and Graafian follicles. The **germinal epithelium** lies over the tunica albuginea and forms the surface of the ovary. Primordial follicles are contained in the ovarian cortex where the formation of primary oocytes proceeds: 100,000 being present in each ovary at birth. During the years preceding puberty some of the primordial follicles begin to mature, but not until puberty do they ripen, come to the surface and rupture to liberate an ovum.

The mature Graafian follicle is about 10 mm in diameter and consists of an outer layer (or theca externa) which is lined with theca interna. Inside the theca interna is a layer known as the membrana granulosa which contains a clear fluid, the liquor folliculi. At one end of the follicle the cells of the membrana granulosa are heaped up to surround the ovum.

## FUNCTIONS OF THE OVARY

**Ovulation,** which consists of the rupture of the ripened Graafian follicle and the expulsion of the ovum, takes place once every month in a normal healthy woman from puberty to the menopause approximately 14 days previous to the first day of the next menstrual period (between the 12th and 16th days after the beginning of the last menstrual period). One follicle matures and comes to the surface of the ovary, ruptures and allows the ovum to escape into the fimbriated end of the tube, cupped underneath it at this time. The corpus luteum or yellow body is formed in the ruptured Graafian follicle. If the ovum is not fertilised, it dies; the corpus luteum degenerates and is gradually replaced by hyaline tissue (the corpus albicans), which allows the ovary to heal where rupture has taken place, without the formation of scar tissue.

**Endocrine action.** The ovary produces progestogens and oestrogens. Oestriol, oestradiol and oestrone are ovarian hormones but oestriol is excreted in the urine in larger quantities than the other oestrogens.

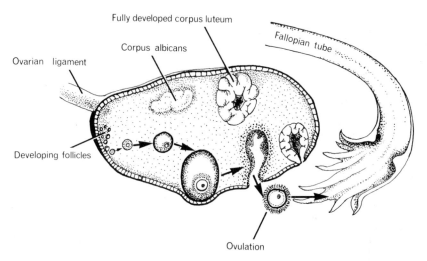

Fig. 2-20   Life cycle of the Graafian follicle.

### OESTROGENS

The oestrogens, under the influence of the follicle stimulating hormone (FSH) of the anterior pituitary gland are produced by the joint action of granulosa cells and theca lutein cells. Oestrogens have widespread metabolic effects; they are also concerned with the proliferative changes in the endometrium, the growth of the breasts, vaginal epithelium, and cervical glands.

During pregnancy the feto-placental unit is intimately associated in the production of oestrogens. In the fetal adrenals a steroid is metabolised and carried to the placenta where it acts as a precursor in the elaboration of oestriol which is essentially a growth hormone concerned with the growth of the fetus, decidua, myometrium and breasts. This hormone is excreted in the urine of pregnant women, and the amount excreted gives some indication of fetal wellbeing.

When conditions exist that could impair fetal growth the termination of pregnancy would be considered after the 34th week in order to promote fetal survival, so assays of urinary or plasma oestriol are made and if low, this signifies that the feto-placental unit is not functioning properly: when below a critical level fetal death may be imminent.

### PROGESTOGENS

Progesterone and related compounds produced by the corpus luteum, under the influence of the luteinising hormone (LH) of the anterior pituitary gland are responsible for the secretory phase—the second two weeks—of the menstrual cycle. Progestogens can only affect tissues that have previously been acted on by oestrogens.

In early pregnancy progesterone is produced by the corpus luteum and by the syncytiotrophoblast under the stimulation of chorionic gonadotrophin. Later the placenta produces increasing quantities; the adrenal cortex may also be involved. Progesterone causes proliferation of the decidua to meet the nutritional needs of the growing embryo and is also concerned with the alveolar growth of the breasts. It may play some part in maintaining fluid and electrolyte balance. Progesterone is thought to be metabolised by the feto-placental unit and excreted in the urine as pregnanediol. Urinary pregnanediol assays reflect functioning of the corpus luteum and are employed in cases of infertility to determine whether ovulation has occurred. They are not of value in later pregnancy.

## THE PITUITARY *(hypophysis)* HORMONES

**The anterior pituitary** *(adenohypophysis)* produces at least six hormones under the influence of the releasing hormones of the hypothalamus. Three are directly concerned with reproduction: (1) the follicle stimulating hormone (FSH) is responsible for the maturation of the Graafian follicles; (2) the luteinising hormone (LH) brings about ovulation and the development of the corpus luteum; (3) prolactin initiates lactation when the breast has been acted on by oestrogens, progestogens and corticotrophin. The anterior pituitary under the influence of the release hormones of the hypothalamus and the ovarian hormones, by a feedback process, interact on each other, stimulating or inhibiting as required and so maintaining an optimal hormonal balance.

**The posterior pituitary** *(neurohypophysis)* produces two hormones the release of which is controlled by the hypothalamus. (1) Oxytocin brings about contraction of smooth muscle fibres of the reproductive tract and the mammary cells during suckling. (2) Vasopressin, the anti-diuretic hormone, plays a major role in the reabsorption of water by the kidney tubules and may be concerned in the production of hypertensive states during pregnancy.

## HORMONES IN PREGNANCY

**Chorionic gonadotrophin** produced by the cytotrophoblast appears in the urine a few days after implantation of the ovum and is the characteristic hormone of the placenta. Its main function, prolonging the life of the corpus luteum during pregnancy, inhibits menstruation. A peak level is reached at about 60 days from the last menstrual period. Finding chorionic gonadotrophin in the urine of a woman is accepted as a sign of pregnancy, in fact this is the basis of the immunological and other pregnancy tests. An excessive amount is present in cases of hydatidiform mole.

**Human placental lactogen,** is produced by the syncytiotrophoblast. The HPL concentration in serum rises steeply during pregnancy until 36 weeks when it drops off. Assays of serum H.P.L. are utilised as a measure of placental function.

## THE BONY PELVIS

**Why is the promontory of the sacrum the most important landmark of the pelvis?**

**Differentiate between** (a) the gynaecoid, android, and platypelloid pelvis, (b) the false and the true pelvis, (c) the obstetric and the anatomical conjugate.

Why is the gynaecoid pelvis so well suited for child bearing?

Describe the following: the diagonal conjugate; pelvic outlet; pelvic joints; true pelvis; pelvic planes; pelvic brim.

**In what way is knowledge of the following facts of value in the practice of midwifery?** (1) The pelvic joints 'give' during labour. (2) the inclination of the plane of the brim is 60°. (3) The antero-posterior is the largest diameter of the outlet.

From the appearance of the woman what would make you suspect abnormality in the pelvis?

**CMB (Eng.) 30-min. question.**—Describe the bony pelvis. What is the obstetric significance of the various parts or landmarks?

## THE PELVIC FLOOR

The main muscle is the .................... Name the three canals which perforate it.

(1) The pelvic floor softens and sags at the end of pregnancy. **Relate this to** (a) lightening; (b) taking the diagonal conjugate.

**(2) What part does the pelvic floor play** in the mechanism of labour? how may it be injured during labour? What damage would be incurred by making a lateral rather than a medio-lateral episiotomy?

**C.M.B. (Scot.) 30-min. question.**—Describe the anatomy of the pelvic floor. What changes may take place as the result of childbearing?

**C.M.B. (Eng.) 30-min. question.**—Describe the anatomy of the pelvic floor. How may a midwife prevent injuries to this structure during delivery?

## THE VULVA

### *Rearrange Correctly:*

| Structure | location | | |
|---|---|---|---|
| (1) Clitoris | pad of fat on pubic area | ( | ) |
| (2) Fourchette | above urethral orifice | ( | ) |
| (3) Vestibule | where labia minora meet posteriorly | ( | ) |
| (4) Mons veneris | posterior wall of urethral orifice | ( | ) |
| (5) Introitus | posterior area of vestibule | ( | ) |
| (6) Skene's ducts | between clitoris and fourchette | ( | ) |

A first degree perineal tear involves the..................................................................................................................

A third degree perineal tear involves the ........................................................................................................

Describe the vulva of a woman who has previously given birth to a child. How would you locate the urethra when much bruising is present after delivery.

Differentiate between the perineum and perineal body.

## THE VAGINA

The anterior wall, lower half, is in contact with ....................................................................................

The anterior wall, upper half, is in contact with ....................................................................................

The posterior wall, lower third, is in contact with ....................................................................................

The posterior wall, middle third, is in contact with ....................................................................................

(a) If difficulty is encountered in passing a catheter during the second stage of labour, what would you do? (b) What is the advantage of the acid medium of the vagina? (c) What types of vaginal discharge should be reported to the doctor? What is a cystocele? What conditions predispose to its formation?

**C.M.B.(Eng.) 30-min. question.** Describe the vagina and perineum. Explain how injuries to these structures can be minimised during labour.

**C.M.B.(Eng.) 30-min. question.**—Describe the anatomy of the female bladder and its relations. Why is this knowledge important in midwifery?

**C.M.B. (Eng.)**—Describe the anatomy of the vagina. What injuries may occur to the vagina during delivery?

### THE UTERUS

**Name.**—The lining of the pregnant uterus...................the part where the corpus and cervix meet.................... the nervous system supplying the uterus.................... the collection of nerves behind the cervix........... the ligament which is a fibro-muscular fold at the base of the broad ligament........... What does the isthmus form?.................... The non-pregnant uterus measures........... weighs........... The uterus at term measures........... weighs........... The uterus lies in a position of........... The uterine artery is a branch of.................. The ovarian artery is a branch of....................

In what way might the woman overstretch the transverse cervical ligaments during labour? What causes the uterus to increase in size during pregnancy and to decrease during the puerperium? Why does a retroverted uterus tend to prolapse?

Differentiate between perimetrium myometrium and endometrium.

**(N. Ireland) 30-min. question.**—Describe the normal non-pregnant uterus, its position and blood supply.

**C.M.B.(Eng.) 30-min. question.**—Outline the anatomy of the body of the uterus. Describe the behaviour of its musculature in the three stages of labour.

**C.M.B.(Eng.)**—Describe the anatomy of the uterus. What changes does the uterus undergo in pregnancy and labour?

### FALLOPIAN TUBES AND OVARIES

**Name** the following parts of the Fallopian tube: The part (a) which passes through the uterine wall.................... (b) in which fertilisation usually takes place.................... (c) immediately adjoining the uterus.................... (d) the widened end....................

**Name** the following structures in the ovary: The functioning part.................. The covering membrane.................. The sac containing the ovum....................

In what way might the Fallopian tubes or the ovaries be responsible for sterility, or infertility? If the tubes are narrowed, what may be the result?........... If they are blocked?....................

**C.M.B.(Eng.) 30-min. question.**—Describe the pathway through which the fertilised egg passes in order to reach the uterus. What may happen if anything obstructs the passage of the fertilised egg into the uterus?

**C.M.B.(Scot.) 30-min. question.**—Describe the anatomy of the Fallopian tube. What abnormalities of the tube may interfere with fertilisation and/or embedding of the ovum?

**C.M.B.(Scot.) 30-min. question.**—Describe the hormonal changes which occur in pregnancy. How can a knowledge of these contribute to diagnosis and management?

**C.M.B.(Scot.) 30-min. question.**—Describe the role of the sex hormones in influencing pregnancy and labour.

### SHORT QUESTIONS

Give function of chorionic gonadotrophic hormone, follicle stimulating hormone, oestrogens, progestogens. What can be assessed from serial estimations of oestriol?

## Oral Questions

**Of what value is your knowledge** that (a) the pelvic canal is curved; (b) the ant.-post. diameter of the outlet is wider than the transverse diameter; (c) the plane of the pelvic brim is at an inclination of 60° with the horizontal; (d) that the lower anterior wall of the vagina is in contact with the urethra.

# 3
# The Menstrual Cycle: the Ovum: the Placenta

*The menopause. Development and embedding of the ovum. Development of the embryo and placenta. The placenta at term, functions, abnormalities. The fetal sac, amniotic fluid. The umbilical cord*

**The menstrual cycle is a series of four phases,** mainly affecting the tissue structure of the endometrium: governed indirectly by the anterior pituitary gonadotrophic hormones and directly by the ovarian hormones, oestrogens and progestogens.

**The regenerative phase** commences by the third day after menstruation ceases. The endometrium is reformed.

**The proliferative phase** begins about five days after the cessation of menstruation and lasts until ovulation takes place 14 days previous to the next menstrual period.

**The secretory phase** corresponds to the luteal phase of the ovarian cycle and commences after ovulation. The endometrial capillaries are distended with blood: this thick soft vascular membrane being admirably prepared for the reception of the fertilised ovum. Should fertilisation not take place, the ovum dies, the corpus luteum disintegrates, and the endometrium shows degenerative changes which are followed by bleeding.

**The menstrual phase,** characterised by vaginal bleeding, lasts for three or four days, and occurs every 28 to 30 days from puberty to the menopause in the normal woman. This is the terminal phase of the menstrual cycle. If the preparations made during the three preceding phases for the reception of a fertilised ovum are not required, they are discarded. The superficial layer of endometrium is shed, along with blood from the capillaries; the unfertilised ovum being discarded as well.

*Although physiologically the menstrual cycle ends with bleeding, it is customary when prescribing contraceptive pills to consider the first day of bleeding to be the first day of the menstrual cycle. This simplifies calculation of the day of starting administration of the pills for the woman concerned.*

## THE MENOPAUSE

The menopause, change of life or climacteric, is the end of the reproductive period: ovarian activity including ovulation ceases. About 50 per cent of women cease menstruating between the age of 45 and 50, but the menopause does rarely occur as early as 35 and as late as 55. The menstrual periods may be scanty and irregular for some months and within one year they usually cease, but the menopause is generally considered to extend over a period of two years. Pregnancy may occur after months of amenorrhoea.

Throughout this period systems of the body other than the reproductive may be disturbed. The effect on the circulatory system may be evident as palpitation. Vaso-motor instability is responsible for one of the most common disturbances, hot flushes. The tendency to obesity is fairly general. The blood pressure may be slightly raised and headaches and noises in the ears may be troublesome. Manifestations of a disturbed nervous system may occur, but they should not arise in a well-adjusted personality: reassurance, sympathetic understanding and much patience are needed in these cases.

Depression, anxiety, insomnia, irritability and tension may be present in slight or severe degrees. When menopausal symptoms are distressing to the patient the doctor may order one of the synthetic oestrogenic substances to be taken: the dose given is the least possible and for the shortest possible time. Good food, fresh air and adequate sleep are very necessary. There is a psychological aspect to this period of life, and women should not be encouraged to expect ill-health. They should lead an active life and maintain an interest in pursuits outside home or employment.

## THE OVUM

### *Early Development*

When ovulation takes place, the ovum, which is about 0·15 mm in diameter (about the size of the point of a fine needle), escapes into the peritoneal cavity and finds its way into the Fallopian tube. It is possible that under the influence of oestrogens at the time of ovulation the Fallopian tube becomes arched so that its fimbriated end is cupped underneath and around the ovary to receive the ovum from the ruptured Graafian follicle. The ovum, having no power of locomotion, is wafted along by the cilia, and by the peristaltic muscular contractions of the tube.

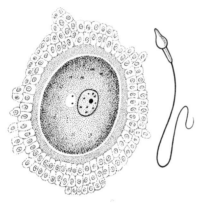

Fig. 3-1   Showing comparative size of ovum and spermatozoon.

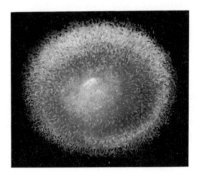

Fig.  3-2  Ovum  in  early  pregnancy covered with chorionic villi.

### Conception

**The fusion of the ovum and spermatozoon is called conception,** fertilisation, or impregnation, and initiates the beginning of a new life. Only one ovum is produced per month by the ovaries, but as many as 300,000,000 spermatozoa each 0·05 mm are deposited in the vagina when coitus takes place. At this time the cervix secretes a flow of alkaline mucus that attracts the spermatozoa. A limited number reach the Fallopian tube; but only one sperm nucleus fuses with the nucleus of the ovum. Almost without exception fertilisation takes place in the Fallopian tube, usually in the ampulla.

By a process of capacitation the spermatozoa are conditioned to fertilise the ovum after they enter the reproductive tract. The sperm head releases an enzyme under the influence of hyaluronidase which dissolves the zona pellucida cells of the oocyte: the cytoplasm of the oocyte then engulfs the spermatozoon. Complex changes in the surface of the oocyte prevent fertilisation by other spermatozoa.

The most likely period for conception to take place is immediately following ovulation which occurs 14 days previous to the next menstrual period. The majority of women conceive between the 10th and 18th day of the menstrual cycle; but fertilisation usually occurs 24 hours after ovulation. Neither ovum nor spermatozoon are thought to be capable of fertilisation for longer than 24 hours.

### Development of the fertilised ovum

While being propelled along the tube, segmentation or cell division takes place and the fertilised cell or zygote divides into 2–4–8–16 and so on until it consists of a ball of cells like a mulberry, known as the morula. (Three to four days are required for the journey along the tube to the uterus, and as the interstitial part of the Fallopian tube through which it must pass has a diameter of 1 mm, the ovum must be very small to pass through it.) A cavity or blastocele forms in the morula which now becomes known as the blastocyst. At one point the cells clump together, forming the inner cell mass; the remainder of the cells are pushed to the periphery.

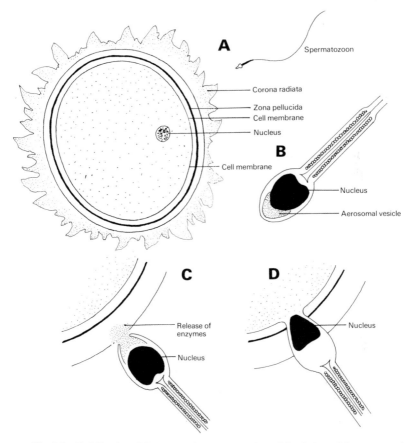

Fig. 3-3   Fertilisation. Diagrammatic representation of the fusion of the ovum and spermatozoon. (B, C and D are highly magnified).

### Embedding of the ovum

Six to seven days may elapse before the fertilised ovum, now at the trophoblast stage is ready for embedding. It comes to rest on the endometrium, and at the area of contact tiny projections or buds appear which could be likened to the sprouting roots of a germinating seed. The outer trophoblastic cells, known as the syncytio-trophoblast, have the power of breaking down tissue, eroding the endometrium and allowing the trophoblast to become embedded. The decidual reaction occurs to limit the invading propensity of the trophoblast.

When the ovum burrows into the implantation cavity, slight vaginal bleeding may occur which might be mistaken for a scanty menstrual period. The endometrial cells heal the opening, and the embedding of the ovum is complete. By the 13th day trophoblastic cells form rudimentary chorionic villi which contain no blood vessels; they absorb nutriment from the disintegrated cells in the implantation cavity.

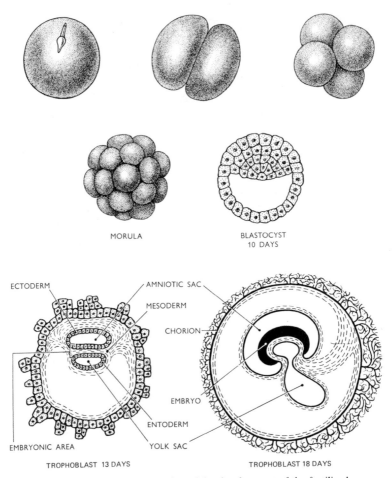

Fig. 3-4   Diagrammatic representation of the development of the fertilised ovum. Enlargement is slight until the trophoblast stage is reached.

## DEVELOPMENT OF THE EMBRYO

Three primitive layers in the ovum can now be differentiated, and from each layer particular parts of the fetus develop.

**The ectoderm** forms the nervous system, skin and certain lining mucosa.

**The mesoderm** forms bone, muscle, the circulatory system, and certain internal organs.

**The entoderm** forms the mucosa of the alimentary tract, the epithelium of the liver, pancreas, lungs and bladder.

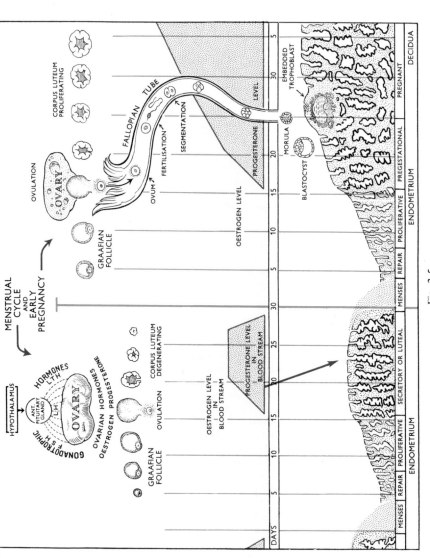

Fig. 3-5

EARLY PREGNANCY.

Diagrammatic representation, showing ovulation, fertilisation, decidual reaction and embedding of the fertilised ovum.

MENSTRUAL CYCLE.

Diagrammatic representation of the action of the gonadotrophic hormones on the ovary and of the ovarian hormones on the endometrium.

*In the Inner Cell Mass two cavities appear:*

(1) **The amniotic sac,** which is filled with fluid, and (2) immediately below it the **yolk sac.** The area between these two sacs is comprised of ectoderm, mesoderm, entoderm, and is known as the embryonic area, from which the embryo develops. The amniotic sac contains and protects the embryo, and as the cavity increases in size the amnion comes in contact with the chorion to which it becomes adherent (about the fourth week). The yolk sac provides nourishment for the embryo, until the trophoblastic cells develop sufficiently to absorb nutriment from the maternal tissues, and later from the mother's blood. The embryo is attached to the placenta by a broad band of mesoderm, the body stalk, which envelops part of the yolk sac and other structures. By a complicated process of 'folding off' the amniotic sac surrounds the embryo; the yolk sac is constricted and eventually atrophies. Primitive blood vessels appear in the embryo and chorionic villi: blood cells develop, and by the 6th week a primitive form of circulation is established, which at the 12th week is functioning completely.

### Formation of the decidua

Every month, from puberty to the menopause, the uterus prepares for a fertilised ovum. If conception takes place this preparation is intensified, and the endometrium becomes known as the decidua. The increased activity of the decidua is brought about by the stimulus of the oestrogenic hormones, which increase structural growth until the endometrium is four times the non-pregnant thickness—from 1·5 to 6 mm.

The hormone progesterone from the corpus luteum, under the influence of chorionic gonadotrophin, stimulates the secretory activity of the endometrial glands and increases the size of the blood vessels. The result is a soft, vascular, spongy bed in which the fertilised ovum can readily become implanted and find nutriment.

### The three layers of the decidua

1. **The compact layer** is made up of closely packed cells and the necks of glands: it is the most superficial of the three layers and is adjacent to the uterine cavity.

2. **The spongy layer** is mainly formed of tortuous dilated glands and of large stroma or decidual cells. This enlargement of the stroma cells during pregnancy is known as the '*decidual reaction*' and is nature's defence against the invading propensities of the syncytiotrophoblast. The function of the decidual reaction in limiting the advance of the chorionic villi to the spongy layer can be appreciated when we consider the method by which the placenta is separated during the third stage of labour. Throughout pregnancy the placenta remains securely embedded in the decidua, but as soon as the baby is born the placenta must be shed. If the placental attachment is limited to the loose spongy layer, it will be possible for the placenta to become separated from the decidua in much the same way as postage stamps can readily be detached at their line of perforation. Should the placenta embed too deeply, it would be morbidly adherent, and so complicate the third stage of labour.

3. **The basement layer** regenerates the new endometrium during the puerperium.

### The three areas of decidua

1. **The decidua basalis** is the area of decidua underneath the embedded ovum.
2. **The decidua capsularis** lies over the developing ovum.
3. **The decidua vera** or true decidua lines the remainder of the uterus.

As the ovum grows, the decidua capsularis distends, and at the 12th week comes into contact with the decidua vera, degenerates and disappears.

### Development of the placenta

During the third week, the ovum is completely covered with chorionic villi; those next to the spongy layer of the decidua grow profusely and are known as **chorion frondosum**, which ultimately form the placenta. These chorionic villi penetrate the blood vessels with which they come in contact, and become bathed in a lake of maternal blood, the opened vessels being known as sinuses and the areas surrounding the villi as blood spaces.

Some of the chorionic villi are attached to the decidua—**the anchoring villi**—the majority float in the slowly circulating maternal blood from which they absorb nutriment. The villi on the remainder of the trophoblast degenerate, leaving the bald chorion—the **chorion laeve**—which on its inner surface is adherent to the amnion and on its outer surface to the decidua capsularis, and after the 12th week to the decidua vera.

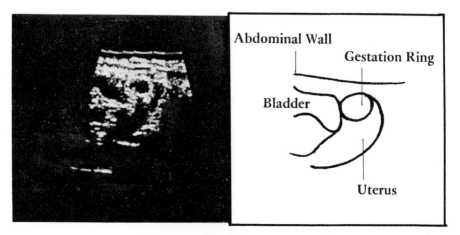

Fig. 3-6   Ultrasonogram of seven weeks' pregnancy.
*Aberdeen Maternity Hospital.*

**A chorionic villus** is a branching structure arising from the chorionic membrane as a single stem, which divides and subdivides until it terminates in the fine filaments that are embedded in the decidua basalis. The outer layer of a chorionic villus, the syncytiotrophoblast, is derived from the cytotrophoblast, the inner trophoblastic layer. By their selective action chorionic villi absorb from the maternal blood the particular substances needed for the developing embryo. The centre of the villus contains mesoderm and blood vessels, within which fetal blood circulates. The fetal heart pumps 500 ml of blood through the placenta per minute.

**The fetus develops its own blood,** just as it develops its heart, brain, eyes, etc., and it must not be thought that maternal blood circulates in the fetus. There are four layers of tissue between fetal and maternal blood, i.e. syncytiotrophoblast, cytotrophoblast, mesoderm and the capillary wall. Unless some breakdown of the placenta occurs, fetal and maternal blood do not mix.

From the 12th to the 20th week the placenta weighs as much as and even more than the fetus, and this is because it must deal with the metabolic processes of nutrition, with which the fetal organs are not sufficiently developed to cope. During the later weeks of pregnancy some of the fetal organs, such as the liver, begin to function, so the cytotrophoblast and the syncytiotrophoblast gradually degenerate.

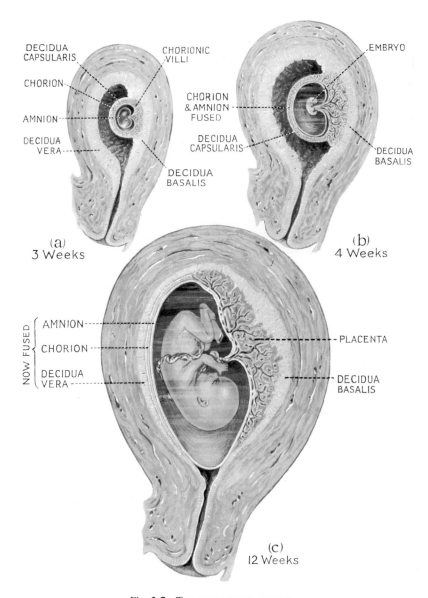

Fig. 3-7 THE DEVELOPING EMBRYO.

(a) (3 weeks).—Showing the amniotic sac, surrounded by chorion which is covered with decidua capsularis. (b) (4 weeks).—Amnion is in contact with chorion: decidua capsularis is growing outwards into the uterine cavity. The placenta is seen embedded in the decidua basalis. (c) (12 weeks).—The decidua capsularis has thinned out and atrophied: the chorion is attached to the decidua vera. (After Williams, *American Journal of Obstetrics and Gynae-cology.*)

## THE PLACENTA AT TERM

The placenta or afterbirth is a round, flat mass, about 20 cm in diameter, 2·5 cm thick at the centre and weighing approximately one-sixth of the weight of the baby at term. It is made up of chorionic villi and blood vessels containing fetal blood. It also consists of the decidua basalis, in which the villi embed, the choriodecidual spaces and the maternal blood contained in them.

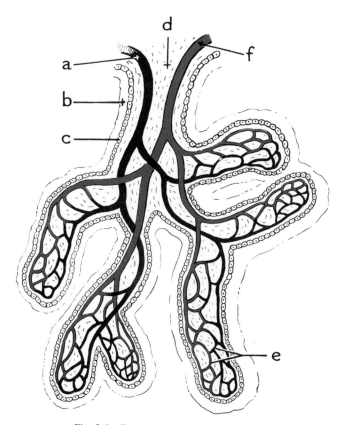

Fig. 3-8   Diagram of a chorionic villus.

(a) Branch of umbilical artery carrying fetal impure blood. (b) Syncytiotrophoblast, the outer layer of the villus. (c) Cytotrophoblast. (d) Mesoderm. (e) Capillaries through which the interchange between fetal and maternal blood takes place. (f) Branch of umbilical vein returning oxygenated blood to the fetus.

**The maternal surface** is made up of chorionic villi, arranged in cotyledons or lobules that are separated by sulci or furrows. Maternal blood gives it a bluish-red colour, and the surface is covered by a thin layer of trophoblastic cells. Frequently the maternal surface is covered with small deposits of lime salts which have no clinical significance.

**The fetal surface** is smooth, white and shiny, and on it can be seen branches of the umbilical vein and arteries and the insertion of the umbilical cord. It is covered with two membranes, the chorion and amnion, which are continued beyond its outer edge to form the sac that contains the fetus and amniotic fluid.

## PLACENTAL CIRCULATION

Blood from the fetal heart circulates through the fetus, and because of the need for oxygenation and replenishment it leaves the fetus and is carried by the arteries of the umbilical cord to the placenta. The umbilical arteries spread over the fetal surface of the placenta and subdivide until they terminate in the chorionic villi, which absorb from the mother's blood the products of digestion; *e.g.* amino-acids,

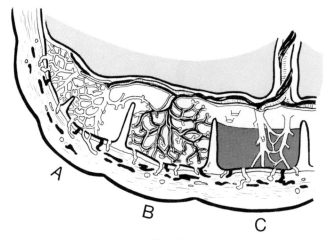

Fig. 3-9

**DIAGRAMMATIC REPRESENTATION OF PLACENTAL STRUCTURE**

Umbilical vein transporting replenished blood from placenta to fetus.
Umbilical arteries transporting impure blood from fetus to placenta.
Three cotyledons separated by septa.
A showing structure of chorionic villi.
B showing villi with capillaries containing fetal blood.
C showing intervillous spaces containing maternal blood which provides $O_2$, nutrients and electrolytes to fetal capillaries in the chorionic villi which are floating in maternal blood.

glucose, minerals, vitamins, and fatty acids. The fetal alimentary tract does not digest food, nor do the lungs inhale oxygen, therefore the placenta carries out the functions of stomach, intestine, liver, lungs and kidneys. Oxygen is taken from the mother's haemoglobin, and carbon dioxide and other waste products are given off into the maternal blood, the interchange of substances taking place by osmosis and diffusion, as well as by the selective action of the cytotrophoblast and the syncytiotrophoblast. The replenished oxygenated blood returns to the fetus via the umbilical vein.

# FUNCTIONS OF THE PLACENTA

The placenta is a metabolic and incomplete endocrine organ as well as the means through which the fetus obtains its needs: it not only selects and transports from the mother's blood the substances necessary for fetal life and growth; it also changes some of these so that the fetus can utilise them. Placenta and fetus are a functioning unit. The fetus is dependant on the placenta for the quality of life *in utero*.

*Placental functions can be classified as:*

**Nutritive**

**The fetus requires amino-acids (proteins) for building tissue;** glucose for growth and energy; calcium and phosphorus for the composition of bones and teeth; water, vitamins, electrolytes, iron and other minerals for blood formation, growth and various body processes.

Until the fetal liver is sufficiently developed to function, the placenta metabolises glucose, stores it in the form of glycogen and reconverts it into glucose as required. The products of digestion which are present in the mother's blood pass to the fetus via the placenta, mainly by enzymatic carriers. Fatty acids pass through the placenta; minerals and vitamins are readily transported across the placenta to the fetus.

It is the mother's food which provides fetal nutriment, and only when her diet is inadequate are her tissues depleted. To meet fetal requirements and avoid maternal depletion a diet rich in the essential foodstuffs is therefore imperative during pregnancy.

### Respiratory

Actual pulmonary respiration does not take place in utero. The fetus obtains oxygen from the mother's haemoglobin by simple diffusion and gives off carbon dioxide into the maternal blood, and although fetal respiratory movements take place there is no pulmonary exchange of gases *in utero*.

### Excretory

Excretion from the fetus is not very great as its metabolism is mainly anabolic or building up. It is the catabolic process of metabolism—the breaking down of tissue—that produces excretory products.

### Endocrine

(*a*) **Human chorionic gonadotrophin** (HCG) is produced in the chorionic villi. This hormone forms the basis of the immunological and other pregnancy tests. Large amounts are excreted during the 7th to 10th week but after the 12th week the peak period has passed and a low level is maintained until term.

(*b*) **Progesterone is produced by the placenta** from about the 12th week; the amount rises steadily throughout pregnancy and falls when the placenta is expelled.

(*c*) **Oestriol is produced by the feto-placental unit** from the 6th to 12th week when the amount rises steadily until term; then, after expulsion of the placenta, it falls and allows prolactin to initiate lactation. The fetus provides the placenta with the vital precursors for the production of oestriol and as both placenta and fetus are concerned in the production of oestriol, the amount excreted in the urine during pregnancy is an index of feto-placental function.

(*d*) **Human** placental lactogen (H.P.L.) is produced by the syncytiotrophoblast. The level of H.P.L. in the blood reflects placental function: a level below 4 micrograms/ml at 38 weeks suggests the possibility of fetal hypoxia during labour. The false positive rate is considerable.

*Every enzyme known to exist in biology has been found in the placenta.*

### Inactivation

The placenta by enzymatic function inactivates a number of undesirable substances. With the exception of certain viruses, few organisms pass through the placenta to the fetus. The treponema pallidum passes readily, more rarely the tubercle bacillus; the protozoa of malaria and toxoplasmosis also reach the fetal blood stream. The virus of rubella passes through the placenta, and if the woman is infected prior to the twelfth week of pregnancy the infant may suffer from cardiac defects, cataract, or deaf mutism.

Sedative drugs and analgesic gases do pass and act on the fetus. If morphine is given to the mother within three hours of the birth of the baby, it could depress the fetal respiratory centre and make the establishment of respiration difficult. Anaesthetics given to the mother pass into the fetal circulation. It is known that antibiotics pass; antisyphilitic drugs given to the mother have the same beneficial action on the fetus. Teratogenic drugs pass through the placenta and cause fetal deformities.

## MALFORMATIONS OF THE PLACENTA

**Placenta succenturiata** is probably the most significant abnormality from the practical point of view, and consists of an accessory lobe of placental tissue, situated in the fetal sac membrane with blood vessels running to the main placenta. It is formed by hypertrophy of some chorionic villi in the chorion laeve, which should have atrophied. Such a lobe is liable to be retained *in utero* and may give rise to profuse puerperal haemorrhage. **If there is a hole in the membrane with blood vessels running to it,** the midwife will know that a succenturiate lobe, and not a piece of membrane, has been retained.

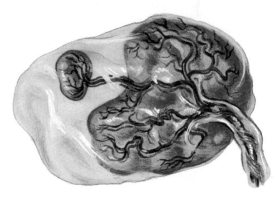

Fig. 3-10  Placenta succenturiata. Fetal surface—showing blood vessels running in the chorion from the main placenta to the accessory lobe.

**Placenta bipartita or tripartita** is one where there are two or three complete, or almost complete lobes. Their blood vessels unite when joining the umbilical cord, whereas the vessels of the succenturiate lobe do not directly join the cord vessels. In twin placentae there are two cords.

**Placenta circumvallata** has a double layer of amnion and chorion which has undergone infarction: this is seen as an opaque ring on the fetal surface. It has little significance.

## DISEASES OF THE PLACENTA

**Hydatidiform mole,** a cystic, degenerative proliferation of the chorionic villi, is considered on page 173.

**Infarcts** are areas of necrosed chorionic villi, red in the early stage and white later with a solid cartilaginous consistency, produced by increased concentration of tissue thromboplastin. They are commonly seen on the maternal surface, but may be present on the fetal aspect.

Calcareous degeneration, characterised by gritty particles that feel like sandpaper and sometimes form plaques on the maternal surface, is not infarction: it is associated with the normal degenerative processes of the placenta at term. The small white areas often present around the periphery of the placenta are fibrin nodes and are not true infarcts.

**Syphilis.** On microscopic examination, changes due to endarteritis—inflammation of the wall of an artery—are seen; syphilitic placentae are not always large, pale or greasy-looking as was once believed.

**Oedema of the placenta.** The large, pale placenta with water oozing from it is associated with hydrops fetalis and is due to haemolytic disease of the newborn, caused by Rhesus immunisation.

At the Simpson Maternity Pavilion, Edinburgh, the following placentae were seen in cases of hydrops fetalis:

Baby 2·38 kg; placenta 2·20 kg.   Baby 1·07 kg; placenta 1·30 kg.

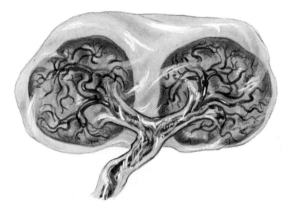

Fig. 3-11   Placenta bipartita. The umbilical vessels bifurcate at the point of insertion of the cord.

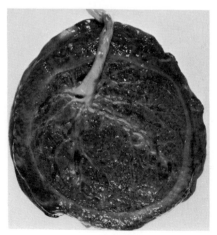

Fig. 3-12   Placenta circumvallata.

### THE FETAL SAC

**The fetal sac** consists of a double membrane; the outer, chorion; the inner, amnion. The fetus and amniotic fluid are contained within this sac, which ruptures during labour to permit the expulsion of both.

**The chorion** is a thick, opaque, friable membrane, adherent to the decidua vera on its outer aspect, until the third stage of labour when it becomes detached during the expulsion of the placenta. As pieces of chorion may be retained *in utero*, it must

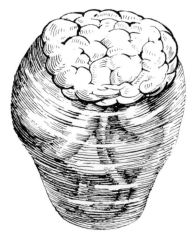

Fig. 3-13    Fetal sac containing 28 weeks' fetus.

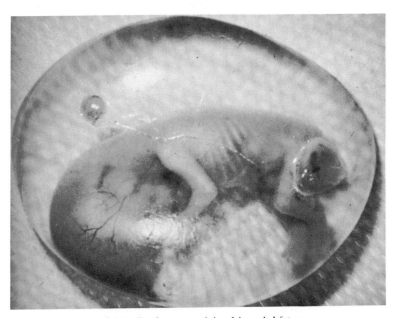

Fig. 3-14    Fetal sac containing 14 weeks' fetus.

always be carefully examined after being separated from the amnion: the chorion cannot be peeled off the fetal surface of the placenta because the placental chorionic villi are growing from it.

**The amnion** is a smooth, tough, translucent membrane, lining the chorion, from which it can be detached up to the insertion of the umbilical cord.

## THE AMNIOTIC FLUID

The clear pale straw-coloured fluid in which the fetus floats is present in the amniotic sac from the earliest weeks of pregnancy: the amount increasing until at term the quantity is from 500 to 1,500 ml. It consists of 99 per cent water, is alkaline in reaction, and various mineral salts are present, including urea, which is derived from urine passed by the fetus. A trace of protein (0·25 per cent) is usually found in the amniotic fluid, therefore a voided specimen of urine from a woman whose membranes have ruptured may contain a trace of protein. If the amount of fluid is over 1,500 ml, the condition is known as **polyhydramnios,** and if less than 300 ml the term **oligohydramnios** is applied.

Epidermal cells and lanugo from the skin of the fetus are usually present, and with vernix caseosa may give it a turbid or milky appearance.

**A green tinge** is due to the presence of meconium and should be taken as a sign of fetal distress, and the fetal heart-sounds investigated. Thick meconium during the second stage of labour in a breech presentation may not indicate fetal distress. Golden coloured fluid is sometimes found in cases of Rh haemolytic disease.

Examination of the amniotic fluid at the 14th to 16th week by abdominal amniocentesis will reveal the presence of chromosomal anomalies and genetic defects. During the third trimester the amount of bilirubin is assessed in cases of Rh immunisation. The possibility of respiratory distress syndrome is likely when the lecithin/sphingomyelin ratio is low after the 34th week.

### Origin

The origin of the amniotic fluid is thought to be both fetal and maternal; the most likely source being the amniotic epithelium covering the fetal surface of the placenta and umbilical cord; also fetal urine from the 10th week of gestation.

The fetus swallows liquor, and in cases where the deglutition centre in the brain is not developed, as in some cases of anencephaly, an excess of amniotic fluid is present.

Fetal malformations, monstrosities, monozygotic (uniovular) twins and diabetes are associated with an excess of fluid.

### Functions

The fluid distends the amniotic sac and allows for the growth and free movement of the fetus. It acts as a shock absorber, protecting the fetus from jarring or injury.

During labour it equalises uterine pressure and prevents marked interference with the placental circulation.

## THE UMBILICAL CORD

The umbilical cord extends from the fetal umbilicus to the fetal surface of the placenta. It is composed of an embryonic form of connective tissue, intermingled with a gelatinous substance known as Wharton's jelly, and is covered with amnion. The cord carries two arteries, which are a continuation of the hypogastric arteries, containing impure blood going to the placenta.

The umbilical vein contains pure blood returning to the fetus after having been oxygenated, and replenished in the placenta. The vein can easily be seen, and in cases where the baby needs urgent treatment at birth, drugs may be injected into the vein and milked into the circulation.

A single artery is present in some cases and is often associated with other fetal abnormalities.

### Length of the cord

The average length of the cord is 56 cm and if less than 40 cm it is said to be short. Cords as short as 15 cm have been known, but fortunately are very rare: if the cord is wound round the fetus it is relatively short. In these cases the descent of the fetus may be retarded, the placenta may be separated prematurely, causing haemorrhage, or the cord may break. Such complications are uncommon.

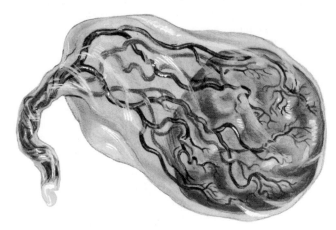

Fig. 3-15    Placenta velamentosa—fetal surface—showing the umbilical cord inserted in the membranes.

A long cord may become wound round the fetus, and cords of 1·5 to 2 m have been reported. It may be wound once, twice or three times round the neck, and this happens during the middle months of pregnancy, when the ratio of amniotic fluid to fetus is so great that it can move about freely.

**True knots in the cord occur** when loops form through which the fetus can pass, and if drawn tight when the fetus descends during labour, will lead to stillbirth due to anoxia. **False knots** are merely a heaping up of Wharton's jelly and are not significant.

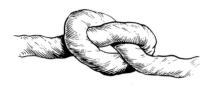

Fig. 3-16    True knot in the umbilical cord.

### INSERTION OF THE CORD

The cord is commonly inserted in the centre of the fetal surface of the placenta—a central insertion—one which is inserted away from the centre yet not at the edge is termed a lateral insertion.

**A battledore insertion** is one in which the cord is situated at the very edge of the placenta.

**A velamentous insertion** exists when the cord is inserted into the membranes of the fetal sac 5 to 10 cm from the edge of the placenta, with the umbilical blood vessels running between placenta and cord. This form of insertion is more dangerous when the placenta is situated in the lower uterine segment because the vessels may then lie over the os. (See vasa praevia below.)

**The term vasa praevia is applied** when the fetal blood vessels traverse the membranes and lie over the os in front of the presenting part during labour. This occurs in some cases of velamentous insertion of cord. The vessels may be

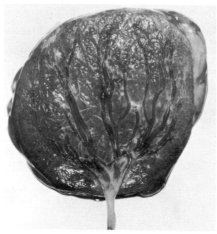

Fig. 3-17  Battledore Placenta. Note the cord inserted at the edge of the placenta.

compressed or may rupture with slight bleeding, and if the bleeding is severe the fetus becomes exsanguinated. The blood passed per vaginam is tested to determine whether it is fetal or maternal, using Singer's alkali-denaturation test. If fetal, delivery would be hastened. The baby's haemoglobin is estimated after birth. In a surprising number of cases the blood vessels do not rupture.

---

## QUESTIONS FOR REVISION
### DEVELOPMENT OF OVUM AND PLACENTA

What term is applied to (1) The ovum: (a) when a ball of cells ..................... (b) when a cavity forms in the cell mass .................... (c) the outer cells of the blastocyst .................... (2) The outer layer of a chorionic villus .................... (3) The chorionic villi which grow profusely and form the placenta ....................

Which conditions might result if the following passed through the placenta? Virus of rubella, morphine; Rh antibodies; teratogenic drugs; treponema pallidum.

Give alternative terms for the following: climacteric; rubella; placenta; conception; zygote.

For which main purpose does the fetus require: calcium; amino acids; iron; vitamins?

By which urine assay can feto-placental dysfunction be assessed.

Describe the following: conception; the fetal sac; amniotic fluid; the decidua; embedding of the ovum.

Differentiate between the terms (a) ovum–embryo: (b) fetus–baby: (c) decidua–endometrium: (d) proliferative and secretory phases of the menstrual cycle.

### Oral Questions

(1) What is the cause of green; golden; turbid amniotic fluid? (2) Name three harmful substances which pass through the placenta, and what the midwife could do regarding prevention. (3) Why should the amnion always be separated from the chorion when examining the placenta? (4) How would the fact that a succenturiate lobe had been retained be evident? (5) How would you recognise:—(a) a velamentous insertion of cord? (b) vasa praevia. Differentiate between (a) true and false knots in umbilical cord (b) amnion and chorion (c) polyhydramnios and oligohydramnios.

## *Rearrange numbers correctly:*

| Description | Term | | |
|---|---|---|---|
| (1) Cord at edge of placenta | velamentosa | ( | ) |
| (2) Accessory lobe of placenta | bipartita | ( | ) |
| (3) Opaque ring on fetal surface | battledore | ( | ) |
| (4) Two lobes of placenta | succenturiata | ( | ) |
| (5) Thrombotic areas of placenta | circumvallata | ( | ) |
| (6) Cord inserted in membrane | vasa praevia | ( | ) |
| (7) Fetal blood vessels lying over os | infarcts | ( | ) |

**C.M.B.(Scot.) 30-min. question.** Describe fertilisation of the ovum and the subsequent development until the 12th week of pregnancy.

**C.M.B.(Scot.) 30-min question.** Describe the functions of the placenta. How may placental function be assessed?

**C.M.B.(Scot.) 30-min question.** Describe the amniotic fluid. How might an examination of this fluid influence the management of a patient during pregnancy and labour?

**C.M.B.(Scot.)** Describe how the placenta is formed. List the abnormalities which may occur during its formation.

**C.M.B.(Scot.)** Describe the processes of ovulation and fertilisation.

**C.M.B.(Eng.)** What are the functions of the placenta? How can placental function be monitored in pregnancy?

# 4
# The Fetus
*Fetal development. Fetal circulation. Fetal skull; bones, sutures, measurements*

It is essential that the midwife should have some idea of how very small the embryo is during the early weeks so that, in cases of abortion, she may know what to look for. Very seldom is the embryo of less than six weeks seen, as it is not readily detected in the blood clot.

**The ovum** is the term used during the first three weeks for the whole structure, including the sac.

**The embryo** is the term used from the 3rd to the 8th week.

**The fetus** is the term used from the 9th week until birth.

It is not always easy to estimate the age of an embryo. Length and weight, the degree of development and the period of gestation are all taken into consideration.

**Three weeks.** The ovum (complete sac) is the size of a small grape and covered with fine shaggy-looking chorionic villi. No human characteristics can be recognised.

**Four weeks.** The sac is 2·5 cm long, about the size of a pigeon's egg. The embryo measures about 1 cm and weighs 1 g. It is curved like a bean so that the head and tail almost meet. The rudimentary eyes are visible and small buds indicate where limbs will develop. Circulation of blood in a rudimentary form exists: the heart is beating. At six weeks the gestation sac can be seen by ultrasound.

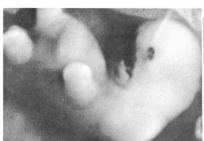 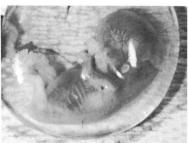

Fig. 4-1 Fetus 5½ weeks.     Fig. 4-2 Fetus 9 weeks in sac.

*Courtesy of Dr T. Baker, Simpson Memorial Maternity Pavilion, Edinburgh.*

**Eight weeks.** The sac is the size of a hen's egg and the chorionic villi will have disappeared, leaving the chorion laeve (bald chorion) except in the area where the villi are deeply embedded. The embedded villi grow profusely and are known as the chorion frondosum which ultimately form the placenta. The embryo is 3 cm long and weighs 4 g. Amniotic fluid 5–10 ml is present. Centres of ossification are apparent in some bones; hands and feet are recognisable. The head is large in proportion to the body. At 10 weeks urine is secreted.

**Twelve weeks.** The sac is the size of a goose's egg and the placenta, which is now well formed, weighs more than the fetus. The length of the fetus is 10 cm and it weighs just under 60 g. Fingers and toes are evident. The fetal head can be seen and measured by ultrasound.

53

**Sixteen weeks.** The fetus measures 15 cm and weighs approximately 170 g. The nasal septum and palate fuse, and if this fails to take place, cleft palate results. There is a good heart beat. Sex can be distinguished: meconium is present in the intestine.

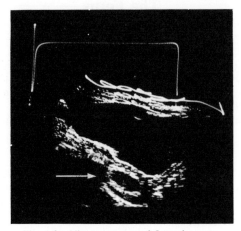

Fig. 4-3  Ultrasonogram of 8 weeks gestation sac. Anteverted uterus containing the sac (arrow) lying behind a very full bladder (black area above).

*Queen Mother's Hospital, Glasgow*

**Twenty weeks.** The fetus is 20 cm long and weighs 400 g. Vernix caseosa is present on the skin and there are fine downy hairs on the head and eyebrows. Finger nails can be distinguished. Fetal movement is felt by the mother (quickening) and the fetal heart can be heard on auscultation.

**Twenty-four weeks.** The fetus measures 30 cm and weighs about 700 g.

**Twenty-eight weeks.** The fetus measures 36 cm and weighs 1 kg. Legally, **the fetus is viable.**

**Thirty-two weeks.** The fetus measures 40 cm and weighs 1·5 kg. The skin is red and wrinkled. Lanugo is less plentiful.

**Thirty-six weeks.** The fetus is 46 cm long and weighs 2·5 kg. There is a little subcutaneous fat. The plantar creases are visible. The nails reach the finger tips and the cartilage of the ears is soft. The survival rate is good.

**Forty weeks.** The fetus measures 50 cm and weighs 3·2 kg but length is a better criterion of maturity than weight. The baby is well covered with subcutaneous fat: the skin is red but not wrinkled.

The figures for length and weight given above are only approximate. Wide variations can occur. The baby born at 40 weeks may weigh from 2·8 to 5·4 kg, male infants being slightly bigger than female. In a series of 40,000 deliveries at the Simpson Memorial Maternity Pavilion, Edinburgh, only six babies weighed over 5·4 kg and one was 6·1 kg.

## THE FETAL CIRCULATION

To understand the fetal circulation, the fact must be appreciated that the fetus develops its own blood and that at no time do the fetal and maternal blood mix unless some pathological process is present in the placenta. The fetus produces its own red and white blood corpuscles. During intra-uterine life the fetal gastro-intestinal and respiratory systems are not functioning, so from the maternal blood the fetus obtains the necessary nutriment and oxygen as explained below.

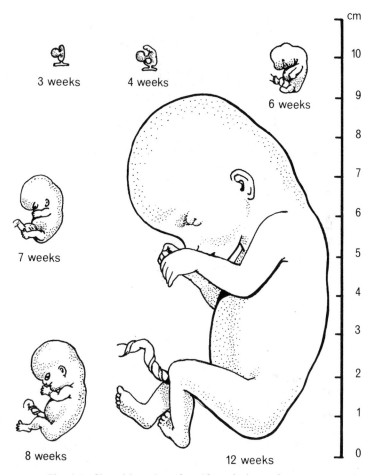

Fig. 4-4  Size of fetus from 3 to 12 weeks in centimetres.

### THERE ARE FOUR TEMPORARY STRUCTURES IN THE FETAL CIRCULATION

1. **The ductus venosus** (*from a vein to a vein*). This vessel from the umbilical vein to the inferior vena cava carries blood, that has been oxygenated and replenished by the placenta, to the heart for circulation throughout the fetus.

2. **The foramen ovale,** a temporary opening between the two atria in the fetal heart to allow the replenished blood to enter the left atrium and be pumped out through the aorta.

3. **The ductus arteriosus** (*from an artery to an artery*). This vessel from the pulmonary artery to the descending arch of the aorta carries the impure blood returned from the head and upper limbs thereby by-passing the pulmonary circulation.

   4. **The hypogastric arteries.** These two vessels branch off from the internal iliac
arteries and are known as the umbilical arteries when they enter the umbilical cord.

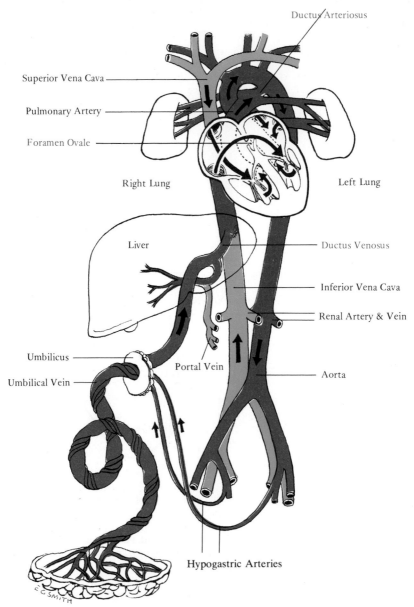

Ductus Arteriosus

Superior Vena Cava

Pulmonary Artery

Foramen Ovale

Right Lung

Left Lung

Liver

Ductus Venosus

Inferior Vena Cava

Renal Artery & Vein

Umbilicus

Portal Vein

Aorta

Umbilical Vein

Hypogastric Arteries

Fig. 4-5   A plan of the fetal circulation. The arrows represent the course which the blood
takes in the heart and vessels.

They return impure blood to the placenta for oxygenation and replenishment.
   Blood which has circulated throughout the fetus requires to be oxygenated and
replenished, so it is carried by the two umbilical arteries in the umbilical cord to the

placenta, where an interchange takes place between the fetal and maternal blood by a process of osmosis and diffusion, as well as by the selective action of the cytotrophoblast and the syncytiotrophoblast. Four layers separate fetal from maternal blood. These are syncytiotrophoblast, cytotrophoblast, mesoderm and the capillary wall. Carbon dioxide and other excretory products are given off into the maternal blood; nutritional substances and oxygen are picked up. It is important to realise that the blood which circulates within the fetal, umbilical and placental vessels is fetal in origin.

The replenished blood returns to the fetus by the vein in the umbilical cord which goes directly to the liver, but, before reaching that organ, a large branch, the **ductus venosus,** is given off and empties the purified blood into the inferior vena cava which is returning the impure blood to the heart from all the vessels below the diaphragm, including the portal vein. The oxygenated blood is therefore mingled with venous blood.

Through the temporary opening, known as the foramen ovale, between the two atria of the fetal heart the oxygenated blood returning from the placenta via the inferior vena cava is shunted from the right into the left atrium and not into the right ventricle, as is the route after birth. The blood then passes from the left atrium to the left ventricle where it is pumped out through the aorta. This blood has the highest oxygen content in the fetal circulation, and the major portion of it goes via branches of the arch of the aorta to the great vessels of the neck that supply the brain, and to the upper limbs. A smaller quantity passes down the descending arch of the aorta. The impure blood from the head and upper limbs returns to the heart via the superior vena cava and passes from the right atrium to the right ventricle (as it does after birth), and leaves the right ventricle by the pulmonary artery.

The pulmonary circulation functions very slightly before birth, the major amount of blood leaving the right ventricle of the fetus is therefore diverted from the lungs via a temporary vessel—the ductus arteriosus which conveys the blood from the pulmonary artery to the descending arch of the aorta, where it is distributed to the abdominal and pelvic viscera and to the lower limbs, but the greater proportion of it is returned to the placenta via the hypogastric arteries, which are branches of the internal iliac arteries. When they enter the umbilical cord they are then known as the umbilical arteries.

### Changes in the Circulation at Birth

The changes which occur are not due to the tying of the umbilical cord, but rather to the establishment of respiration. When the infant cries, the lungs expand and their vascular field is increased: so the blood which has been passing through the ductus arteriosus to the aorta now flows through the pulmonary arteries to the lungs for oxygenation. The ductus arteriosus ceases to function within five minutes after birth and within two months it is closed anatomically; it eventually becomes a cardiac ligament. In a very small number of cases the ductus arteriosus remains patent.

The valve-like foramen ovale closes when the increased flow of blood to the lungs reduces the pressure in the right side of the heart and increases the tension in the left side. If this does not occur, the venous blood in the right atrium will mix with arterial blood in the left atrium of the heart and produce marked cyanosis.

## THE FETAL SKULL

The fetal skull is extremely important in obstetrics, not only because it contains the brain which may be subjected to great pressure while the head is being forced through the birth canal, but because it is so large in comparison with the true pelvis.

Obviously, some adaptation between skull and pelvis must take place during labour. Ninety-six per cent of babies are born head first, and the head is the most difficult part to deliver, whether it comes first or last. Regions of the head may present which increase the hazards of birth for mother and child, but a sound knowledge of the landmarks and measurements of the skull will enable the midwife to recognise malpresentation or disproportion between skull and pelvis and to deliver the baby with the minimal amount of fetal and maternal trauma.

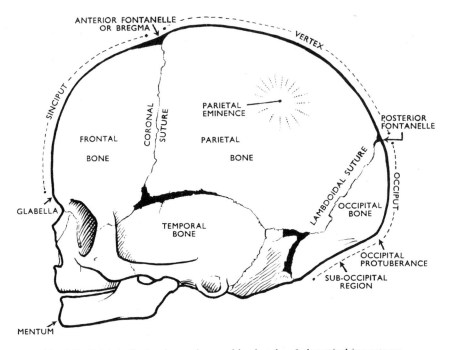

Fig. 4-6   Fetal skull, showing regions and landmarks of obstetrical importance.

## BONES AND SUTURES

The skull bones, having obstetric significance, are the two parietal, the frontal, and the occipital. The skull bones are developed from membrane, whereas most of the skeleton develops from cartilage. The intra-membranous ossification of the skull bones begins as early as the 8th week of intra-uterine life. At term the skull bones are thin and pliable and, as ossification at their edges is not quite complete, areas of membrane persist between the bones. The membranous spaces between the bones of the vault of the skull are known as sutures and during labour considerable overlapping of the skull bones takes place at these membranous spaces. The sutures form very useful landmarks to determine presentation and position when making a vaginal examination during labour.

**The sagittal suture** lies between the two parietal bones.

**The lambdoidal suture** separates the occipital and parietal bones.

**The coronal suture** runs between the parietal and frontal bones, crossing from one temple to the other.

**The frontal suture** separates the two halves of the frontal bone.

## FONTANELLES

Where two or more sutures meet, the membranous space at the junction is known as a fontanelle. There are six fontanelles on the skull, but only two are of obstetrical importance, the anterior and the posterior.

**The anterior fontanelle,** or bregma, is the membranous space at the junction of the sagittal, coronal and frontal sutures. It is diamond-shaped, about 2·5 cm long, 1·25 cm wide, and can be recognised vaginally as the junction of four sutures. Pulsations of the cerebral vessels can be felt through it. The anterior fontanelle

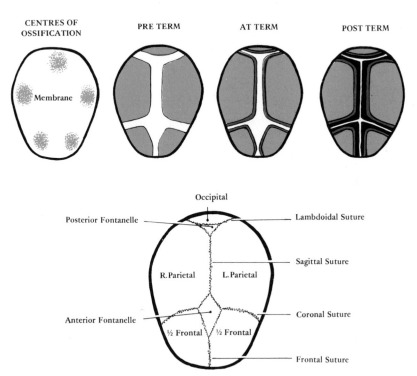

Fig. 4-7 Diagrammatic representation of development of bone in the vertex area of fetal skull showing sutures and fontanelles in the preterm, term and post-term fetus.

should be closed by the time the child is 18 months old, and if not, the possibility of rickets should be considered.

**The posterior fontanelle** is situated at the junction of the sagittal and lambdoidal sutures; it is smaller than the anterior fontanelle and can be recognised vaginally as the junction of three sutures. In shape it is triangular and should be closed about six weeks after birth.

## REGIONS OF THE SKULL

The skull is divided into the vault, face and base. The **vault** is the large dome-shaped compressible part made up of the two parietal, the upper parts of the frontal, occipital and temporal bones, and is the region above an imaginary line drawn from the orbital ridges to the nape of the neck. The **base** is comprised of bones firmly united to afford protection to the vital centres in the medulla.

**The vertex** is the area bounded in front by the anterior fontanelle, behind by the posterior fontanelle and laterally by the two parietal eminences which are seen as two prominent points on the parietal bones. Ninety-five of the 96 per cent of babies who are born head first present by the vertex.

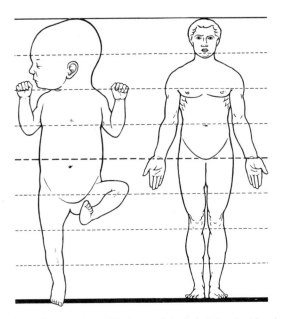

Fig. 4-8   Comparison of proportions of baby to adult. Baby's head wider than its shoulders and one quarter of its length.

**The face,** which in the newborn is very small because of the poorly developed mandible, is the area from the root of the nose to the junction of the chin and neck. The face bones are firmly united at birth and do not permit of moulding. The chin or *mentum* is an important landmark.

**The brow or sinciput** is composed of the frontal bone and is bounded by the orbital ridges and the coronal suture.

**The occiput** is the region over the occipital bone and extends from the posterior fontanelle to the foramen magnum. The suboccipital region is that part under the occipital protuberance, a prominent point on the posterior aspect of the skull.

We are so accustomed to the proportions of a baby that we do not always realise that the head is larger than the width of the shoulders. (The bisacromial diameter of the shoulders measures 11·5 cm; the mento-vertical diameter of the skull measures 13·5 cm.)

### DIAMETERS

**Biparietal**—9·5 cm measured between the two parietal eminences.

**Bitemporal**—8·2 cm measured from the furthest points of the coronal suture (between the temples).

**Suboccipito-bregmatic**—9·5 cm measured from below the occipital protuberance (the nape of the neck) to the centre of the anterior fontanelle or bregma.

**Suboccipito-frontal**—10 cm from below the occipital protuberance to the centre of the sinciput.

**Occipito-frontal**—11·5 cm from the occipital protuberance to the glabella, a point above the bridge of the nose, see Fig. 4–6.

**Submento-bregmatic**—9·5 cm from where the chin joins the neck to the centre of the anterior fontanelle or bregma.

**Submento-vertical**—11·5 cm from where the chin joins the neck to the highest point on the vertex.

**Mento-vertical**—13·5 cm from the tip of the chin to the highest point on the vertex (which is nearer the posterior than the anterior fontanelle).

These measurements should be learned in conjunction with the presentation with which they are associated. It is a distinct advantage for the midwife to be conversant with the most advantageous diameter in each presentation, for by promoting flexion or extension of the head she can often bring more favourable diameters over the perineum with less injury to mother and baby.

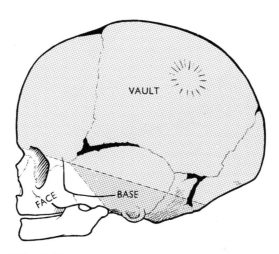

Fig. 4-9 Regions of the skull showing the large compressible vault, the non-compressible face and base.

## CEPHALIC OR HEAD PRESENTATIONS

**Vertex presentation.** When the head is well flexed, the suboccipito-bregmatic and the biparietal are the two diameters of the presenting circular area, the circumference of which is 29 cm. This is the most favourable presentation because of its small size and circular shape. The suboccipito-frontal diameter 10 cm will sweep the perineum.

When the head is deflexed it is erect, as in the military attitude. The engaging diameters are: occipito-frontal, 11·5 cm, and transversely the biparietal, 9·5 cm and bitemporal, 8·2 cm. The circumference measures 34·5 cm, and is ovoid in shape. The occipito-frontal diameter, 11·5 cm, will sweep the perineum.

**Face presentation.** The face presents when the head is completely extended, and the diameter engaging is the submento-bregmatic, 9·5 cm. The submento-vertical diameter, 11·5 cm will sweep the perineum.

**Brow presentation.** When partial extension occurs, the engaging diameter is the mento-vertical, 13·5 cm, with a circumference of 38 cm. Rarely can a baby be born naturally when the brow presents.

## Movement of the fetal head

The fetal head is capable of a wide range of movement, and may be flexed until the chin is in contact with the chest, as occurs in a vertex presentation when the head is well flexed. Complete extension of the head may take place, so that the occiput is in contact with the fetal back, as occurs when the face presents. A certain amount of lateral flexion is possible and the head can also rotate on the neck two-eighths of a circle (90 degrees). These movements are of importance in the mechanism of labour.

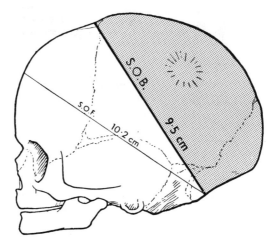

Fig. 4-10    Diameters concerned in a vertex presentation head well flexed. The suboccipito-frontal diameter 'sweeps the perineum.'

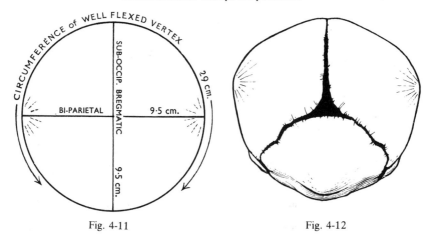

Fig. 4-11                                          Fig. 4-12

Showing the diameters (and circumference) presenting in a well-flexed head.

### MOULDING

Moulding is the term applied to the change in shape of the fetal head that takes place, due to the prolonged compression to which it is subjected, during its passage through the birth canal. This alteration in shape is possible because the bones of the vault, not being well ossified, are somewhat pliable and permit a slight degree of bending, but **the over-riding of the skull bones at the sutures** is the most important factor in moulding.

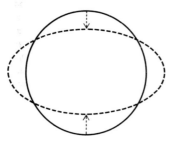

Fig. 4-13 Demonstration of the principle of moulding. The diameter compressed is diminished; the diameter at right angles to it is elongated.

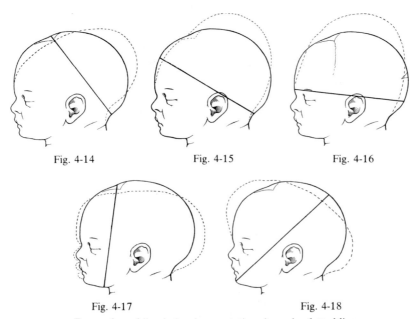

Fig. 4-14          Fig. 4-15          Fig. 4-16

Fig. 4-17                    Fig. 4-18

Types of moulding in head presentation shown by dotted line.

Fig. 4-14   Vertex presentation head well flexed. Fig. 4-15   Vertex presentation, occipito-posterior position (note that the moulding is higher). Fig. 4-16   Vertex presentation head deflexed (the sugar-loaf head). Fig. 4-17   Face presentation. Fig. 4-18   Brow presentation.

A certain amount of moulding is present on every baby's head, except in those born by elective Caesarean section. In breech presentation compression of the head is of short duration so no moulding is evident although over-riding of the skull bones may have occurred temporarily. During moulding the engaging diameter is compressed and may be shortened by as much as 1·25 cm and the diameter at right angles to it will be elongated. In the vertex presentation, L.O.A., the suboccipito-bregmatic diameter is reduced and the mento-vertical diameter is lengthened. It is possible to diagnose what the presentation has been by the shape of the moulded head after birth.

In small preterm babies moulding is excessive; **the soft skull bones and wide sutures afford little protection** to the delicate brain substance. In postmature babies the sutures are almost closed and the head does not mould well; the hardness of the head rather than its increased size tends to make labour more difficult.

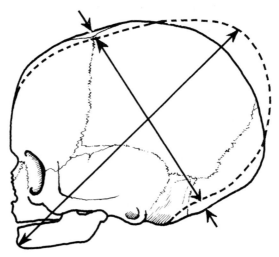

Fig. 4-19  Moulding. Arrows show direction in which the well-flexed head is being compressed. Note how it is elongated in the mento-vertical diameter.

---

## QUESTIONS FOR REVISION

### THE FETUS

How would you recognise the anterior and posterior fontanelles per vaginam? What is the benefit of a well flexed head during labour? When should the anterior fontanelle close?

### *Match term and description by correct numbers:*

|  |  |  |
|---|---|---|
| (1) **ovum:** | fertilised cell from 3rd to 8th week | (        ) |
| (2) **vernix:** | downy hair on newborn skin | (        ) |
| (3) **embryo:** | fertilised cell first three weeks | (        ) |
| (4) **sagittal suture:** | between parietal and occipital bones | (        ) |
| (5) **lanugo:** | creamy substance on newborn skin | (        ) |
| (6) **suture:** | junction of membranous spaces | (        ) |
| (7) **bregma:** | the brow | (        ) |
| (8) **lambdoidal suture:** | between parietal bones | (        ) |
| (9) **cephalic:** | bounded by two fontanelles and biparietal eminences | (        ) |
| (10) **vertex:** | the head | (        ) |
| (11) **fontanelle:** | a membranous space | (        ) |
| (12) **sinciput:** | the anterior fontanelle | (        ) |

Where are the following situated and what are their functions? Ductus venosus; foramen ovale; ductus arteriosus; hypogastric arteries.

Differentiate between cephalic and vertex presentation.

When can the fetal heart sounds be heard on auscultation? When are the plantar creases visible and what is their significance? When is the gestation sac visible by ultrasound? What percentage of babies are born head first?

Which diameters present in the following: vertex presentation—(*a*) head well flexed, (*b*) head deflexed? (2) Face presentation? (3) Brow presentation?

**C.M.B.(Eng.) 30-min. question.** Describe the fetal circulation and the changes that take place at birth.

**C.M.B.(Eng.) 30-min. question.** Describe the vault of the fetal skull. What are the dangers of moulding of the fetal skull?

**C.M.B.(Scot.).** Describe the anatomy of the fetal skull. How does a knowledge of (*a*) the measurements (*b*) the development of the fetal skull assist in the management of pregnancy and of labour.

## C.M.B. Short Examination Questions

**Eng.:** The anterior fontanelle. **Eng.:** Moulding of the fetal skull. **Eng.:** The attitude of the fetus. **Scot.:** The mento-vertical diameter. **Scot.:** Vertex.

PART III—PREGNANCY

# 5
# The Physiological Changes due to Pregnancy

*Uterine growth. Breasts. Blood pressure. Weight gain. Oedema. Nutrition, normal and weight control diet*

A study of the physiological changes that take place in the woman's body during pregnancy will explain many of the phenomena that are regarded as signs and symptoms of pregnancy, as well as affording a sound basis for the intelligent administration of prenatal care. The changes are not confined to the reproductive organs; every tissue and organ reacts to the stimulus of pregnancy, and the metabolic, chemical and endocrine balance of the body is altered.

## THE UTERUS

Changes in the reproductive organs are, of course, predominant. The uterus must enlarge and give nourishment and protection to the growing fetus, so it increases in weight and size. The uterus must also expel the fetus at a viable age, and as this process of expulsion or labour is a muscular feat the muscle coat develops in a remarkable degree: each muscle fibre increases 10 times in length and 5 times in thickness, and new fibres come into being.

**Increase in weight. From 60 g to 900 g.**

**Increase in size. From 7·5 × 5 × 2·5 cm to 30 × 23 × 20 cm.**

### The muscle coat consists of three layers

The fibres of the inner layer are arranged in circular fashion, and as circular fibres guard all the orifices of the body they are plentiful in the lower pole of the uterus, allowing the lower uterine segment to stretch and the cervix to dilate.

The fibres of the middle layer are arranged in every conceivable direction, mainly figure of eight. These fibres contract and retract during labour and because of their constrictive action on the blood vessels during the third stage they control bleeding. and are known as *'living ligatures'*.

The fibres in the outer layer are arranged longitudinally and extend from the cervix, anteriorly over the fundus, down to the cervix, posteriorly. The longitudinal fibres contract and shorten during labour, causing the upper uterine segment to thicken and shorten, and at the same time they draw up and thin out the lower uterine segment.

**The endometrium** (decidua) is described on p. 27.

### Blood supply

The uterus is very richly supplied with blood during pregnancy, particularly in the area of the placental site. The blood vessels increase in size and number and their tortuous arrangement allows for the rapid increase in the growth of the uterus.

### The lower uterine segment

This area of the uterus develops from the isthmus and at term extends upwards for 7·5 to 10 cm from the internal os to the upper uterine segment. The muscle fibres in the lower uterine segment are not as well developed as in the upper segment. Because during the last weeks of pregnancy the lower uterine segment is soft and stretched the fetus sinks further down into the uterus.

66

### The cervix

The cervix becomes softer and cervical racemose glands secrete a tenacious mucus which forms a plug—the operculum—that effectively occludes the cervical canal and provides a barrier against infection.

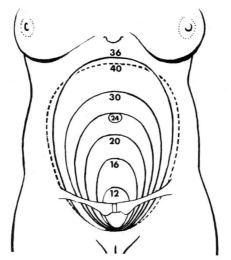

Fig. 5-1    Fundal heights at various weeks during pregnancy.

#### THE GROWTH OF THE PREGNANT UTERUS

The uterus grows at such a regular rate that it is possible, within limits, to estimate the period of gestation by its size. There is, of course, room for error, as the uterus may contain twins, a large fetus or an excessive amount of amniotic fluid.

**Eighth week.** The uterus cannot yet be palpated abdominally. On bimanual examination, it is found to be about the size of a tennis ball but more ovoid in shape.

**Twelfth week.** The uterus fills the pelvic cavity and the fundus reaches just above the summit of the symphysis pubis. It is globular in shape and about the size of a small grapefruit.

**Sixteenth week.** The uterus has risen to just less than half-way between the symphysis pubis and the umbilicus, or 7·5 cm above the symphysis pubis. The shape of the uterus is more ovoid than globular and because it is in contact with the abdominal wall quickening is felt. The uterine souffle can be heard.

**Twentieth week.** The fundus is two fingers breadth below the level of the umbilicus, or 15 cm above the symphysis pubis. The positive signs of pregnancy—fetal heart, fetal parts and fetal movement—can be elicited without ultrasonic aid.

**Twenty-fourth week.** The fundus is at the upper margin of the umbilicus, about 20 cm and the uterus tends to lean and rotate on its axis towards the right side.

**Thirtieth week.** The fundus is midway between the umbilicus and xiphisternum, about 24 cm above the symphysis pubis.

**Thirty-sixth week.** The uterus rises to its highest level and is in contact with the xiphisternum, 30 cm above the symphysis pubis. At the 38th week the fundus sinks down to about the level of a 34 weeks' pregnancy, and this is known as 'lightening'. (See p. 237.)

**Fortieth week.** The uterus is ready to go into labour. The lower uterine segment is relaxed and stretched, the cervix is shortened and soft, and its canal is still closed by the operculum. The fetus lies, usually head downwards, within the amniotic sac.

### THE OVARIES

The corpus luteum in the ruptured Graafian follicle degenerates after the 12th week of pregnancy and its endocrine functions are taken over by the placenta.

### THE VAGINA

There is some degree of hypertrophy of the muscle coat of the vagina in preparation for the distension that will be necessary during labour. The greatly augmented blood supply gives rise to blue discoloration and to increased pulsation in the fornices. All pregnant women have a white vaginal discharge which is due to the action of oestrogens on the squamous epithelium and to venous engorgement.

## THE BREASTS

The breasts are accessory organs of generation and changes in them occur very early, due to the stimulus of the ovarian hormones oestrogens and progestogens, so that even before a woman has missed a period she may be conscious of a prickling, tingling sensation in her breasts. Oestrogens are thought to stimulate the growth of the glandular tissue and ducts, while progestogens activate the secretory function of the breasts. As early as the sixth week, the breasts have enlarged, they have a firm tense feeling and are sometimes tender. The growth of the breasts continues throughout pregnancy with a weight increase of about 450 g. The nipple becomes darker in colour and more erectile.

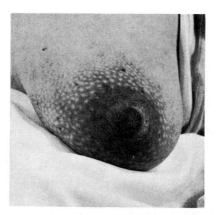

Fig. 5-2  Well-marked pigmentation of the breast during pregnancy. The darker zone extending about 4 cm beyond the nipple is the primary areola. The extensive mottled area is the secondary areola.

**The primary areola.** At the 12th week there is darkening of the area around the nipple and its diameter, which is normally 4 cm, extends until in some instances it may be 7·5 cm. It also looks moist and oedematous in comparison with the flat pink areola of the non-pregnant woman. In reddish fair-haired women the areola may remain pink, but in brunettes it becomes dark brown or even black. At this time a little clear fluid can be expressed from the breasts, but true **colostrum** does not appear until the 16th week.

**Montgomery's tubercles.** From the 8th week onwards, 12 to 30 small nodules appear on the primary areola. They are the pouting mouths of sebaceous glands, and the sebum they secrete keeps the nipple soft and pliable.

**The secondary areola** is seen after the 16th week. It is a mottled zone of pigmentation, extending beyond the primary areola and sometimes covering half of the breast. This breast pigmentation may persist for 12 months after parturition.

Dilated veins can be clearly seen on the chest and breasts from the 8th week.

### BREAST CHANGES IN CHRONOLOGICAL ORDER

| Weeks | | Weeks | |
|---|---|---|---|
| 3 to 4 | Prickling, tingling sensation. | 12 | Darkening of the primary areola. |
| 6 | Enlarged and tense. | 12 | Fluid can be expressed. |
| 8 | Surface veins are visible. | 16 | Colostrum can be expressed. |
| 8 | Montgomery's tubercles appear. | 16 | Secondary areola appears. |

### THE SKIN

Tiny scars, known as striae gravidarum, appear as early as the 16th week on the lower abdomen, thighs and breasts of some pregnant women. They are thought to be due to the rapid stretching of the skin and can occur in cases of adiposity but it has been suggested that hyperfunction of the anterior pituitary gland or adrenocortical activity may play some part in their production. The deeper layer of the dermis ruptures and the epidermis is thinned out, producing little scars of a bluish pink appearance in the present pregnancy. From previous pregnancies, faded silvery striae are seen intermingled with the pink ones.

Pigmentation of the skin is common during pregnancy and is assumed to be due to the action of the melanin stimulating hormone of the anterior pituitary. It is more pronounced in brunettes and is often seen on the breasts and vulva. On the face it can be quite disfiguring and the bronze, blotchy areas seen on the forehead and sides of the face are known as the chloasma or, more commonly, the **mask of pregnancy.** The linea alba, a white line between the rectus muscles, becomes markedly pigmented and can be seen extending from the symphysis pubis to above the umbilicus: when pigmented it is known as the **linea nigra.** Pigmentation is sometimes seen in the striae of multigravid women. The sweat and sebaceous glands are more active during pregnancy.

### THE BLOOD

There is an increase of about 40–50 per cent in blood volume from the 8th week of pregnancy onwards, mainly in the plasma, but there is only a slight increase in red cells. This watery condition of the blood is known as hydraemia, and because of the haemodilution, red cell counts and haemoglobin estimations will be 10 to 15 per cent lower during pregnancy. It should be remembered that the fetus is withdrawing iron for its immediate needs and storing iron in its liver for future use during the lactational period. The fibrinogen content is increased: fibrinolytic factors decreased.

### THE HEART AND LUNGS

During pregnancy the heart is called upon to carry an additional load, but as a rule the healthy heart can cope with this. The increased volume of blood has to be pumped with sufficient force to maintain adequate placental circulation, so the cardiac output is increased from about the 16th week of pregnancy by about 40 to 50 per cent and remains elevated until delivery.

The lungs are displaced slightly upwards when the growing uterus encroaches on the thorax and restricts the free excursion of the diaphragm. Shortness of breath may be due to the deeper respirations which are necessary because of increased oxygen consumption.

### THE BLOOD PRESSURE

There is no physiological rise in blood pressure during pregnancy, in spite of the increased blood volume and cardiac output: in fact it may be slightly lower than normal during the middle trimester. The blood pressure appears to be very labile (unstable) in some pregnant women: a slight drop in pressure, due to emotional or other causes, tends to cause fainting. Conversely, excitement or exertion may produce a transient rise.

### THE URINARY TRACT

Frequency of micturition is common from the 6th to the 12th week: this is not now considered to be due to pressure by the uterus. In the later weeks of pregnancy, when lightening takes place, the lax condition of all the tissues of the pelvic floor may be a contributory cause of the frequency and even of slight incontinence of urine that occurs at this time.

The ureters are liable to be compressed by the uterus when it rises out of the pelvis. After the 16th week laxity in the walls of the ureters renders them subject to compression and more capable of being dilated. Stasis of urine occurs in the dilated part and is believed to predispose the woman to pyelonephritis.

### WEIGHT GAIN (based on Hytten)

A gain of about 12 kg is to be expected in the pregnant woman of average build and can be accounted for by the following.

| | |
|---|---|
| Fetus | 3·4 kg |
| Placenta | 0·6 kg |
| Amniotic fluid | 0·8 kg |
| Increase in weight of uterus | 0·9 kg |
| Increase in weight of breasts | 0·4 kg |
| Increase in blood volume | 1·5 kg |
| Extra-cellular fluid | 1·4 kg |
| Fat | 3·5 kg |
| Total | 12·5 kg |

A pregnant woman gains on the average approximately 2·5 kg during the first 20 weeks of pregnancy. During the second 20 weeks, weight gain amounts to approximately 9 kg (0·45 kg per week). Many factors are involved, including the metabolic rate of the individual, fluid balance, and the uterine contents, *e.g.* twins, polyhydramnios.

**Inadequate weight gain** during the first 20 weeks could be due to poor nutrition often in conjunction with smoking or to conditions such as severe anaemia or pyelonephritis. During the second 20 weeks, it may be due to fetal growth retardation and when fetal death occurs. Oligohydramnios is a less common cause.

### THE SKELETON

A change in the gait of the pregnant woman is noticeable during the second half of pregnancy when the balance of the body is altered because of the enlarged uterus. The shoulders are thrown backwards and the lumbar curve is increased almost to lordosis, which, along with relaxation of the pelvic joints and ligaments during the later weeks of pregnancy, may give rise to discomfort or actual backache.

It is the bones and not the teeth that are the storehouses for calcium, so it is no longer believed that the woman's teeth decay during pregnancy because calcium is being withdrawn from them.

### THE NERVOUS SYSTEM

Pregnancy is one of the three periods in a woman's life when there seems to be a lowering of the ability to cope with the emotional experiences of life. At puberty and the menopause a similar degree of instability may be manifest and in each instance the cause is probably endocrine in origin.

During pregnancy there are emotional as well as physical adjustments to be made and, even in cases where the coming baby is welcome, a mild degree of depression or irritability may be evident during the early months.

Fifty years ago cravings for indigestible foods, and temper tantrums were a common occurrence, but women should be discouraged from the belief that they are a normal accompaniment of pregnancy. Longings for certain sour or tart articles of food may be due to nausea rather than to nervous instability, and the tactful implication that cravings and tantrums are rather old fashioned is usually a sufficient deterrent.

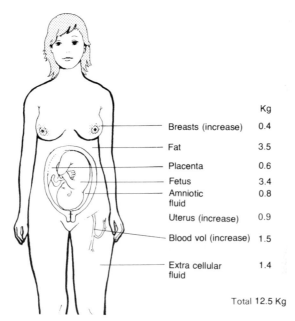

| | Kg |
|---|---|
| Breasts (increase) | 0.4 |
| Fat | 3.5 |
| Placenta | 0.6 |
| Fetus | 3.4 |
| Amniotic fluid | 0.8 |
| Uterus (increase) | 0.9 |
| Blood vol (increase) | 1.5 |
| Extra cellular fluid | 1.4 |
| Total | 12.5 Kg |

Fig. 5-3   Showing disposition of weight gain in pregnancy.

### THE GENERAL METABOLISM

It is well known that once a woman becomes physically and emotionally adjusted to the impact of pregnancy she enjoys a feeling of wellbeing. Her appetite is good, she looks and feels well, but this can only be experienced if she is healthy, well nourished and not overworked. The basal metabolic rate increases during the latter half of pregnancy in response to the demands of the growing fetus and maternal tissues, so the woman's fuel requirements are higher and a diet providing 2,400 calories (10 megajoules) will be necessary unless she is physically inactive.

The metabolism of carbohydrates in pregnancy is not wholly understood. Glycosuria occurs in 10 per cent of women, probably due to a lowering of the renal threshold for glucose. Normal fasting blood glucose is 4.4 to 5.5 mmol/l of blood and the kidney does not excrete glucose in the urine of a healthy individual until the blood glucose rises to 8.9 mmol/l. During pregnancy that threshold may be lowered and the kidney excretes glucose when the blood glucose is 6.6 mmol/l.

### OEDEMA IN PREGNANCY

#### Physiological oedema

About 40 per cent of pregnant women have slight ankle oedema, during the last 12 weeks of pregnancy, which disappears with rest and is rarely present in the morning. This may be due to: (a) the normal reduction of plasma proteins in pregnancy tending by osmosis to draw fluid into the tissues; (b) venous pressure in the iliofemoral veins being intensified when the erect posture is maintained for long periods because the return flow of blood from the lower limbs is slowed down by the greatly augmented venous return from the uterine veins. This may be aggravated by pressure of the enlarged uterus and by the wearing of constricting bands.

#### Pathological oedema

**Pre-eclampsia.** This is the cause for which the midwife must be constantly on the alert, and oedema should never be considered physiological until all pathological causes have been ruled out. Abnormal water retention may cause a marked increase in weight.

**Cardiac disease.** If there is circulatory inefficiency the kidneys do not function well, and when the oedema is generalised it is a sign of serious import.

**Renal disease.** The impaired kidneys do not excrete sodium efficiently and therefore fluid is retained in the tissues.

**Malnutrition.** When nutrition is very poor the plasma proteins become seriously depleted. Low protein diet will therefore cause oedema.

**Varicose veins** in the legs or vulva will give rise to oedema in those regions.

# NUTRITION IN PREGNANCY

It is now widely accepted that fetal growth and subsequent growth and development after birth can be critically influenced by the mothers' diet during pregnancy.

The woman's food requirements are increased during pregnancy, but more so in quality than quantity. More attention should be paid to the inclusion of the vital substances needed for growth and health.

It is essential that pregnant women are given advice to ensure that they partake of the vital nutrients needed for fetal and maternal health. But the mother's nutrition prior to pregnancy has a profound effect on her reproductive efficiency and this influence begins with the fetus in utero who is a potential parent.

Stunting can result from impaired growth in utero when the fetus is deprived of essential substances. The expectant mother's skeletal structure can be conditioned by wrong feeding in infancy as well as by genetic factors or disease. Unwise dietary restrictions during adolescence can result in anaemia and debility, so senior schoolgirls should be made aware of the importance of good food in equipping them for their reproductive role.

Midwives have a unique opportunity to teach health education in the community.

### THE DIET IN PREGNANCY SHOULD PROVIDE FOR:

**The needs of the growing fetus.**
**The maintenance of maternal health.**
**Physical strength and vitality during labour.**
**Successful lactation.**

The expectant mother need not adhere rigidly to any special diet, but the midwife must advise and guide her in selecting proper foods, if it is evident that her diet is defective. Advice on how to teach 'nutrition' to expectant mothers is given in the chapter on preparation for parenthood.

| DAILY REQUIREMENTS | Grams | | | Calories | Megajoules |
|---|---|---|---|---|---|
| Proteins | 80 | × 4 | = | 320 | 1·3 |
| Fats | 90 | × 9 | = | 810 | 3·4 |
| Carbohydrates | 320 | × 4 | = | 1,280 | 5·4 |
| | | | | 2,410 | 10·1 |

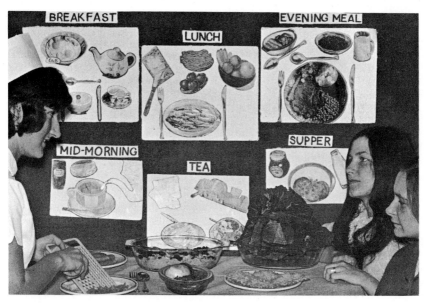

Fig. 5-4  Midwife demonstrates making vegetable salad.
*Maternity Unit, Central Hospital, Irvine, Ayrshire.*

### PROTEINS

These are absolutely essential, because they are the only substances that build tissue, and the mother has to provide for the growth of the fetus, placenta, uterus, breasts and the increased blood volume. The maintenance of a normal red cell count and haemoglobin level is dependent on an adequate dietary intake of proteins.

More attention is now being paid to the nutritional requirements of the fetus: the brain cells being particularly vulnerable to deprivation of nutrient substances essential for growth (proteins) during the third trimester of pregnancy.

A daily intake of 80 g ought to be provided during pregnancy, and 60 per cent should be first class. From the following foods, 80 g of proteins could be obtained daily.

## ONE DAY'S PROTEIN REQUIREMENTS

| | | |
|---|---|---|
| **Milk, 900 ml** | 30 g | **First-class proteins** |
| **Egg, 1** | 6 g | ,,　　　,, |
| **Meat, 100 g (raw weight)** | 20 g | ,,　　　,, |
| **White fish, 100 g (raw weight)** | 15 g | ,,　　　,, |
| **Cheese, 14 g** | 3 g | ,,　　　,, |
| **Wholewheat bread, 4 slices, 100 g** | 10 g | **Second-class proteins** |

Total 84 g

### CARBOHYDRATES AND FATS

Because carbohydrate is cheap and readily available the intake is usually more than adequate, and when that is so, the intake of the vital substances (proteins, minerals, vitamins) may be dangerously low. Abnormal weight gain may be due to an excessive intake of sugar in foods such as cakes, biscuits, jam, ice-cream, sweets and chocolate.

Fat should consist mainly of the animal type, which contains vitamins A and D. A daily quota of 90 g of fat would be a reasonable amount. An excessive fat intake will produce weight gain as when foods such as pastry, fat meat or bacon, and cream are eaten, and where frying is the main method of cooking meat and fish.

Some authorities advocate controlling the weight by dietary measures and limiting the total weight gain to 11 kg. A diet with adequate proteins and containing the essential minerals and vitamins found in fresh fruits and vegetables will help to produce a healthy mother and baby. Sugar and starchy foods should be curtailed, fat foods limited.

### WEIGHT-CONTROL DIET

*(Approx. 7·5 Megajoules, 1,760 Calories)*

**Breakfast.** Orange; porridge or flakes and milk with no added sugar; egg; one slice 28 g wholewheat bread; 7 g butter; coffee or tea ......... milk 180 *ml*

**Mid-morning.** Milk, flavoured if desired .......................... milk 180 *ml*

**Lunch.** 210 ml milk-soup; 100 g lean meat or liver or chicken or kidney or sweetbreads; one average-size potato; cooked green or root vegetable or salad; 7 g butter; raw or stewed fruit .......................... milk 150 *ml*

**Tea.** One slice wholewheat bread; 7 g butter; tomato, lettuce, cress or grated raw carrot; slice plain cake (no icing or cream filling) ....... milk 30 *ml*

**Supper.** 100 g fish or tripe cooked with milk, or egg or 14 g cheese; one slice bread; 7 g butter; apple or other raw fruit ................... milk 180 *ml*

**Bed Time.** Milky drink ............................................ milk 180 *ml*

**At each main meal,** meat, fish, egg or cheese and fresh fruit or vegetable should be taken. Dried and canned fruits contain sugar. By skimming 900 ml milk 225 calories can be removed. *Unfortunately meat and fruit are expensive articles of diet.*

## Minerals

**Iron,** an essential component of haemoglobin, ranks very high in importance for the pregnant woman: the fetus requires iron, not only for its immediate needs but for the lactational period, so iron is stored in its liver during the last 10 weeks of intra-uterine life. The woman's diet should contain 15 mg iron per day. Foods rich in iron are: Liver, kidney, beef, blood sausage, eggs, prunes, raisins, green vegetables, black treacle. Six slices of wholewheat bread provide half the day's iron requirements.

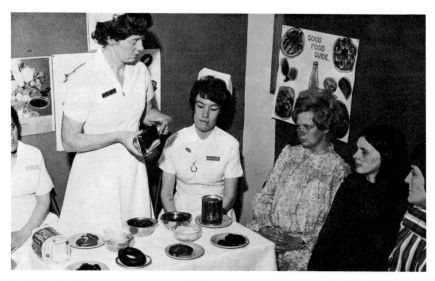

Fig. 5-5   Midwife demonstrates foods rich in iron: brown bread, chocolate, green vegetables, treacle, prunes, blood sausage, meat.

*Maternity Hospital, Stirling*

**Calcium** is needed in the formation of fetal bones and teeth. The teeth are forming as early as the 6th week of pregnancy, but the calcium need is greatest in the last 12 weeks when rapid ossification of the fetal skeleton is taking place. The pregnant woman needs 1·5 g of calcium daily. 600 ml of milk contains 0·68 g of calcium. Cheese is also a good source. The calcium in milk is very readily absorbed and utilised, whereas the calcium in tablet form is not.

## Vitamins

During pregnancy a vitamin deficiency may be due to imperfect absorption, or persistent nausea and vomiting, as well as an insufficient intake. Vitamins are present in nearly all fresh animal and vegetable foods.

**Vitamin A** (Retinol equiv.). The chief sources are butter, milk, liver, egg-yolk and particularly fish-liver oils. A pregnant woman needs 750 micrograms daily (2,250 i.u.).

**Vitamin $B_1$.**—During pregnancy the demand for vitamin $B_1$ is increased fivefold, to about 700 to 800 units, or 2 to 2·5 mg daily. The chief sources are wholewheat bread, meat, liver and yeast.

**Folic acid** and folacinic acid are water soluble vitamins and coenzymes which in conjunction with vitamin $B_{12}$ are concerned with the normal development of blood cells in the bone marrow. Ascorbic acid plays some part in their metabolism. Fresh dark green vegetables and liver are the best sources with other green vegetables, cauliflower, and kidney second best. Insufficient amounts will cause megaloblastic anaemia. During pregnancy larger amounts are required so folates are given prophylactically to pregnant women.

**Vitamin C**—ascorbic acid—is required during pregnancy for the growing fetus. It is also concerned in blood formation and the absorption of iron. The daily intake of ascorbic acid during pregnancy should be 100 mg. Citrus fruits are a good source.

**Vitamin D** promotes the absorption of calcium in the intestine and is the antirachitic vitamin produced by the body when exposed to sunlight. Certain animal products are good sources, e.g. milk, butter, cheese, herring and salmon.

**Vitamin $K_1$** is essential in the formation of prothrombin, which is necessary for the coagulation of blood. The pregnant woman's diet should contain foods which are good sources, such as cabbage, cauliflower, lettuce, carrots.

Vitamin deficiency has been associated with congenital abnormalities such as spina bifida.

### *The Daily Menu should include*

| | |
|---|---|
| **Milk, 900 ml** | **Whole-grain cereal** |
| **Egg 1** | **Orange, grape-fruit, or tomato** |
| **Meat,** average helping | **Two vegetables,** one green (raw) |
| **Fish** | **Potatoes** |
| **Wholewheat bread** | **Butter,** or margarine (fortified) |

If these foods are taken, the woman can make up the remainder of her diet with whichever foods she prefers so long as they are wholesome and digestible. Liver is a valuable food and should be taken once a week if available. All the necessary factors can be obtained within a comparatively small range of well-selected foods; proteins, minerals and vitamins frequently being present in one food. Two glasses of water, in addition to milk, tea, coffee, etc., will provide the necessary amount of fluid.

Whether the baby's birth weight can be lessened by decreasing the mother's intake of food during pregnancy has not yet been satisfactorily proved. It is more likely to result in the birth of an infant of such poor vitality as to be incapable of withstanding the hazards of birth or of surviving the risks of the neonatal period.

---

## QUESTIONS FOR REVISION

### THE PHYSIOLOGICAL CHANGES IN PREGNANCY

**Fundal height—fill in correct week**

| Level | | week |
|---|---|---|
| Midway between symphysis and umbilicus | 12 | ( ) |
| At summit of symphysis pubis | 16 | ( ) |
| When lightening occurs | 36 | ( ) |
| At the umbilicus | 30 | ( ) |
| In contact with xiphisternum | 38 | ( ) |
| Midway between umbilicus and xiphisternum | 24 | ( ) |

When do the following appear in the breast?
　　Darkening of primary areola . . . . . .Surface veins . . . . . .
　　Montgomery's tubercules . . . . . .Colostrum . . . . . .

In which areas is pigmentation seen? What are striae gravidarum?

Which conditions may influence fundal height levels? What is the average weight gain for a pregnant woman?

## Oral Questions

What are the causes of inadequate weight gain during the first 20 weeks and during the second 20 weeks? What can you learn from: The height of the fundus every 4 weeks; the height of the blood pressure; the size of shoes worn; the height of the woman? State the average weekly weight gain. How would you deal with syncope from vena caval occlusion? Why look for oedema in the pregnant woman?

**Differentiate between**—corpus uteri and corpus luteum; physiological and pathological oedema; primary and secondary areola of breast; linea alba and linea nigra.

Which physiological changes are used as probable signs of pregnancy? How soon should a pregnant woman wear a supporting brassière? What can a midwife surmise from seeing silver striae? Why does the haemoglobin fall in pregnancy?

**C.M.B.(Eng.) 30-min. question.** Describe the non-pregnant uterus and the changes that take place in its size and shape during pregnancy.

**C.M.B.(Scot.) 30-min. question.** Describe the physiological changes which occur in the reproductive tract throughout pregnancy prior to the onset of labour.

### NUTRITION IN PREGNANCY

What is the reason why the following are necessary: Proteins—iron—calcium—vitamins?

Name the cheaper forms of proteins. Why is protein such an important food factor? What is the function of folic acid? Why is liver such a valuable food? Give reasons why vitamin deficiency may occur in pregnancy. How many calories are there in one gram of protein, carbohydrate, fat? The fetal brain cells are particularly vulnerable to deprivation of ..........

Differentiate between the functions of vitamins A, B, C, D.

|  | Proteins | Iron | Calcium | Vit. A | Vit. C |
|---|---|---|---|---|---|
| Red meat<br>Milk<br>Liver<br>Butter<br>Fish<br>Cheese<br>Orange |  |  |  |  |  |

*Use + signs to indicate the nutrients contained in the above foods.*

Outline a diet for one day containing at least 80 g protein. Which foods are rich in iron? Which foods cause excessive weight gain? Mention foods you would recommend in language the woman could understand: for breakfast, lunch, supper.

**C.M.B.(Scot.).** What advice would you give to a pregnant patient regarding diet in pregnancy? What are the dangers associated with incorrect diet?

## C.M.B. Short Examination Questions

**Eng.:** Weight changes in pregnancy.

**Eng.:** Significance of glycosuria in pregnancy. **Eng.:** Obesity in pregnancy. **Eng.:** Causes of oedema in pregnancy. **Eng.:** Important points regarding diet for the pregnant woman. **Scot.:** Describe the changes which take place in the uterus during pregnancy. **Scot.:** Striae gravidarum. **Eng.:** Weight loss in pregnancy. **Eng.:** Weight gain in pregnancy.

# 6
# The Signs and Diagnosis of Pregnancy

*Presumptive, probable, positive signs. Immunological pregnancy tests. Signs of previous childbirth. Relationship of fetus to uterus and pelvis, lie, attitude, presentation, position*

When a healthy married woman who has been menstruating regularly misses a period she suspects pregnancy and in 98 per cent of cases she is correct. The use of immunological pregnancy tests and ultrasonic devices has eliminated the need to rely on the more inaccurate presumptive and probable signs of pregnancy. Most women book at about 12 weeks.

## PRESUMPTIVE SIGNS AND SYMPTOMS

| AMENORRHOEA | MORNING SICKNESS | SKIN CHANGES |
|---|---|---|
| BREAST CHANGES | BLADDER IRRITABILITY | QUICKENING |

**Amenorrhoea** almost invariably accompanies pregnancy, and the sudden cessation of menstruation is most significant. Very slight bleeding may take place during the implantation of the ovum, which might be mistaken for menstruation: hence the need to inquire whether the last menstrual period was normal in length and amount. Change of environment; emotional disturbances; serious illness may also cause suppression of menstruation. When the contraceptive pill is discontinued a period of amenorrhoea may ensue so the woman should be told to look for and record the date of breast changes, morning sickness and quickening. At the menopause, because of the increase in body weight and delayed periods, women often erroneously think they are pregnant.

**Breast changes** have been described on page 68, and are only significant in the primigravid woman. Slight tingling may be experienced by non-pregnant women; pigmentation may persist after parturition.

**Morning sickness** occurs in about 50 per cent of pregnant women during the 4th to the 14th week, but other conditions may give rise to vomiting. Although morning sickness is not considered to be a definite symptom, in conjunction with amenorrhoea it is very suggestive of pregnancy.

**Bladder irritability** usually consists of frequency of micturition without pain or burning, occurring before the 12th week.

**Skin changes** include pigmentation, manifest as the chloasma, linea nigra, darkening of the primary areola and the formation of the secondary areola of the breasts. They are useful but not indisputable signs of pregnancy. The presence of striae on the abdomen, thighs and breasts is an equally indefinite sign.

**Quickening** is the term applied to the movements of the fetus in utero when first recognised by the mother; usually felt between the 16th and 20th week. The fetus is, of course, alive from the moment of conception, but in the early months the fetal limbs are not well developed and their movements are sluggish. Not until the uterus has risen out of the pelvis and is in contact with the abdominal wall will any feeling of movement be perceptible by the woman. There is no sense of touch in the uterus, and the kicking must be transmitted to the abdominal wall before the woman is conscious of it. Non-pregnant women sometimes imagine they feel fetal movement, so the symptom is not dependable.

HEGAR'S SIGN                          SOFTENING OF CERVIX
JACQUEMIER'S SIGN                     UTERINE SOUFFLE
OSIANDER'S SIGN                       ABDOMINAL ENLARGEMENT
CHANGES IN UTERUS                     BRAXTON HICKS' CONTRACTIONS
                   INTERNAL BALLOTTEMENT


The majority of these signs are elicited by the doctor, mainly by vaginal examination: the midwife must ensure that the patient's bladder has first been emptied.

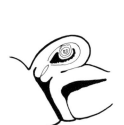 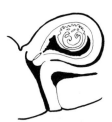 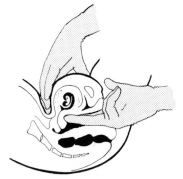

Fig. 6-1  Four weeks pregnancy: uterus anteverted.

Fig. 6-2  Six weeks preg-
nancy: Uterus size of
duck's egg.

Fig. 6-3  Eight      weeks
pregnancy: Uterus size of
medium orange. Hegar's
sign can be elicited.

Figs. 6-1–6-2–6-3  Findings per vaginam in pregnancy.


**Hegar's sign**—*6th to 12th week*—is one of the early signs seldom now employed unless facilities for pregnancy tests are not available. It is mainly done to establish gestation age. Two fingers are inserted into the anterior fornix of the vagina, and the other hand is placed behind the uterus abdominally. The fingers of both hands almost meet, because of the softness of the isthmus which is marked at this period. Rough handling of the uterus should be avoided.

**Jacquemier's sign**—*8th week onwards*—is the violet blue discoloration of the vaginal mucous membrane, and is due to pelvic congestion. It may also be present, in cases of retroversion and pelvic cellulitis.

**Osiander's sign**—*8th week onwards*—is the increased pulsation felt in the lateral vaginal fornices, due to the marked vascularity. It may also be present in pathological conditions that cause pelvic congestion.

**Changes in the uterus**—*8th week onwards*—In size the uterus enlarges: the consistency is soft: the shape globular rather than pear.

**Softening of the cervix**—*10th week onwards*—The consistency of the cervix is comparable with that of the lips, while the cervix of the non-pregnant uterus feels like the tip of the nose.

**The uterine souffle**—*16th week onwards*—is a soft blowing sound, heard on auscultation and synchronous with the mother's pulse. The uterine souffle is also heard when fibroid tumours are present and during the puerperium.

**Abdominal enlargement**—*16th week onwards*—No other condition makes the uterus enlarge so rapidly and so progressively. Abdominal enlargement may, however, be due to fat, gaseous distension of the bowel, a full bladder, tumours or ascites.

**Braxton Hicks' contractions**—*20th week onwards*—are the painless uterine contractions felt on abdominal palpation, occurring about every 15 minutes and increasing in intensity after the 35th week. These contractions facilitate the circulation of blood in the placental site and also play some part in the development of the lower uterine segment.

**Internal ballottement**—*16th to 28th week*—is most useful in cases of obesity during mid-term and is performed with the patient in the semi-recumbent position. Two fingers are inserted into the vagina, and the uterus is given a sharp tap just above the cervix, which causes the fetus to float upwards in the amniotic fluid. The left hand, which is placed abdominally on the fundus uteri, detects the gentle impact of the fetus. The fetus sinks back again and is felt by the fingers in the vagina; this rebound is known as ballottement.

None of these signs is positive, as there are fallacies, mostly gynaecological in origin, that prevent them from being conclusive. The probable signs are more reliable than the presumptive signs.

### IMMUNOLOGICAL TESTS FOR PREGNANCY

The most reliable tests are those which depend upon the presence of chorionic gonadotrophin in the urine. This hormone is excreted soon after the fertilised egg has implanted.

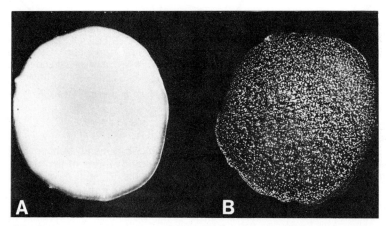

Fig. 6-4   Prepurex pregnancy test. A, The white circle, non-agglutinated pattern is a presumptive positive test. The dark circle B with macroscopic agglutination is presumptive negative.

Immunological tests for pregnancy are of two types, haemagglutination inhibition tests such as Pregnosticon (Organon Ltd.) and Prepuerin (Burroughs Wellcome & Co.) and latex particle tests e.g. Gravindex (Ortho Pharmaceutical Ltd.), Planotest (Organon Ltd.) and Prepurex (Burroughs Wellcome & Co.). These tests are available as kits containing all the reagents needed to do a test. In the Pregnosticon and Prepuerin test the reagents and the urine to be tested are mixed together in a tube or ampoule.

A positive reaction, inhibition of haemagglutination, appears as a brown ring or button at the bottom of the ampoule or tube. A negative reaction, haemagglutination, shows up as a uniformly yellow-brown precipitate at the bottom of the tube. In the latex particle inhibition tests the reagent and urine are mixed together on a glass slide. A positive result is one in which there is no agglutination of particles and a negative result is one in which agglutination occurs within 2 minutes of the reagents being mixed together.

Results are more reliable if the tests are done on urines collected 14 days after the missed but expected period. A positive pregnancy test is not synonymous with the presence of a viable fetus. Immunological tests like biological tests measure chorionic gonadotrophin and will be positive when urines from women who have a hydatidiform mole, invasive mole or choriocarcinoma are tested.

For these tests 15 ml of the first morning specimen of urine is required. The patient should refrain from drinking after 1800 h the previous evening. The specimen must be labelled accurately, kept cool and sent to the laboratory as soon as possible.

## POSITIVE SIGNS

### FETAL HEART, FETAL PARTS, FETAL MOVEMENT, ULTRASONIC AND RADIOLOGICAL EVIDENCE

**Hearing the fetal heart** is a most convincing sign of pregnancy and can with acute hearing be detected as early as the 20th week (usually about the 24th week). When the abdominal wall is thick, the amount of amniotic fluid excessive, or the examining room noisy, the heart sounds may be inaudible; but inability to hear the fetal heart does not necessarily exclude pregnancy or denote fetal death although it may arouse suspicion.

**Fetal parts** can be felt about the 22nd week, but fibroids may be mistaken for fetal parts.

**Fetal movement** felt by the examiner about the 22nd week, should not be confused with movement which is felt by the mother (quickening).

**Ultrasonic evidence** is available as early as 6 weeks amenorrhoea: the gestation sac being seen on the oscilloscope screen or recorded by a polaroid camera as an ultrasonogram.

The Sonicaid and the Doptone ultrasonic detectors pick up the fetal heart beat at 14 weeks and have done so at 10 weeks.

**Radiological** demonstration of the fetal skeleton can be made at the 16th week of pregnancy, but as other diagnostic methods are available X-rays are not used at this early stage because of the radiation hazards.

### SIGNS OF A PREVIOUS PREGNANCY

It is desirable for practical reasons that the midwife should be aware whether the pregnant woman has previously given birth to a child. The second stage of labour may be very rapid in a multiparous woman and if the midwife is under the impression that the woman is a primigravida she may not be 'scrubbed up' for delivery in time. Women do not always admit, for reasons best known to themselves, that they have already had a baby, and the midwife must accept the woman's statement without question and keep her opinion to herself.

*The following signs are suggestive of previous childbirth*

**The breasts are more flabby** and the nipples prominent in women who have breast-fed their infants, and pigmentation of the areola may still persist in brunettes.

**The abdominal muscles** are more lax and the skin loose, so that there may be anterior obliquity of the uterus and bulging of the colon at the sides of the abdomen.

**The uterine wall is less rigid** and the contour of the uterus is broad and round rather than ovoid. The fetus is more easily palpated.

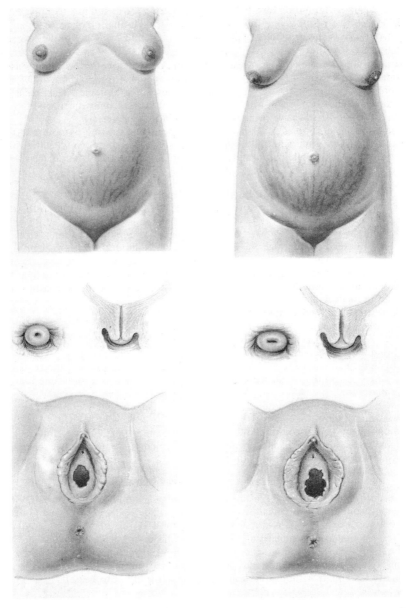

Fig. 6-5 Primigravida. Breasts firm; uterus ovoid; abdominal muscles firm; os, round opening; os admits finger tip; vulva not patulous; hymen partly evident; perineum firm, no scars.

Fig. 6-6 Multipara. Breasts flabby; uterus round; abdominal muscles flabby; os, transverse slit; os one cm; vulva patulous; carunculae myrtiformes present; perineum may be lax; scars may be present.

**Old striae gravidarum** are silvery-white in appearance, but when due to the present pregnancy they are pink. Some pigmentation of the linea alba and striae may be present from a previous pregnancy.

**The vulva gapes** and is more patulous: the labia minora tend to project below the labia majora and are darker in colour and leathery in texture. The vaginal orifice is larger and a cystocele may be evident. Carunculae myrtiformes (*tags of hymen*) are present. A lax or deficient perineum and the *scars* from previous laceration or episiotomy may be seen.

**The vagina** is more roomy and the **cervical os** is a slit which admits one or more fingers, whereas in the primigravida it is a small pinhead opening at the beginning of pregnancy but may admit one finger-tip during the last month.

### PSEUDOCYESIS

Phantom or false pregnancy are terms applied to the condition in which a woman shows several of the signs and symptoms of pregnancy, such as breast changes and enlarged abdomen, firmly believes she is pregnant and yet no pregnancy exists. Such patients are usually infertile married women who have an overwhelming desire to give birth to a baby. Obstetric examination reveals the **absence of any positive signs.**

## THE DURATION OF PREGNANCY

The actual duration of pregnancy is believed to be about 265 days from the date of conception, but there is no accurate method of calculating this. Ovulation usually occurs 14 days previous to the first day of the menstrual period but it may be delayed. The ovum is only capable of fertilisation for 24 h, but conception has been known to take place at various times during the menstrual cycle.

The question sometimes arises as to the length of the period of gestation which can be considered legitimate when a child is born more than 280 days after the death or absence of the putative father. In Gt. Britain and the United States there is no legal limit to the length of pregnancy; each case is considered on its merits. In the English courts, during the year 1921, a gestational period of 331 days was allowed, in 1948 one of 340 days was not allowed. The Scottish courts have allowed a period of 305 days.

### Calculation of the Date of Confinement

For practical purposes the date of the last menstrual period has proved by experience to be a reliable guide. By adding seven days to the first day of the last menstrual period and counting back three months or forwards nine months, **a total of 280 days,** the expected date of delivery is arrived at. But the baby may be born one week before or after that date and yet be at term. It has been estimated that only 5 per cent of women go into labour on the calculated day.

In cases where the menstrual periods are irregular or when the women forgets the date of her last period, 22 weeks are added to the date of quickening. The height of the fundus can also be used as a means of assessing the period of gestation, but the fallaciousness of this method must be kept in mind. When the contraceptive pill is discontinued women may have amenorrhoea for from 6 to 18 months. They should be advised to note and record the dates of the early signs of pregnancy.

## THE RELATIONSHIP OF THE FETUS TO THE UTERUS AND PELVIS

Certain terms are used to describe the relationship of the fetus to the uterus and pelvis, and the student midwife ought to be familiar with them before learning how to palpate the abdomen. This relationship determines which part of the fetus will enter the pelvic brim first, and governs the mechanism by which the fetus will pass through the birth canal.

The terms are:

| LIE | PRESENTATION | POSITION |
|---|---|---|
| ATTITUDE | DENOMINATOR | PRESENTING PART |

### LIE

Lie is the relation of the long axis of the fetus to the long axis of the uterus (not to the abdomen or spine). It should be longitudinal, and is so in 99·5 per cent of cases, but it may be transverse. The fetus and uterus are both longer than they are broad, and when the fetus *in utero* lies with its length parallel to the length of the uterus the lie is longitudinal, and the head or the breech will occupy the lower pole of the uterus.

LONGITUDINAL LIE

Breech            Vertex            Vertex

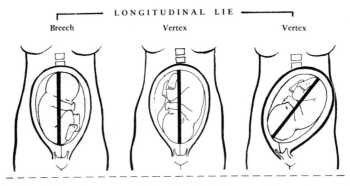

Fig. 6-7, 6-8 and 6-9 depict the longitudinal lie. Confusion sometimes exists regarding Fig. 6-9 which gives the impression of being an oblique lie, but the fetus is longitudinal in relation to the uterus and merely moving the uterus abdominally rectifies the presumed obliquity.

OBLIQUE LIE        TRANSVERSE LIE

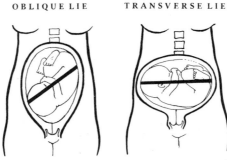

Fig. 6-10 is an oblique lie because the long axis of the fetus is oblique in relation to the uterus.

Fig. 6-11 is the true transverse lie with shoulder presentation.

The longitudinal lie is usual because the uterine cavity is ovoid in shape, but any condition, such as lax uterine walls or an excessive amount of amniotic fluid, making the uterine cavity round instead of ovoid, would reduce the likelihood of the fetus adopting the longitudinal lie. When the lie is transverse, the shoulder occupies the lower pole of the uterus and the long axis of the fetus lies across the long axis of the uterus: a serious state of affairs which must be rectified because normal birth is impossible.

## ATTITUDE

Attitude is the relation of the fetal limbs and head to its trunk, and should be one of *flexion*. It concerns the fetus only. The back is bent, the head is flexed with the chin on the chest, the arms are flexed on, or alongside the chest, the thighs are flexed on the abdomen and the legs on the thighs. The fetus, therefore, forms a snug compact, ovoid mass, which accommodates itself admirably to the uterine cavity and can be expelled en masse during labour. Any deviation from this normal attitude of flexion will give rise to difficulty during labour; e.g. if the head is not well flexed a larger circumference will have to engage in the pelvic brim; if extended, the face presents.

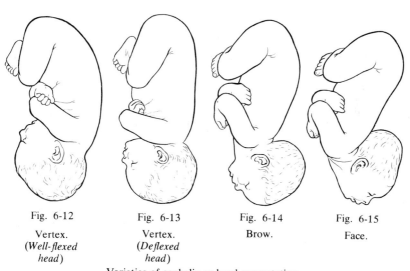

| Fig. 6-12 | Fig. 6-13 | Fig. 6-14 | Fig. 6-15 |
| Vertex. | Vertex. | Brow. | Face. |
| (*Well-flexed* | (*Deflexed* | | |
| *head*) | *head*) | | |

Varieties of cephalic or head presentation.

## PRESENTATION

Presentation refers to the part of the fetus which lies at the pelvic brim or in the lower pole of the uterus. There are five presentations:

1. **The vertex** presents in approx.     96·8 per cent of cases
2. **The breech** presents in approx.     2·5 per cent of cases
3. **The shoulder** presents in approx.     0·4 per cent of cases 1 per 250
4. **The face** presents in approx.     0·2 per cent of cases 1 per 500
5. **The brow** presents in approx.     0·1 per cent of cases 1 per 1000

Vertex, face and brow are all head or cephalic presentations. When the head is flexed the vertex presents: when it is extended the face presents, and when neither well flexed nor properly extended it is midway between vertex and face, so the brow presents (see Figs 6-12 to 6-15). The reason for the greater number of head presentations is explained mainly by the law of accommodation. The uterine cavity is ovoid in shape during the later months of pregnancy and its walls, being contractile, tend to cause the fetus to accommodate its ovoid shape to that of the uterus. The bulky breech of the fetus finds greater space in the fundus which is the widest diameter of the uterus, and the head lies in the narrower lower pole. When the fetal head is unduly large, as in hydrocephaly it may occupy the roomy fundus, causing the breech to present. The tonicity of the fetus also plays a part in maintaining the vertex presentation: a dead fetus has no tone so the normal presentation and attitude are not maintained.

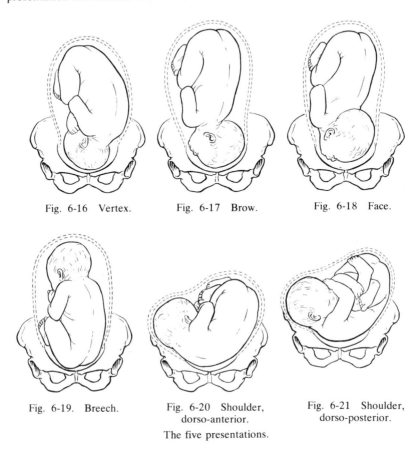

Fig. 6-16   Vertex.          Fig. 6-17   Brow.          Fig. 6-18   Face.

Fig. 6-19.  Breech.          Fig. 6-20  Shoulder,          Fig. 6-21  Shoulder,
                            dorso-anterior.              dorso-posterior.

The five presentations.

### THE DENOMINATOR

The denominator is the part of the presentation that indicates or determines the position of the fetus.

The denominator in vertex presentation is the **occiput.**
The denominator in breech presentation is the **sacrum.**
The denominator in face presentation is the **mentum.**
The denominator in shoulder presentation is the **acromion process.**

### POSITION

Position is the relation of the denominator to six areas of the pelvic brim. The areas of the brim are:

| | |
|---|---|
| **Right posterior** | **Left posterior** |
| **Right lateral** | **Left lateral** |
| **Right anterior** | **Left anterior** |

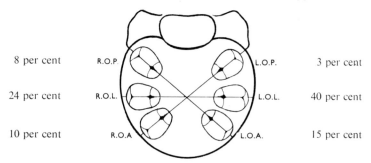

| 8 per cent | R.O.P. | | L.O.P. | 3 per cent |
| 24 per cent | R.O.L. | | L.O.L. | 40 per cent |
| 10 per cent | R.O.A | | L.O.A. | 15 per cent |

Fig. 6-22   Diagrammatic representation of the six vertex positions and their relative frequency.

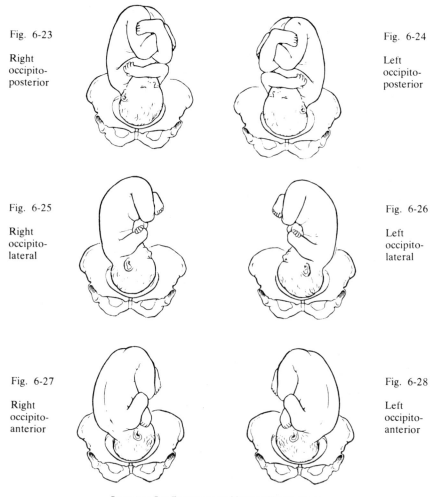

Fig. 6-23

Right occipito-posterior

Fig. 6-24

Left occipito-posterior

Fig. 6-25

Right occipito-lateral

Fig. 6-26

Left occipito-lateral

Fig. 6-27

Right occipito-anterior

Fig. 6-28

Left occipito-anterior

SHOWING SIX POSITIONS IN VERTEX PRESENTATION.

In the vertex presentation the occiput is the denominator. If the occiput points to the left anterior the position is left occipito-anterior.

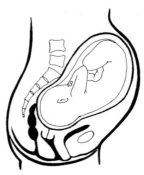

Fig. 6-29   Vertex presentation anterior position. Head well flexed, fetal back conforms to maternal abdominal wall, flexion thus being facilitated.

### Positions in Vertex Presentation

**Left occipito-anterior (L.O.A.)** The occiput points to the left ilio-pectineal eminence on the left anterior area of the pelvic brim; the sagittal suture is in the right oblique diameter of the brim.

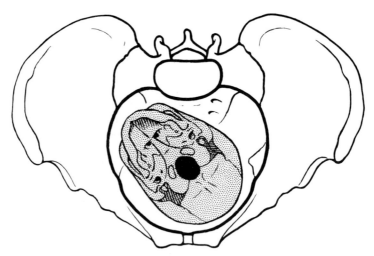

Fig. 6-30   Vertex—left occipito-anterior, showing the advantage of an anterior position. The biparietal diameter occupies the roomy anterior part of the pelvic brim.

**Left occipito-lateral (L.O.L.).** The occiput points to the left side of the pelvic brim midway between the left ilio-pectineal eminence and the left sacro-iliac joint; the sagittal suture is in the transverse diameter of the brim.

**Left occipito-posterior (L.O.P.).** The occiput points to the left sacro-iliac joint, the left posterior area of the pelvic brim; the sagittal suture is in the left oblique diameter of the brim.

**Right occipito-anterior (R.O.A.).** The occiput points to the right ilio-pectineal eminence on the right anterior area of the pelvic brim; the sagittal suture is in the left oblique diameter of the brim.

**Right occipito-lateral (R.O.L.).** The occiput points to the right side of the pelvic brim midway between the right ilio-pectineal eminence and the right sacro-iliac joint. The sagittal suture is in the transverse diameter of the brim.

**Right occipito-posterior (R.O.P.).** The occiput points to the right sacro-iliac joint in the right posterior area of the pelvic brim; the sagittal suture is in the right oblique diameter of the brim.

| | Right ant. | Right lat. | Right post. | Left ant. | Left lat. | Left post. |
|---|---|---|---|---|---|---|
| **VERTEX** | R.OA. | R.O.L. | R.O.P. | L.O.A. | L.O.L. | L.O.P. |
| **BREECH** | R.S.A. | R.S.L. | R.S.P. | L.S.A. | L.S.L. | L.S.P. |

Anterior positions are more favourable than posterior positions, because when the fetal back is in front it conforms to the concavity of the mother's abdominal wall and can therefore flex better. When the back is flexed, the head tends also to flex and a smaller diameter engages. There is also more room in the anterior part of the pelvic brim for the broad biparietal diameter of the head.

### 6. PRESENTING PART

The presenting part is the part that lies over the cervical os during labour and on which the caput forms. The term is often used erroneously, when the word "presentation" is meant.

The practical significance of the presenting part is that, should the baby's head be born before there has been time to diagnose the position of the fetus by abdominal examination, and the caput is situated on the right parietal bone posteriorly, this will indicate that the position is left occipito-anterior. Such knowledge facilitates management of the delivery of the shoulders.

---

### QUESTIONS FOR REVISION
#### DIAGNOSIS OF PREGNANCY

**State whether the following signs are positive, probable, or presumptive:**

Morning sickness .........................................

Amenorrhoea .............................................

Uterine enlargement ....................................

Fetal heart heard ........................................

Quickening ................................................

Fetal movement felt ...................................

Immunological test ....................................

Uterine souffle heard .................................

Braxton Hicks' contractions .......................

Fetal parts on palpation ............................

**At which weeks do the following signs and symptoms occur:**

Quickening ................................................

Colostrum .................................................

Fetal heart ................................................

Uterine souffle ..........................................

Enlargement of breasts ...............................

Abdominal enlargement .............................

Primary aerola ..........................................

Bladder irritability .....................................

Fetal parts felt ..........................................

Tingling of breasts .....................................

Insert the correct week at which the following give a positive sign of pregnancy.

| Weeks | | | Weeks |
|---|---|---|---|
| 2 | Feeling fetal parts | ( | ) |
| 6 | Radiography | ( | ) |
| 10 | Ultrasonogram | ( | ) |
| 16 | Chorionic gonadotrophin test | ( | ) |
| 20 | Sonicaid fetal pulse detector | ( | ) |
| 22 | Hearing the fetal heart | ( | ) |

What is quickening? How can you estimate the expected date of delivery by knowledge of quickening? When does (a) the primigravid (b) the multigravid woman recognise it? On what symptoms does a woman suspect pregnancy? What do you mean by a quantitative gonadotrophin test and when is it used? How many days are there in pregnancy? Differentiate between face and brow presentation: presentation and presenting part.

How would you recognise that a woman was a multipara from:

(a) Abdominal examination?                    (b) Vulval and vaginal examinations?

**C.M.B.(Eng.) 30-min. question.** What is the normal duration of pregnancy and how do you estimate the expected date of delivery? What observations during pregnancy may assist you in estimating the date and how may errors arise?

**C.M.B.(Eng.) 30-min. question.** What are the signs and symptoms of pregnancy? Make a list of those which are definitely diagnostic of pregnancy.

**C.M.B.(Scot.) 30-min question.** Describe methods available for the diagnosis of pregnancy at: (a) 10 weeks, (b) 28 weeks.

### RELATIONSHIP OF FETUS TO UTERUS AND PELVIS

#### *Rearrange numbers:*

| Description | | | Term |
|---|---|---|---|
| (1) Part that lies over os. | ( | ) | Presentation |
| (2) Relation of fetus to the long axis of the uterus. | ( | ) | Attitude. |
| (3) Relation of limbs and head to the trunk. | ( | ) | Lie. |
| (4) Part that lies at the pelvic brim. | ( | ) | Presenting part. |
| (5) Part of presentation that determines position. | ( | ) | Position. |
| (6) Relation of fetus to certain areas of mother's pelvis. | ( | ) | Denominator. |

Why is transverse lie a serious state of affairs? What is the presentation when the lie is transverse? Name two presentations produced by faulty attitude of the head. What are the advantages of the vertex presentation? Why are the anterior vertex positions more favourable than posterior positions? What is the advantage of anterior positions of the vertex during labour.

### *C.M.B. Short Examination Questions*

**Eng.:** Diagnosis of pregnancy. **N. Ireland:** Pregnancy tests. **Scot.:** Immunological pregnancy tests. **Scot.:** Attitude of the fetus. **Scot.:** Position of the fetus. **Scot.:** Internal rotation. **Eng.:** Signs and symptoms of early pregnancy. **Scot.:** The vertex. **Scot.:** Define chloasma. **Scot.:** Define quickening. **Eng.:** Diagnosis of pregnancy.

### *Oral Questions*

The period of amenorrhoea may be in doubt when the contraceptive pill is stopped. What advice does the midwife give to establish the EDD? Can a woman get a pregnancy test done under the NHS? How do you calculate the EDD? How much urine is required for an immunological pregnancy test? What is a pseudocyesis? Why are immunological pregnancy tests presumptive and not positive? Differentiate between: presentation and position: cervix and cervical os: lie and attitude: primary and secondary areola of the breast? How do you calculate the date of confinement? There are 5 presentations, name them.

# 7
# Prenatal Care

*Aims. Psychology. Health Education. Smoking. Counselling. Genetic aspect. Obstetrical aspect. Screening; of fetus, tests. Amniocentesis. Fetal growth. Fetal death.*

The modern midwife may not be aware that until about 1915 few pregnant women came under the care of doctor or midwife until they actually went into labour. The results were often disastrous; maternal and fetal death rates were high.

## THE AIMS OF PRENATAL CARE

1. **To promote** and maintain good physical and mental health during pregnancy. Health education including good nutrition is of primary importance.

2. **To ensure** a mature, live, healthy infant. This also includes the supervision of fetal growth and wellbeing, the prevention of congenital abnormalities due to viral infection, drugs, alcohol and other causes.

3. **To prepare** the woman for labour, lactation and the subsequent care of her child from the physical, psychological, social and educational points of view.

4. **To detect** early and treat appropriately "high risk" conditions, medical and **obstetrical,** that would endanger the life or impair the health of mother or baby.

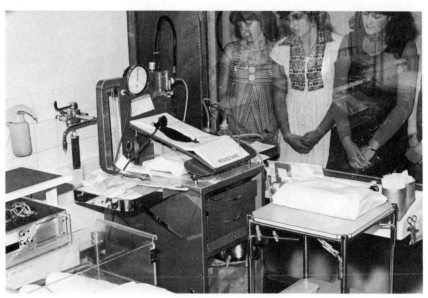

Fig. 7-1 Parenthood Class observing labour ward 'set up'. *Bellshill Maternity Hospital, Lanarkshire.*

## SHARED RESPONSIBILITY

Responsibility for prenatal care in the United Kingdom is shared between the obstetrician, general practitioner and midwife.

**This is an age of team endeavour and specialisation.** No one person practising obstetrics as an individual today can gain enough experience to be expert in every aspect of obstetric care. The concept of continuity of care by one person, i.e. the community midwife may seem admirable but it is very limited in scope and now outmoded. The hospital midwife who has specialised in one branch of obstetrics e.g. prenatal, intranatal intensive neonatal, brings extensive experience and skill combined with knowledge of modern ideas and procedures to bear on her care of mother and child.

**Childbearing women** are entitled to the highest standards of maternity care in all its wider aspects. This can best be provided in the hospital by obstetricians in conjunction with qualified midwives who are receptive to and competent in the practice of modern obstetrics.

The pregnant women has faith in the maternity hospital staff as a whole for her safety and care, not in any one member of staff.

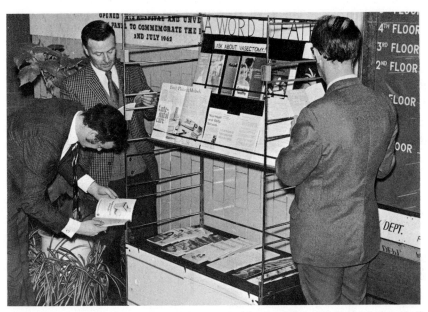

Fig. 7-2    A word to fathers. Books on baby care and family planning on display in front hall of Bellshill Maternity Hospital, Lanarkshire.

## THE PSYCHOLOGICAL ASPECT

It is now accepted that, for the successful practice of obstetrics, understanding of the psychological aspect of childbearing is as essential as knowledge of the physical aspect. Undoubtedly we must concern ourselves with the woman's health and obstetric wellbeing, but we must be equally concerned about her emotional welfare. The tendency to become so engrossed in obstetrics *per se* should be resisted, in case the woman as an individual is relegated to second place. Psychological, educational and social avenues of approach are utilised to provide family centred maternity care that enables the woman to fulfil her maternal role successfully and happily.

The advent of a first pregnancy produces a certain degree of emotional turmoil in the mind of any thinking woman. Emotions, such as mother-love and pride in creation, induce a feeling of tranquillity and gladness, for the woman is about to enter on one of life's most enriching experiences. But these emotions may be counterbalanced by others of a disturbing nature such as fear and resentment. Not all women are well balanced or emotionally mature, and their reactions to pregnancy will depend on such factors as temperament, intelligence and education, health, age and the marital situation. Whether the child is wanted or not dominates almost everything else. All babies are not planned or wanted at the time of conception but the majority of married women adjust to the situation and when born the baby is welcomed.

## The attitude of the husband

Being sustained by the care and consideration of a kindly husband is essential for the happiness and emotional stability of the pregnant woman. It seems reasonable to expect the husband to have some understanding of the physical and emotional demands pregnancy makes on his wife: by taking an active interest in her physical wellbeing, particularly in regard to nutrition, rest and recreation, he is also meeting her psychological needs, because he is demonstrating his protective role and showing his concern for her welfare. The discomforts of pregnancy may make her petulant at times, but the husband should exercise forbearance on such occasions. She needs his steadying influence and will respond to understanding and kindliness rather than logical argument.

Husbands should be encouraged to attend classes on 'preparation for labour' so that they can give emotional support before and during labour.

### The Influence of the Midwife

The midwife must try to appreciate the heightened sensitivity of the expectant mother, and endeavour to inculcate in her patients an attitude of mind that brings the higher emotions into play, for when a woman can anticipate the birth of her baby with courage and serenity, fear is subordinated. She should keep in front of her patients the idea that childbearing is a natural event and try to foster a cheerful outlook.

The midwife must also be aware of the conflicts and fears that can be so disturbing to the expectant mother's peace of mind; her willingness to listen and give sympathetic advice will often help the woman to face and overcome her difficulties. Tact and resourcefulness are needed, so that her approach and advice may be acceptable to all types of women. Invariably the successful midwife is one with certain qualities of character that are apparent in her kindly manner and friendly interest in human beings; she expresses her interest in the woman as an individual as well as a patient.

If by her understanding of the psychological aspect of pregnancy the midwife can bring a woman into labour in a serene, courageous frame of mind, she is making a valuable contribution to obstetrics.

## Fear of labour and how to eliminate it

Even when a woman is delighted at the prospect of motherhood and eagerly awaiting the birth of her baby, her peace of mind may be upset by vague fears, some real, some imaginary, but none the less real to her. These can be counterbalanced by confidence in the hospital, doctor and midwife as well as by education. She dreads the unknown experience, so the process of labour should be explained in simple language, telling her what to expect and in what way she can help herself. Fear of death no doubt crosses the mind of every pregnant woman at some time, but it is not a dominant fear. It could be likened to the fleeting fear that may precede a journey by sea or air. The expectant mother should be reminded that thousands of women give birth to babies, simply and easily, every day, and her thoughts directed away from labour and focused on the baby's birthday—a happier thought.

Fear of pain looms large on the horizon of the pregnant woman. She can be told that everything possible will be done for her comfort, as long as it does not harm the baby or unduly retard labour (see 'Relief of pain,' p. 259). With such assurance, the woman's fear is diminished and she gains confidence in herself and her midwife.

Practically every method of preparation for childbirth includes giving knowledge of labour. When the woman is aware of what is going to happen she gains confidence in her ability to cope with the situation. This must not be interpreted as meaning that the expectant mother will be less afraid if given a detailed description of the anatomy of the pelvic organs and the physiological processes of labour. The pregnant woman is more concerned regarding what she will experience and how she will react than with anatomical details.

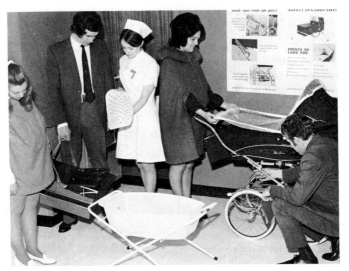

Fig. 7-3 Equipment for baby. Expectant parents are advised on the 'points' to look for when buying baby equipment.

*Maternity Hospital, Stirling.*

## THE EDUCATIONAL ASPECT

No matter how excellent the medical and obstetrical care is, it cannot be completely effective without the active co-operation of the mother. It is she, personally, who will observe the rules of health to keep herself fit during pregnancy and in preparation for labour.

Knowledge of labour must be presented in an elementary fashion and judiciously applied in a practical rather than theoretical way to elaborate some point concerning the management of labour or to explain the processes of labour as they affect the woman's feelings and reactions. What she needs most of all is the assurance that she will be physically safe and psychologically secure under the care of a competent team who are interested in her welfare, willing to alleviate discomfort, mental or physical, and eager to relieve pain.

**Every prenatal clinic should be a school for expectant mothers; every midwife a teacher.** The mother-to-be is eager to do what is best for her baby and this attitude should be fostered; she is in a most receptive frame of mind and midwives should be prepared to talk to mothers individually or in groups.

# HEALTH EDUCATION

The midwife has an excellent opportunity for the promotion of good health, physical and mental: she must motivate as well as teach. The need for inaugurating a programme of health education, over and above what may be included in education for parenthood, is urgent.

### *Pregnant Women Should be Advised:*

**To avoid contact with infectious disease,** particularly rubella and viral infections.

**To refrain from taking drugs** other then a mild aperient unless prescribed by the doctor and limit strictly the intake of alcohol.

**To stop smoking** or reduce the number of cigarettes to under four per day.

**To take foods rich in body-builders,** minerals and vitamins.

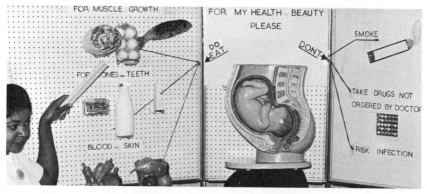

Fig. 7-4 Good health for mother and baby. Student midwife talking to expectant mothers. (Fresh food is attached to the peg board.)

*Bellshill Maternity Hospital, Lanarkshire.*

Unfortunately a number of mothers are not aware that fetal growth can be disturbed during the first 8 to 12 weeks of pregnancy: drugs and infections such as rubella having caused congenital malformations by interfering with the development of the embryo. Alcohol may cause mental retardation of the fetus.

Mothers should be shown how to promote the good health of their families. The maintenance of physical wellbeing, prior to and during pregnancy can foster fetal growth and wellbeing as well as having a profound influence on the health and vigour of the baby.

Anaemia is still more common among childbearing women than it ought to be and an active campaign for its prevention is long overdue. Foods rich in iron are given on page 75.

### COMBATING NICOTINE DEPENDENCE

Twenty per cent of expectant mothers give up smoking during pregnancy so, midwives should feel encouraged to participate in the non-smoking campaign so essential for the health of mother and child. The welfare of the baby is a powerful incentive to give up nicotine addiction. Those who persist in the habit should be warned that when baby is taken home from hospital he will live day and night in a cigarette-smoke-polluted atmosphere. Such babies are liable to recurrent respiratory infections; they look pale and lack vigour.

### The Harmful Effects of Smoking

To talk convincingly to groups of mothers the midwife should be a non-smoker. She must (*a*) be informed regarding the harmful effects of smoking and (*b*) have understanding of how difficult it is to stop; and (*c*) have insight as to how mothers can be persuaded to do so.

As few as five cigarettes per day will adversely affect fetal growth and over ten per day increases the perinatal mortality rate. Smoking is particularly harmful when the mother is 'at high risk' for some medical or obstetrical cause including age over 35 and multi-multiparity. These women must be strongly advised to desist. It has been found that carbon monoxide and nicotine from cigarette smoke pass through the placenta and reduce the oxygen carrying capacity of the blood. Abortion, stillbirth, low birth weight and preterm labour are more common: anaemia is 10 per cent more prevalent. Men who are heavy smokers have a higher incidence of abnormal spermatozoa.

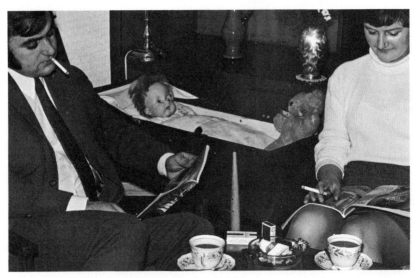

Fig. 7-5 Baby is subject to cigarette smoke in double measure when both parents are nicotine dependent.

*Bellshill Maternity Hospital, Lanarkshire.*

Many women who smoke heavily are undernourished; preferring cigarettes to food. They go out to work or use the housekeeping money to buy cigarettes and the family is deprived of wholesome food. When questioned they allege that smoking soothes their 'nerves' and gives great pleasure. They don't realise that the so-called 'nerves' is a craving by the body for the drug on which they have become dependent—nicotine. The soothing effect of a cigarette comes from satisfying the craving by taking more of the drug of addiction.

Some women can stop at once, others do so gradually, a few of the less responsible have not the will power or even the desire to stop. All need encouragement: discussion groups that include a few who have succeeded in giving up smoking may have a therapeutic effect. Mothers should be advised to do their utmost to persuade their children not to start smoking.

## PROMOTING MENTAL HEALTH

This is just as important as promoting physical health. Not all pregnant women have the emotional stability that is enhanced by being reared in a secure happy home and strengthened further by a tranquil marriage.

Midwives should endeavour to prevent or alleviate some of the factors that give rise to mental strain and emotional tension: for the recorded incidence of psychosis in obstetric patients is considerable. An effort should be made to meet the psychological needs of pregnant women.

### GOOD HUMAN RELATIONSHIPS

Interest should be shown in the woman as a person; not only in her blood pressure, pelvis and fetus, important though they be. Getting to know the woman as an individual is time-consuming but it is an integral part of good prenatal care. Most women approach labour with some degree of apprehension and this aspect deserves more attention. Midwives should be allowed time to give the necessary emotional support:

**During pregnancy**

Giving sympathetic understanding, listening, offering advice, answering questions.

**During labour**

Providing patient, kindly care and companionship: instilling confidence; reducing mental trauma and physical suffering.

**During puerperium**

Proffering guidance and encouragement rather than direction regarding care of the baby. Discussing personal questions such as family planning.

## THE NEED FOR PRENATAL COUNSELLING

Expectant mothers are taking a lively interest in aspects of obstetric care beyond the subjects usually presented to them. Some of the more vocal mothers are critical of procedures that they consider will interfere with the process of childbirth: they also want to participate in decision-making regarding 'where', 'when' and 'how' labour should be conducted.

**Midwives ought to be alert to these trends** and fortified (a) to communicate and explain modern ideas, aided by discussion: (b) to give reasons for the various procedures adopted and the equipment employed. When approached with tact and courtesy expectant mothers are likely to accept new ideas if they are clearly explained to them. Because of their professional qualifications and practical experience midwives are ideally equipped to counsel expectant mothers and ought to do so, otherwise they may be given erroneous, outmoded, or biased information. Certain groups who are neither qualified, experienced, nor licensed to practise as midwives are giving instruction to pregnant women with a fanatical degree of fervour that appeals to and convinces them.

**Pregnant women should be encouraged to ask questions** and to express their points of view: wrong conceptions should be clarified. Young midwives should be taught how to counsel such mothers.

**The reasons for procedures that some mothers object to should be explained to them, such as:**

1. INDUCTION OF LABOUR

When the obstetrician considers that the uterus no longer provides an adequate or a safe environment for the fetus, or that pregnancy jeopardises the woman's health or life, labour may be induced—a meritorious, humane procedure.

2. PUNCTURE OF MEMBRANES

This is done to induce or to accelerate labour. It is also an admirable means of detecting meconium in the amniotic fluid; an early sign of fetal distress.

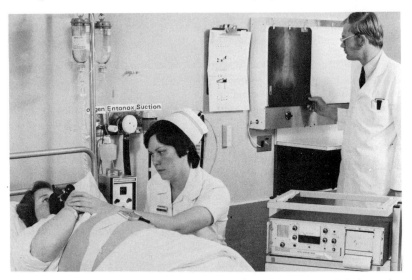

Fig. 7-6 Obstetrician and midwife giving highly specialised care. Ivac infusion unit and Sonicaid monitor in use. Entonox being administered.

*Maternity Unit, Perth Royal Infirmary.*

3. THE USE OF ELECTRONIC EQUIPMENT

Childbearing women may (wrongly) imagine that the use of electronic monitoring equipment deprives them of the personal care and observation of the midwife. In fact the midwife's powers of observation are extended to provide greater safety for mother and child. Vigilant, unceasing supervision is essential to detect early signs of fetal distress, which signifies hypoxia; a condition that can damage fetal brain cells. Electronic equipment provides this protective supervision.

4. EPISIOTOMY

When the baby's head is held up on a rigid perineum he may suffer brain damage. The over stretched pelvic floor does not subsequently support the pelvic organs and uterine prolapse can occur; the bladder and urethra may be bruised and injured. An episiotomy prevents a perineal tear from extending into the rectum; it also heals better than a ragged tear.

5. PROCEDURES THAT SOME MOTHERS WISH TO ADOPT

**(a) Psychophysical methods of pain-relief**

Some of the thirty psychophysical systems of relieving pain in labour involve types of breathing that deprive the fetus of oxygen and are harmful.

### (b) The Leboyer teaching

Leboyer stresses the harmful effect of bright light on the psychological develop-ment of the new born baby, so some mothers are demanding that lights in the labour ward be dimmed during birth; but this is unnecessary, for nature has arranged that babies eyes are tightly shut during and for some hours after birth. The midwife needs light to observe mother and baby and to carry out resuscitative methods when necessary. Leboyer also condemns noise at birth; but the only noise then is the welcome cry of the baby expanding his lungs. Midwives know that 'the violence' deplored by Leboyer is never applied in Britain during labour and can assure mothers of this.

### (c) Natural childbirth

Pregnant women are inadvisedly exhorted by certain groups to demand 'natural childbirth' and to refuse any interference. But when left to nature, labour can be long, painful, exhausting to the mother and lethal to both mother and child. Women today are not aware of the disastrous results of 'natural childbirth' at the beginning of this century and in some underdeveloped countries today.

**Childbirth has been made safer, shorter, and easier by the very scientific procedures some misinformed women object to.** Reverting to primitive methods is a retrograde step which has no justification and should not be condoned.

### (d) Home confinement

It is understandable that some expectant mothers would choose to have their babies at home. In familiar surroundings, with the doctor and midwife she knows, and her family near her, labour would seem to be a natural, simple occurrence.

**But unpredictable complications do arise:** in a recent report it was shown that seven per cent of women who were selected as 'low risk' cases for home delivery had to be transferred to hospital during labour. Some community midwives deliver less than five babies per annum: their experience being minimal compared to hospital midwives. Reliance on the 'flying squad' does not guarantee safety, for there may be delay in their arrival. Should haemorrhage occur, the ambulance journey to hospital could be deleterious to the shocked woman. The reasons in favour of home confinement are emotional and social rather than obstetrical.

In recent years much has been done in hospital to create a more friendly, home-like atmosphere: husbands are made welcome in the labour ward. Midwives do endeavour to be patient, kindly and sympathetic; they give constant supervision and professional companionship as well as striving to provide emotional support and encouragement while attending proficiently to their responsible arduous duties.

If midwives have failed in fully appreciating the woman's point of view this can be remedied by better communication and more sympathetic understanding.

### (e) Should mothers make professional decisions?

To the expectant mother, labour is a very personal experience which engenders the presumption that she ought to participate in professional decisions and dictate regarding her obstetric care. But she may have little understanding of the tremendous amount of knowledge and years of experience needed in the practise of competent obstetrics. If she knew more she would realise the wisdom of having faith in professional experts and allowing them to make decisions regarding her own and her baby's wellbeing and safety throughout labour.

**Obstetricians and midwives have theoretical knowledge, expertise, manual skill, and vast experience,** which they should be given freedom to exercise. They have gleaned wisdom in the application of these professional attributes. As well as saving the lives of mothers and babies they, in co-operation with paediatricians and anaesthetists aided by electronic monitoring equipment and resuscitative techniques, are improving the quality of infant life. Mothers should not choose to deprive themselves or their babies of the modern mechanical techniques now available for their welfare, comfort and safety. They ought to be made aware of the dangers of making professional decisions they are not qualified to sustain and should also be discouraged from doing so.

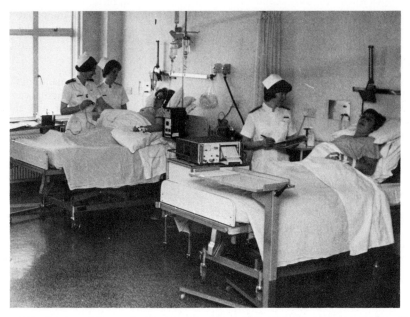

Fig. 7-7 Midwives giving professional care to patients whose condition is being monitored by electronic equipment.

*Aberdeen Maternity Hospital.*

**Expectant mothers need counsel** that will help them to fulfil their maternal role successfully and with satisfaction, even joy. Midwives must co-operate in achieving this aim.

## THE MEDICAL ASPECT

The need for medical, apart from obstetrical, supervision ought to be clearly appreciated. Every effort should be made to maintain maternal wellbeing at a high level, for the good health of the mother has an important bearing on the prevention of obstetrical complications and on ensuring the future wellbeing of the child. It could be argued that it is too late to start a scheme for physical wellbeing during pregnancy, but if we presume that the fetus *in utero* is a potential parent, then we are truly laying the foundations of good health for the next generation.

**The midwife should encourage the woman to be seen early in pregnancy by the doctor,** so that he can assess her general health and give advice before any existing disease has been aggravated by pregnancy. The routine blood and chest examinations provide a means of recognising early such conditions as cardiac disease, anaemia, diabetes, syphilis and tuberculosis, the prompt treatment of which may avert disaster.

# THE GENETIC ASPECT

The diagnosis of genetically transmitted defects or diseases during pregnancy by biochemical, biophysical and other scientific procedures has revealed new dimensions in prenatal care. A number of obstetric units in Britain have established genetic counselling clinics. The obstetrician may suspect a heritable condition from the patient's history: the general practitioner may have knowledge of a genetic disease in the patient's family, e.g. diabetes, essential hypertension and schizophrenia.

Sickle cell anaemia and phenylketonuria are transmitted genetically but not all of the 2 per cent serious congenital disorders are genetic in origin; many of the more common defects such as cleft palate, spina bifida and anencephaly are caused by a combination of genetic and intra-uterine (environmental) factors. Some congenital abnormalities are entirely environmental; midwives being well aware of the teratogenic effect of drugs such as Thalidomide and the virus of rubella on the embryo at the early vulnerable period of gestation. Any maternal condition that deprives the fetus of oxygen can damage the brain cells and cause mental retardation; hypoxia must be avoided or dealt with promptly.

## CHROMOSOMES

The hereditary characteristics of the parents, and their ancestors, are transmitted in the genes of the autosomes (which are non-sex chromosomes), i.e. colour of skin and eyes, blood group and Rh factor, stature and facial appearance, intelligence as well as defects and diseases.

Every cell in the human body has 46 chromosomes (23 pairs). One pair, the sex chromosomes, is responsible for the determination of the sex of the zygote (the fertilised ovum). The pair of sex chromosomes in the ovum is designated XX and they can only produce a female child. The pair of sex chromosomes in the sperm is designated XY; X can produce a female child, Y a male child. Just prior to conception the ovum and the sperm each shed 23 chromosomes (meiosis). When fertilisation occurs the ovum and sperm each contribute 23 chromosomes (one of which is a sex chromosome) so that the zygote will have 23 pairs of chromosomes. The ovum does not determine the sex of the child. An X chromosome from the mother and an X chromosome from the father produces a female: X from the mother and Y from the father produces a male child.

| **Father** | X | Y | |
|------------|----|----|----|
| **Mother** | X | X | |
| Baby girl | XX | XY | Baby boy |

(Statistics show that the sex ratio remains fairly constant—about 106 boys are born to every 100 girls.)

Abnormalities in sex chromosomes can give rise to intersex states, male and female infertility and disturbances in sexual function: hermaphroditism being an abnormality the midwife may encounter. Fortunately nature discards many defective embryos: 30 per cent of first trimester spontaneous abortions are found to have chromosomal anomalies.

## PRENATAL DIAGNOSIS OF GENETIC DEFECTS

Since the liberalisation of the Abortion Act 1967 the diagnosis of an abnormal fetus in early pregnancy has great clinical significance: termination of pregnancy now being permissible if there is a substantial risk that the child when born would be seriously handicapped by a physical or mental disability.

When serum alpha feto-proteins are above the accepted level transabdominal amniocentesis is performed; amniotic fluid being withdrawn from the gestation sac and subjected to biochemical and cytological investigation: detection of Down's syndrome being one of the more common indications for amniotic fluid cell culture. By screening women at 'high risk' of producing a mongoloid child, i.e. those over 40 years of age and others who have previously borne such a child, the pregnancy could be terminated if the fetus was found to be affected and the parents requested this.

**Sex prediction** may be undertaken by chromosomal analysis of cultured amniotic fluid cells after 14 weeks gestation in women who are known carries of disorders such as Duchenne muscular dystrophy or haemophilia which affect males only. If the diagnosis is positive, selective abortion might be considered should the parents desire this.

A rapid method of determining fetal sex by measuring the concentration of testosterone in amniotic fluid during the second trimester is now being used. When the fetus is male the concentration of testosterone is higher than when female.

The enzyme and metabolite content of the amniotic fluid is analysed; a high level of phenylalanine having been found in cases of uncontrolled phenylketonuria in pregnant women.

Ultrasonography and other diagnostic procedures are described on page 107.

## GENETIC COUNSELLING

When counsel is requested regarding a serious hereditary disease or condition, the medical geneticist explains the situation to the parents in elementary terminology and gives an estimate as to the likelihood of its occurrence or recurrence. He may mention some of the implications in caring for a severely handicapped child, particularly beyond the stage of infancy: the facilities available to improve the quality of life for such children should also be enumerated.

Should the prenatal diagnosis of a serious fetal defect be made, the question of allowing the pregnancy to continue, or to be terminated by selective abortion followed by contraception, and rarely sterilisation, is discussed. The parents are given time for reflection; they personally must decide, for it is their lives that will be affected: the counsellor does not urge or advise, even if invited to do so by the parents. Their decision will be influenced by their emotional maturity and the stability of the marriage: financial circumstances are important but above all their compassionate attitude to a child who may inflict restrictions and considerable strain on family life.

The expectant mother may worry unduly about a particular defect or disease that has occurred in her own or her husband's relatives. Such groundless fears are frequently due to ignorance. If the parents are first cousins they may be apprehensive at the possibility of some congenital abnormality but the defect they dread may have been environmental, e.g. caused by drugs such as Thalidomide or by rubella. Unjustifiable guilt feelings, if present, are dispelled.

Adoption societies may seek genetic advice if a parental disorder is suspected of being heritable. Cases of disputed paternity do occur and it can be proved that the man in question is not the father if the child has a blood group substance which is not present in the putative father's blood or the child lacks a blood group substance present in the putative father's blood. But if both have the same blood group this does not prove that the putative father is the true father.

### The Midwives' Role

The midwife is not professionally qualified to express an opinion or to give advice on this difficult and highly specialised subject. Her role is educational and supportive. When an abnormal child is born or if expectant parents have doubts or fears *re* some hereditary trait the midwife should advise them to attend the genetic counselling clinic after having made preliminary arrangements with their doctor. Her main contribution can be in prenatal health education in order to prevent intra-uterine (environmental) congenital defects, e.g. those caused by teratogenic drugs, alcohol and viral infections.

At the genetic clinic the midwife gives the necessary psychological support by allaying anxiety and creating a friendly atmosphere. She explains terms used that the patient does not understand or wishes to know about.

## THE OBSTETRICAL ASPECT

The purely obstetrical aspect of prenatal care cannot be separated from the other aspects, they dovetail into each other and all have obstetrical significance. In the narrow sense, it is concerned with the supervision and management of pregnancy, the making of provision for labour, the puerperium and the newborn child, as well as the prevention, diagnosis and treatment of complications. This involves investigation, examination, supervision, advice and treatment: these are described in subsequent chapters. Education of expectant mothers is potentially preventive.

### Taking the history

It should be kept in mind that the purpose of taking a history is not merely for the recording of facts and statistics; it is a means of assessing the health of the woman and bringing to light any defect which would adversely affect childbearing. History-taking should lead to remedial action as far as is possible.

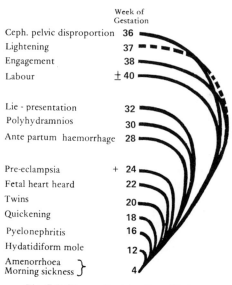

Fig. 7-8 Diagnostic dates for midwives.

### The social history

Taking the social history enables hospital staff to find out whether the expectant mother's home conditions are adequate. If overcrowding exists or the house constitutes a health hazard the environmental health officer should be informed. She may be an unsupported mother or her husband may be unemployed, ill, or disabled. If she is unable to obtain sufficient nourishment, application for free milk and supplementary benefit can be made. Should it be surmised that the expectant mother is incapable of budgeting wisely or of making preparation for the care of the baby, suitable advice should be given or sought.

### The family history

This should be inquired into, as some families have a genetic predisposition to certain diseases such as psychiatric disorders, diabetes and essential hypertension. The tendency to produce twins also runs in families. If parent, brother or sister is dead, the cause should be ascertained without giving rise to distress in doing so.

### The medical history

It is necessary to have some knowledge of the woman's previous health, as former illnesses may have damaged certain structures or organs, and this might give rise to complications during pregnancy or labour. Anterior poliomyelitis, or tuberculosis of the spine and hip may cause deformities; rheumatic infection may leave cardiac impairment. Diseases, such as chronic nephritis, tend to be aggravated by childbearing: diabetes and cardiac disease may seriously complicate pregnancy and labour: syphilis and diabetes both endanger the life of the child. Previous accidents or pelvic operations may affect parturition. Enquiries should be made regarding blood transfusions given at any time, including childhood, because of the possibility of Rh-immunisation occurring in an Rh-negative woman.

## THE OBSTETRIC HISTORY

A record of previous pregnancies, labours and puerperia will often give a clue as to what may be anticipated in the present instance. Certain conditions may recur, and it may be possible to give advice or institute treatment to avert them: an account of any complications should be obtained. Particulars of abortions should be included, with a statement of the time at which they occurred and the cause, if known. Any previous history of excessive sickness, pyelonephritis or pre-eclampsia will necessitate close supervision during this pregnancy.

### Previous labours

Was labour premature or postmature? Spontaneous or induced: date and where delivered?

Most labours are straightforward. The length of labour is important. The baby's weight, and the fact that forceps had been necessary, would give an idea as to whether delay was due to cephalopelvic disproportion. A woman who has previously given birth spontaneously to a baby weighing 3·5 kg is likely to have a normal pelvis.

If a Caesarean section has previously been performed (the scar would be evidence), all subsequent labours ought to be conducted in hospital, on account of the risk of rupture of the uterine scar. A previous third degree perineal tear would suggest the need for an episiotomy to avoid its recurrence. A history of postpartum haemorrhage or adherent placenta would necessitate hospitalisation in case such an accident be repeated.

### Previous puerperia

Progress during the puerperium can best be assessed by asking the woman whether she felt well during this period. Complications, such as venous thrombosis, or puerperal sepsis, usually come to light with shrewd questioning.

### Previous babies

A record of normal-sized babies, born alive and well, is usual, but when the weight of a previous baby is stated to have been over 4 kg it is usual to examine the urine for glucose to rule out diabetes; some do a glucose tolerance test. A history of stillbirth would demand careful questioning if no record was available, and the cause of neonatal deaths should be investigated. If there is no living child, or in cases of repeated preterm births, or in severe jaundice, the doctor should be informed; he will recommend delivery in a hospital where prompt skilled treatment and the facilities available may save the baby's life. Should infant deaths appear to be due to lack of good mothercare, additional instruction ought to be given by the midwife and health visitor.

### HISTORY OF THE PRESENT PREGNANCY

The first question when taking the hisory is usually in regard to (a) the date of the last menstrual period to establish the period of gestation, (b) whether it was normal in length and amount and if the woman had been menstruating regularly. If there is any doubt regarding the last menstrual period, the woman should be asked if she had taken 'the pill' and when she stopped doing so and told to note and record the date of quickening (see p. 78). The length of time married is important in cases of infertility.

Enquiry should be made as to whether she has felt well since becoming pregnant, and if not the cause should be sought and appropriate action taken. Exposure to rubella during or immediately prior to pregnancy is very significant.

'**High Risk**' cases are primigravidae over 30; multipara, 4+ or age over 35, bad obstetric history; medical complications; obstetric complications.

**Drugs taken.** Some authorities enquire regarding drugs taken during pregnancy and six weeks prior to conception because of their possible teratogenic effects. Antidepressant drugs such as phenelzine (Nardil) may potentiate the action of pethidine.

**Diet history** If there is no dietitian, the midwife should inquire into the type of meals the woman is having, in order to make sure she is getting the necessary substances for the baby's and her own wellbeing (*body building foods, minerals, vitamins*). Dietary advice is given when weight gain is excessive, but in cases of gross obesity specialist supervision is essential, also in certain medical complications of pregnancy (*see under appropriate headings*).

### The grande multipara (Fig. 7-9, p. 106)

This term is applied to the woman who has given birth to five or more children, in order to stress the hazards of such a situation. With each succeeding birth after the third the maternal mortality and stillbirth rate rise steeply and even more so when the woman is over 30 years of age. Severe anaemia is common because of repeated childbearing and poor nutrition. Because of their age the cardiovascular system is often impaired: hypertension and obesity accentuate the risks of high parity. Midwives ought to pay special attention to those women, advising them regarding the need for rest and suitable food and referring them to the social worker who will arrange for a home help or other means of lightening the domestic burden. They should be delivered in hospital for the incidence of malpresentation, rupture of uterus and postpartum haemorrhage is very much greater in the grande multipara.

### The older primigravida

Age is important, particularly if this is her first baby and she is over 30. To such a patient the term 'older primigravida' is applied and women of that age often worry regarding their ability to go through the processes of childbearing safely, so much assurance accompanied by careful supervision throughout pregnancy and labour is essential. It may be, if she has been married for a number of years, that she is relatively infertile so special precautions are taken to prevent abortion and to secure a live child. For example, postmaturity is not permitted to develop and Caesarean section is performed four times more frequently than in the younger woman. Pre-eclampsia and prolonged labour increase the dangers to the fetus.

The maternal mortality rate is only slightly increased. But complications may occur such as pre-eclampsia, essential hypertension, venous thrombosis and uterine fibroids: uterine dysfunction and rigidity of the soft tissues of the birth canal accentuate the need for delivery by forceps. The perinatal mortality rate is doubled in woman over 35 and the possibility of Down's syndrome is always present. Midwives should, when the opportunity arises, advise women not to defer their first pregnancy too long beyond the optimal child-bearing age of 18 to 25 years.

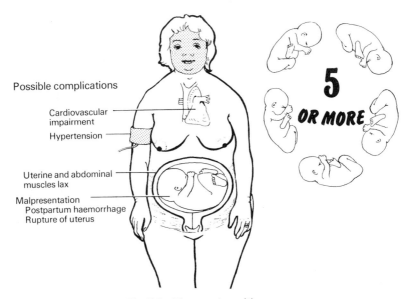

Possible complications

Cardiovascular impairment

Hypertension

Uterine and abdominal muscles lax

Malpresentation
Postpartum haemorrhage
Rupture of uterus

Fig. 7-9   The grande multipara.

### Method of taking the history

Great patience and infinite tact are needed when taking the history of a new patient, especially a primigravida, to whom the experience may seem to be something of an ordeal. The midwife should be kindly in her approach, and by her reassuring manner convey the impression that having a baby is a happy event and a natural process.

The woman's name, address, age and occupation are recorded. Patients are often forgetful in regard to dates and past illnesses; they may even neglect to mention a surgical operation until their attention is drawn to the presence of a scar. Questions should be asked in such a way as to avoid creating the impression that you suspect the woman is suffering from some particular ailment. To ask an expectant mother outright if there is tuberculosis or psychiatric disorders in her family might well alarm her; it would be better to inquire whether her father and mother were in good health and if there had been any serious illnesses in the family.

Simple, non-technical language should be used, as terms very familiar to the midwife may be unknown and even frightening to the woman, and wrong answers may be given because of lack of understanding. By listening to an experienced midwife taking histories the student midwife learns the terminology which suits the mentality of different patients.

# PRENATAL SCREENING

The modern midwife participates in the prenatal screening process to assess maternal health, and to monitor fetal wellbeing, growth and maturity. Screening reveals incipient evidence of conditions that put the pregnant woman or her fetus at 'high risk' before signs of the actual disease are manifest. Confirmatory diagnostic tests are then made to establish the findings.

### TRADITIONAL SCREENING MEASURES

Many routine examinations that midwives make can be classified as screening: they provide information that (a) indicates normal progress, (b) that forbodes harmful developments.

**History taking;** blood and urine testing.

**Physical examination,** weighing.

**Obstetrical examination:** abdominal inspection and palpation: serial auscultation of the FH: assessing pelvic capacity.

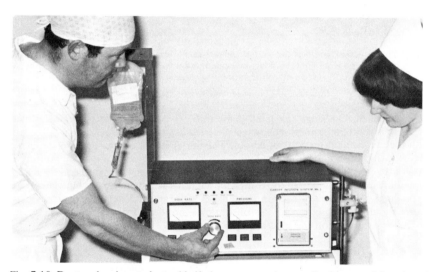

Fig. 7-10 Doctor showing student midwife how to control manually the rate of flow i.v. of Syntocinon. The Pye Dynamics Infusion pump (Cardiff Infusion System) automatically regulates the rate of flow.

*Forth Park Maternity Hospital, Kirkcaldy.*

## THE USE OF ELECTRONIC AND ULTRASONIC EQUIPMENT

Professional skills and mechanical devices both have meritorious obstetric usefulness. The modern midwife welcomes the aid of monitors and ultrasonic scans that extend her supervisory powers, visual auditory and tactile.

**Continuous monitoring of the fetal heart** brings a greater degree of accuracy than the use of the fetal stethoscope when the FH rate pattern is causing concern. Electronic equipment contributes to fetal assessment and wellbeing.

**Ultrasonic scans and the electrocardiograph** will, it has been predicted, be utilised at every prenatal visit in the future to screen fetal wellbeing.

**Ultrasonic scans,** electronic equipment and biochemical tests help to monitor fetal growth and wellbeing as well as detecting genetic, medical and obstetric conditions that put the fetus at high risk.

**Electrocardiography** is employed to determine fetal wellbeing. In 'at risk' pregnancy the fetal heart rate pattern is studied by monitoring the FH continuously for 20 minutes at intervals during a period of 2 or more hours. Acceleration, deceleration, persistent tachycardia, loss of base line variability are among the abnormal traces classified .

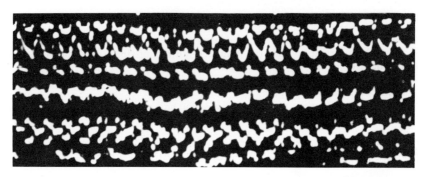

Fig. 7-11 Detection of fetal heart movement at 7 weeks menstrual age using pulsed ultrasound. Echoes from the fetal heart movement are recorded in waveform (rate 165 beats per minute): used for, confirmation of pregnancy and missed abortion.

*Courtesy of Queen Mother's Hospital, Glasgow.*

**The oxytocin challenge (or fetal stress test)** by administering a small dose of oxytocin is sometimes employed when the fetus is at risk to assess how it will cope with the uterine contractions of labour. The initial stage of induction of labour by i.v. syntocinon 0·5 units in 500 ml glucose solution 5 per cent, is usually preferred as a more appropriate time than during late pregnancy. A decision is made depending on the reaction of the compromised fetus as to whether labour is allowed to proceed or Caesarean section should be performed. Observation of the fetal status should be vigilant and the obstetrician notified if an abnormal FH rate pattern is exhibited on the electrocardiotocograph.

### URINARY OESTRIOL

**Assays** are made after the 34th week of pregnancy. When urinary oestriol is diminished to 11–18 micromoles/24 hours, the fetus is at 'high risk'. Levels below 8 micromoles/24 hours indicate fetal death.

KLOPPER

| Weeks of pregnancy | 20 | 24 | 28 | 32 | 36 | 40 |
|---|---|---|---|---|---|---|
| Range of micromoles per 24 hours | 7–28 | 21–45 | 28–63 | 38–83 | 59–132 | 69–170 |

The total amount of urinary oestriol excreted in 48 hours is a guide to the functional ability of the feto-placental unit; the trend of a series of assays having more diagnostic value than the level of one reading. Accurate collection of a 24 hour specimen of urine is imperative; this being done on 2 consecutive days. In some centres a radioimmuno-assay of plasma oestriol is done; the result being obtained more rapidly. Some utilise the oestrogen/creatinine ratio from an early morning specimen of urine.

### Examination of maternal blood

Tests for conditions that compromise the fetus are made, e.g. syphilis, Rh incompatibility, rubella antibodies.

**Serum placental lactogen** is measured to assess placental function: a level of less than 4 micrograms/ml and failure to rise on three or more subsequent examinations after the 30th week, suggests placental insufficiency.

**The role of placental specific proteins** (SP) has been reported in monitoring intra-uterine fetal growth. A steady increase in the plasma level denotes satisfactory fetal growth.

**The alpha feto-protein** level in maternal serum is elevated at 16–18 weeks when a fetal open neural tube defect, such as spina bifida or anencephaly is present.

### Examination of maternal urine

**Detection of pre-eclampsia by finding protein:** and the possibility of diabetes by finding glucose, both of which put the fetus at 'high risk'.

### A SELECTION OF PRENATAL SCREENING TESTS

| DETECTION OF MATERNAL CONDITIONS THAT AFFECT FETAL WELLBEING | | TO OBTAIN EVIDENCE OF FETAL WELLBEING | |
|---|---|---|---|
| **History:** | Family, medical, obstetrical. Present pregnancy. | **Auscultation:** | Intermittent, Doptone, continuous electronic monitoring. |
| **Physical examination:** | Systemic, skeletal, abdominal, vaginal, blood pressure, weight gain. | **Ultrasonography:** | Gestational age; fetal growth; deformity; bi-parietal cephalometry; real-time scan. |
| **Blood:** | Hb, ABO group, VDRL, Rh factor and antibodies, alpha feto-proteins, placental lactogen, rubella antibodies. | **Amniocentesis:** | Chromosomal anomalies; neural tube defects; spectrophotoscopy; lecithin/sphingomyelin ratio. |
| **Urine:** | Protein, glucose, oestriol. | **Electrocardiography** (ECG). | |

## AMNIOCENTESIS

Amniotic fluid is withdrawn by syringe via the anterior abdominal wall; the fluid and exfoliated fetal cells are examined to detect certain fetal abnormalities and conditions such as:

(a) **Chromosomal anomalies:** (after 15th–17th week of gestation): Down's syndrome being the most common indication. Cells present in the amniotic fluid contain fetal chromosomes: with increasing maternal age the incidence of chromosomal anomalies rises (see page 596). Some recommended that all pregnant women over 35 years should be offered amniocentesis.

(b) **Open neural tube defect:** (at 16th–18th week of gestation). When spina bifida or anencephaly has occurred in a previous child or when a significantly raised concentration of alpha fetoprotein is found in maternal serum detected during a prenatal blood-screening programme, amniocentesis is then done to confirm the diagnosis by finding alpha fetoprotein in amniotic fluid.

(c) **Prediction of sex.** This is done in such cases as haemophilia and Duchenne muscular dystrophy in which the condition is transmitted genetically via the male fetus. The parents may wish termination of such a pregnancy.

(d) **Some rare genetic disorders** and inborn errors of metabolism are detected.

(e) **Spectrophotometric scanning of amniotic fluid** is done in cases of Rh haemolytic disease from 24 weeks to estimate the amount of bilirubin excreted by the fetus.

(f) **The lecithin sphingomyelin ratio** in amniotic fluid after 34 weeks gives information re maturity of the fetal lungs. If low—induction of labour may be delayed until fetal lung maturity is reached: the risk of respiratory distress syndrome being thereby reduced. Betamethasone is sometimes administered to the mother to stimulate the production of fetal pulmonary surfactant.

**The fetal heart is monitored** before and after amniocentesis by Doptore or Sonicaid.

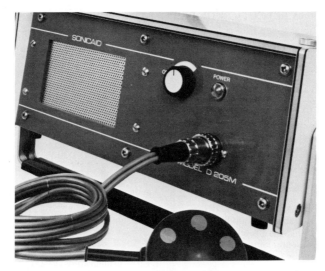

Fig 7-12 Sonicaid ultrasound apparatus. Can be used to locate the placenta prior to amniocentesis.

*Aberdeen Maternity Hospital.*

### Preparation for amniocentesis

**Prior to amniocentesis,** the parents are consulted and given an explanation of the procedure as well as the slight risks involved. They are advised that amniocentesis will only be carried out if they sign a consent form and agree that the pregnancy will be terminated if a serious fetal abnormality is found.

**Maternal blood is examined** prior to amniocentesis for group and Rh type: the Kleihauer test for fetal red cells in maternal blood is done before and 10 minutes after amniocentesis. Placental localisation by ultrasonic scan is carried out immediately preceding amniocentesis to avoid penetrating the placenta and causing a feto-maternal 'bleed'. Rh anti-D immunoglobulin is given to Rh negative women as a prophylactic measure.

**The bladder:** full or empty? The midwife should ascertain the wishes of the obstetrician. After 20 weeks' gestation the bladder is always empty; at 15 weeks' gestation some obstetricians prefer a full bladder to raise the uterus out of the pelvic cavity.

**Amniocentesis involves routine skin preparation** and the usual towels, swabs, gown and gloves. Aseptic technique is mandatory: one 2 ml syringe and needle for lignocaine: one 20 ml syringe and standard sharp lumbar puncture needle and stillette. Two universal containers (dark glass if for spectrophotometry); 2·5 cm micropore tape. The patient is observed for one hour before being allowed home.

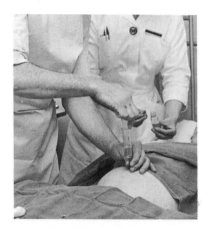

Fig. 7-13 Abdominal amniocentesis.
*Simpson Memorial Maternity Pavilion, Edinburgh.*

## PRENATAL SCREENING OF THE FETUS

A resolute endeavour is being made to improve the quality of fetal life and to reduce the perinatal mortality rate: prevention of preterm labour being high on the list of priorities

**The midwife as a member of the fetal welfare team** has a sentinel role, alert to incipient signs of maternal conditions that could have a deleterious effect on the fetus: vigilant in the detection of fetal growth retardation and diligent in counselling parents re fetal wellbeing.

### FETAL GROWTH

This has recently been studied intensively in order to determine the normal range. Standard rates of fetal growth have been prescribed as a guide, but all fetuses do not develop at the same rate. Genetic influence, intrauterine nutrition and oxygenation affect fetal growth.

### Gestational age must first be established

(a) **Menstrual history,** date of breast tingling, morning sickness, and quickening are helpful but a bi-manual pelvic examination at 6 to 8 weeks is a more definitive aid.

(b) **Abdominal inspection, girth and palpation,** although helpful, are not sufficiently accurate to have reliable diagnostic value.

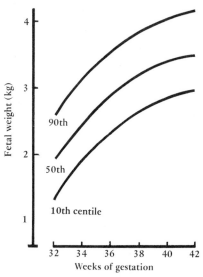

Fig. 7-14 Centile birth weight for gestation scale. A baby below the 10th centile is light for date. At the 50th centile he is the approximate weight for gestational age. At the 90th centile he is large for gestational age.

**By ultrasonography a fetal sac of 5 weeks** has been detected: should the ovum be blighted, it can be identified as having an irregular outline instead of a clearly defined white ring. The fetal head can be seen and measured at 12 weeks; its continued growth can be calculated by serial ultrasonic cephalometry.

**The Sonicaid Blood Flow Dectector,** an ultrasound apparatus that operates on the Doppler principle, is used (a) to detect the fetal heart sounds as early as 10 weeks' gestation to confirm pregnancy, (b) to localise the placenta, e.g. prior to trans-abdominal amniocentesis and when placenta praevia is suspected. The transducer, held in the hand, is placed on the abdomen, the sounds being heard, via a stethoscope plugged in, or amplified through a loud speaker.

**The real-time ultrasonic scanner** detects fetal life as early as 8 weeks by showing fetal heart movements.

### FETAL WELLBEING

**The fetus and placenta function together** as the fetoplacental unit. Fetal wellbeing is dependent on the efficiency of the placenta as a nutritive, metabolic, respiratory, excretory and endocrine organ. The placenta requires adequate intra-uterine blood flow from which to obtain nutrients and oxygen. The feto-placental unit produces oestriol and the amount excreted in maternal urine is an index of feto-placental efficiency.

## Counselling parents on Fetal wellbeing

Midwives ought to utilise their knowledge of maternal and fetal health by advising parents as to how they can help to enhance the growth and wellbeing of their child in utero.

**Adequate maternal nutrition** will contribute to the development of a healthy baby; fewer preterm labours and stillbirths occur when expectant mothers are well nourished. Many expectant mothers are unaware of the need for, and the specific foods that contain body builders, minerals such as iron and calcium, and essential vitamins. They need instruction.

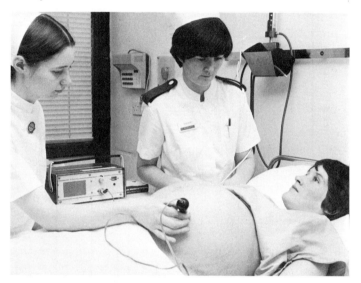

Fig. 7-15 Midwife auscultating the fetal heart using Sonicaid.

**Healthy living** includes simple outdoor activities, such as walking, to provide a well oxygenated intra-uterine environment for the fetus. Sufficient rest and sleep increases the uterine blood flow from which the placenta obtains nutrients and oxygen for the growing fetus. This should be explained to them.

**Expectant mothers should be warned:**

**That smoking over 10 cigarettes** daily will cause smaller babies, a higher incidence of preterm labour and stillbirth. (see p. 95).

**The use of drugs** and contact with infectious diseases such as rubella should be avoided.

**Maternal alcoholism** puts the fetus at risk of mental retardation.

### THE KICK COUNT CHART

#### Daily Fetal Movement Counts (DFMC)

**To assess fetal wellbeing** the activity of the fetus, felt by the pregnant woman as episodes of kicking, is recorded by her at home during the 30th to 40th week of gestation. Over a daily period of 12 hours, or until 10 kicking episodes have

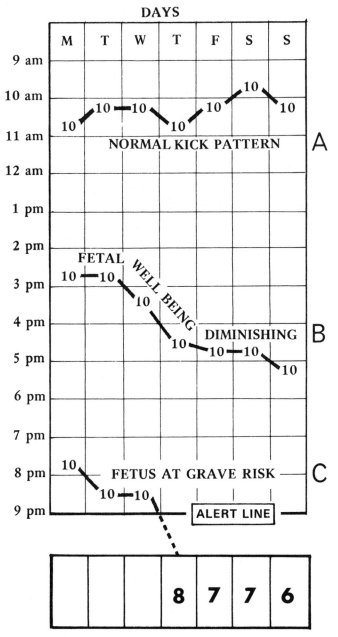

Fig. 7-16 Kick count chart.

occurred from 09.00 hrs to 21.00 hrs, the woman records an 'X' or (10) on the chart at the time of the 10th episode. See Fig. A. If the number of hours required for 10 episodes increases each day this would suggest that fetal activity (and wellbeing) is diminishing (see Fig. B).

**When less than ten kick episodes occur** during the 12-hour period 09.00 hrs to 21.00 hrs this is recorded on the chart area below the alert line (Fig. C) and the total number of kicks during this 12-hour period is recorded daily. When a low count occurs the fetus is at 'high risk' and the woman telephones the hospital, is seen and either assured or admitted for further investigation, e.g. electrocardiography, or delivery as indicated. Fetal movements usually cease 24–48 hours prior to cessation of the fetal heart.

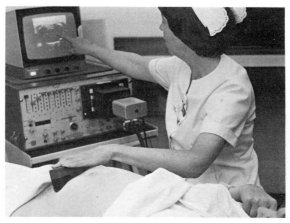

Fig. 7-17 Sister, who has received instruction in the use of the real-time ultrasonic scanner, doing routine scanning at the prenatal clinic.

*Queen Mother's Hospital, Glasgow*

### THE REAL–TIME ULTRASONIC SCANNER

This apparatus detects fetal movements as early as 7 weeks' gestation. Vigorous fetal activity is considered a favourable sign of wellbeing. Later, diminished fetal respiratory activity is believed to denote the likelihood of feto-placental insufficiency. It is now possible to scan fetal breathing, swallowing, hiccups and thumb sucking as well as the usual movements of body and limbs. The real-time scanner is considered to have greater prognostic value regarding fetal health than kick count charts.

## FETAL GROWTH RETARDATION

Genetic influence, intra-uterine malnutrition, deficient oxygenation, and maternal diseases such as severe pre-eclampsia, give rise to placental dysfunction which retards fetal growth. Blood flow in the chorio-decidual space is reduced and the fetus is deprived of the essential substances for growth and life.

**Urinary oestriol radioimmunoassays** are made to determine the degree of placental dysfunction (also human placental lactogen see p. 45).

### *Findings that suggest intra-uterine growth retardation*

(1) **Crown-rump length** is measured by sonar during the first trimester of pregnancy. From 7–14 weeks this method has been used to estimate fetal maturity

to within 3–4 days accuracy: a finding of use when reliable knowledge of the period of gestation is of clinical importance.

(2) **Ultrasonic scanning.** The fetal head can be seen and measured at 12 weeks: its continued growth can be calculated by serial cephalometry; i.e. after the 30th week the biparietal diameter is measured at two weekly intervals in cases of suspected placental dysfunction; normal growth at this time being 1·7 mm per week; after 34 weeks bi-parietal diameter growth is 1·1 mm per week.

(3) **Placental function** tests are below normal.

(4) **On abdominal palpation** fetal size is less than would be expected.

(5) **Maternal weight** loss is greater than 0·5 kg in the last 3 weeks. Girth does not increase as it should.

**Patients with a history of stillbirth associated with retarded fetal growth,** small for date babies, and those suffering from such conditions as pre-eclampsia, essential hypertension, renal disease, diabetes and cardiac impairment are carefully supervised throughout pregnancy for fetal growth and wellbeing.

# FETAL OR INTRA–UTERINE DEATH

**Prior to the 28th week,** IUD would be classified as an abortion: after the 28th week the term 'stillbirth' is used.

**Following mid-term,** fetal death is ultimately due to anoxia; some stillbirths being associated with disease such as pre-eclampsia or with antepartum haemorrhage.

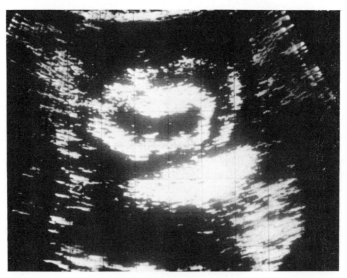

Fig. 7-18 Ultrasonogram of uterine contents less than 6 weeks. 'Double ring' is suggestive of a blighted ovum.

*Aberdeen Maternity Hospital.*

### SIGNS AND DIAGNOSIS OF FETAL DEATH

#### BEFORE MID-TERM

**Signs of pregnancy subside.**
**The uterus is small for date** and does not increase in size.
**Softening of the breasts** occurs.
**A brownish discharge** per vaginam may be present.

**ULTRASONOGRAPHIC EVIDENCE**

(a) *a blighted ovum* with an imperfect blotchy sac;

(b) *fetal heart sounds* not detected at 10 weeks by the sonar blood flow detector;

(c) *fetal heart movements* not seen as rapid regular waveforms during the first trimester of pregnancy.

(d) *fetal head growth* after 12 weeks is stationary.

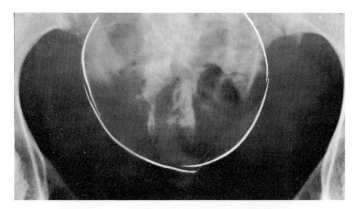

Fig. 7-19 Spalding's sign of fetal death.

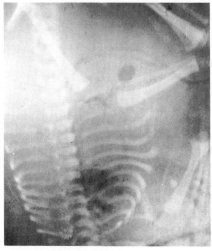

Fig. 7-20 Sign of fetal death. The presence of infra-fetal gas in the blood vessels of the umbilical cord and in the chambers of the heart.

*Simpson Memorial Maternity Pavilion, Edinburgh.*

**AFTER MID-TERM**

**The uterus is small for date;** there is cessation of uterine growth.

**The fetal heart beat is not detected** on successive examinations after the 22nd week, by Pinard's stethoscope, electronic monitor or real-time ultrasonic scanner.

**Fetal movement is not felt** by midwife or mother. The woman may state that she feels movement, but this is the dead fetus moving 'en masse' when the woman alters her posture as in turning over in bed.

**Biparietal cephalometry,** by sonar after the 30th week shows no increase in growth at weekly intervals.

**Urinary oestriol is reduced** below 8 micromoles/24 hours.

### RADIOLOGICAL EVIDENCE

(a) **Intra-fetal gas.** Bubbles of gas form in the heart and large blood vessels 12 hours after fetal death and one week earlier than Spalding's sign.

(b) **Spalding's sign.** There is gross overlapping of the bones of the vault of the skull due to disintegration of the brain substance. Slight overlapping may be seen during labour with a live fetus.

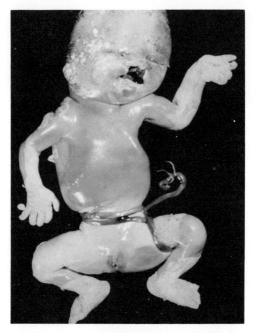

Fig. 7-21 Multiple abnormalities. Umbilical cord round body. Gross maceration.

### *The following are suggestive but not diagnostic radiological signs*

**The thoracic cage collapses:** the ribs fall together.
**Hyperflexion of the spine** with bizarre fetal attitudes.
**Transverse lie** with fetus slumped in the lower pole of the uterus.

### MANAGEMENT

Having ensured that no coagulation defect exists it is usual to induce labour by Prostaglandins, see p. 609.

**Maceration** takes place when the fetus in utero has been dead from 6 to 24 hours, aseptic autolysis produces large skin blebs containing dark-coloured fluid: later, extensive denuded areas show the shiny fascia.

## AIMS OF PRENATAL CARE

**(N. Ireland) 30-min. question.** What are the objects of antenatal care? Give an outline of what you consider to be adequate antenatal care.

**C.M.B.(Scot.).** How may the information obtained from a social, family, medical and obstetric history taken at the first prenatal visit influence the management of the present pregnancy.

**C.M.B.(Eng.) 30-min. question.** Discuss the value of antenatal care in making childbirth safe for mother and baby.

## PSYCHOLOGICAL ASPECT

**C.M.B.(Eng.) 30-min. question.** What anxieties and fears may beset pregnant women? How would you seek to allay them?

**C.M.B.(Eng.) 30-min. question.** Describe the measures which may be employed to allay anxiety and fear during pregnancy and labour. How can the midwife give emotional support to the pregnant woman?

How can the midwife help to abolish fear of labour? What advice should husbands be given on providing emotional support? How would you encourage a pregnant woman to ask questions and to discuss her fears? How would you put a woman at ease in a busy clinic?

## HEALTH EDUCATION

**C.M.B.(Eng.) 30-min. question.** What is the role of the midwife in health education during the antenatal period?

How can the midwife promote good health in pregnant women? Outline a talk to expectant mothers on why and how they can give up smoking. Why is the prevention of anaemia important in pregnancy? How can the midwife promote good mental health during pregnancy?

**Explain how expectant parents** can enhance the wellbeing of their child *in utero*. Explain as to an expectant mother the advantages of suitable food, a daily outing, adequate rest.

## COUNSELLING

**Why should midwives be aware of criticisms** made of certain obstetric procedures e.g. induction of labour, episiotomy, amniocentesis and what assurance can they give?

**What advice would you give** to the woman who wants natural childbirth in her own home? How would you counsel expectant parents regarding improvement of the quality of infant life?

## THE GENETIC ASPECT

**C.M.B.(Eng.) question.** Describe the factors concerned with abnormal development of the fetus.

**C.M.B.(Scot.) question.** Describe the current methods of investigation available to reach a diagnosis of fetal abnormality.

Why should the midwife refrain from expressing her opinion *re* any genetic abnormality? For what reasons do prospective parents attend a genetic counselling clinic? Which women are at 'high risk' of producing a mongoloid child? Differentiate between chromosomes and autosomes; the **XX** and the **XY** chromosomes; genetic and intra-uterine causes of congenital abnormalities.

## *Taking the History*

**C.M.B.(Eng.) 30-min. question.** What questions would you ask a woman early in her second pregnancy who states that her first child was stillborn? How may this information be of value in preventing a further stillbirth?

**C.M.B.(Eng.) 30-min. question.** Discuss the dangers to which the grande multipara is subject in pregnancy, labour and the puerperium.

**C.M.B.(N.Ireland) 30-min. question.** What history should be taken and what examinations and investigations made at the first antenatal visit?

What can be learned from taking (*a*) the social, (*b*) the family, (*c*) the medical histories?

In taking the obstetrical history, why are the following facts significant? (*a*) Length of labour; (*b*) weights of babies; (*c*) stillbirths or neonatal deaths; (*d*) instrumental delivery; (*e*) previous Caesarean section. What do you understand by the terms: Older primigravida: Grande multipara.

## *Prenatal Screening*

**Differentiate between screening and diagnostic procedures.**

**What are the benefits** of using ultrasonic and electronic equipment to screen the pregnant woman and her fetus; what are the following used for? Electrocardiograph. Kick count chart. Real-time scanner. Urinary oestriol assay.

**In which pregnant women are the** following blood tests done. Alpha feto-protein. Serum placental lactogen, HAI Test.

**How would gestational age be assessed.** In what circumstances is this important?

**Why is the Rh-woman given Rh anti D** immunoglobulin after amniocentesis?

**Which pregnant women are offered amniocentesis?**

## FETAL GROWTH AND WELLBEING

By what means can fetal growth by assessed? What is a 'high risk' fetus? Give examples. What are the causes of intrauterine growth retardation? How is fetal gestational age assessed? What is the significance of the lecithin/sphingomyelin ratio in amniotic fluid? How can the midwife help to foster fetal growth and wellbeing? What are the advantages of using electronic equipment to monitor fetal wellbeing? What is intra-uterine growth retardation? Give causes and signs.

**Define:** Crown rump length; ultrasonic biparietal cephalometry; a blighted ovum as seen on a sonar scan.

## FETAL OR INTRAUTERINE DEATH

**C.M.B.(Scot.) 30-min. question.** Give the causes of intrauterine death and indicate how this diagnosis might be established.

What would make you suspect fetal death before and after mid term?

What is (a) Spalding's sign of fetal death? (b) a macerated fetus; (c) intra-fetal gas.

**Why is prostaglandin preferred** to induce labour with a dead fetus?

# 8
# Examination of the Pregnant Woman

*By the doctor. By the midwife. Vena caval occlusion. Pelvic capacity. Abdominal examination: inspection, palpation, auscultation. Cephalopelvic disproportion.*

The examination of the pregnant woman can be carried out entirely by the doctor, or it may be shared by the midwife. There are, however, certain procedures which midwives are not qualified to undertake, and it is only right that every woman should reap the benefit of any investigation or examination that makes childbirth safer for mother and child. A friendly atmosphere should prevail in the prenatal clinic, and scientific investigation, essential though it is, should not obtrusively dominate the situation. The woman needs helpful advice and friendly counsel as well as professional supervision, for her concern is mainly about the minor disorders which make her life miserable and her lack of knowledge regarding labour and the care of babies. The midwife can do much to remedy this. Zeal should not outstrip discretion, for a woman can be upset to the verge of tears when interviewed and examined by too many people; she is so confused that she cannot remember the advice she has been given. The appointment system has reduced waiting time; further organisation will, by postponing some of the investigations to the second or third visit, eliminate much unnecessary emotional and physical stress.

## THE FIRST VISIT

The woman usually goes to her doctor or the clinic when she has missed one or two menstrual periods, and as she walks into the examining room observation begins, for **small stature, deformity or a limp** are more readily detected when the woman is on her feet. An impression of health and vitality can be gained by her bearing; the tired malnourished woman looks apathetic, her shoulders droop and she lacks energy.

### Height

The woman of good physique is unlikely to have a contracted pelvis, and as a general but not infallible rule few women over 1·6 m in height are found to have abnormal pelves. Short stature is more significant when due to disease or malnutrition than when occurring in the petite type of woman with small bones who is more likely to give birth to a small baby.

### Weight

The woman should be weighed early in pregnancy (at her first visit) in order to determine her normal weight; the procedure being repeated on each subsequent occasion. She should be undressed and given a washable dressing-gown to wear, because the difference in the weight of clothing may be considerable during the three seasons over which pregnancy extends. Recording the weight in graph form draws attention to static, poor, or excess gain which should be reported to the doctor. A gain of 12 kg can be accounted for physiologically during pregnancy.

## URINE ANALYSIS

This is carried out at every visit, and includes *inspection*, and testing for protein and glucose. Great importance is attached to finding protein in the urine, as it is one of the signs of pre-eclampsia, a condition which must be treated promptly to avert

121

# Routine at every visit

| Enquire re wellbeing | Urine analysis | Blood pressure | Health and | Abdominal Examination |
| Discuss problems | Protein | Oedema | Parenthood | Fetal growth |
| Answer questions | Glucose | Weight | education | |

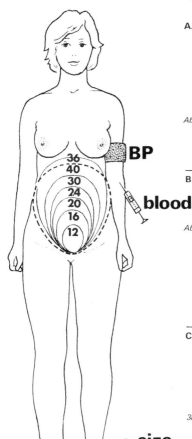

**A. First visit 8 to 12 weeks**

| *History:* | family, medical, social, obstetrical, present pregnancy. |
| *Physical examination:* | heart, lungs, breasts, teeth, height, pelvis. |
| *Blood examination:* | Hgb, group, Rh factor, for syphilis, rubella antibodies, alpha feto protein. |
| *Abdominal examination:* | to confirm pregnancy. |
| *Vaginal examination:* | to confirm pregnancy, period of gestation, cervical cytology. |
| *Enquire re:* | discontinuance of contraceptive pill, minor disorders. |

**B. 16 to 34 weeks**

| *Abdominal examination:* | Fundal height. Fetal growth. Fetal heart 20-22 weeks. Lie presentation position. Twins polyhydramnios. |
| *Uricult:* | For asymptomatic bacteriuria. |
| *Amniocentesis:* | At 16 weeks if A.F.P. raised. |
| *Enquire re:* | quickening 18 to 20 weeks. Blood examination for Hgb: Rh antibodies if necessary: amniocentesis for sphingomyelin lecithin ratio at 34 weeks + |

**C. 36th week**

| *Fundal height:* | lie presentation, disproportion. |
| *Pelvic capacity:* | P.V. |
| *Fetal:* | heartbeat, growth, wellbeing. |
| *Check:* | Hgb. Rh antibodies if necessary. |

*38 weeks.* Is head engaged?

## VISITS TO PRENATAL CLINIC

| WEEKS | 4 | 8 | 12 | 16 | 20 | 22 | 24 | 26 | 28 | 30 | 32 | 34 | 36 | 37 | 38 | 39 | 40 |
|---|---|---|---|---|---|---|---|---|---|---|---|---|---|---|---|---|---|
| | | Every 4 weeks | | | | | Every 2 weeks | | | | | | | Every week until delivered | | | |

Fig. 8-1

more serious developments. **Proteinuria** may also be caused by such conditions as pyelonephritis and chronic nephritis.

Glycosuria is fairly common during pregnancy, and if more than a trace of glucose is present on two occasions a blood glucose test is done after breakfast and if necessary a glucose tolerance test is carried out to diagnose diabetes.

### *Obtaining a Midstream Specimen (at Clinic)*

**Seven per cent of pregnant women have asymptomatic bacteriuria** which is treated to avoid pyelonephritis. If urinary infection is suspected a 'clean catch' specimen of urine is obtained. The woman passes some urine then obtains a specimen directly into a 60 ml universal container with screw top, or a plastic carton; a 300 ml metal measuring jug is convenient for the woman to hold but the urine must then be poured into the laboratory container. Some recommend swabbing without an antiseptic, others, separation of the labia. Unless the urine reaches the laboratory within one hour it must be kept in a cool place at 4·4°C or the bacterial count will be inaccurate. The Uricult dip slide is suitable for large scale screening.

## EXAMINATION BY THE DOCTOR

During the first trimester of pregnancy it is mainly the medical aspect that requires supervision. Obstetrical complications, such as pre-eclampsia, malpresentation and disproportion, occur later. The cardiovascular and respiratory systems, are examined as early in pregnancy as possible: when conditions such as diabetes, tuberculosis or cardiac disease are diagnosed the woman is referred to the appropriate clinic or specialist.

## BLOOD TESTS

The Wassermann test is now being replaced by other serological tests, e.g. The Venereal Disease Research Laboratory (VDRL) slide test: the automated reagent test. Tests are made on all pregnant women (see also p. 221).

**Blood groups ABO** are determined because of the risk of haemorrhage in obstetrics so that compatible blood can be given without delay should transfusion be necessary. Incompatibility between maternal and fetal blood ABO groups may occur and give rise to a less severe form of haemolytic disease of the newborn.

**To determine whether the Rh factor is negative** or positive the blood of every pregnant woman should be examined because of the possibility of immunisation.

**Haemoglobin estimation** is made because child bearing women often suffer from anaemia and if the haemoglobin is below 12·6 g/dl, iron, folic acid and vitamins $B_1$ and C are prescribed. If below 10·3 g/dl further blood investigation is carried out.

**Alpha feto proteins.** Maternal blood serum is examined in many clinics for alpha feto proteins at 15–17 weeks and if raised amniocentesis is done to detect fetal neural tube defects such as spina bifida and anencephaly.

**Human placental lactogen** is detectable in plasma and reflects placental function. Low levels (*a*) in threatened abortion, indicate a poor prognosis; (*b*) in late pregnancy, indicate placental dysfunction and risk to the fetus.

**Screening for rubella antibodies,** the H.A.I. test, is carried out in some centres. Ninety per cent are immune: non-immune (susceptible) women are offered vaccination and contraceptive advice during the early postnatal period but are not vaccinated during pregnancy.

**Maternal blood is tested for phenylalanine** at some prenatal clinics.

**Sickle cell haemoglobin** tests are made on certain immigrant women (see p. 214).

**The hepatitis B (Australia) antigen test** is made at some clinics.

### THE BLOOD PRESSURE

The blood pressure should be estimated at the first visit to find out the usual level and then at each subsequent visit because a rise in blood pressure, manifest during the second half of pregnancy, is one of the earliest signs of pre-eclampsia. The diastolic pressure should be recorded at stage 4 the muffling stage. A blood pressure of 130/80 is viewed with suspicion, and 140/90 is considered to be pathological. But a steadily rising diastolic pressure may be significant so the woman is seen every week. In some pregnant women the blood pressure is very unstable, and excitement or exertion may cause a temporary increase in the systolic pressure which subsides with rest. The woman should be recumbent when the blood pressure is taken, and if her pulse is rapid and her blood pressure raised it may be due to nervousness, but some consider this to be a significant warning rise. The test should be repeated 20 minutes later.

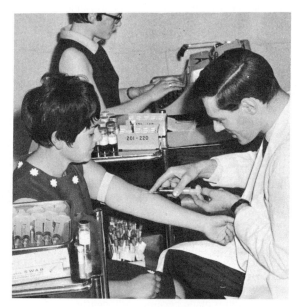

Fig. 8-2   Venepuncture is employed to procure blood for all tests. Secretary types in triplicate lists for the departments of Haematology, Bacteriology and Blood Transfusion Service.

*Prenatal Clinic, Simpson Memorial Maternity Pavilion, Edinburgh.*

### VAGINAL EXAMINATION

At the first visit some doctors make a vaginal examination, not only to confirm the diagnosis and duration of pregnancy but to exclude any pelvic abnormality. In primigravid women pelvic size and shape are assessed at the 34th to 36th week. Conditions such as retroversion, fibroids, ovarian or vaginal cysts, double uterus and septate vagina will be detected. Other authorities consider that the procedure is not warranted because the findings are so often negative. Cervical cytology is done in most prenatal clinics at this visit.

**VENA CAVAL OCCLUSION**

*Supine Hypotensive Syndrome*

A number of pregnant women feel faint when they lie in the supine position (on their backs) during the third trimester of pregnancy. This syndrome is due to a reduction in cardiac output because the blood returning from the lower limbs is impeded by the large heavy pregnant uterus compressing the inferior vena cava. In approximately 96 per cent of women the collateral circulation redirects the dammed up blood: the 4 per cent of women who have an inadequate collateral circulation develop the hypotensive syndrome.

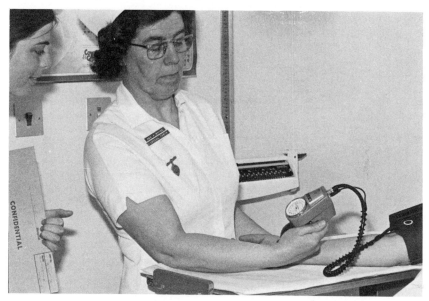

Fig. 8-3   Midwife using electronic sphygmomanometer at midwives clinic.
*Maternity Hospital, Stirling.*

**Signs**

**The woman looks intensely pale:** she feels faint: her blood pressure falls to 80 and sometimes 60 mm Hg. Slight tachycardia is followed by profound bradycardia.

*Treatment*

Any woman in late pregnancy or early labour who exhibits pallor or feels faint should be turned on her side immediately when she will rapidly recover. Women should be encouraged to lie on their side during the first stage of labour. Vena caval occlusion is unlikely during the second stage of labour.

**EXAMINATION BY THE MIDWIFE**

The woman lies comfortably on a firm bed or couch, and before beginning the examination, the midwife should ask her a few simple questions such as, how she is feeling, whether she sleeps well, if she goes out every day, in order to show interest in her as an individual. An enquiry as to whether she is eating well, will lead to the giving of advice about a suitable diet with adequate body building foods, fruit, vegetables and milk. Much helpful advice can also be offered about the minor disorders, such as constipation, heartburn and morning sickness, if necessary.

The examination should be carried out systematically, so that no point is omitted, always beginning at the head.

Facial appearance gives a general impression of physical and mental well-being. The woman may look healthy, well-nourished and happy, or she may be mal-nourished, ill, or apprehensive. Pallor of gums, lips and conjunctiva may denote the presence of anaemia, but a red conjunctiva does not preclude anaemia. Oedema of the face is a grave sign (*not usually seen at the prenatal clinic*) most commonly found in serious cases of pre-eclampsia. The mouth is inspected for dental caries, and arrangements made for the woman to see the dentist when necessary. Signs of ill-health, such as swollen glands of the neck, cyanosis, breathlessness or persistent cough, would be apparent; and if the midwife detects any abnormality at the first or any subsequent examination she must obtain medical advice.

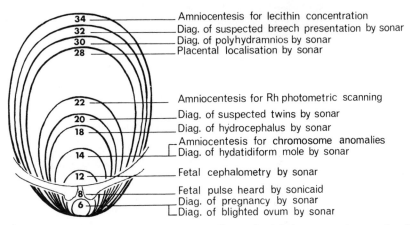

Fig. 8-4   Diagrammatic representation of some diagnostic techniques at various weeks of pregnancy

### The breasts

They are examined for signs of pregnancy (p. 68), and if any condition exists that would create difficulty in lactation appropriate advice should be given.

### The vulva

The presence of a vaginal discharge that is profuse, purulent, irritating, green and frothy or blood-stained should be reported. Oedema or varicose veins, vulval warts, or lesions suggesting syphilis such as chancre or condylomata lata would necessitate getting medical advice.

### The lower limbs

They are examined for deformities; bending of the tibia would be suggestive of rickets. The size and width of the foot may give a clue to pelvic capacity, size three or less in shoes being abnormally small. The tissue over the tibia near the ankle should be tested for oedema (*pre-tibial oedema*) at every visit. Varicose veins, unless very slight, should be reported to the doctor so that suitable advice may be given.

## PELVIC CAPACITY

The majority of pelves are adequate for the safe passage of an average-sized baby, but the midwife must be constantly on the alert for any deviation from normal, so that arrangements can be made for labour and delivery to be conducted in hospital under specialist supervision.

No matter how normal the woman's physique and stature may be, pelvic capacity should be estimated, for a small pelvis may be present in a woman of average proportions. The pelvis must also be considered in relation to the size of the fetus *in utero*. It has been aptly said that 'the fetal head is the best pelvimeter,' for, unless the pelvis is large enough to accommodate the head of the fetus, the fact that the pelvis is of average size and shape is of no value. But not until the 36th week of pregnancy has the fetal head grown sufficiently large to judge whether it will enter the pelvic brim or whether disproportion exists. Some pelves are so small or deformed that a 3·2 kg baby could not be born naturally and Caesarean section would be necessary. A minor degree of pelvic contraction may be difficult to diagnose.

The midwife will, of course, realise that it is not possible by pelvimetry to determine that the fetal head will pass safely through the pelvis. The strength of the uterine contractions, the 'give' of the pelvic joints and the degree of over-riding of the skull bones, all influence the outcome of labour.

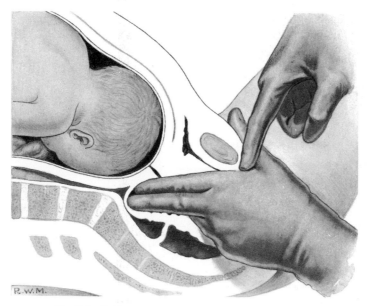

Fig. 8-5   Taking measurement of the diagonal conjugate.

### The Assessment of Pelvic Capacity

**Radiography** is the most precise and accurate method, but X-rays are not employed for pelvimetry unless there are clinical indications of contracted pelvis because of the radiation hazards involved.

**Clinical (digital) pelvimetry** is probably the most widely used method, and an experienced obstetrician can usually give a good estimate of pelvic capacity by digital examination per vaginam. The size of the obstetrical conjugate can be assessed by measuring the diagonal conjugate.

**The diagonal conjugate** is measured from the lower border of the symphysis pubis to the centre of the promontory of the sacrum and is usually 12 to 13 cm. To allow for the depth of the pubic bone 2 cm is subtracted; the result gives the measurement of the obstetrical conjugate. This measurement may be taken in every primigravida and in multiparous women who have had a difficult labour with normal-sized babies. It is usually done between the 34th and 36th week of pregnancy as the vagina and pelvic floor are softer then, causing less discomfort to the women and making it easier for the examiner.

The women lies in the dorsal position with knees drawn up, the bladder having previously been emptied. The vulva is swabbed with antiseptic, e.g. Hibitane 1–2,000 and the thighs draped. The first two fingers of the gloved hand are lubricated with obstetric cream and inserted into the vagina. An effort is made to reach the sacral promontory, and if bone is encountered the fingers should be directed farther upwards. No bone is felt above the promontory because the fifth lumbar vertebra recedes.

The point where the left hand is in contact with the lower border of the symphysis pubis is marked by the forefinger (Fig. 8-5) and after withdrawal the distance between that point and the tip of the middle finger is measured with ruler or calipers. On subtracting 2 cm the measurement of the obstetrical conjugate is obtained.

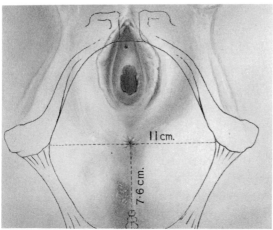 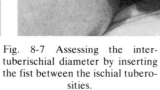

Fig. 8-6   Intertuberischial diameter of the pelvic outlet.

Fig. 8-7 Assessing the intertuberischial diameter by inserting the fist between the ischial tuberosities.

### Assessment of the Pelvic Outlet

The ischial spines are palpated to see if they are unduly prominent, which would indicate diminution of the bispinous transverse diameter of the outlet. Two fingers are placed in the sacro-sciatic notch to determine if it is adequate. The curve of the sacrum is noted, and before removing the fingers the pubic arch is examined to see whether it is acute. Two fingers can usually be accommodated in the apex of the pubic arch.

The intertuberischial or transverse diameter of the lower outlet, the distance between the ischial tuberosities, is 11 cm on the bony pelvis, but the fat and tissue of the buttocks lessen the diameter by at least 1·2 cm. It is practically impossible to measure this diameter with any degree of accuracy but a general impression of size can be obtained by inserting the closed fist between the ischial tuberosities. Fists vary in size, but after the midwife has estimated the size of the outlet in a large series of patients it is possible for her to judge whether the intertuberischial diameter is average, small or large; and, if small, medical advice is necessary.

The patient lies on her left side with her knees well drawn up. The midwife places the knuckle of her middle finger on the posterior border of the anus, and the middle joints of the gloved fist are inserted between the ischial tuberosities and directed slightly backwards.

## ABDOMINAL EXAMINATION

The midwife should be thoroughly proficient in abdominal examination, not only for the purpose of diagnosis during pregnancy but also for intelligent observation in the conduct of labour. Considerable practice is needed in order to acquire precision in manual dexterity and to develop the essential sense of touch.

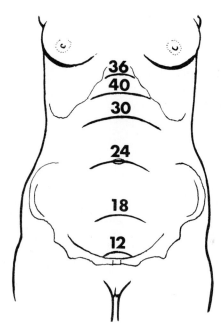

Fig. 8-8   Growth of the uterus, showing the fundal heights at the 12th, 18th, 24th, 30th, 36th and 40th weeks.

### During the first half of pregnancy

Abdominal examination is usually carried out to corroborate the diagnosis of pregnancy and the period of gestation. It is not always easy to palpate the uterus before the 16th week, and the presence of obesity or a rigid abdominal wall exaggerates the difficulty. If doubt exists, the woman should be referred to the doctor who will perform a bimanual examination, when, by feeling the size, shape and consistency of the uterus, it may be possible to substantiate the diagnosis. It is usual to ascertain whether the size of the uterus corresponds with the period of amenorrhoea.

At about the 18th week the fundus will be mid-way between the symphysis pubis and the umbilicus. At this time the woman will detect fetal movements (*quickening*); the multiparous woman, having had previous experience will recognise this one or two weeks earlier than the primigravida. (*Although the umbilicus is usually taken as a landmark to assess fundal height its situation in the abdomen may vary as much as 4 cm in different women, depending on their height and build.*)

**The fetal heart** will sometimes be heard if the stethoscope is placed in the mid-line, half-way between the umbilicus and symphysis pubis. But, unless the room is absolutely quiet and the examiner has very acute hearing, the fetal heart is not likely to be heard until the 24th week. An ultrasonic pulse detector, the Sonicaid or the Doptone, will pick up the fetal heart beat at 10 weeks; sometimes as early as the 8th week. Fetal parts can be felt about the 20th week.

### Method of Abdominal Examination

The woman should be comfortable so that she can relax physically and mentally. Her arms ought to lie limply by her sides and her back should sink into the couch so that she can relax her abdominal muscles. An interested enquiry about her family or her own welfare and a few words of advice on how to relax are usually sufficient to put her at ease. Her bladder should be empty.

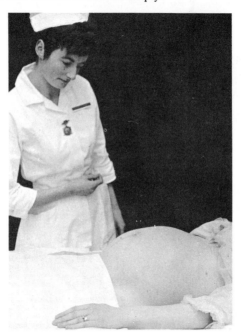

Fig. 8-9   Abdominal inspection.

The blanket should be folded down once to knee level, and the sheet folded in a similar manner to just above the level of the symphysis pubis, as it is impossible to examine the abdomen properly with a mound of bedclothes in the way. Patients should never be exposed unnecessarily. It is a good habit to stand on the patient's right side, for the same reason that all nursing procedures are done on the right: most people are right-handed and become expert when one method is used. From the left side, the procedure is often done in a perfunctory manner.

Three senses are used, visual, tactile, auditory, and the examination should be carried out systematically by (1) **inspection,** (2) **palpation** and (3) **auscultation,** in that order.

### 1. SIZE OF THE UTERUS

**The period of gestation** may be assessed roughly by inspection but not reliably for a distended colon or a thick abdominal wall gives the impression of undue size.

**Multiple pregnancy or polyhydramnios increase the length and breadth of the uterus** whereas a large baby increases the length.

### 2. SHAPE OF THE UTERUS

**When the lie of the fetus is longitudinal** as occurs in 99·5 per cent of cases, the shape of the uterus is ovoid longitudinally (longer than it is broad). When the lie of the fetus is transverse the uterine shape is ovoid transversely (low and broad).

**The multiparous uterus** lacks the snug ovoid shape of the primigravid uterus.

**Position may be diagnosed**. Occasionally it is possible to see the prominent fetal back on one or other side of the abdomen. In posterior positions of the vertex a saucer-like depression is seen at or below the umbilicus.

### 3. FETAL MOVEMENT

**This is evidence that the fetus is alive;** it also aids in the diagnosis of position, as the back will be on the opposite side to that on which movement is seen.

### 4. CONTOUR OF ABDOMINAL WALL

**A pendulous abdomen** is more commonly seen in the multigravid woman and can be more readily detected when she is standing. It is due to laxity of the abdominal muscles which allows the uterus to sag forwards, sometimes known as anterior uterine obliquity. In primigravid women pendulous abdomen is of serious import and necessitates medical investigation as it may be due to pelvic contraction or spinal deformity.

**That lightening** has occurred can be seen, particularly when the woman is standing (see p. 237).

**The umbilicus becomes less dimpled** as pregnancy advances and during the later weeks may protrude above skin level.

**A full bladder** is more evident during the later weeks of pregnancy.

### 5. SKIN CHANGES

**Striae gravidarum** are frequently seen: silvery streaks suggest a previous pregnancy; pink streaks occur in the present pregnancy.

**Linea nigra** is the dark line of pigmentation seen running longitudinally in the centre of the abdomen above and below the umbilicus. It is of interest as a presumptive sign of pregnancy.

**Operation scars.**

## ABDOMINAL PALPATION (after 30th week)
### HOW TO PALPATE THE UTERUS

The hands should be clean and warm: cold hands do not have the necessary acute sense of touch; they tend to induce contraction of the abdominal muscles and the patient resents the discomfort of them. Arms and hands should be relaxed and the pads—not the tips—of the fingers used with delicate precision: the hands being moved smoothly over the abdomen without lifting them. Erratic dipping of the fingers, sudden pressure and rough manipulation are irritating to the abdominal wall and the uterus, causing contractions that make the detection of fetal parts impossible.

### 1. ESTIMATING THE PERIOD OF GESTATION

The following system of assessing the period of gestation is open to fallacy, because the size, number of fetuses and amount of amniotic fluid vary, but it is a convenient, useful method so long as its limitations are appreciated.

### Assessing fundal height

The distance between the fundus and the xiphisternum is estimated in fingers breadth. As many fingers (*not the tips*) of the left hand, as can be accommodated, are laid flat between the upper border of the fundus and the xiphisternum. At 36 weeks no fingers can be inserted. When lightening takes place three or four fingers can be inserted.

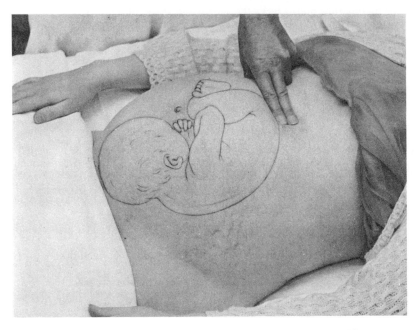

Fig. 8-10    Assessing the fundal height in fingers-breadth below the xiphisternum.

### Size of the uterus

When the uterus is unduly big, multiple pregnancy or polyhydramnios may be suspected: in some cases it might be due to a large fetus. The uterus of the woman of short stature appears to be more prominent than the uterus of the tall woman.

When the uterus is smaller than average the most likely explanation is that the woman is mistaken in the date of her last menstrual period. In cases of pre-eclampsia the fetus may be small due to placental dysfunction.

#### 2. FUNDAL PALPATION

This manoeuvre will help to determine whether the presentation is cephalic or podalic, and the lie longitudinal or transverse. In 95 per cent of cases the breech will be in the fundus and this denotes a cephalic presentation, commonly the vertex. When the head is in the fundus the presentation is podalic (breech). When breech or head is in the fundus the lie is longitudinal. If neither can be palpated in the fundus further investigation is required in case the lie is transverse.

*Method*

The midwife stands on the patient's right with her thighs against the couch and her body, turned at the waist, facing the woman's head. Both hands are laid on the sides of the fundus, fingers held close together and curving round the upper border of the uterus.

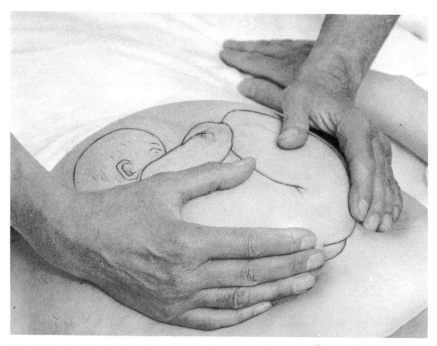

Fig. 8-11 Fundal palpation. Palms of hands on either side of the fundus, fingers held close together palpate the upper pole of the uterus.

Gentle yet deliberate pressure is applied using the palmar surfaces of the fingers to determine the soft consistency and indefinite outline that denotes the breech. Sometimes the buttocks feel rather firm but they are neither as hard, smooth nor well defined as the head. With a gliding movement the position of the hands is changed in an endeavour to grasp the fetal mass, which may be in the centre or deflected to one or other side, and assess its size and mobility. The breech cannot be moved independently of the body as can the head.

The head is much more distinctive in outline being hard and round; it can be ballotted between the finger-tips of the two hands, or between the thumb and finger of one hand, because of the free movement at the neck. If the diagnosis is in doubt the finger-tips should be pressed deeply into the abdominal wall over what is thought to be the head and by giving a sharp tap the bony hardness of head will be readily detected.

### 3. LATERAL PALPATION

This manoeuvre is useful to locate the fetal back as an aid to diagnosis of position. Obesity, and an excess of aminiotic fluid increase the difficulties in palpation.

*Method*

While facing the woman's head (or feet) the hands are placed on both sides of the uterus at about umbilical level. Pressure is applied with the palms of alternate hands to differentiate the degree of resistance between the two sides of the uterus. One hand is used to steady the uterus and press the fetus over towards the examining hand which determines the presence of the broad resistant back or the small parts that slip about under the examining fingers. If the back cannot be palpated readily and small parts are evident over a wide area occipito-posterior position may be suspected. By using a rotary movement of the fingers the back may be mapped out as a continuous smooth resistant mass from the breech down to the neck, where the resistance disappears.

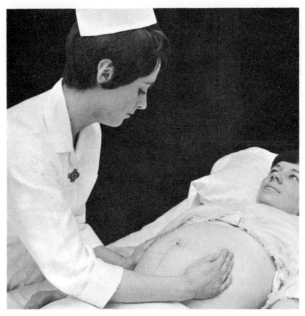

Fig. 8-12   Lateral palpation. Hands placed at umbilical level on either side of the uterus. Pressure is applied alternately with each hand.

'Walking the finger tips' of both hands over the abdomen from one side to the other is an excellent method of locating the back (see Fig. 8-14). The fingers should be dipped into the abdominal wall deliberately and fairly deeply and the firm back can be distinguished from the fluctuating amniotic fluid and the receding knobbly small parts. To make the back more prominent fundal pressure can be applied with the left hand, and the right hand used to 'walk' over the abdomen.

The back in an L.O.A. will be felt 2·5 cm left of the midline.
    ,,    ,,  L.O.L.    ,,    7·5 cm left of the midline.
    ,,    ,,  L.O.P.    ,,    10 cm left of the midline.

The anterior shoulder can be located by palpating from the neck upwards and inwards. When the head is high the shoulder will be about 12 cm above the symphysis pubis; about 5 cm when the head is engaged, and just above the symphysis when the head is engaged deeply in the pelvis.

#### 4. PELVIC PALPATION

This is the most important manoeuvre in abdominal palpation because of its value in the diagnosis of presentation of the fetus, position, engagement of the fetal head and disproportion between head and pelvis.

| $\frac{5}{5}$ | $\frac{4}{5}$ | $\frac{3}{5}$ | $\frac{2}{5}$ | $\frac{1}{5}$ | $\frac{0}{5}$ |
|---|---|---|---|---|---|
| Sinciput & Occiput above | Sinciput prominent Occiput descending | Sinciput rising Occiput can be tipped | Sinciput not so prominent | Sinciput Occiput not felt | Head on pelvic floor |

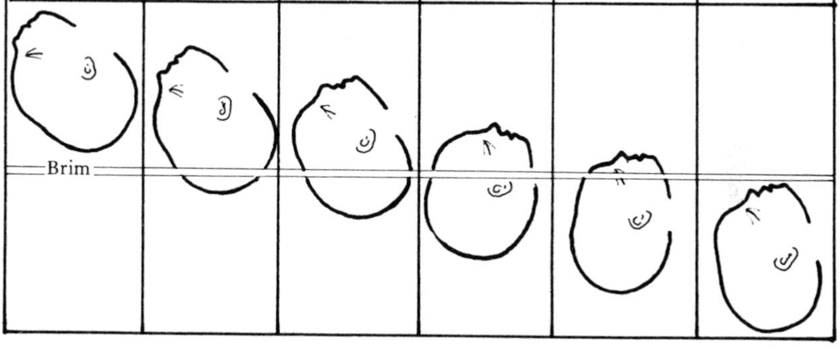

**Abdominal palpation in fifths to determine descent of the fetal head.**

Fig. 8-13

5/5 **The whole head is palpable above the brim.** It is 'high' or 'free'. Sinciput and occiput easily felt.

4/5 **Four fifths of the head are palpable** one fifth has entered the pelvic brim. The occiput is lower but can readily be felt.

3/5 **Three fifths of the head are palpable** above the brim. The head has flexed and occiput can be tipped by dipping the fingers down into the brim. The sinciput rises somewhat because of head flexion. The parietal eminences will have entered the brim which is said to be the stage of engagement.

2/5 **Two fifths of the head are palpable** above the brim. The sinciput is descending but can still be felt: occiput not palpable.

1/5 **One fifth of the head is felt** above the brim. Nearing the end of labour the occiput reaches one lateral half of the pelvic floor and rotates forwards: the sinciput goes into the hollow of the sacrum and cannot be palpated abdominally.

#### Method

To relax the abdominal muscles the woman's knees should be slightly raised: she can assist still further by opening her mouth and breathing steadily and quietly. The midwife stands with her thighs against the couch, her body, turned at the waist, facing towards the woman's feet. The sides of the uterus just below umbilical level are grasped snugly between the palms of the hands; the fingers, held close together, pointing downwards and inwards. If the hands are placed correctly the first joints of the little fingers will be on a level with the anterior superior iliac spines, and the outstretched thumbs will meet at about the level of the umbilicus (see Fig. 8.15).

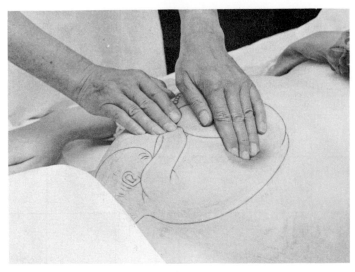

Fig. 8-14  'Walking' the finger tips across the abdomen to locate the position of the back.

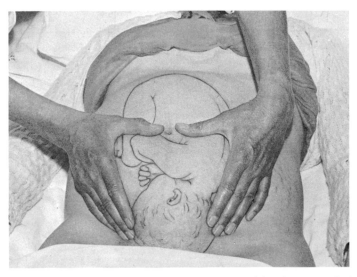

Fig. 8-15  Pelvic palpation. If the hands are in the correct position the outstretched thumbs will meet at about umbilical level. The fingers are directed inwards and downwards.

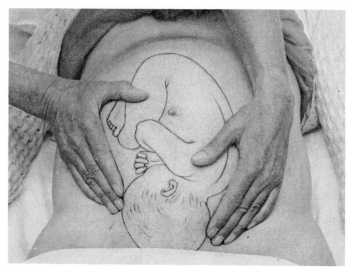

Fig. 8-16 Method of pelvic palpation to determine position in a vertex presentation. The higher cephalic prominence (the sincipital) will be on the opposite side to the back; on the right in an L.O.A.

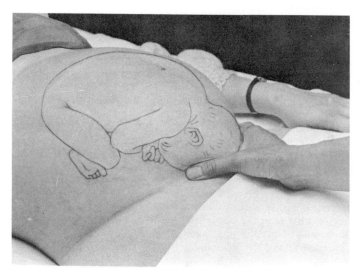

Fig. 8-17 Pawlik's manoeuvre. The lower pole of the uterus is grasped with the right hand, the midwife facing the woman's head.

### Diagnosis of cephalic presentation

The fingers are directed inwards and, if the head is presenting a hard mass with a distinctive round smooth outline will be detected. To determine if the vertex is presenting the two cephalic prominences, the occipital and sincipital, are located. The higher one will, if on the opposite side from the fetal back, be the sincipital and this denotes a vertex presentation, head flexed. In face presentation the higher cephalic prominence will be on the same side as the fetal back.

### Diagnosis of position

With the hands grasping the lower pole of the uterus, the finger tips palpate both sides of the head and are arrested on the higher cephalic prominence which may be at a level of 5 to 7·5 cm above the prominence on the other side. The higher cephalic prominence is the sincipital and, in vertex presentation, it is always on the side of the woman's abdomen opposite to that on which the fetal back is located. The lower and less definite cephalic prominence is the occipital and the position of the fetus in relation to the pelvic brim is determined according to which of the six areas of the brim the occiput points.

*The position will be one of the following*

| | |
|---|---|
| **Right occipito posterior** | **Left occipito posterior** |
| **Right occipito lateral** | **Left occipito lateral** |
| **Right occipito anterior** | **Left occipito anterior** |

### Pawlik's manoeuvre

This method of palpating the lower pole of the uterus is most effective when the head is not engaged. By this manoeuvre it is easy to locate the round, hard head and to judge its size, flexion and mobility. The midwife, standing on the patient's right, faces the woman's head and, using the right hand, grasps the lower pole of the uterus with the thumb on the woman's right side and the fingers on the left side of the uterus (Fig. 8.17). Fingers and thumb must be sufficiently far apart to accommodate the fetal head. The woman is asked to take a deep breath and let it escape slowly through her open mouth. In carrying out this manoeuvre great gentleness should be exercised.

*An excellent diagnostic procedure is falling into disrepute because it is being done roughly and therefore causing pain. No matter where the head is situated or how it is grasped undue pressure applied to it will be painful for the expectant mother.*

**The combined grip** can be used when there is doubt regarding whether head or breech is presenting. It is an excellent method of comparing the contour and consistency of what is in the upper and lower poles of the uterus. While facing across the woman's body the right hand grasps the lower pole of the uterus as in Pawlik's manoeuvre and the left hand grasps the fundus in a similar manner.

## ENGAGEMENT OF THE HEAD

An engaged head is one in which the bi-parietal diameter has passed through the pelvic brim. Deciding whether the head is engaged or not requires, as well as manual dexterity, judgment in assessing the clinical findings for no one manoeuvre or observation is conclusive.

The head should be engaged in a primigravid woman at the 38th–39th week of pregnancy and, if not, the cause must be investigated so medical aid should be sought. Engagement does occasionally occur in multiparous women who have firm abdominal muscles but more commonly not until after the onset of labour.

**The greater bulk of the head** is not palpable above the brim.

**The head is not mobile.**

**The higher cephalic prominence** will be felt less than 5 cm above the brim.

**The anterior shoulder** would be little more than 5 cm above the symphysis pubis.

### Method

When grasping the head as in pelvic palpation it cannot be moved from side to side nor can the fingers displace it upwards. The amount of head accommodated within the two hands is less than with a non-engaged head. While the woman is breathing out, the fingers are directed further down because more of the head is in the pelvis. To reach the lower cephalic prominence the finger tips, descending steeply, are dipped well down, in a somewhat backward direction, depending on how deeply the head has descended into the pelvic cavity. The higher cephalic prominence will be less pronounced than in the non-engaged head.

### Head Engaged Deeply in the Pelvis

**On rare occasions the head is not palpable abdominally because it is engaged so deeply** in the pelvis that the vertex has reached the level of the ischial spines. The finger tips are dipped well down into the pelvis while the woman 'breathes out' and by giving a sharp tap the hard head may be detected. The anterior shoulder in these circumstances will lie immediately above the symphysis pubis and may be thought to be a breech presentation. When doubt exists a vaginal examination will reveal the deeply engaged head.

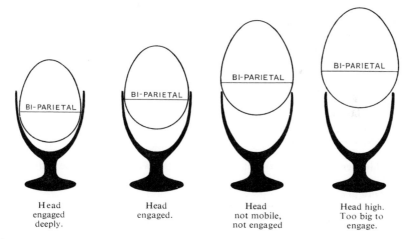

| Head engaged deeply. | Head engaged. | Head not mobile, not engaged | Head high. Too big to engage. |

Fig. 8-18  Diagrammatic representation of engagement of the fetal head by the use of egg-cups and eggs.

### Terminology that should be abolished

The word 'fixed' is sometimes used to designate an engaged head. It is true that the engaged head is fixed but conversely the fixed head is not necessarily engaged. This has given rise to misunderstanding and confusion. If the student midwife considers a fixed head to be engaged cases of minor degree disproportion will be missed. The word 'fixing' or 'engaging' is used by some to describe cases in which the head is neither mobile nor considered to be engaged; but the head is either engaged or it is not engaged and no intermediate stage should be countenanced diagnostically. **The midwife must seek medical advice if the head is not engaged when it ought to be.**

## FINDINGS WHEN HEAD IS NOT ENGAGED

**The head may be high and freely movable.**
**The higher cephalic prominence**—the sincipital—may be 7·5 cm above the brim.
**The greater bulk of the head is above the brim.**

There is no difficulty in diagnosing a non-engaged head that is high because it will be mobile. But the non-engaged head is not always high and movable: it may partly settle into the pelvic brim and be immobile although the parietal eminences have not passed through the brim. The hydrocephalic head could mould during labour and partially enter the brim: it would not be mobile, but it may not engage. A duck's egg could partly enter an ordinary egg-cup; it would not be movable yet its largest presenting diameter could not pass through the rim of the egg-cup.

### Method

The mobile head is most easily detected by using Pawlik's manoeuvre (Fig. 8-17). When the head is not mobile and the question of engagement is in doubt the midwife should make an attempt to find out whether the head will engage temporarily or not. While grasping the head with the two hands, as in pelvic palpation, steady yet gentle pressure is applied in a downward, backward direction, keeping in mind the inclination of the plane of the pelvic inlet. If a feeling of 'yield' or 'give' is experienced the outlook is good. The left hand grip (p. 144) can also be used. If doubt still exists the woman must be seen by a doctor.

### Causes of non-Engagement of the Head

**Failure of the lower uterine segment and lower birth canal to soften** and so allow the head to sink into the pelvis.

**Larger diameters of the deflexed head** which present in posterior positions of the vertex.

**Faulty assessment of period of gestation:** dates probably wrong.

**Cephalo-pelvic disproportion** due to contracted pelvis, large head, or a combination of both: brow presentation; hydrocephalus.

**Twins and polyhydramnios.**

**Full bladder.**—This case ought not to exist: the woman should be required to empty her bladder prior to abdominal examination.

**Placenta praevia.**

**Tumours and ovarian cysts** are uncommon but significant causes.

**Pelvic brim inclination of 80°** instead of the usual 60° occurs in some African women and the head does not engage until labour has been in progress for some hours.

## AUSCULTATION

The fetal heart-sounds are heard over the area at which the fetal left scapula and ribs come in contact with the uterine wall. They should be listened for at every visit after the 20th week of pregnancy. Fetal heart-sounds have been likened to the ticking of a watch under a pillow but the suggestion of the dull thud of a small motor is also helpful. Other sounds may be heard, such as fetal movement, intestinal rumbling, uterine and, rarely, funic souffle. A rate of 120 to 140 is usual and the novice should count the mother's pulse rate for comparison. (*Confusion in rates is more likely in cases where the mother's heart-beat is rapid.*)

**The Sonicaid or the Doptone,** ultrasonic fetal pulse detectors, will pick up the fetal heart sounds as early as the 10th week.

### DIAGNOSTIC VALUE OF HEARING THE FETAL HEART

**A positive sign of pregnancy.**
**Proof that the fetus is alive.**
**Corroboration in the diagnosis of presentation and position.**

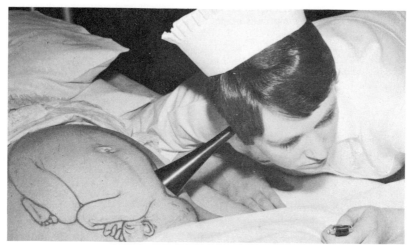

Fig. 8-19  Auscultation of the fetal heart. Vertex left occipito-anterior.

### *Method*

Pinard's stethoscope is commonly used and the hand should not touch it while listening, or extraneous sounds are produced. Electronic bin-aural stethoscopes are now available. Closing the eyes is an aid to concentration. The ear must be in close, firm contact with Pinard's stethoscope and care taken that it is held at right angles to the point over which it is directed, otherwise the abdominal wall moves causing the stethoscope to slip sideways. The area on the mother's abdomen on which the fetal heart is heard most clearly is known as the point of **'maximal intensity'** and the fetal stethoscope should be moved about until that point is located. The point of maximal intensity varies according to fetal presentation and position, and is high or low depending on whether the fetal head is engaged or not.

### *Locating the Fetal Heart-sounds*

From the 20th to 28th week of pregnancy the fetal heart is heard most clearly in the midline well below the umbilicus.

### From about the 30th week onwards

**Vertex L.O.A.** The heart-beat will be best heard at a point midway between the umbilicus and the left anterior superior iliac spine.

**Vertex L.O.L.** The heart-beat will be heard about 5 cm further to the left than in the L.O.A.

**Vertex R.O.A.** The point of maximal intensity is on the right but nearer the midline than in an L.O.A. (*By placing the doll in the pelvis this can be demonstrated.*)

**Vertex R.O.P.** The heart-sounds will be heard in the mother's right flank and as the muscles there are thick the sounds may be muffled. Should the fetus be in the military attitude with the chest thrown forwards the fetal heart will be heard in the midline (through the fetal chest wall) and just below umbilical level, because the head will be high.

**Breech presentation.** The heart-sounds will be heard at or above the level of the umbilicus but if the breech is engaged as may occur when the legs are extended, the heart-sounds will be lower than in the complete breech, and a mistaken diagnosis of vertex presentation is sometimes made.

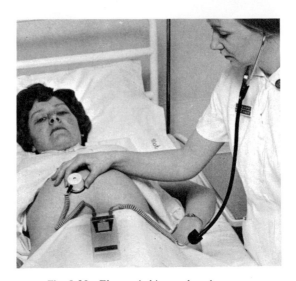

Fig. 8-20   Electronic bin-aural stethoscope.

### The Uterine Souffle

This is a soft blowing sound which is synchronous with the maternal pulse, heard mainly on the lower lateral borders of the uterus where the large uterine vessels are.

### The Funic Souffle

This high-pitched sound synchronous with the fetal heart-beat is believed to be caused by interference with the circulation in the umbilical cord. Occasionally it may be heard during the latter weeks of pregnancy or during labour, if the cord is in such a situation that the stethoscope can be placed directly over it.

### Is the Fetus Alive?

The absence of fetal heart-sounds, or the woman not feeling fetal movement when previously having done so, is suspicious but not diagnostic of intra-uterine death. The mother need not be told, as it may be possible to hear the fetal heart one week later and if not medical aid should be sought. Cases are known in which the woman states that she feels fetal movement and the baby is subsequently born in a macerated condition. The movement experienced by the woman was probably due to the shifting of the dead fetus *en masse* that occurred when she altered her posture.

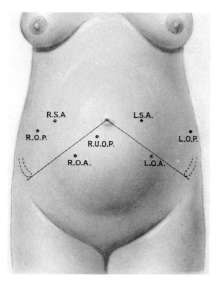

Fig. 8-21   Showing the points of maximal intensity of the fetal heart-sounds in vertex and breech presentation.

## CEPHALO-PELVIC DISPROPORTION

Disproportion means that the head is too big for the particular pelvis through which it must pass: there is a misfit. It is a relative term, and disproportion can be pelvic or cephalic in origin, due to a small pelvis, a large fetus or a combination of both. It cannot be diagnosed until the 36th week, because before then the fetal head is too small for comparison with the pelvis.

### THREE DEGREES OF DISPROPORTION:

**Minor degree.** The anterior parietal bone is level with the anterior border of the symphysis pubis.

**Moderate degree.** The head slightly overlaps the anterior edge of the symphysis pubis.

**Major degree.** There is a pronounced bulge of head over the anterior edge of the symphysis pubis.

It is considered to be a fairly good working rule that if there is no disproportion at the 36th week the head will engage during labour, but this is not infallible so the patient should be seen every week to make sure. The circumference of the head increases by about 2 mm per week from the 36th to the 40th week, but this additional growth is compensated for during labour by head flexion, over-riding of the skull bones, good uterine contractions, as well as by the 'give' of the pelvic joints. It is not the duty of the midwife to determine the degree of disproportion but to obtain medical assistance when any condition exists which suggests disproportion between head and pelvis.

## Methods of Determining Disproportion

### By pelvic palpation

The head is grasped, as described for pelvic palpation (Fig. 8-15), and pressure exerted on it, in a downward and backward direction, remembering that the plane of the brim makes an angle of about 60° with the bed. If a sense of 'give' is experienced and there is no overlap, cephalo-pelvic disproportion is not present.

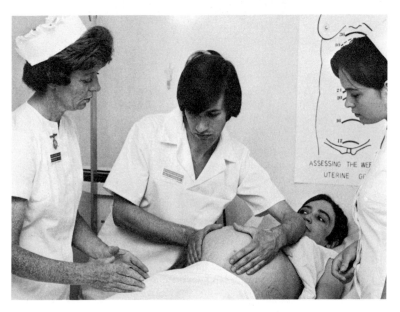

Fig. 8-22   Sister showing male student midwife the method of pelvic palpation.
*Maternity Hospital, Stirling.*

### Left hand grip

While facing the woman's feet, the left hand grasps the fetal head, the thumb being on the patient's right side, and when the head is pushed in a downward-backward direction 'give' can be recognised. The first two fingers of the right hand assess any overlap at the symphysis pubis.

### By sitting the patient up

The midwife grasps the fetal head using her right hand as in Pawlik's manoeuvre, with the ulnar border of that hand resting on the symphysis pubis. The woman is asked to sit up without assistance and to lean forwards for a short time. Her diaphragm and abdominal muscles tend to press the fetus downwards, and sitting forwards enlarges the antero-posterior diameter of the pelvic brim. The right hand, grasping the fetal head and resting on the symphysis pubis, acts as a brace directing the head into the pelvic inlet. As the woman lies down again, pressure may be applied to the fundus in a further endeavour to cause the head to engage temporarily. The right hand remains in position throughout the procedure and when no cephalo-pelvic disproportion exists no overlap is palpable. If the head remains above the brim, the patient is referred to the doctor who will estimate the degree of disproportion.

**Chassar Moir's Method**

While facing the patient's feet the midwife straightens her left arm until it is rigid and, using the ulnar border of her hand, presses the head in a downward and backward direction in the axis of the pelvic inlet. The first two fingers of the right hand are used to estimate the degree of overlap at the symphysis pubis (see Fig. 8.23).

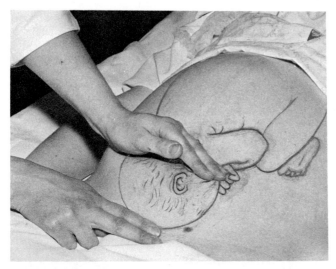

Fig. 8-23    Chassar Moir's method of determining the degree of overlap.

**Munro Kerr's Method**

This modification of Müller's method is employed by the doctor to determine the degree of disproportion when there is doubt as to whether vaginal delivery is possible. The patient is placed in the lithotomy position. Two fingers of the gloved hand are inserted into the vagina, with antiseptic precautions. The other hand grasps the head abdominally and applies downward pressure to it: the amount of descent being detected by the fingers in the vagina. The thumb of the hand in the vagina assesses the degree of overlap at the summit of the symphysis pubis.

### FUTURE VISITS

To provide good prenatal care the woman should be seen frequently during the period of the possible onset of pre-eclampsia, the 20th to 30th week.

**Every four weeks** until the 20th week ⎫
**Every two weeks** until the 36th week ⎬ **and more frequently if necessary.**
**Every week** until she is delivered ⎭

A number of pregnant women do not book early or attend regularly because clinics are situated inconveniently. The expense and effort of bus travel are detrimental. This could be remedied.

Under the General Practitioner Cooperation Scheme normal patients who attend the hospital prenatal clinic may be referred to their family doctor for routine care until the 34th week.

**Follow up on non-attenders**

A letter is sent to each non-attender within 24 hours asking her to attend the clinic the following week. If the letter is ignored a home visit is paid. When the woman is a diabetic or has a cardiac or any other condition requiring close supervision and she fails to attend the clinic her family doctor is requested by telephone to visit her. The welfare of the woman and her unborn child depends on close cooperation between family doctor, clinic and midwife.

## SAFE CHILDBEARING

**Childbearing today is safer and easier** than at any other period in history. Improved health, socio-economic status, scientific advances in obstetrics, paediatrics and other medical disciplines have all contributed to this admirable state of affairs. Previous circumstances, both genetic and environmental, greatly affect the woman's reproductive performance. If, as a fetus, infant or adolescent, she has been subjected to sub-standard living conditions, poor nutrition, or diseases that inhibit skeletal growth, her pelvic architecture may be defective, her general health impaired: both will have an adverse effect, maternal and fetal.

**Second and third pregnancies are the safest;** the first being the least predictable. Age over 18 and under 30 years: height above 1·6 m. Medical history and general health good, Hb over 12·6 g/dl, blood pressure under 130/80; no medical or obstetric abnormalities present.

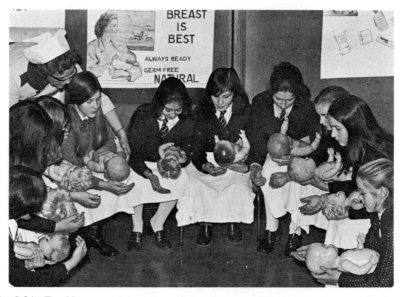

Fig. 8-24   Teaching potential mothers. Tutor showing schoolgirls 'bathing positions' in a course of parentcraft teaching.

*Maternity Section, Central Hospital, Irvine, Ayrshire.*

**The midwife can by health education** help to reduce maternal and fetal risks, via (*a*) senior schoolgirls, who should be made aware of how they can, by good nutrition, healthy living and knowledge of baby care prepare for their future reproductive role. They should also understand why early prenatal supervision is essential and know of the avoidable dangers caused by drugs and viral infections; (*b*) a programme of talks, illustrated by modern teaching aids, followed by discussion, could be arranged for potential as well as expectant mothers in the catchment area.

## EXAMINATION OF THE PREGNANT WOMAN

As a midwife how would you conduct a physical examination?

**What would you suspect from:** (1) small stature, limp or deformity; (2) oedema of hands or face; (3) breathlessness on slight exertion?

**Name the various blood tests:** why are they carried out? What do you consider to be an abnormal rise in blood pressure? What reasons would you give women to encourage them to attend the prenatal clinic early and regularly?

**Which investigations are made at every visit?** For what type of vaginal discharge would you seek medical aid? If pregnancy was in doubt what test would be made?

**What is the purpose** of cervical cytology? Why should the bladder be empty prior to abdominal examination?

**What is the value** of routine urine testing during the prenatal period? What can be learned from examination of: the head; the breasts; the vulva; the lower limbs?

**How would you palpate the abdomen:** (a) fundal; (b) lateral; (c) pelvic; (d) Pawlik's manoeuvre; (e) for disproportion.

**How would you diagnose:** (a) vertex, L.O.A., R.O.P.; (b) an engaged head; (c) location of FH in R.O.A., L.O.P.; (d) well-flexed head.

**Differentiate between** the diagnosis of: (a) multiple pregnancy and polyhydramnios; (b) vertex and breech presentation; (c) three degrees of disproportion.

**Define** (a) asymptomatic bacteriuria; (b) digital pelvimetry; (c) glycosuria; (d) proteinuria; (e) auscultation; (f) causes of a high head in a primigravida at term.

**What is the value of:** Weighing the pregnant woman; obtaining a clean-catch specimen of urine; taking the blood pressure; examining the lower limbs?

**State when or why**

The head engages in a primigravid woman. A clean catch specimen of urine should reach the laboratory. Fetal heart is first heard with Pinard's stethoscope. Fundus reaches the (a) umbilicus; (b) xiphisternum. Disproportion can first be diagnosed. Digital pelvimetry is carried out. The patient is seen from 30–36 weeks. The patient is seen from 36–40 weeks.

**What arrangements could a midwife make** to teach 'preparation for labour'?

## PRENATAL SCREENING

**Give 10 examples** during pregnancy in which the midwife participates. How is fetal growth and wellbeing assessed?

**Give reasons** why the following tests are carried out: H.A.I.; Kleihauer; spectrophotometric; lecithin/sphingomyelin. What is the significance of a feto-maternal 'bleed'?

**Give examples** of an open neural tube defect.

**Give reasons** why amniocentesis is carried out. Which mothers are classified as 'high risk'? Which maternal conditions put the fetus at 'high risk'?

## C.M.B. QUESTIONS

**C.M.B.** (Eng.) 30 min. question. Enumerate the causes of non-engagement of the head in a primigravida 38 weeks pregnant. Discuss the possible investigations of this condition.

**C.M.B.** (Eng.) 30 min. question. Describe your antenatal examination of a primigravida at 36 weeks. To what points would you pay particular attention at this stage in pregnancy?

**C.M.B.** (Eng.) 30 min. question. At what intervals should a pregnant woman be examined? What special observations should be made in the last month of pregnancy and what advice may be needed?

**(N. Ireland)** 30 min. question. Protein is found in the urine at the 32nd week of pregnancy. What may be the cause of this and what investigations should be made?

**C.M.B.** (Eng.) 30 min. question. In what ways may the results of urine tests influence the subsequent management of a pregnancy?

**C.M.B.** (Eng.) 30 min. question. Discuss the significance of the sounds which you may hear from the pregnant uterus and the importance of listening to them.

**(N. Ireland)** 30 min. question. What conditions may cause excessive size of the uterus at 34 weeks of pregnancy? Describe the possible dangers associated with these conditions.

**C.M.B.( Scot.) 30-min. question.** Describe the brim of the pelvis. What do you understand by the engagement of the head? What investigations should be carried out when this fails to occur?

**C.M.B. (Scot.) 30-min. question.** Describe the value of the investigations which may be carried out on the urine during the antenatal period.

**C.M.B. (Scot.) 30-min. question.** What information may be obtained from abdominal examination of the pregnant woman?

**C.M.B. (Scot.) 30-min. question.** Describe the antenatal care of a patient in the last 12 weeks of pregnancy.

**C.M.B. (Eng.) 30 min. question.** What antenatal haematological investigations are carried out today? Explain why they are necessary.

## *C.M.B. Short Examination Questions*

**Eng.:** Oedema of the ankles.

**Eng.:** Weighing the antenatal patient.

**Eng.:** Proteinuria in pregnancy.

**Eng.:** Engagement of the fetal head.

**Eng.:** Routine blood tests in pregnancy.

**Eng.:** Causes of non-engagement of the fetal head.

**Eng.:** Weight gain in pregnancy.

**Eng.:** Maternal haemoglobin levels in pregnancy.

**Eng.:** High head at term.

**N. Ire.:** 'Free head' in a primigravida at term.

**Scot.:** Cephalo-pelvic disproportion.

**Eng.:** Abdominal examination at the 38th week of pregnancy.

**Eng.:** Diastolic blood pressure.

# 9
# Advice to the Pregnant Woman

*Recreation: suitable clothes: personal hygiene: minor disorders, morning sickness, heartburn, backache, varicose veins, fainting*

A woman pregnant for the first time has much to learn, and is usually eager and willing to do what is best for her baby. Advice may be given to individual women or to groups, and should be presented in a simple attractive manner, the matter being sound as well as practical. Expectant mothers should be encouraged to ask questions and to discuss obstetric or parentcraft subjects regarding which they are in doubt or worried.

### Fresh air and sunshine

The pregnant woman should be advised to spend two hours a day in the fresh air, if possible away from the busy streets and preferably walking or sitting in the garden or park. If reminded that baby needs a daily airing before birth as well as after, she will be more likely to go out when she might not otherwise do so.

### Exercise and recreation

Exercise out-of-doors is, of course, ideal, and pregnant women need to be encouraged to continue with such out-door recreation as they have been accustomed to, so long as it does not cause jolting as would occur with riding or tennis. Games should not be strenuous nor should they be carried to the stage of exhaustion. A good brisk walk is excellent. It provides a change of scene, stimulates the circulation, and gives a feeling of wellbeing besides whetting the appetite, aiding elimination and inducing sleep. During the later months the woman's activities will be curtailed to some extent by her ungainliness, so that she is unlikely to indulge in any harmful pursuit. Housework, such as making beds, sweeping and polishing brings many, but not all, muscles into play, so exercises have been devised to keep the muscles to be used during labour in good trim and the pelvic joints flexible. At some clinics, classes are held where keep fit exercises are practised and the women shown how to maintain good posture.

The pregnant woman should not lift heavy weights, as this may predispose to abortion in susceptible cases. Constant standing may aggravate any predisposition to varicose veins. The woman should not climb to reach high shelves, because of the likelihood of over-balancing and her tendency to faint.

### Travel

The majority of international airlines do not permit pregnant women to fly after the 34th week, domestic air lines after the 35th week. After the 28th week a statement of fitness to fly and of the EDD must be obtained from the woman's doctor.

### Rest and sleep

During the second half of pregnancy the expectant mother is carrying a constant load, which increases to 11 kg or more, and towards the end of the day she becomes fatigued and her legs may ache. She should be advised to have short rests with her feet up throughout the day, and to lie down and relax or sleep for one or two hours during the afternoon. This is not always easy where there is a family to be looked after, but, if overworked, she will only become exhausted and irritable.

The ability to relax at will is of inestimable value, both during pregnancy and labour: if a woman can relax completely she will obtain more benefit from her rest periods. By conserving nervous energy she will be able to keep calm in times of stress, and sleep will be more easily induced; all of which will be invaluable during labour.

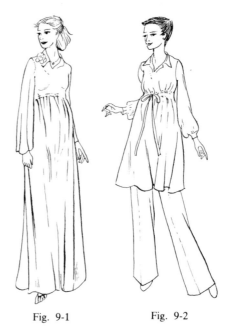

Fig. 9-1          Fig. 9-2

*Courtesy Vogue pattern service.*

At least nine hours sleep should be obtained every night, and some women need more than that. The minor disorders and the petty frustrations of life are felt more acutely at this time, and nervous exhaustion should be avoided at all costs. Sleep is the great restorer. The gentle tiredness induced by outdoor recreation, a warm bath and a glass of hot milk are natural sedatives. The weight of the uterus may create discomfort and sleeplessness, but a small pillow tucked under the abdomen when lying on the side usually gives relief. Near term, sleep may be disturbed by false pains, and, if persistent, it may be necessary to see the doctor so that a sedative can be prescribed.

**Suitable clothes**

These are a necessity, not a luxury. When dressed in comfortable, becoming, maternity garments, the woman has a feeling of assurance that combats her inclination to be self-conscious about her figure. She can be just as feminine and elegant as at any other time and there is is no reason why she should not enjoy a normal social life throughout the whole of pregnancy, as long as it does not interfere with rest and sleep. It is essential that the expectant mother goes out every day for fresh air and change of environment, so she ought to have clothes to wear in which she feels inconspicuous and happy.

An uplifting brassière, reinforced on its under-surface and with broad shoulder straps, should be worn as early as the 12th week because of the enlargement of the breasts which may increase the bust measurement by as much as 8-10 cm. The brassière ought not to be tight enough to depress the nipples. A maternity belt need not be worn until after the 20th week and, although many primigravidae have good abdominal muscles and do not require support, they appreciate the comfort of a maternity roll-on during the last twelve weeks. Tight corsets are harmful and must not be worn. Multiparous women frequently have lax abdominal muscles which allow the uterus to lean forwards. The shoulders have then to be held back to counteract the anterior obliquity, so the lumbar curve of the spine is increased, giving rise to backache and fatigue which could be eliminated by wearing an adjustable supporting belt or corset. Women should be advised not to wear constricting bands on the legs; they impede the venous circulation and increase any susceptibility to varicose veins and oedema.

Sensible shoes should be worn, with a 4·5 cm heel having a broad base. Narrow high heels cause fatigue in maintaining good posture, and increase the likelihood of stumbling or overbalancing which is common in pregnancy.

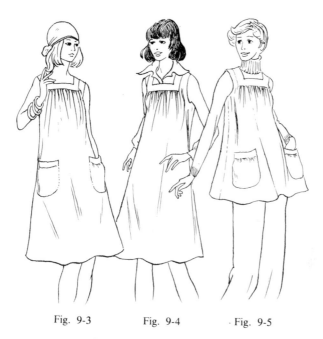

Fig. 9-3        Fig. 9-4        · Fig. 9-5

*Courtesy Vogue pattern service.*

**The bowels**

The bowels should move every day without having to resort to laxatives. Simple wholesome remedies, such as a glass of warm water on rising in the morning and the regular habit of defaecation after breakfast will often help matters. Adequate fluid should be taken between meals and drinking two glasses of water daily, either plain or flavoured with orange juice, may promote bowel action. Strong tea is better avoided because of the constipating effect of tannin. Plenty of roughage ought to be included in the diet, and wholewheat bread, fruit, vegetables, prunes, raisins and figs are excellent for the purpose.

### Care of the Teeth

It was previously believed that the withdrawal of calcium from the mother's teeth occurred because of the fetal demands for calcium, but it is from the mother's bones and not her teeth that calcium is withdrawn during pregnancy. For tooth extraction a local analgesic is administered to avoid cyanosis. **(Dental treatment in Great Britain is free during pregnancy.)**

*Care of the breasts is discussed under lactation.*

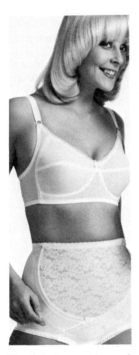

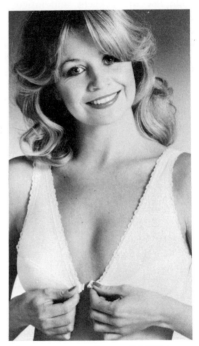

Fig. 9-6    Prenatal bra and pantie girdle.      Fig. 9-7    Sleep bra model 692 in soft stretch nylon.

*Courtesy Balance Maternities.*

### Bathing

**The skin is an excretory organ which should be kept active during pregnancy.** A daily tub-bath or shower is ideal, but hot baths are exhausting and may cause fainting. Unless the patient is very vigorous and accustomed to sea-bathing, it is better that she should not indulge in this round the north-east shores of Great Britain where the water is very cold.

### Marital relations

In women who have a history of abortion, coitus should be prohibited during the early months of pregnancy.

*Vaginal deodorants* should not be used. They alter the pH of the vagina and further the growth of organisms.

### Warning without frightening

It is necessary to tell pregnant women to report any unusual symptoms promptly because, if treated in the early stages, a major complication may be averted. This should be done in a matter-of-fact, almost casual, manner without giving the impression that their occurrence is anticipated. The woman should be told to go to her doctor or midwife if she thinks things are not quite right, or to send for her doctor if she feels ill or has any vaginal bleeding, swelling of her face or hands, or severe headache.

Pregnant women should be warned regarding taking drugs unless prescribed by the doctor. The embryo is at risk during the first 12 weeks. Alcohol should be limited.

## THE MINOR DISORDERS OF PREGNANCY

Although the minor disorders do not endanger life, they must not be ignored or treated lightly, for by interfering with nutrition, sleep and outdoor recreation they may undermine the woman's health. They can make life very miserable and often distress the woman far more than the more serious disorders of pregnancy. The midwife should ensure that women do not accept the minor disorders as an inevitable accompaniment of pregnancy and she should endeavour to cure or alleviate them.

### MORNING SICKNESS

About 50 per cent of pregnant women vomit between the 4th and the 14th week of pregnancy. It usually occurs immediately after getting up in the morning, when retching and the vomiting of mucus, sometimes bile-stained, takes place. The sickness is usually accompanied by nausea which may persist throughout the day and impairs the appetite. If the vomiting of food continues, the mother's nutrition suffers. The condition should never be ignored, for if 'nipped in the bud' hyperemesis gravidarum would seldom occur.

Vomiting is more common in women who have a 'sensitive' nervous system, but there appears to be some disturbance in the metabolism of glucose with increased production of ketone bodies. The ensuing ketosis causes vomiting and this is likely to occur when the intake of glucose is low, as occurs during the night.

#### Treatment

To maintain the glycogen supply, a light sweet meal should be eaten before retiring: a glass of milk and biscuits would be suitable. Extra sugar should be taken. Foods with a high fat content, like butter, cream, pastries and those that are fried ought to be restricted. The woman should have a cup of tea and toast with marmalade-jelly or a biscuit before getting up in the morning, and although a thermos flask could be utilised it seems to be more efficacious if freshly made tea is brought to her, preferably by the husband. Nausea may be extremely troublesome, and the avoidance of hunger by having some easily digested food every two hours may help. It is important that the woman should eat food, and a savoury may tempt the appetite when sweet foods are refused. Vomiting may deplete the blood chlorides and reduce the intake of vitamin $B_1$, so Marmite, which is usually acceptable will help to replace both. An adequate fluid intake is essential and in mild cases treated at home the woman should be told to report if her urine is dark in colour. Constipation results because of dehydration and the lack of food. The doctor only should prescribe drugs for morning sickness.

### HEARTBURN

**This is probably the most usual and the most intractable minor disorder of pregnancy;** being more troublesome at night when the recumbent position is adopted. The burning sensation is due to irritation caused by the reflux of gastric juice into the oesophagus or bile regurgitation. The cardiac sphincter of the stomach is relaxed and reflux oesophagitis may occur.

### *Treatment*

Greasy, highly seasoned, or indigestible foods should be eliminated from the diet.

Raising the head of the bed 30 cm and an extra pillow may help. No infallible cure exists, although many simple remedies seem to give relief. Sips of milk or hot water, peppermint, and the proprietary alkaline lozenges are reputed to be efficacious. Five ml of Aludrox or milk of magnesia may be beneficial, also Nulacin; and 4 ml of magnesium trisilicate may be prescribed. The practice of ingesting repeated doses of sodium bicarbonate is neither rational nor advisable: it inhibits digestion, causes flatulence, hinders the absorption of vitamin B, and in some women may produce oedema.

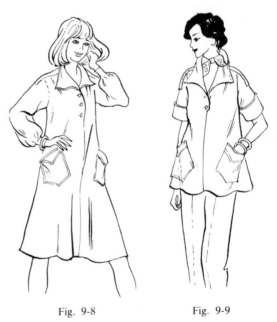

Fig. 9-8            Fig. 9-9

*Courtesy Vogue pattern service.*

## BACKACHE

Slight backache may be due to faulty posture and is more common in tired multiparous patients whose muscle tone is poor. Lax abdominal muscles produce anterior obliquity of the uterus and this causes the woman to hold her shoulders too far back in order to support the uterus and to keep her balance. The increased lumbar curve amounts to lordosis and gives rise to strain of the muscles of the back, resulting in fatigue and backache.

A firm supporting maternity corset and a reasonable amount of rest are needed. Good posture, sensible shoes and a comfortable bed that does not sag will do much to prevent backache. Sacro-iliac strain may be troublesome during the last months when the uterus is heavy and the joints are relaxed, and it may be necessary to provide firm support in the sacro-iliac region. If backache is severe and persistent medical advice must be sought.

## VARICOSE VEINS

The tendency to varicose veins is increased during pregnancy, and about 10 per cent of pregnant women are found to have varicosities of the legs in greater or lesser degree. The venous return from the lower limbs is impeded in the common iliac veins by the increased flow of blood from the uterus. The woman complains of a dull aching pain in her limbs, and the superficial veins are often seen to be in a state of engorgement. The limbs may be oedematous in severe cases.

Medical advice must be obtained when varicose veins are troublesome or serious. Injury may lead to haemorrhage or to ulceration of the skin, but the most vital risk is that varicose veins predispose to vein thrombosis. Varicose veins tend to subside after parturition, but are aggravated by each succeeding pregnancy.

### Treatment

No tight bands that would impede the circulation of the lower limbs should be worn. The woman is advised to avoid long periods of standing and when reading or knitting to sit with her feet raised; the ankle joints should be moved freely while sitting. If the aching causes her to be disinclined for walking out of doors, she should be advised to lie down for an hour, with her feet higher than her head before going out to relieve the congestion and the pain. The wearing of elastic stockings or tights for pregnant women supports the column of blood, relieves the aching and gives considerable comfort. Before putting on the stockings, the legs should be elevated at right angles to the body for a few moments previous to getting out of bed in the morning. In serious cases absolute rest in bed, the foot of which is raised, may be necessary.

### Varicose veins of the vulva

They can be very painful and if so the doctor may inject them but, as a rule, wearing a firmly applied perineal pad for support, and resting with the hips raised, give relief.

### Haemorrhoids

External haemorrhoids are varicose veins on the anal margin. Constipation should be avoided. The application of a soothing cream such as Anusol may be sufficient in mild cases; when painful, Nupercainal ointment is effective. Ice packs may be tried and in some instances a warm sitz bath to which magnesium sulphate crystals have been added will reduce the engorgement. Prolapsed haemorrhoids should be lubricated and an attempt made to replace them gently.

### Constipation

There is a tendency to constipation during pregnancy which may be due to the pressure of the enlarged uterus. Drugs will have to be resorted to if increasing the amount of fruit and vegtables in the diet is not sufficient to treat the condition; Senokot, Dulcolax or any mild vegetable laxative being suitable.

### Itching of the skin

Itching of the skin of the abdomen and breasts may be intense and occasionally the itching is generalised over the whole body (scabies, of course, should be kept in mind and can usually be diagnosed). The cause is not understood and may be endocrine, toxic, or due to some nervous element. Simple remedies such as the application of lanoline or cold cream, can be tried. Soothing substances, such as calamine lotion are useful. The clothing worn next to the skin should be non-irritating; water should be taken freely and the bowels kept open.

### Pruritus vulvae

Itching of the vulva may be very distressing. If due to irritation from vaginal discharge or lack of cleanliness, the remedy is soap and water. The itching may be due to glycosuria and, if so, further investigation is necessary to rule out diabetes. *Vaginal thrush* gives rise to intense itching of vagina and vulva, accompanied by a white flaky discharge (see p. 220). The application of Nystatin ointment is helpful.

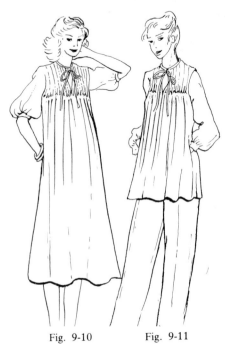

Fig. 9-10          Fig. 9-11

*Courtesy Vogue pattern service.*

### Fainting

This is a frequent source of anxiety to the patient and her relatives, but if cardiac impairment is absent she can be assured that the condition is not serious. Fainting in pregnancy is thought to be due to the instability of the vaso-motor centre in the medulla which controls arterial tone, and if a rapid fall in blood pressure takes place the woman faints. It may also be due to pressure of the uterus on the inferior vena cava (see supine hypotensive syndrome, p. 125). Sudden changes in posture, as from the recumbent to the upright, or standing for long periods, particularly in hot weather, may cause fainting. Fatigue or excitement may instigate an attack, as well as stuffy rooms or crowded halls. Tight corsets should not be worn and meals that overload the stomach or cause flatulence should be avoided.

**When the woman's complaints suggest more than a minor disorder she must be referred to the doctor.**

If a pregnant woman sought your advice on the following matters what reasons would you give to convince her:

(a) **Entering** a strenuous sports contest; (b) **travelling** by air; (c) **the amount** of rest and sleep needed during pregnancy; (d) **the benefit** of attending relaxation classes; (e) **how to treat** morning sickness, heartburn. **Excessive** aching in her legs, backache. (f) **Is fainting** a sign of heart disease?

Why should a pregnant woman (a) have a daily walk out of doors? (b) be told to report any vaginal bleeding?

Give reasons why the following are not advisable: high heels, tights that are too small, baths that are too hot, anti-emetic drugs for morning sickness.

What would you recommend for (a) itching of the skin of the abdomen? (b) constipation? (c) pruritus vulvae? (d) haemorrhoids?

What points would you stress in the selection of: (a) a brassière, (b) maternity dresses, (c) maternity girdle, (d) shoes? Why should expectant mothers be advised to procure maternity clothes? Why should vaginal deodorants not be used?

What serious condition can be avoided by treating morning sickness?

**C.M.B. (Eng.) 30-min. question**. Mention some of the commoner minor disabilities of pregnancy and the advice you would give for their relief. What would make you decide to advise medical aid?

**C.M.B. (Scot.) 30-min. question.** What advice would you give a primigravid woman in regard to (a) diet (b) clothing (c) exercise (d) care of the breasts?

**C.M.B. (Scot.) 30-min. question.** What advice and guidance would you give to a young primigravida at her first attendance at an antenatal clinic?

# 10
# Conditions associated with Bleeding in Early Pregnancy

*Implantation bleeding: Cervical lesions: Abortion, types and treatment: counselling: Cervical incompetence: The Abortion Act: Ectopic pregnancy: Bacteraemic shock: Hydatidiform mole: Choriocarcinoma*

All vaginal bleeding during the prenatal period should be reported to the doctor, for prompt treatment will often save the pregnancy and prevent serious loss of blood. The midwife should instruct her patients to report any bleeding, however slight, but such advice should be given in a matter-of-fact way, without creating the impression that bleeding is anticipated.

### Implantation bleeding

**Slight vaginal bleeding may occur when the trophoblast erodes the endometrium** during the process of embedding. This may simulate the menstrual period that would be anticipated at about this time and if the implantation bleeding is erroneously thought to be a menstrual period calculation of the expected date of delivery will be incorrect.

### Cervical lesions

**Erosion** may produce a slight blood-stained mucoid discharge; treatment is seldom required during pregnancy.

**Mucous polypus** is a tiny growth, rather like a small cherry with a short stalk. It can be very readily snipped or twisted off.

**Carcinoma of the cervix** is a rare but very serious condition.

## ABORTION

The commonest cause of vaginal bleeding in early pregnancy is abortion, which can be defined as 'the interruption of pregnancy before the 28th week of gestation', after which period the fetus is viable (capable of living a separate existence).

### FETAL CAUSES

Maldevelopment or disease of the fertilised ovum, and in 30 to 40 per cent of spontaneous, first trimester abortions chromosomal anomalies are present.

The normal development of the embryo may be affected by hypoxia resulting from separation of and damage to the placenta.

### MATERNAL CAUSES

*General Conditions*

**Infections.** Acute febrile conditions such as influenza may cause death of the fetus.

**Disease** such as chronic nephritis.

**Effect of drugs.** The large doses necessary to induce abortion are poisonous.

**Endocrine dysfunction.** No convincing proof. (Progesterone deficiency is the secondary effect of feto-placental damage, not the cause.)

**ABO incompatibility** between mother and embryo.

*Local Conditions*

**Conditions that interfere** with the embedding, development and nutrition of the ovum.

Implantation of the ovum in the lower uterine segment.

**Trauma.** Criminal interference; accidents; violent exercise; stimulation of the uterus such as might be due to some necessary abdominal operation.

**Incompetent cervix** (see p. 165). **Uterine malformations;** fibroid tumours.

## TYPES OF ABORTION

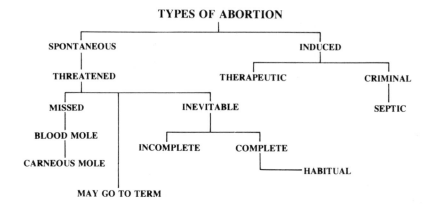

### SIGNS AND SYMPTOMS

**Vaginal bleeding,** the earliest sign, is due to partial detachment of the embedded ovum.

**Pain,** which is usually felt low in the abdomen, intermittent in character and often accompanied by backache, is due to uterine contractions.

**Dilatation of the os** is present when the abortion is inevitable.

## THREATENED ABORTION

Threatened abortion is one in which the disturbance is so slight that it is possible for the pregnancy to continue to term. Bleeding is not severe. Backache may be present, the os is closed and the membranes intact. Very occasionally, intermittent pain is felt low in the abdomen.

### *Possibilities in the Outcome of a Threatened Abortion*

**The pregnancy goes to term** if the signs and symptoms subside.

**The abortion becomes inevitable** when free bleeding continues, and painful uterine contractions are present.

**Missed abortion** occurs when the fetus dies and is retained *in utero* (p. 165).

### *Treatment of Threatened Abortion*

**The patient is put to bed,** reassured, and kept quiet. Maternal placental lactogen is assessed to predict the outcome by radio immunoassay; if low, abortion may be inevitable: an ultrasonic scan may be made to detect a blighted ovum.

**Medical assistance is obtained.**

**All vaginal discharge, pads, stained clothing and linen are kept** for the doctor's inspection. (The relatives should be instructed to save everything passed vaginally during the midwife's absence.)

**Vulval swabbing** is carried out twice daily while the brownish discharge persists.

Analgesics are usually ordered. **Panasorb,** tabs 2, for slight pain. **Pethidine,** 100 mg if pain is troublesome or promazine (Sparine) 25 mg. Amylobarbitone sodium (Sod. Amytal) 200 mg may be ordered for night sedation.

If constipation exists, the doctor may order small doses of a mild aperient: suppositories may be employed.

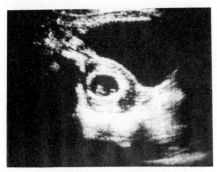

Fig. 10-1   The gestational sac being irregular in outline denotes a blighted ovum

The pulse and temperature are taken and recorded twice daily in non-febrile cases; otherwise every four hours.

The patient is allowed up after bright red bleeding has ceased for 3 days.

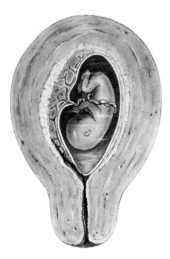 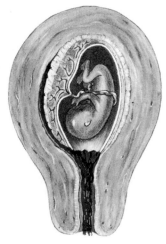

Fig. 10-2   Threatened abortion. Slight placental separation: slight bleeding: membranes intact: os closed.

Fig. 10-3   Inevitable abortion. Placental separation: moderate bleeding: membranes ruptured: os dilated.

A speculum examination is made to exclude cervical lesions. The opportunity is taken to detect early cancer by taking a Papanicolaou smear.

In all cases of abortion the Rh negative woman is given Rh anti-D immuno-globulin 50 micrograms if under 12 weeks and 100 micrograms if over 12 weeks.

**Advice on discharge**

The patient is advised to take extra rest, to restrict her activities within reasonable limits and to avoid heavy lifting, strenuous exercise, fatigue and excitement. Coitus is contra-indicated for 2 or 3 weeks. She should go to bed immediately if bleeding starts again and call her doctor.

## INEVITABLE ABORTION

In this case it is not possible for the pregnancy to continue.

Free bleeding usually means that a considerable part of the placenta has become detached.

Intermittent uterine contractions, accompanied by pain, constitute a reliable sign.

If the membranes rupture and the ovum protrudes through the dilating os, abortion must take place.

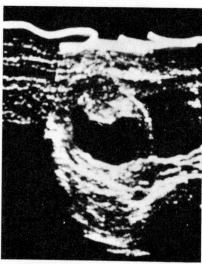 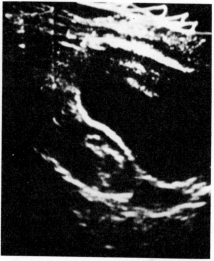

Fig. 10-4   Small sac situated near cervix, 11 weeks amenorrhoea, inevitable abortion.

Fig. 10-5   Empty gestational sac. No fetus developed, 12 weeks amenorrhoea, finally aborted.

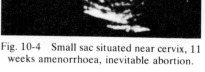

*Courtesy of Queen Mother's Hospital, Glasgow.*

### *Treatment*

The midwife should treat an inevitable abortion as 'threatened', until the arrival of the doctor, unless the bleeding is severe when she should give ergometrine 0·5 mg or Syntometrine 1 ml intramuscularly. Everything passed vaginally is kept for the doctor's inspection. Pethidine 100 mg may be given for pain.

In hospital extra-ovular prostaglandin or an oxytocin drip is usually given, especially after the 16th week. If not successful, the uterus is evacuated by suction under general anaesthesia: blood transfusion may be necessary for profuse bleeding. Some consider it advisable to explore the uterus in all cases, unless the abortion appears to be complete, to ensure that no placental tissue has been retained. Preparation for evacuation of the uterus is described on page 163. Ergometrine,

0·5 mg, is usually administered when the evacuation is completed. (See foot of page 160, re administration of Rh anti-D immunoglobulin.)

## COMPLETE ABORTION

Before the 8th week an abortion is more likely to be complete because the fetal sac is expelled intact. When an abortion is complete, bleeding is reduced to a mere staining, pain ceases, the cervix closes and involution of the uterus takes place.

After the 20th week milk may come into the breasts; if so, a firm uplift bra should be worn.

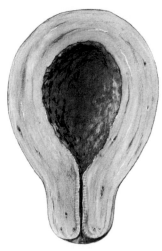

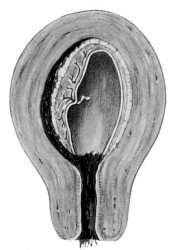

Fig. 10-6  Complete abortion. Fetus and placenta expelled: bleeding scanty: os closed.

Fig. 10-7  Incomplete abortion. Fetus expelled: placenta partially separated: free bleeding: os dilated.

## INCOMPLETE ABORTION

The fetus has been expelled, but the whole or part of the placenta and membranes has been retained *in utero*. The patient is usually more than 12 weeks pregnant because then the placenta is firmly embedded and the slender cord breaks.

**Lochia** continue and bleeding may be profuse.

**Pain** may or may not be present.

**The os** partly closes, but not completely; the cervix is patulous.

**Involution** does not take place.

### *Treatment of Haemorrhage by Midwife on District*

The midwife must immediately send for the doctor.

When medical aid is not readily available the midwife should give Syntometrine, 1 ml, or ergometrine, 0·5 mg, intramuscularly: this can be repeated in 10 minutes or even in 5 minutes if haemorrhage is profuse, but the second dose is seldom necessary. Pethidine, 100 mg, is given if pain is severe.

**If bleeding is profuse** the midwife should send for the 'flying squad' who will deal with the emergency. Resuscitative measures are always employed prior to removing the patient by ambulance. A blood transfusion, and 5 to 10 units oxytocin in glucose 5 per cent will probably be given. Subjecting a shocked or exsanguinated woman to an ambulance journey may be the cause of her death. The midwife will, of course, accompany her patient to hospital and report on treatment and drugs administered.

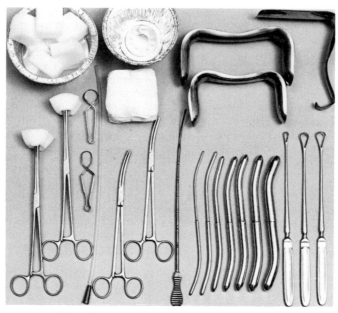

Fig. 10-8   Instruments for evacuation of uterus.
*Aberdeen Maternity Hospital.*

### *Prepacked*

**INSTRUMENTS**
2 Swab holding forceps
2 Towel clips
1 Disposable catheter 14 FG
2 prs. Volsellum forceps
1 Uterine sound
1 set Hegar's dilators
3 Uterine curettes
2 Sim's speculae
1 Goodwin's retractor

**LINEN: DRESSINGS**
Cap, mask, hand towel, gown
1 pr. Lithotomy leggings
1 Perineal towel
10 Foam sponges
10 Gauze swabs
Foil bowl with Savlon
Foil bowl with obstetric cream

**MISCELLANEOUS EQUIPMENT**

Tray with syringes and needles
Prepacked disposable gloves
Kidney basin for urine
Central venous pressure manometer i.v. fluid to combat
circulatory failure. Cross-matched blood.

Drugs:
  Ergometrine
  Syntometrine
  Syntocinon
  Hibitane Cream

## TREATMENT OF INCOMPLETE ABORTION IN HOSPITAL

If the patient is not suffering from the effect of blood loss Syntometrine, 1 ml, or ergometrine, 0·5 mg, is given intramuscularly; the blood is typed and haemoglobin estimated; a high vaginal swab is taken. The uterus is evacuated vaginally. Some use vacuum aspiration. The woman may be discharged 24 hours later if there are no reasons for further treatment. See foot of page 160 re Rh anti-D immunoglobulin.

**Woman collapsed from loss of blood**

She is received into a warm bed, the foot of which is then elevated. Ergometrine, 0·5 mg, is given intravenously. While waiting for cross-matched blood, dextrose 5 per cent with Ringers lactate solution is given to combat circulatory failure; Syntocinon 10 units may be added to the glucose drip.

The pulse is taken and recorded every 5 minutes, the blood pressure every 15 or 30 minutes. The central venous pressure is monitored. When the patient's condition is satisfactory the uterus is evacuated under general anaesthesia. Pentothal may be adequate. To ensure against further haemorrhage, a gauze pack may be inserted into the uterus; the remainder fills the vagina, thus stimulating good uterine contractions. Syntometrine, 1 ml, or ergometrine, 0·5 mg, is given intramuscularly. Pulse and blood pressure are recorded every half-hour until satisfactory—temperature 4 hourly. The pack is removed in 6 hours. Anaemia if present is dealt with. The woman is discharged, if her condition warrants this, on the 4th or 5th day after evacuation.

WHEN NO MEDICAL AID IS AVAILABLE

In desperate cases when bleeding endangers life and the home is in a remote area the midwife will have to cope with the situation alone. A second dose of Syntometrine or ergometrine is given as mentioned on page 162.

Retained products must be removed as bleeding will continue otherwise, so hands and vulva must be cleansed quickly: antiseptic obstetric cream is applied to the gloved right hand. With her left hand on the abdomen the midwife will antevert and press the uterus downwards. With the right index finger the retained products are removed.

To treat shock the foot of the bed is raised and 300 ml of tap water given rectally.

### Packing may be Necessary in Remote Areas

Packing could be condemned as an out-of-date measure and if the uterus has been evacuated properly it should not be necessary but it may be the only means of controlling severe haemorrhage in the absence of medical aid in remote areas. A pack made of 90 cm folded gauze: perineal pads smeared with obstetric cream could be used. The number inserted must be recorded to ensure their entire removal.

The bladder should always be emptied before inserting a vaginal pack. With the patient in Sims' left lateral position and the fingers of the left hand used as a perineal retractor the fornices are packed firmly and the vagina tightly filled until the pack protrudes at the vulva. A perineal pad attached to a belt will increase the pressure. The pack should be removed within six hours.

## HABITUAL OR RECURRENT ABORTION

When a woman has had two consecutive spontaneous abortions, the term 'habitual abortion' is used. The cause is obscure in many cases. A very thorough investigation is carried out between pregnancies, to exclude diseases such as nephritis, hypothyroidism. A pelvic examination is made to diagnose uterine abnormalities, displacements or fibroids. Cervical erosion, laceration, incompetence or infection are dealt with, if present.

### Management

Husband and wife are both advised to take a well balanced diet, especially proteins, minerals and vitamins (see p. 75), and another pregnancy may be started as soon as the woman is in good health. She reports to the clinic when she thinks she is pregnant, and is given the same advice as on discharge following threatened abortion (p. 161). The fact is stressed that coitus should not take place during early pregnancy.

Adequate rest is essential; women with home responsibilities should not undertake outside employment or heavy work in the home. Psychological support is needed by certain personality types: any emotional stress should be enquired into and suitable advice given. A mild sedative may be necessary.

## Cervical suture

Abortions occurring at about mid-term may be due to incompetence of the cervix allowing the membranes to rupture. A purse-string suture of heavy non-absorbable material is inserted about the 8th week, e.g. braided Mersilk. Mersilene (5 mm) is non-irritating but expensive. Cervical assessment is made by some authorities prior to suture and, if a No. 8 dilator passes easily into the cervix it is incompetent.

**Midwives should be aware** that the cervical suture must be removed at the 38th week, or sooner if the woman goes into premature labour, otherwise severe damage will be inflicted on the dilating cervix.

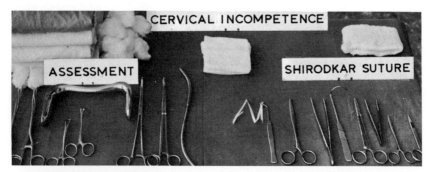

Fig. 10-9    Prepacked requirements for cervical assessment and modified Shirodkar's suture.
*Bellshill Maternity Hospital, Lanarkshire.*

### FOR ASSESSMENT
**Instruments**
2 sponge forceps. 2 Towel clips.
1 Sims' speculum. 2 Ring forceps.
1 cervical dilator No. 8.

**Linen and dressings**
1 Doctor's gown and cap. 1 Waterproof paper sheet.
1 Lithotomy sheet or leggings.
20 Wool swabs; 5 gauze swabs; 1 perineal pad.

### FOR SUTURE
**Instruments**
1 Blunt, 1 Sharp aneurysm needle
2 Spencer Wells forceps.
2 Non-toothed dissecting forceps.
1 Needle holder. 1 Stitch scissors.
Braided mersilk or Mersilene.

### MISSED ABORTION

*This term is used when the fetus dies and is retained in utero.*

Signs of threatened abortion arise and then subside; the uterus does not increase in size. The breasts become soft and the other signs of pregnancy disappear.

The woman has a brownish vaginal discharge, but no pain.

The ultrasonic Doppler cardioscope has been used to confirm the absence of fetal heart beat.

Blood coagulation disorders may develop in cases of missed abortion which persist for over six to eight weeks, therefore plasma fibrinogen level estimations are made weekly.

The uterus may retain the fetus for long periods, in one case for as long as 14 months. Certain authorities do not believe in interfering because of the risk of sepsis, but few women are willing to suffer the discomfort of a constant vaginal discharge, and they also object to having a dead fetus *in utero*. Prostaglandin by the extra ovular route may be used to induce abortion. Fresh compatible blood should be available to combat haemorrhage.

## BLOOD MOLE

Rarely does a blood mole form. This is a brownish red mass, about as big as a medium-sized orange, that arises in cases of missed abortion when the decidua capsularis remains intact and permits the ovum to be surrounded with layers of blood. The mole forms before the 12th week and if it is retained *in utero* for a period of months, the fluid is extracted from the blood and the fleshy firm hard mass is known as a **carneous mole**. When cut, it resembles a miniature placenta at first glance, but what appear to be cotyledons are raised blebs of amnion with blood underneath. A tiny embryo, less than 1·25 cm long, may be seen hanging by a short cord.

### *Treatment*

Prostaglandin E$_2$ may be administered by the extra-ovular route (between the fetal sac and uterine wall):

A high dosage oxytocin drip may be given: **10 units Syntocinon in 540 ml glucose 5 per cent at 1·2 ml per minute.** Increase by 0·3 ml every 30 minutes until 2·4 ml are being given.

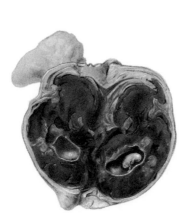

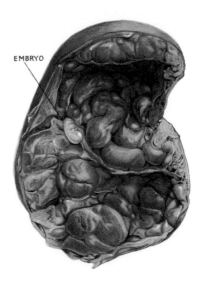

Fig. 10-10  Tubal mole. Tubal pregnancy, in which the embryo has died and is surrounded with blood clot. The distended Fallopian tube is opened lengthwise. Ovary attached.

*Simpson Memorial Maternity Pavilion, Edinburgh.*

Fig. 10-11  Carneous mole cut open shows the embryo and the blebs formed by blood collected between the amnion and chorion. The outer surface is smooth. Measurement (unopened) 7·5 × 9 cm.

*Simpson Memorial Maternity Pavilion, Edinburgh.*

**If no response:** start a new bottle with double the amount of Syntocinon = 20 units at 1·2 ml per minute and increase by 0·3 ml every 30 minutes to 2·4 ml.

**If no response:** double the number of units to 40, start with 1·2 ml and increase to 2·4 ml per minute.

**If no response:** the doctor may review the situation before giving 80 and 160 units. Some give as much as 200 units.

Vigilant observation is essential. A careful collection of urine is made and if the output is low the infusion should be stopped.

Transplacental haemorrhage occurs in many cases of abortion, particularly when surgical evacuation is employed. Rh negative women, who have no antibodies, are liable to immunisation if their fetus is Rh positive. It is now usual to give these susceptible women an i.m. injection of 50 micrograms anti D immunoglobulin after an abortion less than 12 weeks gestation and 100 micrograms after 12 weeks.

## THERAPEUTIC ABORTION

Therapeutic abortion consists in the evacuation of the uterus, carried out by a qualified medical practitioner as treatment in the interest of the mother's life or of her total wellbeing. The abortion may be legally carried out in Great Britain only in a National Health Service Hospital or a Nursing Home recognised for this purpose.

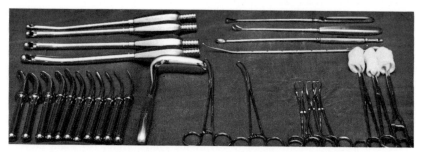

Fig. 10-12   Instruments for vacuum aspiration of embryo and placenta.

### THE ABORTION ACT, 1967

The provisions of the Act are briefly as follows: If two registered medical practitioners are of the opinion that a pregnancy should be terminated under the following conditions they shall not be guilty of an offence under the law relating to abortion: That the continuance of the pregnancy would involve a risk to the life of the pregnant woman or of injury to her physical or mental health, or any existing children of her family; or a substantial risk that the child when born would suffer from such physical or mental abnormalities as to be seriously handicapped. The woman's actual or reasonably foreseeable environment may be taken into account when determining the risk of injury to health should the pregnancy be allowed to continue. The termination must be reported to the Chief Medical Officer, Dept. of Health and Social Security (Eng.) The Home and Health Department (Scot.).

Husband and wife must both give written consent, and the duty of obtaining such signatures as well as permission to operate is usually delegated to the ward sister to avoid unnecessary delay. In certain religious beliefs therapeutic abortion is not sanctioned, but the priest should be informed when the question arises.

### VACUUM ASPIRATION

First trimester abortions are frequently carried out by vacuum aspiration, using the Karman-type catheter, a flexible polyethylene tube 6 or 8 mm in diameter: near the tip are two eyes with convex upper borders that act as a curette. Otherwise the Friedman curette is used after suction to ensure complete evacuation. There is less bleeding at 7 than at 10 weeks and some do not consider an injection of ergometrine to be necessary; others give 0·25 mg ergometrine i.v. prior to suction or on completion of the operation.

A cervical smear and high vaginal swab are taken; an intra-cervical block is given using 1 per cent lignocaine. The patient is told to report to the hospital any bleeding in excess of the menstrual flow, feverishness or pain. Contraceptive advice is given.

Prostaglandin $E_2$ may be used for mid-trimester abortion (15–21 weeks) using the extra-amniotic route. The average injection-abortion interval is 14 hours. Vomiting may occur. The Central Midwives Board (Scotland) permits midwives to 'top-up' Prostaglandin $E_2$ via an extra-amniotic catheter if they have received instruction. They may refuse on conscientious grounds.

'See page 160 re administration of Rh anti-D immunoglobulin'.

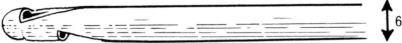

Fig. 10-13　Karman aspiration catheter—6-8-10 mm; length 24 cm.

*Courtesy Rocket Ltd., Watford, England.*

### MENSTRUAL REGULATION (*ASPIRATION*)

**When the menstrual period is less than 14 days** overdue and the woman has reason to suspect that she is pregnant, menstrual regulation is carried out. She may or may not be pregnant, and a negative pregnancy test at this early stage is not reliable. Thirty per cent are not pregnant.

The usual investigations are made: general diseases, Hb, Rh factor, cervical cytology; permission forms are signed. Some inject lignocaine 12 ml of one per cent into the cervix. The procedure confirms that no pregnancy exists or terminates an existing one. A sterile polyethylene Karman catheter, diameter 4 to 6 mm is inserted into the uterus and an adequate source of vacuum for suction used: a 50 ml syringe being commonly employed. The woman is usually fit to leave within two hours.

Written instructions are given re (a) taking temperature, (b) slight bleeding, (c) slight pain, (d) reporting back in one week or earlier if necessary, (e) refraining from sexual intercourse for one week.

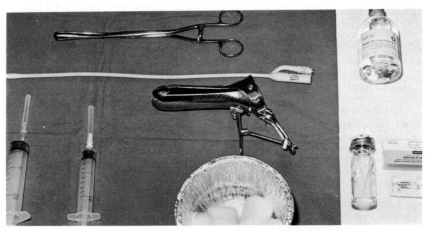

Fig. 10-14　Prostaglandin in $E_2$ for extra-amniotic infusion.

*Royal Maternity Hospital, Glasgow.*

### CRIMINAL ABORTION

A criminal abortion is one performed when the conditions set out in the Abortion Act, 1967, as described on page 167, are not fulfilled. As the name implies, the procedure is illegal and is punishable by imprisonment. Abortionists usually resort to vaginal interference: many are unqualified persons having little knowledge of asepsis.

The midwife must, under no circumstances give advice or information which could result in an illegal abortion; neither should she assist any person to perform an illegal abortion.

Injuries such as perforation of the pouch of Douglas and laceration of the uterus have been known to be inflicted. Sudden death can occur due to the introduction into the uterus of soap solutions, pastes, and from air embolism. Sepsis and acute renal failure may cause death. Acute renal failure has resulted from forcible douching with soap solution as an abortifacient; this causes blood haemolysis and destruction of the tubular epithelium of the kidney.

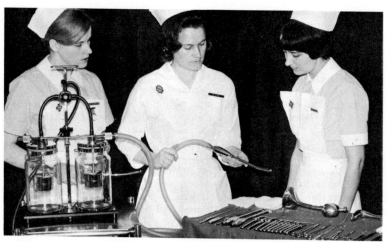

Fig. 10-15  Non-sterile set up for clinical instruction. Electric vacuum pump for evacuation of uterus.

*Simpson Memorial Maternity Pavilion, Edinburgh.*

## SEPTIC ABORTION

This serious condition is usually associated with incomplete abortion, and particularly if it has been induced criminally. The condition is similar to *puerperal sepsis* following childbirth and is a *notifiable disease* in Scotland. Infertility and ill health may ensue; the mortality rate is high. In some of these cases the doctor is not called until sepsis is well developed, therefore antibiotics are not given early enough to combat the infection and prevent complications.

### SIGNS AND SYMPTOMS

**Uterus.** Tender on palpation.          **Pulse.** Rapid.

**Lochia.** Offensive and profuse.          **Temperature.** Raised.

**Abdominal pain** may or may not be present.

### *Management*

When a patient who is in the process of aborting develops an elevated temperature or rapid pulse, or is admitted to hospital with these signs, barrier nursing should be instituted immediately, or, better still, she should be removed to a single room until the diagnosis is confirmed, when she will be transferred to an isolation hospital. Clinical, bacteriological and haematological investigations, including the degree of leucocytosis, are made as in puerperal sepsis. A blood culture is made in serious cases. *Cl. Welchii* or *E. Coli* may be the causal organism. A specimen of urine is sent for bacteriological examination. Vaginal interference is usually avoided, unless severe bleeding occurs, until the infection is controlled.

**Ampicillin, 500 mg,** may be given, followed by 250 mg 6 hourly. A blood transfusion is given if necessary. (*After 24 hours when the bacteriological report is received the appropriate antibiotic is administered.*)

**Metronidazole** (Flagyl) has been used with success in anaerobic infections.

**Electrolyte control** is necessary, daily.

The medical and nursing treatment is similar to what is necessary for puerperal sepsis.

After the first 12 hours the main concern is kidney function. A careful watch must be kept on renal function: the fluid balance being accurately recorded. (See acute renal failure, p. 219.

### BACTERAEMIC (ENDOTOXIC) SHOCK

In obstetrics endotoxic shock is most frequently associated with septic criminal abortion. When a patient suffering from severe septicaemia exhibits a low cardiac-output-state this is usually due to the endotoxins released into the circulation from Gram-negative organisms, commonly *E. Coli.*

#### SIGNS AND SYMPTOMS

The degree of hypotension is always greater than any blood loss warrants: the blood pressure may be unrecordable.

**Tachycardia, cyanosis,** cold moist skin.

**The temperature** may or may not be high.

**Oliguria** is a serious sign. **Mental confusion and coma** are terminal manifestations.

#### *Treatment*

**Blood and urine are cultured:** cervical and throat swabs are taken.

**Blood gases and electrolytes** are monitored.

**A wide spectrum antibiotic** in full doses is prescribed.

**Intravenous infusion of fresh blood and glucose** 5 per cent is administered to maintain cardiac output.

**Electrolytes are given** to correct the metabolic acidosis. **The amount of urine secreted** is monitored.

**Corticosteroids** may be given for a few days to combat circulatory failure.

**The central venous pressure** is noted.

### ABORTION COUNSELLING (BY MIDWİVES)

**The counselling process is a humane service,** supportive and informative rather than advisory or directional: no attempt being made to influence the pregnant woman by persuasion or coercion. After the various alternatives have been explained to her she personally, must make the decisions.

The midwife's approach to termination of pregnancy should be unbiased: therefore those with religious, moral or conscientious objections should not become counsellors. It is almost certain that the woman will be in a state of emotional anguish and this is more likely in the unsupported expectant mother: forty-nine per cent of whom are single, many under 15 years of age: 8 per cent are widowed, separated or divorced: 43 per cent are married.

#### THE UNWED EXPECTANT MOTHER

**For the single girl an unwanted pregnancy creates a very complex situation.** She is distressed regarding the disclosure of a sexual relationship: the putative father may not be free to marry; if single he may be deeply concerned; on the other hand he could be indifferent, hostile, even deserting her. Her parents are likely to be disturbed and disapproving; they may use pressures regarding marriage or adoption which are not acceptable to the girl; some are unsupportive. She is concerned that her education might be curtailed, her career jeopardised and her future matrimonial prospects diminished. Some are depressed and threaten to commit suicide.

To gain the girl's confidence she should be interviewed in a quiet private room, encouraged to talk and to ask questions. By making sympathetic enquiries about her parents and home life, leading on to whether she is cohabiting, the relationship stable and the putative father's response helpful. Her reaction to pregnancy should be sought and what she feels about the situation, the baby and its future. Her fears, problems and tentative plans should be discussed and in so doing a solution may emerge. Alternative arrangements, their advantages and disadvantages could be considered, e.g. marriage; a one parent family, the baby being cared for by herself, by her parents or fostered.

**If adoption is proposed** the 1976 Children Act whereby the adopted child at 18 years may try to trace his parents, should be mentioned. What is best for the baby could be proposed as a basis for the final course of action.

**Termination of pregnancy may be what she is determined to have:** her reasons for this should be examined closely but, the agonising decision must be made by the girl herself. The counsellor should be aware of the need for quick action so that if the decision to terminate is made, this can be carried out before the 10th or 12th week.

### THE COUNSELLOR

**An abortion counsellor should have a mature personality** and kindly disposition: she should be tactful and uncensorious. Her attitude to abortion should be impartial and pressure for or against should not be applied. The midwife-counsellor should be aware of adolescent behaviour in the permissive society today: she may not approve of the lax trends in sexuality nor the practice of cohabitation but her counsel must be non-judgmental, her outlook tolerant. Understanding of human nature and all its frailties is needed when dealing with persons having differing intelligence, social background, maturity and emotional stability.

Midwives who wish to undertake the role of counsellor to women with unwanted pregnancies should have specific knowledge of counselling, suitable personal attributes and advanced knowledge of all aspects of the situation and the facilities available, medical and social.

**Skill in handling people successfully is of vital concern** not only to the counsellor but to the hospital midwife who attends the girl before and after termination of pregnancy: the sophisticated type may resent the humiliation of the situation and adopt a blasé, almost belligerent attitude. Mature, married, midwives are usually capable of handling such girls judiciously and sympathetically.

**Additional knowledge and deeper insight** into the varied aspects of the situation are needed over and above what has been attained during the midwife's nursing and midwifery education. She would be well advised to attend a course in counselling.

**The following are some of the subjects that need further study.** The role of the Health Visitor and Social Worker; psychology of sexuality; the permissive society; marriage and the nuclear family; the one parent family; fertility control; schoolgirl pregnancy and its effects; the unmarried father, his reaction and responsibilities; pressures exerted by the putative father and the parents; facilities for unwed mothers; statutory and voluntary agencies; mother and baby homes; fostering; state benefits; legal aid; affiliation order; alimony; adoption procedures and societies; abortion procedures including 'menstrual regulation,' all aspects of termination of pregnancy; emotional trauma after abortion and more permanently, after adoption.

# ECTOPIC GESTATION

If the fertilised ovum embeds outside the uterus, the condition is known as an ectopic or extra-uterine pregnancy. Most commonly it is tubal, but it may occasionally be abdominal and very rarely ovarian. If the passage of the zygote is delayed by the effects of previous salpingitis, or by spasm, or the kinking of a long tube, it will embed in the Fallopian tube. When the chorionic villi penetrate tubal blood vessels the haemorrhage that occurs greatly distends the tube.

## *Three Possible Terminations of a Tubal Pregnancy*

### Tubal abortion

The lining of the tube ruptures, the ovum and blood escape into the lumen of the tube and are then expelled through the fimbriated end into the peritoneal cavity.

### Tubal mole

It is similar to a uterine blood mole (p. 167) and develops when the ovum in the tube dies and becomes surrounded by layers of blood clot.

### Tubal rupture

Rupture may occur into the peritoneal cavity, or more rarely between the folds of the broad ligament, and usually take place between the sixth and tenth week. When the zygote embeds in the ampulla, any of the three terminations just mentioned may take place, but when embedding takes place in the narrow isthmus, rupture of the tube usually occurs about the sixth week.

### SIGNS OF TUBAL PREGNANCY

The early signs of tubal pregnancy are very similar to those of threatened abortion, but in abortion, bleeding precedes pain and is more profuse than in ectopic gestation. Recurrent spasmodic pain, low on one side of the abdomen, which is increased during defaecation and often accompanied by nausea and faintness. A history of having missed one or two periods is elicited in 60 per cent of cases; the early signs of pregnancy such as breast changes and morning sickness may be present. Slight dark brown vaginal discharge (which comes from the decidua). Laparoscopy may be used when the diagnosis is in doubt.

It is the midwife's duty to get medical assistance for any abnormality in pregnancy, and if these early warning signs are overlooked the prognosis will be more grave.

### SIGNS OF TUBAL RUPTURE

The general condition of the patient is always worse than the slight vaginal bleeding warrants. Severe abdominal pain. Signs of internal haemorrhage.

## *Treatment*

Should such a catastrophe occur, the midwife will send for medical aid, treat the patient for shock by the application of blankets: some raise the foot of the bed. If the need for blood transfusion is obvious the 'flying squad' should be called. The patient will be transferred to hospital for immediate salpingectomy, blood transfusion being given before, during and following operation as is necessary.

*In only 60 per cent of cases will tubal rupture give rise to the acute signs described above; when rupture is gradual, signs of internal haemorrhage and shock may not be obvious.*

### Abdominal pregnancy

Abdominal pregnancy is very rare, and occurs when the intact fetal sac is expelled from the tube into the abdominal cavity and the chorionic villi become attached to omentum, intestine, or perimetrium and re-embed. If the fetus subsequently dies, it may become surrounded with lime salts and form a lithopaedion or stone fetus. Should the fetus live, the abdominal pregnancy may go to term, when an abdominal section will be necessary. A few cases have been recorded in which the baby was born alive. In view of the grave risk of haemorrhage as there are no 'living ligatures' to control bleeding from the placental site, it is usual to leave the placenta *in situ*, where it will be absorbed by the lymphatics and peritoneum.

### Ovarian pregnancy (very rare)

The spermatozoon fertilises the ovum before it has been expelled from the ruptured Graafian follicle—bleeding into the substance of the ovary occurs. The signs and symptoms are similar to those of tubal pregnancy, but the Fallopian tube is found to be intact at laparotomy.

# HYDATIDIFORM MOLE

## Molar Pregnancy: vesicular mole

A hydatidiform mole is a mass of vesicles resulting from cystic proliferation of chorionic epithelium. Some moles are simple, a few are malignant. The distended villi form vesicles varying in size from a pin-head to a small grape. This process begins about the sixth week of pregnancy, and the embryo is absorbed. The exuberant growth of the chorionic villi gives rise to the production of excessive quantities of chorionic gonadotrophin, and large amounts are excreted in the urine.

#### SIGNS AND SYMPTOMS

Vaginal bleeding, beginning about the 12th week, is the earliest sign, and the discharge may be bright red and profuse, or brown due to the presence of old blood. The vesicles, which have been likened to 'white currants in red currant juice', are rarely found until actual expulsion of the mole is taking place.

Undue enlargement of the uterus occurs in the majority of cases and a woman with 12 weeks' amenorrhoea may have a uterus the size of a 24 weeks' pregnancy. But if the mole becomes detached from the uterine wall the uterus may be normal in size or even less than normal. The uterus has an elastic consistency; pain and tenderness, if present, are due to its excessive distension by the mole or blood clot.

Fetal movement will not have been felt. The fetal heart-beat is not heard.

Fetal parts will not be detected on palpation.

Vomiting is often present. Pre-eclampsia occurs in about 30 per cent of cases.

#### DIAGNOSIS

A quantitative chorionic gonadotrophin test is a valuable aid to diagnosis, and when the Pregnosticon test is positive in urine dilutions of 1 in 500, this is diagnostic.

An ultrasonic scan at 15–17 weeks is used with greater certainty than any other method (see Fig. 10-17). The Doppler effect cardioscope has also been used to rule out the presence of a live fetus.

#### Treatment

The patient is admitted to hospital and kept in bed.

Routine blood examination and urine analysis are carried out.

Cross-matched blood should be at hand.

Vulval swabbing carried out twice daily: pads carefully inspected.

Moles may be removed by hysterotomy or suction curettage, but many are evacuated with the aid of Syntocinon infusions. Some use prostaglandin $E_2$.

Hysterectomy is sometimes performed in women over the age of 40.

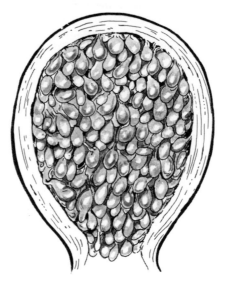

Fig. 10-16    Uterus with hydatidiform mole *in situ*.

If intravenous ergometrine does not control severe haemorrhage a gauze pack may be inserted into the uterus and removed within six hours. After operation the midwife must keep a close watch on the patient's pulse and also for vaginal bleeding.

### DANGERS

**Haemorrhage** which, before, during and after evacuation, may be sudden and profuse.

**Sepsis,** which is combated by strict aseptic technique and prevention of blood loss.

**Erosion of the uterine wall.** After evacuation of a mole, chorionic villi may remain deep in the uterine wall forming an invasive mole. Occasionally these perforate the uterus causing internal haemorrhage.

**Choriocarcinoma.** This tumour ensues in about 3 per cent of cases but their development as well as that of dangerous invasive moles can be detected by measuring chorionic gonadotrophin in the serum or urine by radioimmunoassay. Tests are done every two weeks till the tests are normal, then monthly for a year, then 3 monthly for a second year. Curettage and arteriography are used to confirm a diagnosis of choriocarcinoma. Hysterectomy is not usually necessary but if so is deferred till after cytotoxic chemotherapy.

### CYTOTOXIC CHEMOTHERAPY

About 95 per cent of these tumours are now cured by drugs. Early diagnosis is important. Methotrexate with folinic acid, cures some patients but others require treatment with actinomycin D, vincristine, cyclophosphamide, hydroxyurea,

6-mercaptopurine, VP 16213 and other drugs. Treatment is continued till chorionic gonadotrophin values have been normal for many weeks.

Patients may be registered with a central laboratory for follow-up. If the radioimmunoassay urinary test for chorionic gonadotrophin is positive the woman is referred to Charing Cross Hospital (Fulham). The Jessop Hospital, Sheffield and the University of Dundee are also collaborating.

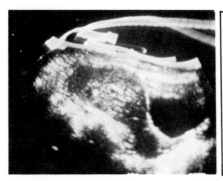
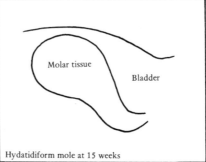

Hydatidiform mole at 15 weeks

Fig. 10-17   Hydatidiform mole. Ultrasonogram. White speckled area indicates the mole (left arrow). (Lower arrow indicates the cervix.)

*By courtesy of Queen Mother's Hospital, Glasgow.*

## QUESTIONS FOR REVISION

### VAGINAL BLEEDING

Mention the various causes of bleeding early in pregnancy: From the **Cervix** (3); **Moles** (3); **Abortion** (6); **Other Causes** (3).

Define ectopic gestation and describe the signs of tubal pregnancy before and after rupture of the tube.

**C.M.B.(Scot.) 30-min. question.** A patient who is two months pregnant complains of vaginal bleeding. Outline the possible causes.

Give reasons why the following procedures are necessary in cases of threatened abortion: (*a*) No enema is given for 48 hours; (*b*) All vaginal discharge is saved for inspection. Give three general and three local causes of abortion. What are the signs and dangers of hydatidiform mole? What drugs and equipment would you anticipate might be used in cases of: (1) missed abortion; (2) ruptured ectopic; (3) insertion of Shirodkar's suture; (4) hydatidiform mole; (5) evacuation of uterus for incomplete abortion.

**Differentiate between:** inevitable and incomplete abortion; blood mole and carneous mole; uterine, ectopic and abdominal pregnancy: therapeutic and criminal abortion.

**Give alternative names for:** abortion; fleshy mole; tubal pregnancy.

What special investigations are made in: (*a*) missed abortion; (*b*) septic abortion; (*c*) hydatidiform mole; (*d*) habitual abortion.

Define cervical incompetence; therapeutic abortion; bacteraemic shock; choriocarcinoma.

What questions would you ask a woman who has slight vaginal bleeding in early pregnancy? What first aid treatment would you give for serious bleeding from an inevitable abortion? What are the midwife's responsibilities: (*a*) when a Shirodkar's suture has been inserted? (*b*) in dealing with severe haemorrhage from an incomplete abortion in a remote area?

**C.M.B.(Scot.).** A patient gives a history of 16 weeks amenorrhoea. On abdominal examination the size of the uterus corresponds to 24 weeks gestation. What are the possible causes of this discrepancy? How is a differential diagnosis made?

**(N. Ireland).** (*a*) Describe the vagina and its anatomical relations. (*b*) What are the causes of bleeding per vaginam during pregnancy?

**C.M.B.(Scot.) 30-min. question.** Describe the clinical features of a case of inevitable abortion at the third month of pregnancy. In the presence of severe bleeding while the patient is still at home, what emergency treatment would you carry out pending the arrival of medical assistance?

**C.M.B.(Scot.) 30-min question.** Give an account of the causes of vaginal bleeding before the 28th week of pregnancy. How would this be investigated?

**(N. Ireland) 30-min. question.** What clinical signs and symptoms would make you expect a hydatidiform mole? Describe the investigation and possible complications of such a case.

*C.M.B. Short Examination Questions*

**Eng.:** Bleeding per vaginam in the first 12 weeks of pregnancy. **Scot.:** Inevitable abortion. **Eng.:** Ectopic pregnancy. **Scot.:** Threatened and missed abortion. **Eng.:** Incompetent cervix. **Eng.:** Hydatidiform mole. **Scot.** Habitual abortion. **Eng.:** Inevitable and Incomplete Abortion. **Scot.:** Cervical incompetence. **Eng.:** Termination of pregnancy before the 24th week. **Scot.:** Therapeutic abortion.

## Counselling

How would the midwife prepare to undertake counselling? What is meant by the nuclear family? The putative father? Menstrual regulation? What agencies are available to assist the unwed mother? What is an unsupported mother? Describe the personal attributes and mode of approach of the good counsellor.

# 11
# Polyhydramnios—Uterine Abnormalities

*Chronic and acute polyhydramnios. Oligohydramnios. Uterine malformations and displacements. Fibromyomata. Ovarian cysts.*

In polyhydramnios the amount of fluid in the amniotic sac exceeds the normal quantity of 500 to 1,500 ml but is not as a rule clinically apparent until the amount is over 3,000 ml. During a period of 10 years in the Simpson Maternity Pavilion five patients had over 12 litres of fluid, the maximum being 15·6 litres. Polyhydramnios occurs in about 1 in 200 pregnancies. The cause is unknown, but the condition is associated with monozygotic (uniovular) twins and with pathological conditions, both fetal and maternal.

**Monstrosities and malformations** such as anencephaly and spina bifida are common, and it is possible that in these conditions transudation of cerebrospinal fluid, through the exposed meninges, occurs into the amniotic sac. The fact that polyhydramnios occurs when the oesophagus is imperforate, gives credence to the idea that the inability of the fetus to swallow amniotic fluid may be a causative factor. About 25 per cent of pregnant diabetic women have marked polyhydramnios; a number having it in lesser degree.

## CLINICAL TYPES OF POLYHYDRAMNIOS

**Acute polyhydramnios** is very rare. It usually occurs just prior to mid-term, comes on suddenly, and in three or four days' time the uterus is so excessively distended that the fundus reaches the xiphisternum. Monozygotic twins or some fetal abnormality is usually present but the uterus may be so tense that it is impossible to detect fetal parts. Abdominal pain may be severe, vomiting troublesome and if pressure symptoms are causing distress the membranes are punctured. The most common outcome is spontaneous abortion.

**Chronic polyhydramnios** is the common type, which comes on slowly, usually about the 30th week. When the amount of fluid is excessive, the term 'gross polyhydramnios' is applied, and in such a case it is usual to find a severe fetal malformation.

### SIGNS AND SYMPTOMS

**On inspection**

The uterus is large, and at term the girth is over 1 m (the author having seen a case in which the girth was 1·37 m).

The shape of the uterus is globular rather than ovoid.

The abdominal wall is thin and tense, the skin shiny with prominent veins and marked striae gravidarum.

**On palpation**

Palpation of the fetus is difficult, because it recedes from the examining fingers, but can be ballotted between the two hands. To facilitate palpation the woman may be turned on her side or placed in the knee-elbow position, and by deep percussion of the dependent part of the abdomen, fetal parts can be detected.

A fluid thrill can be elicited by laying the palm of the left hand in close contact with one side of the uterus, and on giving a sharp flick or tap on the other side of the uterus with the fingers of the right hand the wave of fluid transmitted is felt by the left hand. It is desirable to use a third hand to interrupt the fluid wave along the abdominal wall (see Fig. 11-2).

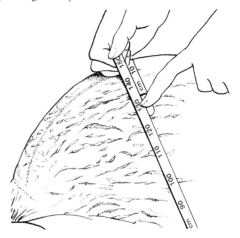

Fig. 11-1    Measuring abdominal girth in a case of polyhydramnios.

## On auscultation

The fetal heart-beat is muffled and may be inaudible because of the density of fluid.

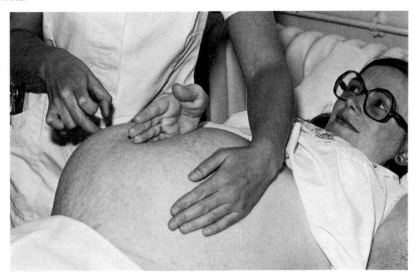

Fig. 11-2    Eliciting the fluid thrill. Patient's hand used.
*Royal Maternity Hospital, Glasgow.*

## Diagnostic aids

An ultrasonic scan reveals polyhydramnios as clear areas containing blob-like echo complexes (floating fetal limbs).

**On X-ray** after the 30th week twins or fetal monstrosities may be diagnosed. If there are twins the mother will want to know, so that she can prepare for two babies; if a monstrosity is present the doctor will almost certainly induce preterm labour. The excess of fluid makes the film milky or blurred in appearance; the large uterine outline can be seen.

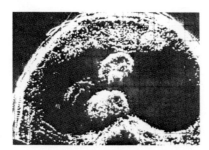

Fig. 11-3   Polyhydramnios. Ultrasonogram.
*Aberdeen Maternity Hospital.*

## THE EFFECT OF POLYHYDRAMNIOS ON PREGNANCY

Pressure symptoms may be intense and distressing.

**Oedema of the vulva** and lower limbs is present in severe cases. Dyspnoea and palpitation may be disturbing, especially at night, interfering with rest and sleep. Extra pillows will give some relief, but a sedative may be necessary. Vague abdominal discomfort and pain in the region of the lower ribs may be complained of: if distension is severe, extra rest in bed should be advised. **Indigestion,** heartburn and constipation are more troublesome. **The urine is examined for glucose** because of the association with diabetes.

**Abdominal amniocentesis** is rarely carried out to relieve extreme discomfort, but unfortunately the fluid accumulates again very rapidly and in some cases the procedure tends to induce labour. A 50 ml syringe, two-way stop-cock and spinal needle are required; as much as 3,000 ml may be withdrawn, but 600 to 1,200 ml is more usual. **The bladder must first be emptied.**

### EFFECT ON LABOUR

**Prolapse of cord.** If the membranes are allowed to rupture spontaneously the cord is usually swept down with the rush of fluid. A vaginal examination should be made immediately.

**Malpresentations** although common, because the fetus can move freely *in utero*, can be easily corrected.

**Preterm labour** is likely to increase the danger to the fetus.

**Postpartum haemorrhage** may take place because of the over-stretched and ineffectual uterine muscle. (*Some doubt this.*)

### *Treatment of Polyhydramnios*

Treatment is directed towards avoiding or dealing with the complications. In view of the risks involved and the high perinatal mortality rate, the woman should be delivered in an obstetric hospital, and it is advisable to admit her for complete rest during the last two weeks of pregnancy, or earlier if possible.

The membranes are punctured prior to or when labour starts (*any malpresentation having first been rectified*) for the following reasons: in order to reduce the size of the uterus so that contractions will be more effective and to allow the presenting part to sink into the lower pole of the uterus, in order to stimulate the cervical nerve endings.

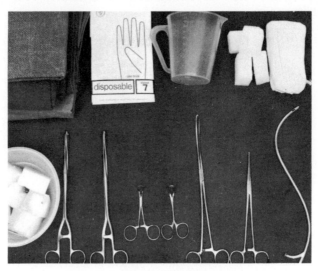

Fig. 11-4    Puncture of membranes.

**LINEN: DRESSINGS**

Lithotomy sheet or towels.
Foam swabs: perineal pad.
Measuring jug: lotion bowl.
Gloves: gown: hand towel.

**INSTRUMENTS: METAL WARE**

2 Swab holding forceps.
2 Towel clips.
1 Drew Smythe's catheter.
1 Stiles' or Goodwin's
   amniotomy forceps.

**NON-STERILE**

Fetal stethoscope: obstetric cream and lotion.

*Aberdeen Maternity Hospital.*

The woman empties her bladder. A sedative is usually given. After cleansing the vulva amniotomy forceps are used to puncture the fore-waters: some puncture the hind waters, taking care to avoid a low-lying placenta. Others insert a metal catheter to drain the amniotic fluid into a measuring jug; or they insert the hand to surround the cervix and stem the rush of fluid *for the following reasons.*

Prolapse of cord is less likely to occur. Fetal and maternal distress are avoided; the fetal heart being carefully noted. Premature separation of the placenta (antepartum haemorrhage) does not occur so readily when the size of the uterus is slowly reduced.

**An oxytocin drip is given simultaneously;** starting cautiously with 0·5 units in 540 ml glucose, 5 per cent, at 1·2 ml per minute and increasing 0·3 ml every half hour to 2·4 ml. If no response a new bottle with 2 units is begun and increased as formerly. When labour is established no increase in rate or dosage is made.

The baby should be held upside down at birth for a few seconds to drain the fluid from the respiratory passages; a No. 14 F.G. oesophageal catheter is passed into the stomach and fluid is aspirated with a syringe to avoid its regurgitation and inhalation. The passage of the oesophageal catheter is a necessary means of diagnosing the oesophageal atresia which may be present.

## OLIGOHYDRAMNIOS

In this rare condition there is a gross deficiency in the amount of amniotic fluid, the total being probably less than 60 ml. It is associated with congenital absence of the kidneys and with intra uterine fetal growth retardation. Certain deformities, such as talipes, may develop because of pressure on the fetus: amputation of limbs due to adhesions between the amnion and the tiny embryo are sometimes attributed to this cause. The baby's skin is dry and leathery in appearance.

## UTERINE MALFORMATIONS

The bicornuate or double uterus is a rare malformation due to a developmental error, and in some cases there is complete duplication of uterus, cervix and vagina. When pregnancy occurs in one horn, the other also enlarges and forms a decidua. Abortion is common. If the septum extends only part way down the centre of the uterus, a transverse lie may be present, the fetus lying with its head in one horn, breech in the other. Attempts at external version do not succeed in such cases.

The condition is usually diagnosed on vaginal examination during pregnancy, but the author recalls one case being diagnosed during labour, in which the cervix was said to be 'fully dilated' by one midwife and cervix 'not taken up' by the other; each having inserted her fingers into different halves of a septate vagina. The labour was completed spontaneously.

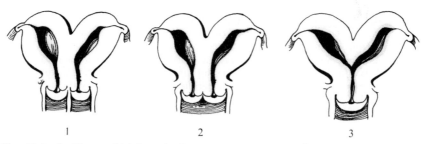

Fig. 11-5  1, Uterus didelphys, duplication of body of uterus, cervix and vagina. 2, duplication of uterus and cervix, single vagina. 3, Duplication of uterus, single cervix and vagina.

**The course of labour may not be affected,** but if the non-pregnant horn fills the pelvic cavity it will obstruct labour. In order to avert such an outcome Caesarean section would be performed.

## DISPLACEMENTS OF THE PREGNANT UTERUS

**Retroversion** may be congenital or it may be a sequela of previous childbearing, during which the uterine ligaments and the pelvic floor have been over-stretched. No attempt is made to rectify a backwardly displaced uterus during pregnancy unless it is giving rise to discomfort or pain.

*There are two possibilities in the outcome of retroversion in pregnancy:*

**Spontaneous rectification** is the more likely. At the 12th week the uterus, now globular in shape, rises above the pelvic brim, and becomes anteverted.

**Incarceration** of the retroverted gravid uterus is a rare condition in which the backwardly displaced pregnant uterus becomes imprisoned in the pelvic cavity and does not rise above the pelvic brim after the 12th week.

The chief complaint is of some disturbance of bladder function between the 12th and 16th weeks of pregnancy. Retention of urine gives rise to low abdominal pain, and the woman states that she cannot pass urine. The bladder can be palpated as a tense fluctuating swelling, which may reach well above the umbilicus. But when paradoxical incontinence (the overflow of retention) is present, the inexperienced midwife may not associate it with an over-distended bladder.

### *Treatment*

The midwife should send for medical assistance. While awaiting his arrival, she ought to pass a fine plastic disposable catheter to withdraw the urine slowly: if the rectum is loaded an enema should be given. The doctor will manually correct the displacement and insert a Hodge pessary, which is worn for four or six weeks. Except in the very mild cases, the woman is admitted to hospital for a few days; a self-retaining catheter is inserted for 48 hours (with closed drainage system or air-sealed polythene bag to reduce the risk of infection).

**The results of incarceration,** i.e. sacculation of the anterior wall of the uterus, exfoliative cystitis, rupture of bladder are extremely rare and would only occur in areas where doctors and qualified midwives were not available to recognise and deal with incarceration.

#### ANTEVERSION AND ANTEFLEXION

In multiparous women, the abdominal wall may be so lax, because of repeated childbearing, that it fails to provide the necessary support for the pregnant uterus. When the fundus leans forwards and the abdomen is unduly prominent this is known as anterior obliquity of the uterus. Sometimes the rectus muscles are widely separated and the uterus leans so far forwards that it hangs downwards, giving rise to a *pendulous abdomen*. To relieve pain and discomfort in walking, and to support the weight of the uterus, a well-fitting maternity corset should be worn. **Anteversion of the uterus in a primigravida is a serious matter,** usually indicating pelvic contraction or spinal deformity which so limits the accommodation for the pregnant uterus that it is forced outwards. In such a case the woman should be seen by an obstetrician.

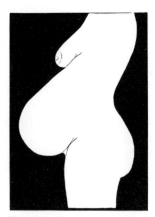

Fig. 11-6   Pendulous abdomen.

Such obliquity may give rise to malpresentation during labour. The force of the uterine action will also be misdirected and labour will be prolonged. To avoid this a firm binder should be worn during labour and the woman advised to lie on her back propped up until the fetal head has entered the pelvis.

### Prolapse of the pregnant uterus

This type of displacement is very rare because the woman with a prolapsed uterus does not usually become pregnant. A ring pessary is inserted, and worn until the uterus rises out of the pelvic cavity. In cases where the cervix protrudes outside the vulva, the woman should be confined to bed and any cervical abrasions treated. Strict aseptic precautions must be observed because of the risk of sepsis.

## THE EFFECT OF FIBROMYOMATA ON CHILDBEARING

Fibroids are most commonly found in older primigravidae. The situation of these tumours has an important bearing on the outcome, depending on whether they are in the upper or lower uterine segment and into which of the three coats of the uterus they permeate. From 5 to 50 small fibroids may be scattered throughout the uterine wall and infertility may exist when they encroach on the endometrium. The large fibroid can be palpated as a firm mass during pregnancy and after the expulsion of the baby.

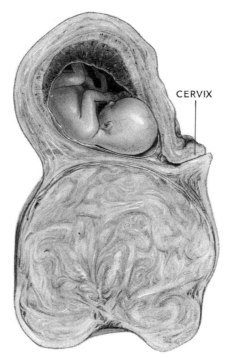

CERVIX

Fig. 11-7 Fibroid tumour in pregnant uterus. The fibroid being in the lower segment of the uterus and measuring 11 to 12 cm, would have filled the pelvic cavity and obstructed labour.

*Simpson Memorial Maternity Pavilion, Edinburgh.*

Abortion may take place. Red degeneration of the fibroid may occur and give rise to pain and uterine tenderness: palliative measures are often successfully employed—rest in bed and sedatives. Very rarely in pregnancy is a fibroid so large as to cause real distress, and if so, myomectomy is sometimes performed; unfortunately the operation tends to induce abortion. During labour a fibroid in the lower pole of the uterus may cause malpresentation. Very rarely does a fibroid tumour obstruct labour; when situated in the corpus, it rises out of the true pelvis with the growing uterus, but if situated in the lower pole, obstruction may occur. Subendometrial fibroids may cause postpartum haemorrhage if situated in the placental site area. During involution the fibroids become reduced in size, but if they have been bruised during labour they may cause subinvolution and profuse red lochia.

## OVARIAN CYSTS

The presence of a fluctuating swelling alongside the uterus would necessitate seeking medical aid. Pressure symptoms will exist if the cyst is large, and torsion may occur during pregnancy or the puerperium, giving rise to acute pain and vomiting. Very rarely a *pedunculated ovarian cyst* will occupy the pelvic cavity, preventing engagement of the head, and if not diagnosed will obstruct labour.

---

## QUESTIONS FOR REVISION

### POLYHYDRAMNIOS

**Give the term for:**

Insufficiency of amniotic fluid; an excessive amount of amniotic fluid; withdrawing fluid through the abdominal wall; retroverted uterus imprisoned in the pelvic cavity.

**Why is it advisable?**

To examine the urine for glucose in cases of polyhydramnios?
To make a vaginal examination when the membranes rupture?
To drain off the amniotic fluid slowly?
To puncture the membranes at the onset of labour?
How could the midwife help to alleviate the discomforts of polyhydramnios? Why should delivery take place in hospital? How would you differentiate between polyhydramnios and multiple pregnancy?

**C.M.B.(Scot.) 30-min. question.** Discuss the differential diagnosis of undue enlargement of the abdomen in the latter part of pregnancy.

**C.M.B.(Scot.) 30-min. question.** Describe the diagnosis and management of polyhydramnios at the 32nd week of pregnancy.

**(N. Ire.) 30-min. question.** What conditions are associated with polyhydramnios? Describe how this condition may affect the course of labour.

**C.M.B.(Eng.) 30-min. question.** How can polyhydramnios be recognised in the antenatal period? What is the significance of this condition?

**Retroversion**

Give the causes of retroversion of the uterus, and state which symptoms would indicate the necessity for medical assistance. What complications may arise when pregnancy occurs in a retroverted uterus?

**C.M.B.(Eng.) 30-min. question.** What conditions may cause retention of urine during pregnancy and the puerperium? What dangers may result from it?

# 12
# Disorders due to Pregnancy

*Hyperemesis gravidarum, management, nursing care. Pre-eclampsia: Eclampsia, obstetric management and nursing care: Essential hypertension*

## HYPEREMESIS GRAVIDARUM

Hyperemesis differs from morning sickness in that the vomiting persists throughout the day and the woman's health becomes impaired. The combination of vomiting, nausea and anorexia can produce an undesirable state of malnutrition, which results in a profound metabolic disturbance that may be fatal. **Women are very apt to neglect morning sickness** and many cases of hyperemesis might have been 'nipped in the bud' had the woman sought advice sooner. The midwife may treat cases of morning sickness, but refers cases of hyperemesis to the doctor.

In women who have a 'sensitive' nervous system, morning sickness is more likely to develop into hyperemesis. It is known that the emotions stimulate the sympathetic nervous system which in turn probably influences the endocrine system.

All the pathological changes which take place in the liver, kidneys, heart and brain can be explained as being due to deprivation of certain constituents of food, as well as the ketosis, dehydration, avitaminosis and electrolyte imbalance that are present. Potassium deficiency causes muscle weakness particularly of the cardiac muscle. Vomiting produces potassium deficiency and this induces further vomiting.

### SIGNS AND SYMPTOMS

These vary according to the length of time vomiting has persisted, and the severity of the condition. In a moderately severe case the woman usually gives a history of persistent nausea and vomiting for a week or more, and in some cases, intermittently for three or four weeks. Loss of weight is a reliable sign of persistent vomiting.

**The patient is apathetic,** weak and miserable. **The eyes are dull** and sunken.

**Pulse rapid: blood pressure low.**

**The skin is dingy** and inelastic. **The tongue is brown,** thickly coated or red and raw.

**The teeth are covered with sordes,** the lips cracked and sore.

**The breath is offensive** and smells of acetone.

**The urine:—dark in colour,** high specific gravity, contains ketones, low chlorides.

**Constipation is present,** due to starvation and dehydration.

### Admission to Hospital

All but the mildest cases should be admitted to hospital, and this appears to have a beneficial effect: the home surroundings being associated with nausea and retching, and relatives may have been too sympathetic or too indifferent. On admission the doctor takes her history and carries out a physical examination: plasma electrolytes are estimated. Other causes of vomiting are excluded, such as urinary tract infection or hydatidiform mole.

## MANAGEMENT

The vital substances of which the woman has been seriously depleted—fluid, glucose, sodium chloride and vitamins B and C must be replaced. No food is given by mouth for at least 24 hours, in order to rest the stomach.

Fluid is urgently needed, and the intravenous route is preferred. Glucose is essential to counteract the ketosis, protect the liver and overcome the prostration. Salt is required to replenish the blood chlorides. Potassium is added to the i.v. drip if the plasma potassium is low. When marked dehydration or ketosis is present, it is usual to give 2,500 to 3,000 ml of 5 per cent glucose and isotonic saline intravenously daily for two or three days: the amount necessary being assessed by the urinary output.

A fluid balance record is kept and vomitus should not be charted under output, but recorded in a separate column.

### Drugs

The vitamin B complex is required in the metabolism of carbohydrate and for the health of nerve tissue. Parentrovite can be given intramuscularly once daily when food is not retained. Aneurine 100 mg daily is recommended.

Promazine (Sparine), 50 mg, administered 8 hourly has proved effective. Meclozine (Ancolan), cyclizine (Valoid), buclizine hydrochloride (Vibazine), prochlorperazine (Stemetil), promethazine theoclate (Avomine), pyridoxine (Benadon) are sometimes used.

Certain antihistamine and anti-emetic drugs are not given because of the possible harmful effects on the developing embryo during the first twelve weeks of pregnancy.

The patient is usually worn out with retching and from lack of sleep, but the opium derivatives tend to induce vomiting, so should not be used.

### Nursing care

The psychological aspect is important: the idea of vomiting being banished from her mind, and the best way to do so is to remove the vomit bowl. Subtle suggestion is needed, and the personality of the midwife in charge is of paramount importance, for a judicious blending of kindness, firmness and optimism is needed. The cooperation of the husband and the advice of the social worker may be needed to solve family problems.

Temperature and pulse should be taken and recorded twice daily, and in serious cases four-hourly, as the slightest increase may be significant. The blood pressure is taken twice daily, but it is low blood pressure that is being watched for—a sign of myocardial weakness.

The urine is examined on admission and twice daily for specific gravity, ketones, chlorides, and once daily for protein and bile. In serious cases these tests are done more frequently. The patient is weighed on admission, and if able to be out of bed, every second day.

### Diet

If nausea and retching persist, 48 hours may elapse before food is retained, and an effort should then be made to get the patient to take some solid food. The secret of success lies in pushing up the diet quickly, for the stomach is more likely to retain solid food than fluids. Meals should be served every two and a half hours or so, because an empty stomach contracts more violently than one which contains food.

The first meal given is a cup of tea with crisp toast or a water biscuit and marmalade jelly or honey. Tinned orange juice is preferable, being high in potassium; but too many cold sweet drinks are irritating to the stomach. Milk puddings, fruit jellies, steamed white fish are suitable.

**When the pulse is over 100,** this is a warning sign, and when over 120, weak or irregular, it denotes serious myocardial weakness.

**Temperature over** 37·2°C (99°F). Persistent proteinuria.

**Jaundice** or the presence of bile in the urine.

**Cerebral signs:**—dimness of, or double vision, nystagmus, squint, low muttering delirium and loss of memory. Drowsiness may supervene and the patient sinks into coma.

Hyperemesis gravidarum is amenable to early treatment. Fortunately, therapeutic abortion is seldom necessary and a fatal outcome rare because patients are now sent to hospital in the early stages when the prognosis is good.

# PRE-ECLAMPSIA

**Pre-eclampsia** is peculiar to pregnancy, usually becoming manifest after the 30th week, and rarely prior to the 24th week. It occurs more commonly in primigravidae, and the incidence is increased in cases of multiple pregnancy, essential hypertension, diabetes and hydatidiform mole. Pre-eclampsia is associated with placental dysfunction and if so, intra-uterine growth retardation is likely to occur. Reduced uterine blood flow is a feature of pre-eclampsia.

## The Cause is still Unknown

Increased resistance in the arterioles, due to vasospasm, is characteristic: this produces hypertension which affects the brain, liver and kidneys. Theories as to its causation are so manifold as to be outside the scope of this book: endocrine, metabolic, physiological, haematological, immunological and obstetrical investigations having been made. Recent research suggests disorders of blood coagulation associated with high levels of fibrin breakdown products.

### SIGNS

| *Mild* | *Severe* |
| --- | --- |
| **Blood pressure,** 140/90 mmHg | **Blood pressure,** 160/100 mmHg and over |
| **Proteinuria** under 0·5 g/l | **Proteinuria** over 1 g/l |
| **Oedema** may be present | **Oedema** marked |

The figures given above as mild and severe are only generalisations and not strict criteria of the severity of the condition. Individual variations occur, e.g. eclampsia or fetal death can occur with proteinuria 0·5 g/l or moderate hypertension.

HYPERTENSION

**Raised blood pressure is one of the cardinal signs of pre-eclampsia,** therefore to detect an incipient rise the woman's blood pressure should be taken early in pregnancy in order that her usual pressure is known. The height of the diastolic pressure is of greater prognostic significance than the systolic, because the diastolic pressure is not affected by posture or excitement. The diastolic pressure should be recorded at the muffling stage which is more accurate than the disappearance of sounds: when over 160/100 the fetus is in danger. An increase of 15 mm Hg is an indication for close supervision: the doctor should be notified.

PROTEINURIA

**Proteinuria is a serious sign of pre-eclampsia.** All pregnant women with proteinuria, however slight in a mid-stream specimen of urine should be admitted to hospital for investigation, close supervision, and complete rest. The amount of protein is frequently taken as an index of the severity of the condition, and when eclampsia supervenes the urine may contain as much as 12 g of protein per litre. But eclampsia may occur with only 0·5 g/l of protein in the urine.

OEDEMA

Oedema is an unreliable sign and is not now assessed in judging the severity of pre-eclampsia. Occult oedema may be suspected when there is a marked increase in weight, but this may, of course, be due to causes other than tissue-fluid retention. All pregnant women should be weighed every two weeks from the 16th to the 30th weeks of pregnancy, and if, during this critical period, 1·3 kg or more is gained in any two weeks, the increase is excessive. This should be an indication for close supervision; the woman being weighed and examined weekly.

Oedema of the ankles of slight degree, may be confused with the ankle oedema seen in about 40 per cent of pregnant women which tends to disappear with rest over night. Oedema extending up the leg, can be taken as a more serious sign. In more severe cases, the backs of the hands are massively swollen; the wedding ring is almost submerged. Puffy eyelids and bagginess under the eyes may be present in the morning only; the features are coarse and bloated. Pinard's stethoscope leaves a deep indented ring on the abdominal wall. Labial swelling is not common but can be excessive. In one case seen by the author each labium was the size of a large clenched fist. (No delay occurred during the perineal phase of delivery.)

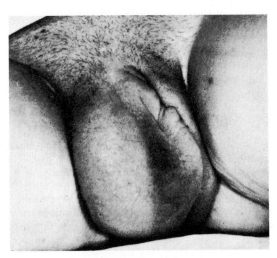

Fig. 12-1   Oedema of the vulva.

**PROPHYLAXIS**

**Prenatal visits are now made more frequently** and greater vigilance directed toward detecting early manifestations of pre-eclampsia. Women with a weight gain over 0·5 kg per week between 20–30 weeks, should be seen every two weeks to detect any rise in blood pressure and proteinuria. Particular attention is paid to cases of multiple pregnancy, diabetes and essential hypertension as these patients are more liable to develop pre-eclampsia.

*The Midwives Responsibility*

Modern prenatal care requires that urine analysis is carried out, blood pressure estimated and the woman weighed and examined for oedema at each prenatal visit. Midwives must co-operate in encouraging women to attend regularly for the frequent examinations now considered essential. Merely visiting a pregnant women in her home to enquire about her health, without carrying out the measures mentioned above, does not constitute competent prenatal care. The necessary examinations must be made, and in remote areas the midwife can transport bathroom scales in her car. Albustix reagent strips for the detection of proteinuria are available. Uristix strips detect protein and glucose simultaneously.

## DANGERS OF PRE-ECLAMPSIA

**Maternal:**

Eclampsia. Placental abruption occurs in 8 per cent of cases.

**Fetal:**

Intra-uterine growth retardation. Fetal death due to placental dysfunction. During labour insufficient placental oxygen reserve may cause anoxia. Neonatal death is more likely when the baby is preterm or light for date.

## MANAGEMENT OF PRE-ECLAMPSIA

*The Principles of Treatment are:*

1. **Hospitalisation for expert care.**
2. **Adequate sedation and rest.**
3. **Prevention of convulsions and reduction of hypertension.**
4. **Diligent observation.**

### Admission to Hospital

Mild cases may be allowed to remain at home if the diastolic blood pressure is not above 90 mm Hg and there is no proteinuria. The woman is required to spend at least 12 of the 24 hours in bed: a suitable night sedative being prescribed. She returns to the clinic every week or is seen by her own doctor. All other cases are admitted to hospital for treatment and the close supervision which is essential.

**Serious cases are admitted** or transferred to an intensive care unit or a quiet single room with the essential equipment for dealing with eclampsia should it occur. The room should not be darkened; sufficient light is needed to observe the woman's colour and the onset of twitching. Dentures are removed; the ears plugged. A midwife should be on constant 'special' duty. The semi-prone or the lateral position is recommended, to increase kidney output including sodium.

**There is no special diet** for pre-eclampsia other than high minerals and vitamins as for any pregnant woman. A low carbohydrate, low fat diet reduces calories and controls excessive weight gain which is advantageous.

**Rest in bed** is one of the most important measures in the management of pre-eclampsia. The blood pressure is reduced, oedema is diminished: improvement in uterine blood flow has a beneficial effect on fetal wellbeing. To facilitate rest, sedatives are usually prescribed. Ambulation for toilet facilities may be permitted after one week, if there is no proteinuria and the diastolic pressure does not exceed 100 mm Hg. Freedom from worry is essential and the social worker will give helpful advice re domestic problems.

## ADMINISTRATION OF SEDATIVES, ANTI-HYPERTENSIVES AND ANTI-CONVULSANTS

### Mild Cases:

Sedatives such as chlordiazepoxide (Librium) 5 mg tabs or diazepam (Valium) 2 mg tabs or chlormethiazole (Heminevrin) 500 mg tabs 8-hourly. Lorazepam (Ativan) is also recommended.

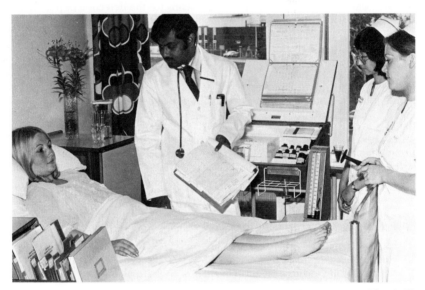

Fig. 12-2   Chart holder, sphygmomanometer and medicine cabinet are portable. Ankles exposed for oedema.

*Bellshill Maternity Hospital, Lanarkshire.*

### Severe Cases:

Sedatives may be combined with anti-hypertensive and anti-convulsant drugs (see below). Diazepam (Valium) is sedative and anti-convulsant and is sometimes given with hydrallazine (Apresoline) which is anti-hypertensive. See also treatment of patient in labour (p. 194).

#### ANTI-HYPERTENSIVES

These drugs are used when eclampsia is imminent; also during induction of and throughout labour. They do not prevent intra-uterine death; some are difficult to control and have undesirable side effects.

**Hydrallazine** (Apresoline) 20 mg is given i.v. The midwife should watch for and report the tachycardia which sometimes occurs.

**Protoveratrine** (Puroverine) is given in 5 per cent glucose by slow infusion pump. If bradycardia occurs the dosage should be reduced.

**Methyldopa** (Aldomet) is given i.v. 250 mg 6-hourly.

#### ANTI-CONVULSANT DRUGS

**Chlormethiazole** (Heminevrin) is anti-convulsant, sedative and hypnotic. It is not anti-hypertensive so a drug such as hydrallazine is also given. It is not analgesic so pethidine is usually prescribed for labour pains, if an epidural analgesic is not being administered. Heminevrin is administered as an i.v. infusion of 0·8 per cent, 60 drops per minute for the first 10 minutes then 10–15 drops per minute to maintain sleep from which the patient can be roused on command. Respiratory depression may occur with heavy dosage, so the airway must be supported in such circumstances. Heminevrin potentiates the phenothiazines and the barbiturates so they are not prescribed.

**Diazepam** (Valium), a phenothiazine being anti-convulsant, 10–20 mg may be given slowly i.v. with anti-hypertensives such as hydrallazine. Caution in dosage should be exercised during labour as it is hypothermic and hypotonic to the newborn baby.

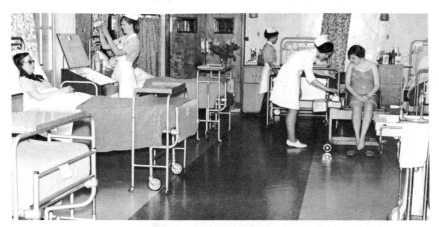

Fig. 12-3   Prenatal ward, armchair bedside scales.
*Simpson Memorial Maternity Pavilion, Edinburgh.*

### DIURETICS

Diuretics do not improve the pre-eclampsia or the prognosis for the fetus so they are now used less frequently. Frusemide or chlorothiazide are sometimes prescribed when massive oedema is present.

## OBSERVATION

### Urine

On admission a mid-stream specimen of urine is examined for protein and if present an Esbach or Biuret quantitative test is made. All urine is collected and a 24-hour specimen examined daily.

### Blood

In addition to the routine tests, potassium, sodium, urea and plasma proteins are assessed in severe cases.

### Blood pressure

This is recorded twice daily in mild cases and one, two or four hourly depending on the severity of the condition: a rising diastolic pressure should be reported to the doctor.

**Weight**

Every second day the woman is weighed on special bed-side scales.

**Oedema**

The amount of oedema is assessed and recorded daily as slight, moderate or gross: the sacral region being examined in recumbent patients.

**Fluid balance**

The fluid intake and output is measured and recorded daily. When inducing labour by i.v. infusion, the amount of fluid is carefully controlled by slow infusion pump or Cardiff infusion unit.

**Temperature, pulse and respiration** are recorded twice daily.

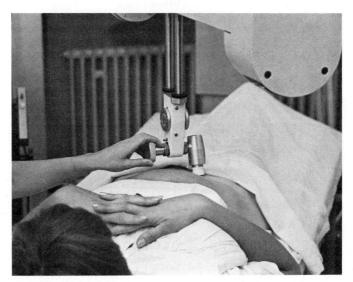

Fig. 12-4   Taking an ultrasonogram to assess fetal growth.
*Queen Mother's Maternity Hospital, Glasgow.*

### Monitoring Feto-placental Function

(*a*) **The fetal heart** rate pattern is monitored twice daily.

(*b*) **Plasma placental lactogen** level is assessed.

(*c*) **Ultrasonic cephalometry** is utilised to determine fetal head growth.

(*d*) **Lecithin/sphingomyelin ratio** is assessed after 34 weeks to determine fetal lung maturity.

(*e*) **Urinary oestriol assays** are made on two consecutive days every one or two weeks after the 30th week to estimate the degree of feto-placental dysfunction and so to determine whether labour should be induced. In serious cases, oestriol is estimated twice weekly. If the urinary excretion of oestriol is below 18 micromoles/24 h. at 30 weeks and 36 micromoles at 38 weeks, the fetus is in danger. Blood plasma oestriol tests give quicker results but their reliability is under question.

### Abdominal Pain

1. **Epigastric pain** is a significant symptom. See serious signs (below).

2. **Placental abruption.** This serious condition is associated with pre-eclampsia in 8 per cent of cases. The uterus is board-like and tender: the pain constant and excruciating.

3. **Labour may have commenced.** The onset of pain is gradual, pain is intermittent; other signs of labour are present.

## SERIOUS SIGNS AND SYMPTOMS

**The midwife must be constantly on the alert** for any of the serious signs. They are signals of the onset of eclampsia so the doctor must be notified at once so that sedative and anti-convulsant therapy can be initiated without delay.

| | |
|---|---|
| **Sharp rise in blood pressure.** | **Vomiting.** |
| **Increase in proteinuria.** | **Drowsiness.** |
| **Severe headache.** | **Urinary output diminished.** |

**Visual disturbances:** Dimness or blurring of vision; flashes of light; coloured spangles.

**Epigastric pain** is a particularly ominous symptom and one frequently misinterpreted as the woman may describe the pain as acute indigestion.

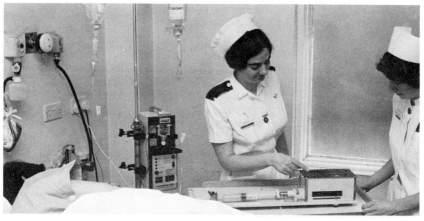

Fig. 12-5   Patient having protoveratrine by Palmer slow infusion pump and Syntocinon by infusion pump.

*Aberdeen Maternity Hospital.*

### Termination of Pregnancy

This may be necessary prior to 30 weeks when serious signs are manifest and no improvement takes place with sedative and anti-hypertensive treatment. After 34 weeks if proteinuria and hypertension persist, fetal lung maturity will be assessed by the lecithin/sphingomyelin ratio test prior to induction of labour or Caesarean section. Pregnancy is not permitted to continue beyond term because of feto-placental dysfunction: induction at 37 weeks is likely. Pre-eclampsia and post-maturity are a bad combination. Caesarean section may be preferred for the older primigravida.

**To induce labour** by puncture of membranes and i.v. oxytocin drip, a slow infusion pump should be employed because of the anti-diuretic effect of oxytocin and the need to limit the amount of fluid administered.

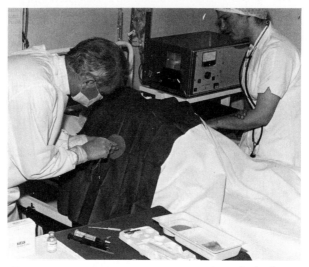

Fig. 12-6   Epidural analgesia. Cardiff infusion unit also in use.
*Maternity Hospital, Stirling.*

### LABOUR IN SERIOUS PRE-ECLAMPSIA

**Adequate sedation should be maintained** throughout labour. Sedatives are sometimes combined with anti-hypertensive and anti-convulsant drugs to minimise the likelihood of convulsions. Epidural analgesia is employed with increasing frequency; the hypotension that occurs being beneficial to mother and fetus.

The midwife should know the action of all the drugs administered and note whether the desired effect is attained. It is essential to report all serious signs and untoward results as well as recording them.

**Constant supervision is essential** because the risk of convulsions is great and to provide the meticulous observation that is necessary: mother and fetus both being at high risk.

**Blood pressure** is recorded hourly.

**Every specimen of urine is measured and tested** for protein.

**Equipment needed for eclampsia** should be at hand. For position of patient, provision of light, removal of dentures, see (p. 197).

**The midwife must auscultate the fetal heart** if electronic monitoring equipment is not available, even more frequently than in normal labour. Loss of base line irregularity must be reported to the doctor.

**Forceps are usually applied** and an episiotomy made to shorten the second stage; this being an advantage to the high risk fetus; and to avoid the effort of 'pushing' which may raise the blood pressure and instigate a convulsion. Ergometrine is not administered during the third stage in the absence of haemorrhage (less than 300 ml) because of its hypertensive action: Syntocinon 5 units being preferred.

### AFTER LABOUR

**The blood pressure is recorded** at the completion of labour and if too high (or too low), every half hour; then every four hours for 24 hours.

**Effective sedation is maintained** after delivery and prior to being transferred to the post-natal ward, to eliminate the risk of postpartum eclampsia. The drug administered during labour being continued, e.g. chlormethiazole. (Heminevrin) is continued for 24–48 hours and thereafter by oral administration of the drug. The patient is nursed in a single, quiet room with a midwife in constant attendance for 12 or more hours.

# ECLAMPSIA

Eclampsia, an acute condition characterised by convulsions and coma, is a more advanced stage of serious pre-eclampsia. Eclampsia can be prevented to a great extent by vigilant prenatal care and the competent management of pre-eclampsia.

20 per cent of cases occur antepartum.

45 per cent occur intrapartum.                                          } *approx.*

35 per cent occur postpartum, usually during the first 12 hours.

### SIGNS AND SYMPTOMS

The prodromal signs of eclampsia are those described as 'serious signs' of pre-eclampsia (p. 193); the more immediate precursors of eclampsia being: **vomiting, intense headache, epigastric pain.** These prodromal signs may be absent in the fulminating type of eclampsia which comes on suddenly but is very rare.

### *The Stages of an Eclamptic Fit*

**Premonitory stage** (lasts from 10 to 20 seconds)

The patient is restless and her eyes roll sideways or upwards, the head may be drawn to one side and twitching of the facial muscles occurs.

**Tonic stage** (lasts from 10 to 20 seconds)

The body is rigid, in a state of muscular spasm, and may be arched in the opisthotonos position. The teeth are tightly clenched, eyes staring, and because the diaphragm is in spasm, **respiration is checked and cyanosis ensues.**

**Clonic stage** (lasts from 60 to 90 seconds)

Violent contraction of the muscles produces convulsive movements, which may be so severe as to throw the patient out of bed. The rapid movement of the jaw churns up the profusely secreted saliva and causes foaming at the mouth, which may be bloodstained if the tongue is bitten. **The face is congested and horribly distorted.** The woman is unconscious, her breathing stertorous and the pulse full and bounding. Gradually the convulsion subsides.

**Stage of coma**

Stertorous breathing continues and coma may persist for minutes or hours; further convulsions sometimes occur without the patient regaining consciousness.

### TREATMENT OF ECLAMPSIA

**The main principle of treatment is to prevent the occurrence of convulsions** and if this can be achieved, recovery is more likely.

The 'flying squad' is sent for. When the patient is first seen, it may be essential to administer sedatives i.v. to bring the convulsions quickly under control and to induce sound sleep during the ambulance journey. Morphine 15 mg may be given intravenously 'on district' if a more suitable sedative is not available, but should not be repeated because of producing vomiting, diminished secretion of urine and respiratory depression with cyanosis.

**Chlormethiazole (Heminevrin) an anti-convulsant,** is favoured at present, 0·8 per cent solution, 15 drops per minute i.v. for sedation, increased during convulsion to 60 drops per minute and stopped during coma. When consciousness returns, 15 drops per minute are given. Over sedation must be avoided (see p. 190).

**Diazepam** (Valium) 10 mg i.v. is sedative and anti-convulsant (see p. 191).

## Other Drugs that may be Prescribed

**Magnesium sulphate** i.v. is used in the U.S.A. but is not popular in Britain. It has a diuretic action, lowers blood pressure and is anti-convulsant. When oliguria is present, it has a toxic effect, with cyanosis, dyspnoea and thready pulse.

**The lytic cocktail** is much favoured in India. 50 mg chlorpromazine (Largactil), 50 mg promethazine (Phenergan) and 50 mg pethidine in 250 ml 5 per cent glucose, i.v. 30–60 drops per minute until sedated; then 15 drops per minute. It is an effective anti-convulsant, but has a respiratory depressant effect on the newborn.

*Anti-hypertensive* and diuretic drugs are considered on p. 190.

*Antibiotics* are administered (a) for early rupture of membranes (b) to combat respiratory infection.

**Bupivacaine** (Marcain) will be required for epidural analgesia.

**Cardiac and respiratory stimulants** may be needed. Digoxin 0·5 mg. Frusemide (Lasix) for pulmonary oedema.

**Mannitol** given by i.v. infusion may be prescribed when renal function is suspect.

## Transfer of the Patient to Hospital

**The woman should be deeply under the effect of a sedative** and anti-convulsant before being transferred. Lack of equipment, sedation and warmth may prejudice the woman's chance of recovery. Oxygen is provided in the ambulance. The pillows and blankets should be brought indoors to warm them: the ambulance doors closed and the heater turned on during this time. Dentures and hairpins are removed: the woman's ears plugged. The driver is instructed to drive carefully over rough roads. The midwife takes with her a rubber wedge or padded spoon, a basin and towels in case vomiting occurs and her delivery bag.

No-one can absolve the midwife from accompanying her patient to hospital: it is a moral as well as a professional duty.

### ADMISSION OF AN ECLAMPTIC PATIENT

No treatment should be carried out until the patient is under the influence of sedatives and anti-convulsants. The blood pressure, temperature, pulse and respirations are recorded. The fetal heart is auscultated. A specimen of urine is examined for protein, bile casts and red cells: an Esbach or Biuret Test is done.

**A self retaining catheter is inserted** with closed drainage system or air sealed polythene bag.

**The mouth is cleansed.**

**No enema or suppository is given** until the acute convulsive stage is under control which is usually within 48 hours.

### Preparations and equipment that may be required

**Oxygen** and polythene face mask: suction apparatus; tracheostomy set.

**Anaesthetic tray** with Guedel airways, spatula, rubber wedge to protect teeth, gauze swabs and swab holders. Kidney basin and wipes for vomitus.

**Intravenous pack:** sterile syringes and needles for giving large and small injections: intravenous fluids: syringe pump or clockwork machine.

**Self retaining catheter** and air sealed drainage bag for urine.
**Oral hygiene tray.**
Blocks for foot of bed if a 'tilt' bed is not provided.
**A trolley with emergency supplies for delivery** and resuscitation of the baby.

## OBSTETRIC MANAGEMENT OF ECLAMPSIA

The administration of sedatives, anti-convulsants and anti-hypertensives, is similar to that described under the management of severe pre-eclampsia (p. 193). Other details are described under Nursing Care (below). Many patients go into labour spontaneously after the onset of eclampsia: others need induction by amniotomy and Syntocinon drip accurately controlled by the Cardiff or other infusion unit.

**Caesarean section may be considered advisable.**

**The total fluid intake** in 24 hours should not exceed 2,000 ml, but in oliguric patients and in the presence of pulmonary oedema, it should be restricted to 500 ml.

**The anaesthetic commonly administered** is nitrous oxide and oxygen given if possible by an obstetric anaesthetist. Continuous epidural analgesia is preferred by many obstetricians because of its hypotensive action.

### AFTER DELIVERY

**The woman is deeply sedated** for 48 hours. (See care in serious pre-eclampsia, p. 194.) A midwife is in constant attendance until the acute stage is past and serious signs have abated; the woman should also be conscious, 48 hours having elapsed with no convulsions. Mental confusion and impairment of vision may exist for a few days.

**The urinary output** is recorded.

**Breast feeding** is contraindicated.

**The period of convalescence** is extended until proteinuria and blood pressure are much reduced but both may persist for some weeks.

## NURSING CARE

**Good nursing is an important factor in saving the patient's life,** and in few instances are experience, efficiency and devotion to duty more necessary than in nursing the woman with eclampsia. Quietness is essential. A single room should be provided and properly equipped; it must be well removed from the telephone bell and other noises. The locker top and all trays are covered with towels. The midwife must work and speak quietly. Cotton wool plugs in the patient's ears will help to exclude noise until adequate sedation is achieved.

**Sufficient light for observation of changes in the patient's condition should be provided.** If the room is too dark, lights must be flashed on in order to carry out treatment, and this is likely to provoke fits. The unconscious or sedated woman is not disturbed by ordinary light nearly so much as by noise.

### PROTECTION FROM INJURY

The top of the bed is padded with two firm pillows, held securely in position with a draw-sheet pinned at the back. If the midwife is alone, it would be advisable for her to push the bed alongside the wall and to place pillows down that side. Any attempt to limit the convulsive movements should be by guiding rather than forcibly restraining them. The woman must never be left alone for one instant, in case she might take a fit; she may also roll out of bed while in her confused state of mind.

**To prevent biting of the tongue,** a rubber wedge is useful, and should be placed between the back teeth during the premonitory phase of the fit and before the jaws are clenched. Rubber has sufficient elasticity to prevent jarring. Two wooden spatulae, bound with a gauze bandage, make a useful substitute; in an emergency the handle of a spoon wrapped in a towel can be used. An unpadded metal spatula or spoon is too hard, and care must be taken to avoid breaking the patient's teeth by not forcing them apart while clenched. A pencil, cork, or substance that can be bitten off should not be used, in case part of it is inhaled into the trachea. It is not advisable to pull the tongue forwards with forceps, as it will then be bitten; neither should a mouth gag be used, in case the jaw might be dislocated, and because when the mouth is wide open, saliva cannot be swallowed and may be inhaled. Dentures should have been removed; pins in the hair taken out.

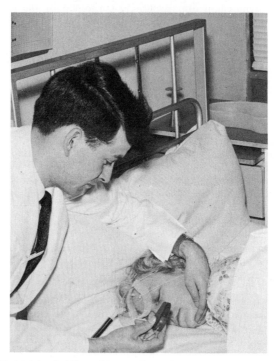

Fig. 12-7    Obstetrician holding rubber wedge to insert when a convulsion threatens.
*Maternity Hospital, Stirling.*

### Keeping the airway clear

During and after a convulsion the woman may inhale saliva, so she should be propped over on the right semi-prone position (using a rubber foam wedge), to allow the saliva to drain out of her mouth. If on her back, her tongue may block the larynx and produce asphyxia; cyanosis must also be avoided for the sake of the fetus. Suction apparatus is excellent and a Guedel airway facilitates the removal of mucus: if not available a swab on a swab-holder is used to mop out the fluid that collects between cheek and teeth.

## SUMMARY OF CARE DURING A FIT

**Place a rubber wedge or substitute between the patient's teeth.**
**Send for medical aid** without leaving the patient.
**Turn the woman on her side;** a foam rubber wedge behind shoulders.

**Keep a clear airway;** use suction apparatus to remove saliva.
**Do not forcibly restrain the convulsive movements.**
**Oxygen should be given.**

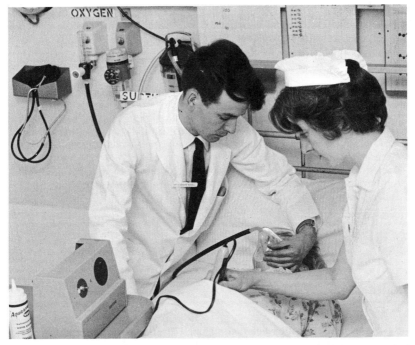

Fig. 12-8   Obstetrician giving oxygen, midwife listening to the fetal heart sounds by
Doptone.

*Photographed at Maternity Hospital, Stirling.*

### NURSING CARE AFTER A FIT

**Oxygen is given for five minutes after each fit,** or longer if cyanosis persists, to
meet the needs of the fetus and to relieve the right side of the heart. Any necessary
treatment ought to be carried out immediately after a fit, while the patient is
unconscious, or postponed until half an hour after a sedative has been administered. Incessant handling is not good nursing. The midwife should not (unless
specifically told to do so) take the blood pressure oftener than every hour, the fetal
heart rate oftener than every one or two hours. Work should be carried out
expeditiously yet gently. The mouth and nostrils should be cleansed after each fit,
or every three hours, because a septic mouth increases the risk of aspiration
pneumonia. No fluid is given by mouth to an unconscious patient; not even 2 ml to
moisten the tongue. The swallowing reflex may be absent and the fluid runs into the
trachea. Any necessary fluid is given intravenously.

The woman is drowsy, dazed, or comatose, so she is placed in the right
semi-prone position, obliquely across the bed, with her head at the edge of the
mattress. In this position saliva can drain out, for with deep stertorous breathing
there is grave danger of the inhalation of mucus and saliva. The jaw is held forwards
if necessary. The patient is turned at intervals of at least 2 hours to avoid hypostatic
congestion of the lungs.

## Pulmonary Oedema

Pulmonary oedema is due to failure of the heart and of the pulmonary circulation. The woman is propped up. If necessary a tracheostomy is performed, an endotracheal tube passed and fluid withdrawn by very brief periods of suction (short sharp sucks). Oxygen may be given by intermittent positive pressure. Frusemide (Lasix) 20 mg i.v. is efficacious in acute pulmonary oedema: digoxin may be given to support cardiac action.

## Bladder and Bowels

A self-retaining catheter (with water seal or air-sealed polythene bag) may be inserted for the following reasons:

It causes less disturbance to the patient than repeatedly passing catheters, changing wet beds, or trying to get a semi-conscious woman to pass urine. The kidney output can be accurately measured. A specimen of urine can be obtained for analysis as required.

An Esbach's or Biuret quantitative test for protein is carried out daily.

Neither enema, suppository nor laxative is given until the acute convulsive stage is under control, which is usually within 48 hours.

## OBSERVATION

*The midwife must note the following:*

### (a) Signs of an eclamptic fit

These are described on page 195. The number, length, severity and time of occurrence must be recorded.

### (b) Signs of labour

Restlessness or moaning when accompanied by uterine contractions can be taken as a sign of labour.

Show, and rupture of the membranes.

On vaginal examination, the cervix will be dilated. (It is usual for labour to start soon after convulsions occur, unless the woman is very heavily sedated.)

### (c) The vital signs are monitored.

The pulse should be taken every 15 minutes, as this can be done without disturbing the patient. The temperature is usually taken every four hours and may rise to 38·8°C (102°F) after a succession of fits or if respiratory infection is present. The respirations are charted every 15 minutes: slow respirations (below 12) may be due to cerebral haemorrhage; rapid respirations associated with rising temperature and pulse may indicate pulmonary infection: moist respirations may be a sign of pulmonary oedema.

### (d) The general condition of the woman

**The colour of the woman** may be dusky, due to cyanosis, and is an indication for the administration of oxygen. An icteric tinge may be due to liver damage.

**The urine** may be dark brown in colour because of its high concentration and the presence of haemoglobin.

### (e) Blood pressure.

—Every one or two hours would seem a reasonable time, but when a drug is given which causes the blood pressure to fall, or when it is very high, estimations may be made more frequently. The arm band can be left loosely in position. A fall in blood pressure may denote an improvement in the woman's condition, and this often follows death of the fetus. If accompanied by cyanosis and cold extremities, it indicates cardiac failure.

(*f*) **The fetal heart rate** may be taken every one, two or three hours, but the woman should not be disturbed unnecessarily to do so, as very little can be done if fetal distress occurs. Continuous electronic monitoring is recommended.

(*g*) **Fluid balance.** An exact record of kidney output must be kept, as well as the intake by mouth or intravenously, and when gross oedema is lessening, the output may be double or treble the amount of the intake for a few days. A mannitol infusion i.v. may be needed to stimulate diuresis. Bladder distension should be looked for at this period of diuresis. An output of 800 ml in 24 hours is considered to be a favourable sign. Anuria is a serious sign, and may indicate the onset of acute renal failure. For treatment, see page 219.

(*h*) **The midwife must report if the sedative prescribed** does not have the desired effect or as in Heminevrin the dose administered causes respiratory depression.
The effect of anti-hypertensive and anti-convulsant drugs must be noted.

(*i*) **Oedema** is recorded as slight, moderate, gross.

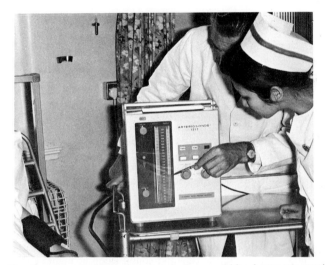

Fig. 12-9   The Arteriosonde 1216. Automated ultrasound blood pressure monitor. A cuff placed on the arm in the usual manner with transducer over the brachial artery inflates and deflates at a preset rate. Monitoring is automatic; measurements being made as often as once every minute.

*Royal Maternity Hospital, Glasgow.*

**SERIOUS SIGNS OF ECLAMPSIA**

Over 20, or rapid fits. (Patients have recovered who have had 40 fits.)
Pulmonary oedema.   Jaundice.

Pulse over 120—thready.
Temperature over 39·4°C (103°F).
Anuria.

## *Summary of Complications of Eclampsia*

**Cerebral:** haemorrhage, thrombosis, mental confusion.
**Hepatic:** liver damage.
**Injuries:** to tongue, fractures.
**Cardiac:** myocardial failure.

**Renal:** acute failure.
**Visual:** temporary blindness.
**Respiratory:** asphyxia, pulmonary oedema, broncho-pneumonia.
**Fetal:** hypoxia; stillbirth.

**The cause of death**

Death is most commonly due to cerebral haemorrhage, myocardial failure, respiratory or hepatic disorders, or acute renal failure.

**The maternal mortality** rate depends on the severity of the condition and whether treatment is started promptly. With expert care the death rate will be as low as 2 per cent, but when prenatal supervision is perfunctory and the treatment of eclampsia unsatisfactory the mortality will range between 12 and 15 per cent.

**The perinatal mortality rate** in Britain is 6·2 per cent.

# ESSENTIAL HYPERTENSION

Essential hypertension may be defined as an elevation of blood pressure over 140/90 present on two or more occasions prior to the 20th week of pregnancy, which is not due to any apparent pathological condition. It seems to be an inherited characteristic in about 80 per cent of cases. The hypertensive woman is liable to develop pre-eclampsia. Fetus and placenta may both be small.

## MANAGEMENT

**Mild cases**

When the blood pressure is not over 150/90 the woman may be treated at home. She is advised regarding the great need for additional rest, i.e. two hours during the day and 10 hours at night. To ensure sound sleep a sedative is usually prescribed: the necessity for salt restriction and for weight control is explained. The woman ought to be seen and weighed every week, a careful check on blood pressure being maintained. The development of signs of pre-eclampsia or a sudden rise in blood pressure would indicate the need for admission to hospital. All patients with essential hypertension are admitted to hospital not later than the 38th week of pregnancy.

**Severe cases**

The woman may have to spend long periods in hospital to ensure complete bed rest, weight control and salt restriction. Sedatives are prescribed to promote emotional tranquillity during the day and sound sleep at night. Phenobarbitones may cause depression.

Anti-hypertensive drugs may benefit the patient but they do not reduce the perinatal loss: **methyldopa** (Aldomet), dose 250 mg t.i.d., is useful when the blood pressure is unduly high.

Blood plasma or urinary oestriol assays are made weekly in some centres on two consecutive days after the 30th week, to detect feto-placental dysfunction: ultrasonic cephalometry is used to assess fetal growth.

The older primigravida may be delivered by Caesarean section at 36 or 37 weeks to ensure a live infant.

*Induction of Labour*

The likelihood of intra-uterine death is kept in mind when the blood pressure remains persistently high. For the multiparous woman with a bad obstetric history, labour is usually induced at the 36th week: puncture of membranes and oxytocin intravenous drip usually being employed.

Care during and after labour is similar to what is given in pre-eclampsia (see p. 194).

## HYPEREMESIS GRAVIDARUM

Differentiate between morning sickness and hyperemesis gravidarum. What could a midwife do to prevent hyperemesis.

State why the following substances are prescribed in hyperemesis: fluid; glucose; promazine hydrochloride; vitamin B. Why should vomitus not be recorded under 'output'?

Outline a suitable diet for the first day when feeding is recommended. Give five serious signs.

**(N. Ire.) 30-min. question.** Define hyperemesis gravidarum. Indicate the signs and symptoms which would cause concern. Outline the treatment.

**C.M.B. (Scot.) 30-min. question.** Give the management of a case of hyperemesis.

## PRE-ECLAMPSIA—ECLAMPSIA

Give the three cardinal signs of pre-eclampsia.

Give six sites where oedema may be detected. Give six prodromal signs of eclampsia.

Name three conditions in pregnancy often associated with pre-eclampsia.

What effect does placental dysfunction have on the fetus? How do you set up an Esbach's test for proteinuria?

What precautions would you take prior to transferring a patient suffering from eclampsia to hospital? What nursing care may be necessary in cases of pulmonary oedema?

Pre-eclampsia may occur prior to the .......... week; more commonly from the .......... to the .......... week.

Urinary oestriol assays are made after the .......... week on .......... consecutive days over .......... or .......... weeks.

State why the following are prescribed: rest in bed, .......... ; sedation .......... , low carbohydrate diet .......... ; oestriol assay .......... .

What should be reported to the doctor when the following drugs are being administered: methyldopa; morphine; chlormethiazole (Heminevrin); hydrallazine.

## State 'Why'

You would suspect that an unconscious woman was in labour. An eclamptic patient should not be nursed in a dark room. Postmaturity is dangerous in cases of pre-eclampsia. Oxygen is given following a convulsion; the semi-prone position is preferred after a fit; the patient's ears are plugged; a mouth gag should not be used; rubber is an ideal substance for a wedge to place between the teeth.

Describe the care of an eclamptic patient during (a) the journey by ambulance; (b) immediately after labour; (c) immediately after a convulsion.

**C.MB.(Scot.) 30-min. question.** Describe an eclamptic fit. How would you manage a case of eclampsia pending the arrival of a doctor?

**C.M.B.(Eng.) 30-min. question.** What are the signs of pre-eclampsia? Give an account of the management of a patient with this condition.

**C.M.B.(Eng.) 30-min. question.** What is meant by pre-eclampsia? What are its dangers and how may they be reduced by good midwifery practice?

**C.M.B.(Eng.).** Define pre-eclampsia. What could be the complications to the mother and fetus? How may antenatal care help to prevent these complications?

**C.M.B. Scot.** Describe an eclamptic fit. What is (a) the immediate management of a patient who is having an eclamptic fit; (b) the continuing care and treatment of such a patient.

Give the emergency treatment of eclampsia: Describe an eclamptic fit. Give the prodromal signs of eclampsia.

What precautions would you take (a) to keep a clear airway? (b) to avoid injury during a fit? (c) to avoid pneumonia?

Give the nursing care of a patient during an eclamptic fit.

What is the significance of hypertension in pregnancy?

**Why are the following tests made?** Urinary oestriol; Ultrasonic cephalometry; Esbach's; Hourly blood pressure.

**Why are the following not recommended?** High carbohydrate diet; oral diuretics; bearing down during the second stage; nursing the patient in a dark room; using cork as a teeth wedge; post-mature labour.

**Give reasons** why the following drugs are prescribed: Aldomet; Valium; Heminevrin; Syntocinon.

**Explain how** you would (a) exclude noise; (b) keep the airway clear; (c) avoid aspiration pneumonia.

**What are the advantages** of using (a) a self-retaining catheter? (b) epidural analgesia in eclampsia? (c) a syringe slow infusion pump? (d) the semi-prone position?

Discuss the blood pressure readings you would consider suggestive of pre-eclampsia. What are the dangers of pre-eclampsia?

Which foods are high in salt?

# 13
# Diseases associated with Pregnancy

*Cardiac disease. Diabetes. Pulmonary tuberculosis. Anaemia. Infections (rubella, urinary tract). Renal disease. Acute renal failure. Sexually transmitted diseases (trichomoniasis, candidiasis, syphilis, gonorrhoea)*

## CARDIAC DISEASE

The number of cases of cardiac disease in pregnancy declines every year; congenital lesions now being the major cause. Since rheumatic fever has decreased in paediatric practice consequent rheumatic cardiac lesions are now less commonly seen in women of childbearing age.

During pregnancy the increased blood volume and cardiac output impose a severe strain on an impaired heart, so a certain amount of deterioration may be anticipated in the majority of cases.

### DIAGNOSIS AND ASSESSMENT

**No longer are the four grades of functional capacity relied on** as a prognostic criterion or a guide to management. With modern surgery and to some extent with drugs, patients of childbearing age should seldom, if ever, reach the more advanced stages of incapacity. Some patients with mitral stenosis have practically no symptoms before suddenly developing acute pulmonary oedema, possibly fatal, and functional grading gives no guidance regarding this serious possibility.

In assessing the cardiac status of the pregnant woman, clinical symptoms, radiological and electrocardiographic evidence are utilised as well as the severity of the lesion and the woman's age. Those with a minor cardiac lesion may make no complaint; breathlessness and ankle oedema commonly occurring during normal pregnancy. Some are breathless on moderate exertion, others on slight exertion: the woman may complain of fatigue, palpitations, dyspnoea and anginal pain. The diagnosis is made by the doctor at the initial visit.

### MANAGEMENT OF PREGNANCY

**Prenatal supervision should be first class:** this being facilitated when cardiologist and obstetrician are closely associated in caring for the woman. The patient's co-operation should be fostered, otherwise good results are not likely to be achieved.

**Cardiac patients are seen at frequent intervals** and the degree of disability estimated at every visit. Those with a minor degree of impairment attend every one or two weeks: transport being provided to eliminate undue exertion. No heavy work should be attempted and exercise that induces breathlessness or exhaustion avoided. Work outside the home should be given up. They may be admitted to hospital one week prior to term.

**In more severe cases** the woman is admitted to hospital when signs and symptoms warrant this. Her ordinary activities should be curtailed and the social worker will arrange for a home help if necessary. Some require complete bed rest when the strain on the heart is greatest, i.e. from the 23rd to the 32nd week: they remain in hospital for delivery.

**Weight control is essential in all cases.** Ample rest and sleep is mandatory for ambulant patients, i.e. 12 hours at night and 2 or 3 hours during the afternoon. Anaemia is treated vigorously and if the Hb level is below 10 g/dl, admission to hospital is recommended: the vitamin B complex is prescribed for cardiac patients. The woman is advised to stay in bed for the common cold to avoid more serious respiratory complication. Dental extractions should only be made when absolutely essential, and with full antibiotic protection.

The main causes of deterioration in cardiac patients are anaemia, respiratory infections, overwork, overweight, insomnia and the development of atrial fibrillation or other arrhythmias which may require urgent treatment.

**Induction of premature labour is not advocated** as no additional cardiac stress occurs during the last four weeks of pregnancy. Mitral valvulotomy has been successfully performed in certain patients, the pregnancy having subsequently continued to term.

### ACUTE HEART FAILURE

The onset of pulmonary oedema is sudden with tachycardia, intense dyspnoea, bronchospasm, cough and frothy mucus.

#### SIGNS AND SYMPTOMS

| | |
|---|---|
| **Intense breathlessness.** | **Cold sweating extremities.** |
| **Cyanosis.** | **Cough with blood-stained sputum.** |
| **Rapid or irregular pulse.** | **Pulmonary oedema.** |

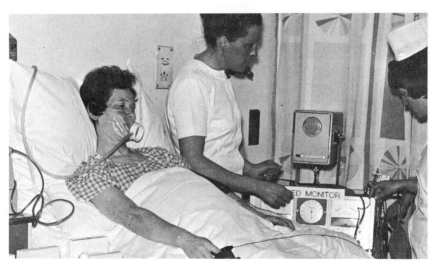

Fig. 13-1   Vital signs Bed Monitor in use, oxygen being administered.
*Bellshill Maternity Hospital, Lanarkshire.*

### Management of acute heart failure

**The patient should be propped up without delay to increase vital capacity.** Morphine 15 mg or heroin (diamorphine) 5 mg is administered i.v. to relieve anxiety and restlessness. Oxygen is given for cyanosis. A diuretic such as frusemide (Lasix) is prescribed to increase fluid excretion. In serious cases venesection carried out promptly may be life-saving by reducing right ventricular output and pulmonary congestion: 300 to 600 ml of blood being withdrawn. Aminophylline 250 mg given slowly relaxes the bronchioles and relieves dyspnoea. Intermittent positive pressure respiration may be of value. Mechanical suction is utilised to remove frothy mucus and maintain a clear airway. For atrial fibrillation full digitalisation would be indicated, followed by maintenance doses.

Obstetrical operative treatment is never carried out during acute heart failure; Caesarean section is rarely advocated unless indications other than cardiac disease are manifest; sterilisation, if indicated, is usually performed during the puerperium.

*Nursing Care*

**This is similar to what is given to non-pregnant patients** in congestive heart failure and includes suitable diet, warmth and the avoidance of any exertion. A single room is an advantage, and two midwives should assist with all major nursing procedures; a back-rest and arm-pillows are usually necessary but the woman should be allowed to adopt the position in which she is most comfortable.

**Sedatives are imperative,** such as nitrazepam (Mogadon) 5–10 mg, to ensure sound sleep at night. To produce mental calm and physical comfort during the day diazepam (Valium), 5–10 mg, is useful.

Fluid may occasionally be restricted to 1,200 ml daily, and a fluid balance chart kept; a salt-poor diet is served when oedema is present.

The apex beat is recorded hourly or as directed by the physician. To prevent venous thrombosis the physiotherapist gives gentle massage and encourages leg movement in long-term cases. Simple remedies are often efficacious in treating the minor ailments which add so much to the woman's discomfort, i.e. nausea, heartburn and flatulence.

## MANAGEMENT OF LABOUR

At the onset or induction of labour in cases where valvular disease is present an appropriate antibiotic is given such as penicillin with streptomycin to prevent the risk of infective endocarditis.

### The first stage

Diazepam (Valium) 5–10 mg, is given early in labour to allay anxiety, but morphine, 15 mg, or Cyclimorph, 1 ml, may be necessary to relieve pain. Continuous epidural analgesia is used with success. Overhydration should be avoided and a slow pump used to control the i.v. fluid intake. Serious signs should be reported; such as severe breathlessness or increased cyanosis, a pulse over 110 and respirations over 24. (*The pulse and respirations should be recorded every 15 minutes in graph form.*)

### The second stage

The patient should adopt the position she prefers, but should be sitting up if she is distressed, and given oxygen continuously. Pushing will embarrass the heart, so it should not be permitted; an episiotomy is made under local analgesia to shorten the perineal phase. The doctor will use the vacuum extractor or apply low forceps for distress or delay, preferably under pudendal nerve block or perineal infiltration. The lithotomy position increases the load on the heart, so ought to be avoided. Nitrous oxide and oxygen should be administered by an obstetric anaesthetist.

### The third stage

Drugs such as nikethamide and digoxin should be at hand. **Collapse may occur when the retracted uterus returns blood to the general circulation** and temporarily overloads the heart. Ergometrine is usually only administered when needed to control haemorrhage. (Many believe that the administration of 0·25 mg ergometrine i.m. is less hazardous than severe blood loss.) If a blood transfusion is necessary packed cells are preferred to avoid overloading the circulation.

**Sedatives are essential after labour** and morphine, 15 mg, is usually given. In order to procure rest and quietness the woman should be nursed in a single room; further sedation and vigilant, skilful, nursing care are necessary.

### The puerperium

To avoid bacterial endocarditis, antibiotics are continued for 3 to 4 days or longer if pyrexia occurs. The temperature should be taken four-hourly during the first few days in order to detect sepsis early. Movement of the legs is encouraged as soon as possible and graduated exercises are given by the physiotherapist.

Mild cases are ambulant in 4 or 5 days to minimise the risk of thrombo-embolism, and when heart failure is present, one week after it has cleared up. A period of convalescence should be arranged and help provided with domestic duties when they are resumed. Contraceptive advice is given to allow the lapse of two years (or longer) between pregnancies. The contraceptive pill would be undesirable in patients with systemic hypertension and those with a history of venous thrombosis and pulmonary thromboembolism. The IUCD presents a slight risk of endocarditis in patients who have valvular disease. Sterilisation may be recommended.

# DIABETES

**Diabetes may appear for the first time during pregnancy;** in fact, pregnancy is one of the factors that may precipitate the onset of diabetes in women genetically predisposed to the condition. The diabetic woman can go through pregnancy and labour in comparative safety, provided she is under the combined care of an obstetrician and a diabetic specialist. Unfortunately the perinatal mortality rate still remains high, but when there is strict supervision of the diabetes during pregnancy and carefully planned delivery by induction or Caesarean section after amniocentesis has shown the fetal lungs to be sufficiently mature, the mortality should not exceed 6 per cent, granted optimal obstetric, paediatric, and nursing care. Delivery is usually induced before term but seldom before 37 weeks gestation.

#### GRADES OF DIABETES

### Potential

As indicated by various criteria, e.g. one or both parents diabetic or history of having borne a baby unduly heavy for maternal height and stage of gestation, chronic marked obesity, glycosuria to Clinistix in a second fasting urine specimen in pregnancy.

### Chemical

Abnormal glucose-tolerance test but without symptoms. It is six times more common than overt diabetes in pregnancy.

### Overt or clinical

Abnormal glucose-tolerance test with symptoms and a raised fasting blood glucose level.

### Latent

No diabetes at present but history of diabetes in the past, e.g. when pregnant, obese or during stress.

### Pre-diabetes

Used only retrospectively to refer to the period before a known diabetic develops an abnormal glucose-tolerance test.

### Gestational Diabetes

Develops during pregnancy and may continue after the pregnancy is over. If the woman reverts to the normal non-diabetic state the term 'latent gestational diabetes' is applied.

#### DIAGNOSIS

**Obstetric history**. When a woman has given birth to one or more babies of unduly large size, e.g. over 4·5 kg, or has had one or more stillbirths, neonatal deaths or a history of polyhydramnios, a glucose-tolerance test is made.

The woman may eventually develop clinical diabetes.

**This potential diabetic state** may indicate that the woman will eventually develop clinical diabetes.

**Glycosuria** after meals is so common in pregnancy as to have little diagnostic value. A rough test of diabetes is to measure the blood glucose level two hours after a meal containing 100 g carbohydrate. If the result exceeds 6·7 mmol/l (120 mg/dl) a full glucose-tolerance test is indicated.

**Polyuria and thirst are diagnostic symptoms.** (The woman should be asked if she requires to drink during the night or has a dry mouth in the morning.) Pruritus vulvae is suggestive, but not diagnostic.

## THE EFFECT OF DIABETES ON CHILDBEARING

**Polyhydramnios** of slight degree is evident in a large number of cases and of marked degree in about 25 per cent: when severe the fetal prognosis is poor, so close supervision in hospital is essential.

**Pre-eclampsia** is an important factor responsible for the increased intra-uterine death rate in diabetic pregnancies, and if pre-eclampsia is severe, pregnancy is usually terminated.

**Large babies** over 3·6 kg occur in 30 to 40 per cent of cases. A main causative factor is probably the raised blood glucose level of the mother which controls that of the fetus and induces excessive secretion of fetal insulin. This in turn stimulates growth and excessive formation of fat. Good control of diabetes in pregnancy results in fewer obese babies.

**Small babies** under 2·7 kg are also common due to placental dysfunction.

**Intra-uterine death of the fetus** occurs in a number of cases after the 36th week. The perinatal mortality rate is 10 per cent. The incidence of fetal abnormalities is said by some to be 5 times higher than normal.

**Neonatal death** is a risk to be taken in relation to early delivery of the mother but respiratory distress syndrome has become a less common cause now that a low lecithin sphingomyelin ratio in the amniotic fluid obtained by amniocentesis can be used to predict immaturity of the fetal lungs. Thus delivery is induced only after the test is favourable, unless there are over-riding conditions for induction such as severe pre-eclampsia.

**Vaginal candidiasis** may be present and should be treated.

**Ketosis** may occur more rapidly in the pregnant than in the non-pregnant state and is likely to produce death of the fetus in utero. Ketosis must therefore be avoided by meticulous attention to the insulin and carbohydrate requirements of the pregnant diabetic woman.

## MANAGEMENT OF PREGNANCY

The best control of the pregnant diabetic woman is achieved at a combined diabetic prenatal clinic staffed by a diabetic specialist and obstetrician. Sonar scanning of the uterus is of great value in establishing accurately the stage of gestation. Most insulin-dependent diabetics have twice daily injections of quick acting insulin and are required to test their urine frequently for glucose and for ketones if much glucose is present. The blood glucose level is measured at each clinic visit. The patient is admitted urgently to hospital if diabetic ketosis occurs; perhaps initiated by a urinary infection or troublesome morning sickness. Strict control of the blood glucose throughout pregnancy, especially in the last trimester, is the factor most likely to produce a successful result. A good protein intake is required.

In many units the woman is admitted to hospital at not later than the 32nd week or earlier if required for pre-eclampsia, hypertension or polyhydramnios. If a decision has to be made about the viability of the fetus, various assays such as plasma levels of oestriol or of human placental lactogen (HPL) may prove helpful, although not wholly reliable. An abrupt fall of insulin requirements between the 30th–37th week is an ominous sign; i.e. of impending or actual fetal death.

### Caesarean section

The operation is performed at the 37th to 38th week in the older primigravida, in the multiparous woman with a bad obstetric history, or if the fetus is unduly large. On the day of the operation, breakfast and the usual insulin dose are omitted. An intravenous drip with 10 per cent glucose is set up: then soluble insulin is given subcutaneously; the blood glucose being kept at 5·5–8·3 mmol/l (100–150 mg/dl). Alternatively, soluble insulin can be given continuously i.v. at a rate of 1–2 units per hour diluted in 0·9 per cent sodium chloride by a clockwork or electrical pump. Ketosis must be avoided. A paediatrician is present to take charge of the baby. The mother's blood glucose concentration is determined and during the period between completion of the operation and next morning 120 to 150 g carbohydrates is given as fluid and light meals. If unable to take food by mouth a 10 per cent glucose intravenous drip is administered at the rate of about 500 ml in 4 hours.

**The insulin requirement falls steeply after delivery,** possibly due to the removal of the placenta, which contains insulin destroying enzymes and anti-insulin hormones; the renal threshold for glucose rises rapidly.

### LABOUR

**Induction of labour is usual at the 37th to 38th week** in the young primigravida and in the multiparous woman whose past and present obstetric history is satisfactory.

**Procedure**—No breakfast is given. At 8.00 hours the membranes are punctured and an oxytocin drip started. A second drip (in the other arm) administers the prescribed amount of glucose. Soluble insulin is given subcutaneously (to insulin-dependent patients) the dose depending on readings by Dextrostix, preferably using the reflectance meter. Hypoglycaemia must be avoided. Long-acting insulin is not given at the time of induction because the insulin requirement falls often by about 50 per cent once the baby has been delivered.

**Sedatives and analgesics that depress the fetal respiratory centre should not be used.** Epidural analgesia is preferred in some centres: fetal metabolic acidosis being reduced is one advantage.

**Delay in labour,** i.e. over 12 hours is more serious in the diabetic woman. Should the woman not be approaching delivery after 8 hours the situation is reassessed and Caesarean section considered.

**On discharge**

Diabetic women are usually advised to have not more than 3 children. The standard contraceptive pills have a diabetogenic effect in many women and are best avoided in favour of alternative methods of contraception. (*Care of the Baby (see p. 538)*.)

# PULMONARY TUBERCULOSIS

The number of pregnant women found to have pulmonary tuberculosis requiring observation or treatment is now below 0·1 per cent. Routine radiography of pregnant women has now been abandoned in many centres, but if chest radiography is indicated, a large film is to be preferred because of its smaller radiation exposure.

## DURING PREGNANCY

These patients should be under the care of an obstetrician and a chest physician who will supervise the chest condition and give such advice as is indicated. A combination of streptomycin, para-aminosalicylic acid (PAS) and isoniazid used to be the recommended standard anti-tuberculosis treatment. However, two new drugs—rifampicin and ethambutol—have been shown to be non-toxic to the fetus, and nowadays the most effective regimen is recognised to be an initial period of eight weeks' treatment with rifampicin, ethambutol and isoniazid, followed by rifampicin and isoniazid to a total period of nine months. For secondary anaemia, present only in acute cases, the woman is given the appropriate treatment. A home help will be arranged for and food supplements provided if necessary. The modern tendency is to allow pregnancy to continue. It has been proved that pregnancy, labour and the puerperium very rarely have any adverse effect on pulmonary tuberculosis, and modern methods of treatment prevent any deterioration. If the disease is infectious (i.e. sputum smear positive) the woman in hospital should be isolated. Therapeutic abortion is exceedingly rarely advocated even in advanced cases; severe dyspnoea due to gross destruction of lung tissue, squalid home conditions and exceptional circumstances in which the woman is grossly over-worked looking after her family may sometimes be taken into consideration.

## DURING LABOUR

An endeavour should be made to provide maximal rest with the minimum of effort.

Exhaustion must be avoided. Pethidine may be given, but inhalational analgesia must not be administered by midwives without permission from the chest physician in charge. Special anaesthetic care is required if bronchitis or bronchiectasis is present. Epidural analgesia may be employed if a difficult forceps delivery is anticipated. To eliminate the need for strenuous pushing, an episiotomy is performed under local analgesia, and, if necesary, forceps are applied under pudendal nerve block, or perineal infiltration. Blood loss during the third stage should be minimal.

**B.C.G. vaccination**

**If the mother is infectious she should not handle her infant,** and he should be segregated until B.C.G. (Bacille Calmette-Guerin) vaccination has been successful or until the mother is non-infectious. The baby is rarely infected with tuberculosis *in utero* so he will be Mantoux negative. After vaccination a small superficial nodule appears on the arm (which should not be bandaged) in two or three weeks' time. The presence of a papule is sufficient evidence of successful vaccination, but it is wise to carry out a Mantoux test at six weeks; the infant being discharged if successful vaccination has taken place. In situations where separation of mother and baby is impossible, the infant may be given isoniazid, 25 mg in syrup once daily and immunised with isoniazid-resistant B.C.G. vaccine.

### The social aspect

Tuberculosis is a social and economic problem. Although the woman may give birth to two or three children without deterioration in her condition, the hard work involved in child-rearing may prove to be even more detrimental than childbearing. Extra help in the home is necessary for 3 months. It may be desirable that contraceptive advice is given until the disease has been quiescent for 2 years or sterilisation may be performed after the birth of 2 or 3 children depending on the extent of the disease. The possibility of infection of the baby when the father at home suffers from active pulmonary tuberculosis is a problem that requires attention.

# ANAEMIA

Anaemia is common in childbearing women, and particularly in multiparae of the lower income group. Many are anaemic before they become pregnant, so it is essential that the condition is diagnosed at the beginning of pregnancy and treated effectively.

**Haemoglobin estimation is made** (a) when the woman first comes to book and at each subsequent visit if necessary, and (b) at the 32nd week and the 36th week as a check that the haemoglobin is at a safe level for labour. A haemoglobin below 11 g/dl is now considered the standard for anaemia. A 10 per cent reduction in haemoglobin occurs during pregnancy because of the physiological increase in blood plasma; the pregnant woman also loses 500 mg of iron to the fetus and placenta. Many authorities consider that all pregnant women should receive iron, e.g. ferrous sulphate, 180 mg t.i.d., throughout pregnancy, others give iron when the haemoglobin level is below 12·6 g/dl and repeat the haemoglobin test at each subsequent visit until a satisfactory level is reached. Some consider the indiscriminate administration of iron to be unphysiological.

## CAUSES OF IRON DEFICIENCY ANAEMIA

Menstrual loss between pregnancies, especially if profuse.
Dietary deficiency, e.g. low iron, protein, and vitamin intake.
Withdrawal of iron by the fetus for its immediate and future needs.
Ante and post partum haemorrhage.
When anaemia is persistent a mid-stream specimen of urine is examined for urinary tract infection as a possible cause.

### Hook worm infection

This contributory factor to anaemia is found in immigrants from tropical countries. The hook worm enters the tissues through the sole of the foot (when shoes are not worn) and the larvae find their way to the intestine. When ova are found in the patient's stool Alcopar is prescribed: one sachet, (5 g) in water by mouth, repeated on three successive days if necessary. Food is withheld for 2 hours after giving Alcopar. Oral iron is continued for 3 months after the haemoglobin has reached normal levels.

### Folic acid deficiency

Minor degrees of folic acid deficiency occur in 26 per cent of pregnant women particularly multiparae over 30 years of age and in cases of multiple pregnancy. Folic acid is necessary for the normal development of red blood cells in bone marrow; liver, kidney and green vegetables in the diet are good sources. At many prenatal clinics folic acid, 0·5 mg daily, is prescribed in addition to iron throughout pregnancy as a prophylactic measure. FeFol contains ferrous sulphate, 150 mg, and folic acid, 0·5 mg, one capsule daily. Slow Fe-Folic contains ferrous sulphate 160 mg and folic acid 400 micrograms, and one tablet daily is well tolerated.

### EFFECTS OF ANAEMIA

It undermines the woman's general health, saps her vitality and deprives her of the energy needed for her household duties and outdoor recreation.

Other complications of pregnancy are rendered more severe.

Oxygen transport at placental level is impaired.

Signs of exsanguination ensue after normal blood loss, and collapse occurs more readily following moderate haemorrhage. Shock, whatever the cause, is more severe.

Venous thrombosis is predisposed to.

The morbidity rate is increased; anaemia is a contributory cause of maternal deaths in underdeveloping countries.

### SIGNS AND SYMPTOMS OF ANAEMIA

**Pallor of mucous membranes.** **Palpitation** and rapid pulse in some cases.
**Lassitude** (always tired). **Poor appetite,** gastro-intestinal upsets.
**Breathlessness.**

### *Treatment*

Mild cases of anaemia respond well to the oral administration of medicinal iron but digestive disturbances and constipation may occur. *All iron tablets should be taken after meals with a little water.* A diet rich in first class proteins, vitamins C and $B_{12}$, iron and other minerals should also be partaken. The need for fresh air and sunshine ought to be stressed.

Ferrous sulphate tablets, 180 mg t.i.d., are effective and cheap: some give one daily dose of folic acid, 300 micrograms throughout pregnancy. Ferrous iron 40 mg, folic acid 200 micrograms tablet t.i.d. ferrous succinate (Ferromyn) and ferrous fumarate (Fersamal) are readily absorbed, and well tolerated. Rarical contains iron, calcium and aneurine. Pregfol contains ferrous sulphate 200 mg and folic acid 0·5 mg: one daily = prophylaxis. Pregamal and Pregaday both contain ferrous fumarate and folic acid; they are given as a prophylactic measure for folate deficiency in some centres throughout pregnancy.

When the haemoglobin is below 10·3 g/dl more detailed expert blood investigation is required and the woman admitted to hospital.

A transfusion of whole blood or packed cells is always given when the haemoglobin is dangerously low, especially when the time of labour is approaching, i.e. at about the 34th week of pregnancy. Slow administration and careful supervision is necessary.

### Jectofer

Occasionally when the Hb level is below 10·3 g/dl, the response to oral iron poor and time limited, Jectofer an iron sorbital/citric acid complex stabilised with dextrin is administered intramuscularly. It is not given during pregnancy to patients with pyelonephritis.

### *The Midwives' Reponsibility*

Midwives have an important part to play in the prevention of anaemia by explaining to pregnant women some of the reasons why they become anaemic: how they can try to prevent this by taking a diet with adequate amounts of body-building foods and those rich in iron such as liver, meat and brown bread, as well as vitamin C in citrus fruits and green vegetables: urging them to take regularly the tablets prescribed by the doctor. Midwives should avoid excessive blood loss during the third stage of labour and encourage puerperal women to continue taking iron pills for one month.

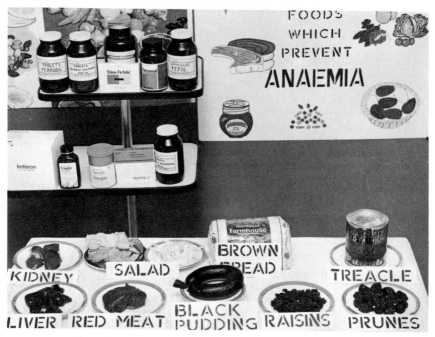

Fig. 13-2 Foods rich in iron. Ferrous preparations in common use. Ferrodic, Ferrous sulphate, Ferro-Redoxin, Slow Fe-Folic, Fersamal, Imferon, Feospan, FeFol, Pregtol, Ferrous gluconate.

Set up for student midwives.

*Maternity Hospital, Stirling.*

## MEGALOBLASTIC ANAEMIA OF PREGNANCY

This severe form of anaemia, due to insufficiency of folic acid, results from the demands of the fetus or some factor interfering with the absorption or metabolism of folic and folinic acid. It tends to occur when the haemoglobin is below 7 g/dl, therefore the administration of iron prophylactically should significantly reduce the incidence of megaloblastic anaemia. Patients with anaemia that fails to respond to iron therapy in four weeks and cases in which the haemoglobin is less than 10·3 g/dl should have blood investigations made to determine if megaloblastic anaemia is present. Pallor is marked, the woman complains of extreme weakness, vomiting, dyspnoea and sometimes diarrhoea and persistent swelling of the ankles.

### *Treatment*

**A striking improvement is evident following the administration of folic acid 5 mg** three times daily with iron throughout pregnancy and continued six weeks postpartum. Rest in bed, and a light diet, high in proteins, iron, and other minerals, are essential. A blood transfusion will be necessary if anaemia is severe, or if in untreated cases delivery is imminent: extreme care is exercised with this procedure.

## SICKLE CELL ANAEMIA

This condition is found in immigrants from tropical Africa and the West Indies; the sickle cell trait being inherited from one or both parents. An abnormal haemoglobin S changes the shape of the red cells, many of which are destroyed by haemolysis. Alarming haemolytic crises take place in the last trimester of pregnancy; pyrexia, jaundice and haematuria sometimes being manifest. Bone pain crises occur in the last weeks of pregnancy and first few days of the puerperium, due to marrow infarction: pulmonary thromboembolism taking place in some cases.

### Treatment

Analgesics and antibiotics are prescribed. The anaemia is treated by an expert. Fetal demands for folic acid are met by giving large doses of folic acid during pregnancy otherwise megaloblastic anaemia may develop. No response to the administration of iron is evident. The fetus is at high risk of hypoxia during labour. The healing process is impaired so a Caesarean section wound or an episiotomy is liable to break down.

**The woman's haemoglobin genotype is ascertained so** that if the Hb is below 7 g/dl, suitable blood for transfusion can be obtained. During crises and when under undue strain with severe anaemia, cardiac failure is an additional risk.

## THALASSAEMIA MAJOR OR MINOR

This is a severe form of anaemia found mainly in immigrants from the Mediterranean area and South East Asia. It is an inherited cause of hypochromic anaemia which occurs even when there is adequate iron in the blood. Iron therapy is therefore not indicated. Red cells are destroyed before release from the bone marrow as well as by haemolysis of circulating red cells. Infection such as pyelonephritis increases the severity of the anaemia. Folic acid is administered and blood transfusion in severe cases. In certain severe types, fetal death from haemolytic anaemia and hydrops takes place.

### Anaemia in Tropical Countries

**Anaemia is one of the most important complications of childbirth in the tropics** and is a major cause of maternal and fetal mortality. Haemoglobin levels below 8·5 g/dl are quite usual and in some instances levels as low as 4·5 g/dl have been seen: life being endangered when below 6·5 g/dl. Iron deficiency anaemia is common, being mainly due to dietary deprivation of iron, folic acid and protein. Haemolysis as occurs in sickle cell anaemia and P. falciparum infections increases the demand for folic acid. Parasites such as hookworm and diseases such as malaria and dysentery are contributory factors.

**Midwives in tropical regions have a grave responsibility** in teaching pregnant women which of the foods, that are available in their area, are rich in iron, folic acid and protein. They must collaborate in the early detection and treatment of anaemia. The treatment depends on the cause. More rapid improvement is achieved by the total dose i.v. infusion technique which ensures that a greater amount of iron is given than by the oral route.

**The third stage of labour and 12 hours postpartum are particularly dangerous:** even a small blood loss can exsanguinate a severely anaemic woman. When the placenta is expelled the retracted uterus returns blood to the general circulation;

the anaemic hypoxic heart muscle is unable to cope with the increased action needed. A transfusion given at this time even if small in amount and infused slowly, can seriously embarrass the heart.

# NEURITIS

Neuritis may occur, both during pregnancy and the puerperium; the woman complaining of pain, numbness and loss of power, usually in one limb. It may be due to deficiency of the vitamin B complex, but is occasionally of cerebral origin. The response to proprietary preparations of vitamin B is usually very good.

**Carpal tunnel syndrome** is fairly common during pregnancy. Tingling, numbness and pain are felt in the thumb and fingers during the night, due to compression of the medial nerve in the carpal tunnel at the wrist. The fluid retention of pregnancy is believed to give rise to pressure on the nerve. Rest and night-splinting may help. The condition disappears spontaneously after delivery.

# ACUTE INFECTIONS

**Pneumonia** and severe influenza of the respiratory type are serious complications during the later months of pregnancy. The disease is treated as in the non-pregnant woman; oxygen is essential to counteract cyanosis. Fifty per cent will go into premature labour, but induction of labour is contra-indicated. Forceps, if required, are applied under pudendal nerve block or perineal infiltration.

**Smallpox** vaccination is not recommended during pregnancy unless contact with smallpox has or will occur: babies of vaccinated mothers have been stillborn or born with generalised vaccinia.

**Poliomyelitis** is considered to be more severe during pregnancy, so polio immunisation of expectant mothers is advocated but not before the 16th week of pregnancy when the embryo is at risk. The Sabin-type vaccine is commonly used. The dangers of poliomyelitis are similar to those in the non-pregnant woman and 75 per cent of deaths occur in the over-15 age group. Spontaneous delivery of the baby is possible even when the abdominal and pelvic floor muscles are paralysed.

## RUBELLA

This disease is a menace when contracted by the pregnant woman, because of its disastrous effect on the fetus *in utero*. If infection occurs during the first 12 weeks of pregnancy, and even more so during the first eight weeks, cell division is inhibited in the embryonic organs: the eyes, ears, heart and brain being particularly vulnerable. The child may be born with one or more of the following defects: cataract, heart disease, mental subnormality. Deafness frequently accompanies the other abnormalities but may occur singly. The diagnosis of rubella is established by virological tests. Therapeutic abortion is considered justifiable by some authorities if the woman develops rubella during the first 12 weeks of pregnancy.

### Prophylaxis

**Rubella is preventable by vaccination** and non-immune girls of 13 to 14 years of age may be vaccinated, using Cendevax or Almevax but it is not known how long the immunity lasts. Adolescents should be made aware of the dangers of rubella so that if non-immune and in contact with children or liable to become pregnant they accept vaccination. The staff in obstetric units are 'at risk' (*a*) from being infected from a baby with congenital rubella, (*b*) they may be incubating rubella and infect women in the early stage of gestation. They should be requested to undergo the haemagglutination antibodies inhibition (H.A.I.) test and offered Cendevax or Almevax vaccine if non-immune.

At many prental clinics blood screening for rubella antibodies is carried out on all women at their initial visit: (a history of having had rubella is unreliable). Demonstration of haemagglutination inhibition antibodies in the serum (H.A.I. test) shows that she is immune to rubella. If antibodies are not demonstrated the woman is susceptible to rubella (10 per cent are). She must not be vaccinated during pregnancy or within two months prior to becoming pregnant but she is offered vaccination during the first week of the puerperium. A reliable contraceptive must be used for 3 months after vaccination in case the baby, conceived during this period, is born with rubella.

## Congenital rubella

The baby is highly infectious and should be isolated; the rubella virus having been recovered from the nasopharynx, blood, urine and stool. He may harbour the virus for one year or longer. Low birth weight, a purpuric rash, eye and heart defects may be obvious. On discharge arrangements are made for the infant to attend an audiometric clinic after 6 months.

# URINARY TRACT INFECTION

Pyelonephritis occurs in about 2 per cent of pregnant women, especially primigravidae, from approximately the 16th to the 26th week of pregnancy. During pregnancy the ureters lack tone and are therefore more readily dilated, kinked or compressed, and this causes stasis of urine with subsequent risk of the multiplication of organisms; the right ureter being more commonly affected because the pregnant uterus leans and rotates on its axis towards the right side. Compression by the pregnant uterus on the ureter where it enters the pelvic brim is most marked from the 16th to the 24th week.

## Source of Infection

The predominant infecting organism in about 80 per cent of cases is the *Escherichia coli*, but the staphylococcus, streptococcus or *ps. aeruginosa* may also be the causal organism. There is some doubt as to how the *E. coli* gains access to the kidney, probably due to vesico-ureteric reflux. Recent work suggests ascending infection, so catheterisation should never be used for diagnostic purposes: midstream (clean catch) specimens of urine are obtained. The use of vaginal deodorants and 'bubble baths' should be discouraged.

## Asymptomatic bacteriuria

Seven per cent of pregnant women have asymptomatic bacteriuria (a count of $10^5$/ml or more organisms in urine on two occasions). Detection and treatment will prevent 60 per cent of all cases of acute pyelonephritis during pregnancy, e.g. amoxycillin 500 mg twice daily for 7 days. The Uricult dip slide system of bacterial culture is useful for screening programmes.

### SIGNS AND SYMPTOMS OF PYELONEPHRITIS

In mild cases the most pronounced features may be loss of appetite, nausea and vomiting which are sometimes mistaken for hyperemesis gravidarum. The onset in acute cases is usually sudden, and abdominal pain, commonly on the right side, is severe. Abdominal tenderness and rigidity are sometimes present and in conjunction with the other signs and symptoms the condition is somewhat similar to appendicitis. In other cases the patient complains of dull backache and pain radiating down to the groin. The temperature ranges from 38·3 to 38·8°C (101° to 102°F) and the pulse from 110 to 130. The patient complains of feeling shivery and sometimes actual rigors occur. The urine looks turbid, and is commonly acid. It contains protein and has a high specific gravity.

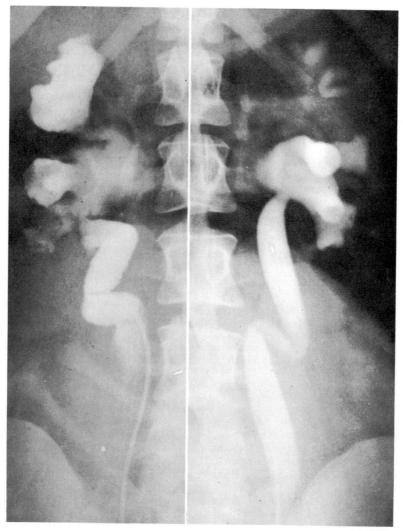

Fig. 13-3   Case of pyelonephritis of pregnancy showing dilatation and marked kinking of ureters.

### Diagnosis

Medical advice must of course be obtained, and the doctor will make the diagnosis. Eliciting tenderness in the loin of a patient with pyrexia, whose urine contains over $10^5$/ml organisms, suggests that active urinary infection is present; finding pus cells is diagnostic but the absence of pus cells does not rule out pyelonephritis.

*Treatment*

The patient is put into a warmed bed, and as she will usually perspire freely, chilling must be avoided, so bathroom privileges are not allowed until the temperature has been normal for some days. Before treatment is begun and 48 hours after a course of antibiotics is completed a mid-stream specimen of urine is obtained, sent for culture and bacteriological investigation. Specimens should reach the laboratory within one hour of passing urine or be kept at a temperature of 4·4°C (40°F), otherwise the organisms multiply and give an excessively high bacterial count. The laboratory may give a tentative report in six hours, causal organism in 15 hours and antibiotic sensitivity in 24 hours.

A fluid balance chart is kept and an adequate intake maintained.

Micturition every two or three hours and complete emptying of the bladder is advisable.

Temperature and pulse are taken and recorded every four hours.

These patients are usually constipated so an enema or suppository is given on admission. Only mild laxatives should be employed.

*Drug Therapy*

The appropriate broad spectrum antibiotic will be prescribed as indicated by the bacteriological sensitivity tests, e.g. ampicillin (Penbritin), 500 mg, six to eight hourly for 10 to 14 days.

Cephalexin (Keflex) (Ceporex) cephaloridine (Ceporin) 250–500 mg i.m. two or three times daily.

Nalidixic acid (Negram) 1 g four times daily has been used with some success against Gram-negative organisms, especially *E. coli* and *B. proteus vulgaris*: relapse may occur. Kanamycin (Kannasyn) is occasionally given in staphylococcal infections resistant to other antibiotics. Nitrofurantoin (Furadantin), 100 mg, four times daily is favoured by some.

*Sulphonamides are rarely used as many organisms are sulphonamide resistant. Whatever drug is used recurrence is common, so follow-up is desirable.*

**The relief of pain**

Heat is usually effective in relieving pain, and as it is advisable to have the patient lying on the non-affected side to encourage good drainage; an electric pad, hot water bottle or Kaolin plaster can be conveniently maintained in position; flexing the knees may also give relief. If the pain is acute the prone position can be adopted and it may be necessary to give an analgesic such as dihydrocodeine (D.F. 118), 30 to 60 mg or Buscopan, 20 mg, Codis tablets (2) or pentazocine (Fortral) tablets 25–50 mg.

The nutritional needs of the pregnant woman must not be forgotten, and her general health should be built up as soon as possible.

**Urological investigation** is made if the infection recurs or bacteriuria persists: radiological examination, cystoscopy, renogram and renal function tests are necessary: these are usually postponed until twelve weeks after delivery.

## RENAL DISEASE

When patients with established renal disease become pregnant, features such as proteinuria, hypertension, oedema, or an elevated blood urea level are present prior to the 20th week. Primary renal disorders complicate about 1 in every 1,000 pregnancies, and pre-eclampsia may be superimposed on the pre-existing disease. If kidney dysfunction is slight, the pregnancy is allowed to continue; the patient being seen weekly; adequate protein and low salt diet is recommended. When renal function is impaired, or where sudden deterioration takes place, termination should be considered. Intra-uterine death may occur, so admission to hospital at 30 weeks and delivery at 36 weeks by Caesarean section may be resorted to for primigravidae and induction of labour for multiparae. Oestriol assay and ultrasonic cephalometry may be utilised to monitor fetal wellbeing.

## ACUTE RENAL FAILURE

This serious condition, when it occurs in obstetric practice, more commonly follows septic abortion, severe abruptio placentae and postpartum haemorrhage with profound shock. Oliguria is the oustanding sign (less than 500 ml urine daily) and this must be reported to the doctor without delay. It is mandatory that an accurate fluid balance record is kept in patients who have been subjected to the above predisposing causes: blood urea estimations and potassium determinations being carried out for 3 days.

### *Management*

The patient is treated if possible in a renal intensive care unit with single rooms to limit the possibility of extraneous infection. Fluids must be carefully regulated, a fluid balance record is kept and 400 ml per 24 hours plus the volume lost in urine and vomitus during the previous 24 hours is given. A 30 g protein diet with 3,000 calories should be given orally. If this is not tolerated intravenous fluid 20 per cent fructose is administered. Parentrovite is given daily. Overhydration is avoided during the oliguric stage and dehydration during the diuretic stage. (Recovery has taken place in patients who have had oliguria for 4 weeks.)

The dietary intake of sodium and potassium is restricted because these ions are excreted by the kidneys; daily estimations of serum, potassium and sodium as well as urea and bicarbonate are made. Hycal glucose syrup (flavoured) is useful being high calorie, low fluid, low electrolyte. Calcium resonium is specific in removing potassium from the body and may be given, 30 g rectally, when the potassium level is found to be rising. If the blood urea or serum potassium rises rapidly—as is the case in most infected and hypoxic patients with acute renal failure—conservative measures will not be sufficient to maintain life until kidney function returns. In these circumstances dialysis therapy will allow a patient to survive even if renal function takes several weeks to return. If the oliguric phase lasts for more than four or five days the use of dialysis with a 50 g protein diet may be safer than the rigorous starvation involved in prolonged conservative therapy.

# SEXUALLY TRANSMITTED DISEASES

## TRICHOMONIASIS

The trichomonas vaginalis, a protozoon, thrives when the vaginal secretion is less acid. The woman complains of a profuse greenish yellow discharge, with burning and irritation of the vulva. The vagina looks red, and a profuse purulent discharge, sometimes frothy with a stale offensive odour, is seen exuding from it. A high vaginal swab is sent to the laboratory in Stuart's transport medium. The organism is identified by direct or dark-ground microscopy and can be easily cultured.

### *Treatment*

Metronidazole (Flagyl) oral tablets, 200 mg, t.i.d., for seven days is usually effective. Nitrimidazine 250 mg night and morning for six days is an equally efficacious remedy. These drugs should not be given while the embryo is at risk, i.e. the first 12 weeks of pregnancy.

The vagina is mopped dry with wool swabs, which in severe cases are moistened with sodium bicarbonate solution to remove the discharge. The doctor may paint the vagina and vulva with an aqueous solution of gentian violet, 1 per cent, to allay irritation but the staining of linen is a disadvantage. Penotrane pessaries have been found to be effective in relieving irritation and counteracting the offensive odour of the discharge. They are inserted into the upper part of the vagina at night, and the woman should lie with her buttocks elevated on two pillows for at least half an hour after their insertion. Conotrane cream, containing penotrane and silicone is suitable for local application to excoriated areas.

## CANDIDIASIS

### Vaginal Thrush

This yeast infection is caused by the candida (monilia) albicans, a fungus found in the vagina of 28 per cent of all pregnant women, and if the vaginal flora is slightly more acid than normal, thrush may develop. The woman complains of intense itching of the vulva and vagina and a thick white or yellow vaginal discharge, which may not be profuse. On the insertion of a speculum, the vagina is seen to be coated with a grey, whitish or yellow curd-like substance which is adherent to the epithelium and on removal leaves an abraded area. The condition is suspected when yeast spores and branching filaments are seen on slides prepared from the plaques of white substance on the vaginal walls and is confirmed by culture.

### Treatment

The vagina is swabbed, as described for trichomoniasis. Two Nystatin pessaries are inserted as high as possible into the vagina at bed-time for 14 nights. Vulval candidiasis responds to Nystatin cream applied night and morning for 14 days. Pruvagol pessaries two or three times weekly may be used. The husband should also be treated.

Many infected women also have infestation of C. albicans in the gastrointestinal tract, which can be a source of re-infection. The oral administration of Nystatin one tablet four times a day will clear this up.

#### GENITAL WARTS

Genital warts are not due to syphilis or gonorrhoea, although they are sometimes seen in such cases. They are caused by a virus and may spread extensively in the vulval region during pregnancy, particularly if the woman has a trichomonal discharge. It is important to find out whether the husband has penile warts as the disease can be spread sexually. A few lesions, ranging from the size of a pinhead to that of a walnut, may be present, and in rare cases they grow profusely to form a large, foul-smelling, fungating mass, which covers the entire vulva and may extend to the thighs and the pubes.

### Treatment

The first essential is the diagnosis and treatment of any accompanying discharge and the maintenance of strict genital hygiene. Resistant and extensive genital warts may have to be removed with the electro-cautery under local or general anaesthesia.

## SYPHILIS

The syphilitic woman who becomes pregnant usually presents few signs or symptoms and the diagnosis of syphilis is made by the routine serological tests for syphilis which should always be carried out during prenatal supervision. These tests should include the Venereal Disease Research Laboratory (V.D.R.L.) test and the Reiter Protein Complement Fixation test (R.P.C.F.T.). Cases with doubtful serological tests require further investigation which include the Fluorescent Treponemal Antibody test (F.T.A.) and/or the Treponema Pallidum Immobilisation test (T.P.I.). These tests are carried out at the V.D. Research Laboratories which give top priority to sera submitted from pregnant women.

**Skin rashes,** yellowish, rose-coloured, becoming dull brown (non-itchy) may be manifest. The rash may form moist papules, on or near the vulva, deep pink in colour with a greyish surface. When they grow exuberantly they are known as condylomata lata; teeming with treponema pallidum and highly contagious.

Student midwives should be warned that false positive serological reactions do occur in pregnancy and that the term 'syphilis' or 'V.D. clinic' should not be used when talking to patients. The doctor only should inform the woman of the result of such tests or discuss their implications.

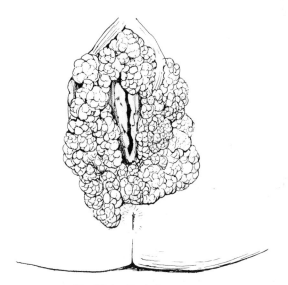

Fig. 13-4   Genital warts.

*The Effects of Untreated Syphilis on Childbearing*

**Abortion may occur after the 20th week.    Labour may be preterm.**
**The fetus may be stillborn (macerated).    The child may be born with syphilis.**
The untreated syphilitic baby who shows clinical manifestations of the disease at birth usually dies, but the less severe cases may recover.

### *Treatment*

Prophylaxis is the best form of treatment, and the routine examination of the blood of all pregnant women by serological tests is one of the finest examples of preventive medicine. Penicillin therapy is used almost exclusively; ideally treatment should begin before the 20th week but results are good even when the treatment is started as late as the 28th week. The woman may be admitted to hospital, though out-patient treatment is adequate in the latent stage of the infection. Triplopen 1·25 mega units daily for 14 days is adequate. If the patient is sensitive to penicillin, Cephaloridine is the alternative. When treated as an in-patient, crystalline penicillin 1 mega unit 8 hourly for 10 days will produce levels adequate to cure.

When infective lesions are present the midwife takes the necessary precautions to protect herself by wearing gown and gloves, and the other patients by segregation of dishes and equipment. Care in the disposal of dressings is necessary until the lesions are non-infectious, which is within 48 hours after intensive penicillin therapy is begun.

Surveillance following treatment for syphilis in the mother must be carried out for two years. Blood tests are carried out monthly for the first six months, then three monthly for the next six months and two blood tests at six monthly intervals should be carried out in the second year.

## CONGENITAL SYPHILIS

An infant with strongly positive serological tests may appear to be normal in every way. Midwives seldom see a newborn baby with signs of syphilis, as these do not usually develop until after the first month of life, neither is the placenta always large and unhealthy-looking, unless the infant is stillborn and macerated. Jaundice may occur. Skin lesions, if present at birth, give rise to suspicion, especially when there are blebs on the palms and soles (syphilitic pemphigus). Various skin rashes may develop during the first month, and the napkin area is particularly vulnerable. If the larynx is affected the cry has a peculiar, cracked or hoarse quality. Fissures in the centre of the lips, the angles of the mouth and around the anus leave permanent scars known as rhagades.

The baby is not born with a saddle nose; such a deformity becomes apparent later in life, due to necrosis of the nasal bones, and is preceded by a profuse purulent blood-stained nasal discharge, syphilitic rhinitis.

### Diagnosis

Cord-blood may contain maternal antibodies which make the interpretation of the infants' serology difficult. Not until the infant is six weeks old can a positive or negative result be accepted as such; a heel stab is made and sufficient blood obtained for the test. The presence of specific IgM detected by the FTA-IgM test is very strong evidence of infection.

#### *Treatment*

Isolation of the infant is wise until penicillin has been given for 48 hours.

If the mother was untreated or inadequately treated, the infant is given procaine penicillin, 150,000 units, by intramuscular injection daily for 10 days. If blood tests are not negative within six months a second course is given.

## GONORRHOEA

The diagnosis and treatment of gonorrhoea during pregnancy is important because of the risk of the baby's eyes being infected by the gonococcus during birth. In the majority of cases the symptoms are slight. Most pregnant women have leucorrhoea, but when the vaginal discharge is greenish, profuse, offensive, or irritating, the midwife should inform the doctor, who will investigate the cause. Gonorrhoea may co-exist with other vaginal infections, such as trichomoniasis and candidiasis, or in conjunction with syphilis. Acute gonorrhoea is infrequently found, and in such a case the vaginal discharge is greenish or yellow and profuse, giving rise to oedema of the labia. The woman complains of frequency and burning pain on micturition.

### Investigation

The woman is told not to pass urine for two hours prior to examination and the vulva must not be swabbed. The patient is placed in the lithotomy position. A platinum loop is used to collect discharge from the urethra, cervix and from Bartholin's ducts; smears and cultures are then made for detection of the gonococcus.

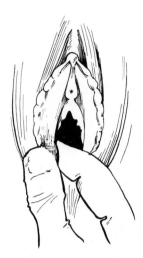

Fig. 13-5 Showing chronic infection of Bartholin's gland. This is not always due to the gonococcus.

### Diagnosis

A history of infection. The clinical findings. The detection of Gram-negative intra-cellular diplococci in smears from the urethra and cervix. Cultures from cervix and urethra (sent to the laboratory in Stuart's medium). Thayer and Martin medium contains antibiotics which suppress other organisms and allow the gonococcus to grow more rapidly.

### *Treatment*

*Procaine penicillin* 1·2 mega units by intra-muscular injection for three consecutive days. For those allergic to penicillin, cephaloridine, 1 g, daily for three days or Kanamycin (Kannasyn), 2 g, in one injection or as 1 g daily intramuscularly for three days are effective remedies. It is most important to examine the patient frequently taking smears and cultures weekly for the first four weeks then monthly for two months to ensure that treatment has been successful. Cases of penicillin resistant gonorrhoea are occurring in Britain.

Serological tests for syphilis should be taken monthly for three months to exclude syphilis which may have been masked by the penicillin given.

# QUESTIONS FOR REVISION

### Cardiac disease

Name the important points in the care of pregnant women with cardiac disease. In what position is she delivered? What signs should be reported to the doctor during labour? Why are the following drugs prescribed: Frusemide, Digoxin, Aminophylline?

Give 3 main causes of deterioration in pregnant patients with cardiac disease.

How would you manage each of the 3 stages of labour?

Why is the lithotomy position not advisable? How would you cope with acute heart failure in the absence of medical assistance?

**C.M.B.(Scot.) 30-min. question.** What are the risks to a patient with cardiac disease who becomes pregnant? Describe the management during pregnancy and labour.

### Diabetes

What signs and symptoms would cause a midwife to suspect diabetes in pregnancy? Name the conditions which may arise during pregnancy because of diabetes. Describe the duties of a midwife during labour, from the diabetic aspect.

Give the causes of glycosuria in pregnancy. Describe the effects of diabetes on childbearing. The management of the pregnant diabetic. The management of labour in diabetes. Discuss in relation to diabetes: (a) polyhydramnios; (b) intra-uterine fetal death; (c) the obstetric history. Differentiate between potential, latent and prediabetic.

Discuss the management of pregnancy in a patient with diabetes mellitus.

**C.M.B.(Scot.) 30-min. question.** In what way may diabetes in the mother complicate the pregnancy? Outline the management of the case and immediate care of the baby.

**C.M.B.(Scot.).** A diabetic woman insulin dependent since childhood has become pregnant for the first time. What information should be given by the midwife to this patient concerning her pregnancy and her baby.

**C.M.B.(Scot.) 30-min. question.** Describe the methods used to reduce fetal loss in pregnancy complicated by diabetes.

### Anaemia

Give (a) the role of the midwife in the prevention of anaemia. (b) Causes of iron deficiency anaemia. (c) The effects of anaemia on childbearing.

Underline the foods that are rich in iron: chocolate; wholewheat bread, green vegetables; milk; butter; oranges; liver; fish; treacle; prunes; eggs.

What is the connection between anaemia in pregnancy and the following; folic acid deficiency; hook worm infection; the sickle cell gene?

Why and how are the following substances administered: ferrous fumarate; ascorbic acid; Alcopar; folic acid; packed red cells. Give an account of the prevention and management of anaemia in pregnancy.

What advice would you give re administration of iron tablets? In which patients might hook worm infection be present? How frequently are haemoglobin estimations made in pregnancy?

**(N. Ire.) 30-min. question.** Anaemia is noted at 34 weeks in a primigravida. Describe the possible dangers, investigation and treatment.

**C.M.B.(Eng.) 30-min. question.** Anaemia still occurs during pregnancy. How may it be prevented and what are the dangers?

**C.M.B.(Scot.) 30-min. question.** What factors are responsible for the high incidence of anaemia in pregnancy? Describe the prevention and treatment of this condition.

**C.M.B.(Scot.).** What changes take place in the blood during pregnancy? What forms of anaemia may currently occur in the United Kingdom? How may anaemia affect the outcome of pregnancy for the mother and the fetus?

### Tuberculosis

Discuss Pulmonary Tuberculosis as a social problem: the modern outlook regarding pulmonary tuberculosis and childbearing.

**(N. Ire.) 30-min. question.** What is 'B.C.G.'? Which babies are especially likely to benefit from its use and what precautions must be observed?

### Rubella

Rubella virus vaccine is recommended for girls before child-bearing age and not for pregnant women, or those liable to become pregnant within three months—why? How long does the virus persist in cases of congenital rubella?

**C.M.B.(Scot.).** Describe in each case the investigations and management if a pregnant woman is known to have been in contact with: (a) Rubella; (b) Pulmonary Tuberculosis; (c) Syphilis; (d) Gonorrhoea.

### Pyelonephritis

Which is the most common invading organism? Describe the signs and symptoms.

What is? (a) asymptomatic bacteriuria; (b) factors that predispose to pyelonephritis; (c) nursing care in acute pyelonephritis.

Which factors predispose to urinary tract infection in pregnancy?

The following drugs may be prescribed in pyelonephritis: stage dose and purpose: kanamycin, papaveretum, ampicillin.

(N. Ire.) 30-min. question. Describe the symptoms and signs, diagnosis and management of a case of urinary tract infection occurring in pregnancy.

C.M.B.(Scot.) 30-min. question. What changes occur in the urinary tract during pregnancy? Give the management of a patient with acute pyelonephritis.

C.M.B.(Eng.). Describe the diagnosis of acute pyelonephritis and the management of a patient with this condition.

### Sexually transmitted diseases

What signs of venereal disease may be evident on examination of the vulva?

State how you would (a) insert a penotrane vaginal pessary; (b) relieve vulval itching due to candidiasis; (c) recognise: (1) condylomata lata, (2) vulval warts.

Signs of congenital syphilis are rarely present prior to the ............................ month.

C.M.B.(Scot.) 30-min. question. How may untreated venereal disease in a pregnant woman affect her baby? Describe in detail the conditions that may be found in the baby. How may they be prevented?

(N. Ire.) 30-min. question. What are the signs and symptoms of gonorrhoea? Describe the treatment and state the dangers to the infant if the condition is untreated.

C.M.B.(Eng.) What are the common sexually transmitted diseases? Discuss the factors which contribute to the increased incidence of such diseases.

### Vaginal discharge

C.M.B.(Scot.) 30-min. question. What are the causes of non-haemorrhagic vaginal discharge in pregnancy? Give the usual treatment of one of the conditions you mention.

C.M.B.(Eng.). What are the causes and dangers of vaginal discharges in pregnancy? What investigations and treatment may follow the discovery of vaginal discharge?

## C.M.B. Short Examination Questions

Eng.: What are the common vaginal discharges in pregnancy and how are they treated? N. Ire.: Candidial vaginitis (Thrush). Eng.: Trichomonal vaginitis. Eng.: The latent diabetic in pregnancy. Eng.: Anaemia in pregnancy. Eng.: Iron-deficiency anaemia. Eng.: Rubella (German measles) in pregnancy. Eng.: Are there any dangers immunising against Rubella? Eng.: The reasons for rubella immunisation. Scot.: Asymptomatic bacteriuria. Eng.: The diagnosis of urinary tract infections in pregnancy. N. Ire.: Bacteriuria. Scot.: Why is the rise in incidence of gonorrhoea of concern to midwives? Scot.: Risks of rubella infection in pregnancy. Eng.: Correction of iron deficiency anaemia in pregnancy. Eng.: Sexually transmitted diseases. Eng.: Gonorrhoea in pregnancy.

# 14
# Antepartum Haemorrhage

*Type undiagnosed; treatment. Placenta praevia; management. Placental abruption; management. Blood coagulation disorders*

Although any vaginal bleeding prior to the birth of the baby might be considered to be antepartum, it is expedient to limit the source of bleeding to that from the placental site, and the time of occurrence to the period of fetal viability. (***Prior to the 28th week of pregnancy, bleeding from the placental site would be a sign of abortion.***)

Some authorities include bleeding from other sources, such as lesions of the cervix (see p. 158) and vasa praevia (see p. 51). Bleeding from cervical lesions can be recognised by speculum examination. Haemorrhage from the placental site constitutes an urgent threat to mother and child which demands immediate admission to hospital for supervision and treatment. The midwife must appreciate the seriousness of placental site haemorrhage.

## DEFINITION

### Antepartum haemorrhage

This is bleeding from the placental site due to premature separation of the placenta after the 28th week of pregnancy and prior to the birth of the baby (the first and second stages of labour are therefore included). Antepartum haemorrhage is classified according to the situation of the placenta, i.e. whether it is implanted in the upper or lower uterine segment.

### Unavoidable haemorrhage

Bleeding due to the premature separation of a placenta which is situated partly or wholly in the lower uterine segment, i.e. a placenta praevia.

### Placental abruption (Abruptio placentae) accidental haemorrhage

Bleeding due to the premature separation of a normally situated placenta.

### Incidental haemorrhage

Bleeding from other sources usually cervical.

## ANTEPARTUM HAEMORRHAGE *(Type undiagnosed)*

Patients with antepartum haemorrhage have to be dealt with on district and in hospital before the haemorrhage has been diagnosed as due to placenta praevia or abruptio placentae. In both types the initial treatment is the same, but when, after admission to hospital, the diagnosis is made, the appropriate treatment is instituted.

*To avoid unnecessary repetition the initial treatment of antepartum haemorrhage is not given when the management of placenta praevia or abruptio placentae is described. Midwives must therefore when deliberating on the treatment of these refer back to initial treatment of antepartum haemorrhage (type undiagnosed).*

## MANAGEMENT

Hospitalisation is imperative whether the bleeding is slight or severe. Every woman who bleeds *per vaginam* after the 28th week of pregnancy must be transferred to hospital as soon as possible. She is in danger of further and more serious haemorrhage; fetal death may occur, so all the facilities provided in a modern maternity hospital to preserve maternal and infant life and health should be made available.

Vaginal examination to determine the situation of the placenta is dangerous and should only be made in an operating theatre. Inserting a finger into the cervical canal or applying pressure through the vaginal fornices may induce profuse haemorrhage, immediately or within a few hours, which may be almost uncontrollable. Two units of cross-matched blood should be available prior to vaginal examination.

### OBSERVATION

**General condition.** Note pulse rate, blood pressure, oedema, pallor.

**Blood loss.** The amount of blood should be assessed (pads and sheets set aside for inspection by the doctor). Enquiry is made as to previous bleeding and whether the onset of the present loss is related to undue physical exertion or emotional stress.

**Abdominal examination** must be carried out with the greatest gentleness, noting pain, tenderness, uterine consistence, malpresentation, high head, fetal heart rate.

**Recording.** A record is made of name, age, parity, week of gestation, blood loss, blood pressure; pulse every 5 to 15 minutes depending on the severity of the condition; amount of urine passed, fetal heart rate, drugs administered.

### Treatment by Midwife on District

Prophylaxis is the midwife's first duty. If the woman has been instructed to report any vaginal bleeding at once, is transferred to hospital promptly without vaginal examination, the prognosis is much better for mother and child.

The woman is put to bed, reassured, and kept flat.

Medical aid is sent for without delay. If the doctor is not available and the situation is urgent, e.g. severe bleeding, or shock and abdominal pain with or without slight bleeding, the midwife should summon the 'flying squad' or communicate with a maternity hospital at once.

The doctor will arrange for the woman to be transferred to hospital after a sedative such as pethidine, 150 mg or papaveretum (Omnopon), 20 mg or morphine, 15 mg is administered. If the woman's condition does not warrant the journey the doctor will summon the 'flying squad' who will give a blood transfusion before transferring her to hospital. The midwife, taking with her the records she has kept, accompanies the woman, having applied two perineal pads and wrapped a linen and a plastic sheet round the woman's hips.

## TREATMENT IN HOSPITAL

### (Type of Haemorrhage undiagnosed)

Certain routine investigations are made on all unbooked patients when admitted to hospital with antepartum haemorrhage, whether the bleeding is slight or severe. Booked patients will have had their blood examined previously, a procedure which saves valuable time when blood transfusion is urgently needed.

### Preparations to be made for Investigation and Treatment

For ABO blood grouping and cross matching, haemoglobin, Rh factor, clotting time, plasma fibrinogen, and serological test for syphilis (if not already done).

For intravenous administration of blood, glucose, Ringer's lactate solution, oxytocin drip, fibrinogen.

For injection of pethidine, papaveretum. Urine analysis. Esbach's test.

Sphygmomanometer, Stethoscope, Fetal stethoscope. Sonicaid. Cylinder of oxygen. Polythene face mask. Central venous pressure manometer.

*Prepare the Following Charts in Graph Form if Possible*

**Pulse,** 5 to 15 minutes.          **Blood pressure,** 15 minutes.
**Fetal heart,** continuous or          **Fluid balance.**
every 10 to 20 minutes.

Have a 'permission for operation and anaesthetic' form ready for signature.

### Treatment of Slight Bleeding

The woman is put into a warmed bed and not allowed to get up.
No vaginal or rectal examination is made.

**Observation**

Note blood loss, pallor, oedema. Vital signs are recorded.

Gentle abdominal examination, noting pain, tenderness, uterine consistence, high head, malpresentation, fetal heart rate.

Sedatives such as diazepam (Valium), 5–10 mg or nitrazepam (Mogadon) 5–10 mg, are administered if necessary.

Blood is obtained for the necessary tests.

Routine vulval preparation is carried out. A specimen of urine is obtained and examined for protein.

No enema on admission (a small enema, Dulcolax suppository or mild laxative may be ordered after 48 hours). Perineal pads are kept for inspection by the doctor if the loss becomes more than slight.

A speculum examination is made after two or three days to rule out cervical causes of bleeding. A Papanicolaou smear may be taken.

The patient is allowed up after five days if there is no bleeding during that time. If after a further two days there is no bleeding, no pre-eclampsia, essential hypertension, and no placenta praevia on X-ray or ultrasonic localisation the woman may be permitted to go home, and told to return if bleeding occurs and for delivery.

### Treatment of Severe Bleeding

The woman will be in a dangerous state of collapse due to profuse or prolonged haemorrhage. Immediate resuscitation is imperative and no time should be lost in obtaining and administering blood. The woman is admitted to the special resuscitation unit and the procedures as for slight bleeding are carried out (see above).

Maternal pulse and blood pressure are taken and recorded. Plasma fibrinogen and clot tests are made.

Sedatives are given for apprehension, analgesics for pain.

Glucose, 5 per cent, and Ringer's lactate solution are given intravenously while compatible blood is being procured. A transfusion of fresh blood is administered.

The fetal heart is auscultated every 10 or 15 minutes or monitored continuously.

Further treatment will depend on whether the haemorrhage continues, and if so a vaginal examination may be made, as outlined on page 232 to determine if bleeding is due to placenta praevia. The appropriate treatment is then given.

## PLACENTA PRAEVIA (*unavoidable haemorrhage*)

The premature separation of a placenta praevia is inevitable and bleeding unavoidable because when stretching of the lower uterine segment occurs during the latter weeks of pregnancy the anchoring chorionic villi are torn across, the venous sinuses in the placental site are exposed and blood escapes. The initial bleeding may be very slight, but, as further stretching of the lower segment proceeds, the bleeding recurs at intervals of hours or days. When the placenta lies over the internal os the seriousness of the situation is intensified because massive separation with profuse haemorrhage must occur while the cervix is being taken up and the os dilating.

### Causes

It occurs more commonly in multiparous women, and may be due to some abnormal condition in the endometrium of the upper uterine segment which does not provide a suitable nidus in which the fertilised ovum can embed.

The placenta may have developed from chorionic villi in the lower part of the decidua capsularis which should have atrophied before the decidua capsularis fused with the decidua vera at the 12th week; these villi then embed in the lower pole of the uterus.

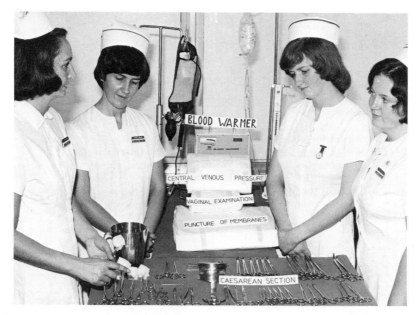

Fig. 14-1   Non-sterile set up for clinical instruction on placenta praevia including Fenwal blood infusion pump. Midwifery forceps are wrapped separately.

*Bellshill Maternity Hospital, Lanarkshire.*

## SIGNS AND DIAGNOSIS

The only sign is vaginal bleeding. A reliable method of diagnosis is by feeling the placenta through the cervical canal, but the risk of instigating massive haemorrhage is so great that a vaginal examination is never made except when the patient is in the operating theatre set up in readiness for Caesarean section.

*Factors which are Suggestive in making the Diagnosis*

### Type of bleeding

Painless vaginal bleeding, for which no obvious cause is apparent; the bleeding often occurring during rest or sleep. The initial loss is usually slight, becoming more and more profuse. Occasionally the first bleeding is sudden and severe.

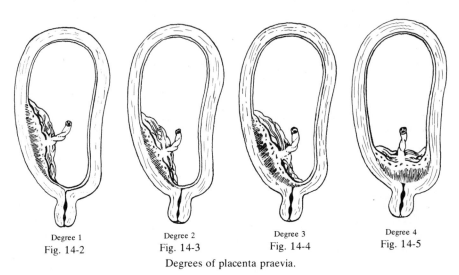

Degree 1
Fig. 14-2

Degree 2
Fig. 14-3

Degree 3
Fig. 14-4

Degree 4
Fig. 14-5

Degrees of placenta praevia.

1—**The edge of the placenta dips into the lower segment.**
2—**The edge of the placenta is at the margin of the internal os.**
3—**The placenta lies completely over the os** when closed and until 4 cm dilatation.
4—**The centre of the placenta lies over the centre of the os.**

Some authorities classify placenta praevia = degree 1 as minor: degrees 2, 3, 4, as major.

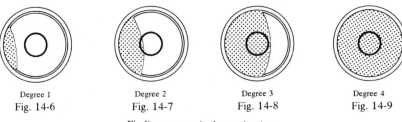

Degree 1
Fig. 14-6

Degree 2
Fig. 14-7

Degree 3
Fig. 14-8

Degree 4
Fig. 14-9

Findings on vaginal examination.

1—**Membrane over os. Placenta may be felt on exploration of lower uterine segment.**
2—**Membrane over os. Placenta felt at margin of os.**
3—**Placenta may be felt over os until about 4 cm dilatation.**
4—**Placenta lies over os until full dilatation.**

## Abdominal findings

Transverse lie occurs because the placenta encroaches on the lower pole of the uterus and prevents the fetus from adopting the longitudinal lie.

Malpresentation particularly breech.

The head is high and slips to one or other side when an attempt is made to make it enter the brim.

The uterus is of normal consistence, being neither hard nor tender on palpation. No abdominal pain is experienced.

## Localisation of placenta

(*a*) **Sonar (ultrasonic technique)** is now being used with over 94 per cent accuracy. The level and margins of the placenta can be defined from the 26th week onward. The bladder should be partially filled or a low lying placenta may not be diagnosed.

(*b*) **Placentography.** After the 33rd week the location of the placenta can be determined on soft tissue X-ray (lateral view, woman erect, bladder empty).

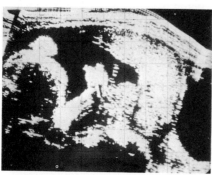 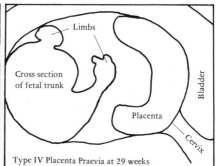

Limbs

Cross section
of fetal trunk

Bladder

Placenta

Cervix

Type IV Placenta Praevia at 29 weeks

Fig. 14-10   Ultrasonogram of placenta praevia.
*Queen Mother's Hospital, Glasgow.*

(*c*) **Radioactive isotopes** injected intravenously are used to locate the vascular placental site which has a high count rate.

(*d*) **Arteriography** is occasionally used from the 28th to the 32nd week. After sedation and local analgesia Conray aqueous solution is injected via a catheter which is inserted into the femoral artery. In 6 seconds the X-ray will show the radio-opaque substance in the intervillous spaces.

## MANAGEMENT IN HOSPITAL

*Initial treatment of antepartum haemorrhage is described on page 227.*

Treatment is aimed primarily at controlling haemorrhage and saving infant life and will be active or expectant depending on the amount of blood loss and the week of gestation.

### ACTIVE TREATMENT

## Severe bleeding

(*a*) Resuscitative measures as for severe antepartum haemorrhage (p. 228).

(*b*) Preparations are made for Caesarean section which is performed immediately if, on admission or subsequently, bleeding is profuse.

### Moderate or persistent bleeding

If the woman is over 37 weeks pregnant, vaginal examination is carried out in the theatre set up for immediate operation. The treatment adopted (1) Puncture of membranes to induce labour, (2) Caesarean section, will depend on the findings as in expectant treatment (see below).

### Slight bleeding

The treatment is expectant.

#### EXPECTANT OR CONSERVATIVE TREATMENT

An attempt is made to prolong pregnancy until the fetus is sufficiently mature to have a reasonable chance of survival. Any interference, such as exploring the cervical canal or puncturing the membranes is postponed until the 38th week.

The woman is kept in hospital, closely supervised and usually confined to bed.

Routine blood tests are made (p. 227). Further bleeding should be reported immediately: perineal pads kept for inspection if blood stained.

A speculum examination is made after two or three days to exclude cervical or vaginal lesions as sources of bleeding.

Blood transfusion is administered if the haemoglobin is low or further bleeding occurs. Food rich in iron, as well as iron supplements, are given.

The doctor is notified if labour starts.

#### At the 38th week the Woman is taken to the Operating Theatre

All equipment is set out, patient's skin prepared, bladder emptied: theatre staff 'scrubbed up' in readiness for immediate Caesarean section.

Cross-matched blood, 1,200 ml (at least), should be at hand. A slow drip of Hartmann's solution and glucose 5 per cent may be started, and facilities for resuscitation of a collapsed patient ready. Central venous pressure manometer at hand.

### Puncture of membranes

A separate trolley is set up for this purpose.

A vaginal examination is made under general anaesthesia by the obstetrician to determine the degree of placenta praevia. For degree one the membranes may be punctured and when labour ensues the baby is usually born spontaneously.

Two sterile gauze vaginal packs 2 m × 10 cm should always be in readiness to control the massive haemorrhage which may occur.

### Caesarean section is performed

(a) If profuse haemorrhage occurs. (b) When placenta praevia degree 2, 3 or 4 is diagnosed.

(c) If in degree 1 the fetus lies transversely, or the woman is an older primigravida.

The baby's haemoglobin level should be estimated at birth because on occasions fetal blood is lost. If within four hours it is below 14·8 g/dl a blood transfusion is given.

Student midwives should note that central placenta praevia does not obstruct labour. The reason why Caesarean section is performed is to avoid massive haemorrhage and so to save mother and baby. The midwife is reminded that serious bleeding is usually due to the unjustifiable digital exploration of the cervical canal or ill-advised attempts to puncture the membranes.

*Active Treatment of Placenta Praevia (summarised)*

**Puncture of membranes** for slight bleeding. (Degree 1).
**Caesarean section** for severe bleeding. (Degrees 2, 3, 4).
**Blood transfusion** for severe or persistent bleeding.

#### DANGERS OF PLACENTA PRAEVIA

**Severe haemorrhage** particularly following vaginal examination.
**Postpartum atonic haemorrhage** because the lower segment does not contract and retract efficiently.
**Stillbirth** due to fetal anoxia.

# PLACENTAL ABRUPTION
## (*Accidental haemorrhage*)

The term 'abruption' means to tear asunder.
Any strenuous physical effort or acute emotional stress that temporarily raises the blood pressure may precipitate the occurrence of placental abruption. The condition is more common in multiparous patients and in those with poor nutritional status. A fall or a blow on the abdomen, or traction on the cord, as might take place during external version, is the cause in a minority of cases.

## TYPES OF HAEMORRHAGE

### (1) EXTERNAL OR REVEALED HAEMORRHAGE

Blood escapes from the vagina; this being the most common type. Slight bleeding may become severe: abdominal pain and tenderness may or may not be present.
Delivery of the fetus should be accomplished within 6 hours if possible. The longer the delay, the greater is the likelihood of coagulation failure developing.

#### *Treatment of severe bleeding*

As for severe antepartum haemorrhage (type undiagnosed) (p. 228).
**Adequate blood transfusion.** When the plasma fibrinogen is below normal, fresh rather than stored blood is used, because of its higher fibrinogen content.
**A careful fluid balance record is kept.**
The woman should lie in the left lateral position until delivered to facilitate more efficient kidney secretion. In the dorsal position shock may occur due to vena caval occlusion.
**The membranes are punctured** and the amniotic fluid drained off, as it is high in thromboplastin; the procedure being carried out in the theatre set up for Caesarean section.
**Caesarean section** is usually performed when haemorrhage persists, and in severe and sometimes moderate bleeding or if during labour fetal distress occurs.
An oxytocin drip is given by some authorities if labour does not commence within a few hours: a syringe i.v. pump being used. If the fetus is dead prostaglandin may be preferred.

### (2) COMBINED HAEMORRHAGE

The haemorrhage is primarily concealed, and then becomes revealed. A degree of shock is exhibited which is always greater than the blood loss warrants, and is usually associated with blood coagulation disorders.
**Treatment** is similar to that for concealed haemorrhage.

### (3) CONCEALED HAEMORRHAGE

This is a desperately serious condition with high maternal and fetal mortality rates. Fortunately it is the least common type of placental abruption.

No vaginal bleeding occurs, but a retroplacental blood clot forms which may weigh as much as 1·5 kg, the placenta when expelled showing a crater-like area, or circumscribed depression on the maternal surface, containing dark old blood clot. Blood coagulation disorders develop in many of these cases (see p. 235).

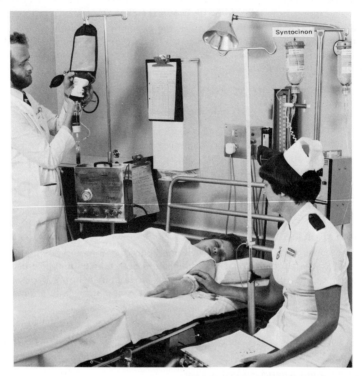

Fig. 14-11 Patient with placental abruption receiving blood via Fenwal BD4 pressure infuser. Grant blood warmer, CVP manometer in use. Syntocinon being administered i.v.
*Maternity Department, Royal Infirmary, Perth.*

### *The following signs and symptoms are those of a severe case:*

**Shock** is the outstanding feature but the blood pressure may not fall to (90/60) in the hypertensive patient, even when hypovolaemia exists.

**Abdominal pain** is excruciating and constant: never intermittent.

**The uterus** is exquisitely tender to touch. The fetus cannot be palpated because of uterine and abdominal wall rigidity; no fetal heart-beat is heard.

**The pulse,** which may be slow at first, becomes rapid and thready.

**Urine**—very little is secreted.

Protein always appears in the urine after concealed accidental haemorrhage occurs and does not necessarily indicate the presence of pre-eclampsia.

### *Treatment in Maternity Hospital (intensive care unit)*

*Measures to combat shock and blood loss should be quickly initiated.*

Routine blood investigations are made (see p. 227). Plasma-fibrinogen and clotting-time tests are performed. The Fi-test, Baxter-Hyland, for hypofib-rinogenaemia is useful when laboratory facilities are not available. The Fibrindex thrombin test is made. Expert haematological advice is essential.

**Pethidine,** 200 mg, or morphine, 15 mg, may be given for pain.

**Blood transfusion of at least two litres** of fresh blood is administered rapidly within one hour then more slowly, depending on the central venous pressure (normal being 8–12 cm of water).

**Fibrinogen,** 4 to 6 g, may be administered intravenously, followed by 1 g at half-hourly intervals until the clotting mechanism is restored to normal, but fresh blood is a rich source of fibrinogen and other factors.

**Renal secretion** is carefully observed and ought to be at least 30 ml per hour. The fluid intake is recorded. Each specimen of urine is examined for volume and protein.

Caesarean section is performed (when the clotting defect is controlled).

Postpartum haemorrhage is a possible danger if the uterus is atonic and any blood coagulation defect has not been corrected.

*(The weight of the retroplacental clot should be recorded.)*

**Postnatal care**

The hazard of acute renal failure is very great indeed so the woman must be observed carefully. The daily fluid intake should be restricted to 1,000 ml for a few days and the diet low in protein, sodium and potassium. Blood urea estimations and potassium determinations are made for 3 days. An accurate fluid balance record is kept and signs of oliguria (less than 500 ml urine daily) reported without delay. Anaemia if present should be treated and further blood transfusion may be indicated.

### *Adoption of the Lateral Position*

Patients whose kidneys are likely to be adversely affected, i.e. in pre-eclampsia, placental abruption and chronic renal disease, should lie on their sides to promote kidney function and prevent vena caval occlusion. In some women there is no collateral drainage from the renal vessels to cope with the impeded blood flow that occurs when they adopt the supine position.

## BLOOD COAGULATION DISORDERS IN OBSTETRICS

Serious haemorrhage in obstetrics may be due to blood clotting failure, the most common cause being abruptio placentae (placental abruption).

**(1) HYPOFIBRINOGENAEMIA, (2) EXCESSIVE FIBRINOLYTIC ACTIVITY or (3) A COMBINATION OF BOTH.**

(1) **Hypofibrinogenaemia.** This is usually due to consumption of available maternal fibrinogen because of the abnormal entry of thromboplastin into the circulation (*a*) from the placental site in abruptio placentae, (*b*) from amniotic fluid (which is rich in thromboplastin), (*c*) from tissue juice from a retained macerated fetus.

*Tests.* The Fibrindex (Ortho) and the Baxter Fi test are available for bedside diagnosis.

Expert haematological advice is needed in the differential diagnosis and treatment.

### *Treatment*

This includes giving intravenous human fibrinogen 4 g to 6 g with, in severe blood loss, adequate whole blood replacement. Dextran is definitely contra-indicated.

(2) **Excessive fibrinolytic activity.** This is due to excessive tissue plasminogen activator entering the maternal circulation and producing substances that inhibit normal blood coagulation. The maternal blood, in a test tube, may clot but rapid lysis follows at once.

### Treatment

This may (rarely) require the administration of a fibrinolytic inhibitor intraven-ously; fibrinogen and/or whole blood as in (1), and heparin.

### (3) **Excessive fibrinolytic activity and hypofibrinogenaemia.**

### Treatment

This includes giving whole blood (as fresh as possible), fibrinogen and other clotting factors if required and sometimes in combination with intravenous heparin therapy to spare further consumption.

Fresh blood contains about 3·3 g fibrinogen in 1,800 ml as well as other factors and is now preferred to fibrinogen. The successful outcome in many cases, where the more sophisticated products are not available, is often no doubt due to the prompt administration of adequate fresh blood.

Serious postpartum haemorrhage may have to be dealt with should the uterus be atonic in the presence of blood coagulation disorders.

---

## QUESTIONS FOR REVISION

### ANTEPARTUM HAEMORRHAGE

Give a list of the equipment you would have at hand for the reception of a patient with moderately severe antepartum haemorrhage and for the investigations to be carried out in such a case.

### Oral Questions

How could you help to reduce the number of cases of serious antepartum haemorrhage?

Why is bleeding from the placental site more serious than from other vaginal sources?

Why must a vaginal examination not be made outwith a theatre equipped for a Caesarean section?

The active treatment of placenta praevia can be summarised for slight and severe cases as (a) . . . and (b) . . . Why is the woman required to lie on her side in cases of placental abruption. Why is Caesarean section performed in placenta praevia?

What observation would you make in a case of antepartum haemorrhage: (1) general condition; (2) history; (3) blood loss; (4) abdominal examination?

State 4 blood tests; 4 charts; 4 intravenous solutions; 4 methods of diagnosis that might be utilised. Define the four degrees of placenta praevia.

Differentiate between: blood coagulation defect and retroplacental clot; active and expectant treatment of placenta praevia; combined and concealed haemorrhage.

(**N. Ire.**) **30-min. question.** What is placenta praevia? When is this condition suspected? What is meant by conservative treatment?

(**Eng.**). Kleihauer test. Vaginal bleeding in late pregnancy. **Scot.** Hypofibrinogenaemia.

**C.M.B.(Eng.).** A patient, 32 weeks pregnant, is admitted to hospital with vaginal bleeding. Describe the management of this case.

**C.M.B.(Eng.).** Define antepartum haemorrhage. Describe the management of a patient with this condition occurring at the thirty-sixth week of pregnancy.

# 15
# Normal Labour

*Cause of onset. Signs. Duration. Mechanism. Physiological changes in first and second stages*

Labour is described as the process by which the fetus, placenta and membranes are expelled through the birth canal. It involves more than the expulsive muscular effort of the uterus, being a strenuous ordeal in which the woman's whole body participates, and demanding physical stamina and emotional control. The term 'labour' is used after the 28th week of gestation: before then the process is called 'abortion'.

### Normal labour occurs when

The fetus is born at term and presents by the vertex.

The process is completed spontaneously **(by the natural unaided efforts of the mother).** The time does not exceed 18 hours. No complications arise.

### CAUSES OF THE ONSET OF LABOUR

The onset of labour appears to be the result of a combination of factors in which hormonal and mechanical elements predominate. It is possible that some signal is given from the fetoplacental unit which plays a major role in oestrogen metabolism depending on changes in fetal pituitary-adrenal activity. The fetal adrenal cortex produces precursors for the synthesis of oestrogen which rises rapidly during the last week.

**Oxytocin** from the posterior pituitary gland has a stimulating action on the pregnant uterus and can be used to induce labour.

**Progesterone** has a sedative action on uterine muscle so its withdrawal at the end of pregnancy may facilitate the onset of labour.

**Prostaglandins** are thought to be synthesised in the decidua at term in response to the release of oestrogens by the fetoplacental unit. The local release of prostaglandins from the uterus may be a major element in the onset of labour.

**Mechanical elements.** As pregnancy advances, there is an increase in the contractibility of the uterus, which becomes more susceptible to stimulation as term approaches. The pressure of the presenting part on the nerve-endings in the cervix may play some part; experience shows that labour is more likely to start on time when the head is engaged than when it is high. Overdistension of the uterus, as occurs with twins or polyhydramnios, tends to induce preterm labour.

### THE PREMONITORY SIGNS OF LABOUR

During the three weeks previous to the onset of labour, certain changes take place which, when manifest, are useful to determine the approach of labour.

| | |
|---|---|
| **Lightening.** | **False pains.** |
| **Frequency of micturition.** | **Slight taking up of the cervix.** |

### Lightening

This is the sinking of the uterus, which takes place about two or three weeks before term. Because the fundus no longer crowds the lungs, breathing is easier, the heart and stomach can function better and the relief experienced by the woman is described as lightening. It occurs because the symphysis pubis widens, the softened, relaxed pelvic floor sags by as much as 4 cm allowing the uterus to descend further into the true pelvis. The lower segment stretches and the fetus sinks further down into the uterus.

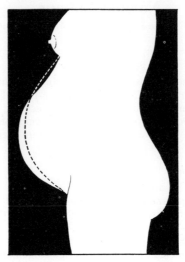

Fig. 15-1   Lightening. The dotted line shows the shape of the uterus prior to lightening.

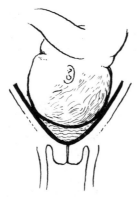
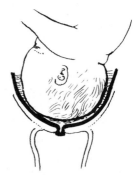

Fig. 15-2   Note 'V' shaped lower uterine segment prior to labour, cervix not ripe os not dilated.

Fig. 15-3   Lower uterine segment soft and 'U' shaped, head has descended, cervix taken up. Bag of waters in the dilating cervix. Vagina stretching.

The fundus is therefore at a lower level; the uterus becomes more prominent and if the abdominal muscles are in good tone, as is found in primigravid women, and no disproportion exists, the head will enter the pelvic brim and become engaged. In multiparous women the bracing action of firm abdominal muscles may be absent, and the uterus will then sag further forwards, the abdomen becomes somewhat pendulous and the fetal head does not as a rule become engaged. Walking is more difficult at this time. Relaxation of the pelvic joints may give rise to backache or pain in the region of the symphysis pubis. Vague discomfort may be experienced in the lower abdomen, groins and thighs. The vaginal secretion becomes more profuse.

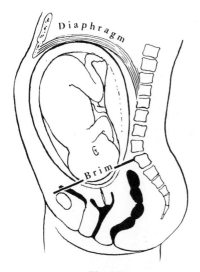 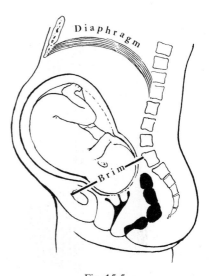

| Fig. 15-4 | Fig. 15-5 |
|---|---|
| Prior to lightening. | After lightening. |

The fundus crowds the diaphragm. The lower uterine segment is not soft and has not stretched to accommodate the fetal head which therefor remains high. The lower segment is 'V' shaped.

The fundus sinks below the diaphragm and breathing is easier. The lower segment is 'U' shaped: it has softened and dilated so the fetal head sinks down into it and may partly enter the pelvic brim.

**Frequency of micturition**

This may be due to pressure of the fetal head on the bladder limiting its capacity and requiring it to be emptied more often. But sometimes there is a state of mild incontinence or poor control of the urethral sphincter, which may be accounted for by the lax condition of the softened pelvic floor at this time.

**False pains**

These are erratic and irregular, causing the uterus to contract and relax, whereas in true labour the uterus contracts and retracts. They may be unduly troublesome and some consider this to be a mild form of inco-ordinate uterine action.

**Taking up of the cervix**

Taking up of the cervix occurs because it is being drawn up and merged into the lower uterine segment. Shortening of the cervix is usually looked for, when, in the interest of mother or child, labour must be induced.

## SIGNS OF TRUE LABOUR

**Painful rhythmic uterine contractions.**     **Dilatation of cervix.**     **Show.**

**Uterine contractions** are now felt by the woman as tightening, discomfort or actual pain. During a contraction the uterus feels hard to the touch. Each contraction begins painlessly; the pain gradually increases in intensity until it reaches its acme, then diminishing and ending painlessly. Slight backache may also be present. These signs are explained in detail on page 246 and the diagnosis of true labour on page 273.

**Dilatation of the cervix.** *The physiology of this is explained on page 249 and diagnosis on page 281.*

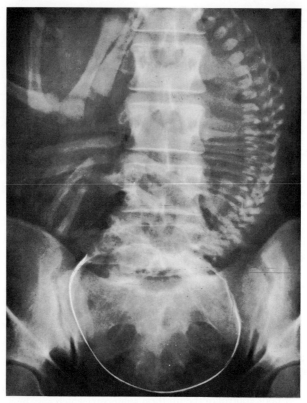

Fig. 15-6 X-ray photograph, showing vertex left occipito-anterior position (head re-touched).

*Simpson Memorial Maternity Pavilion, Edinburgh.*

**Show** is explained on page 250.

Rupture of the membranes cannot be accepted as a sign of true labour, as this sometimes occurs a few days before labour begins, or may not occur until the end of the second stage.

### THE THREE STAGES OF LABOUR

**The first stage** is that of dilatation of the cervix, and lasts from the onset of true labour to complete dilatation of the cervix.

**The second stage** is that of expulsion of the fetus. It begins when the cervix is fully dilated and ends when the baby is born.

**The third stage** is that of separation and expulsion of the placenta and membranes and is also concerned with the control of bleeding. It lasts from the birth of the baby to the expulsion of the placenta and membranes.

**A fourth stage** is described by some in order to stress the continued vigilance which is necessary because of the risk of postpartum haemorrhage, the period of one hour following the birth of the placenta.

### THE DURATION OF LABOUR

There are wide variations in the duration of labour, depending on whether the woman is a primigravida or multipara and on the time that has elapsed since the birth of her last child. The type of pelvis, size and presentation of the fetus and the strength and frequency of the uterine contractions, all influence the length of labour.

The greater part of labour is taken up with the first stage. Seldom is the second stage less than half an hour in a primigravida and the multiparous woman may have a second stage of 15 minutes or less. The duration of the third stage is usually between 5 and 20 minutes.

The consensus of opinion is that during the past 20 years the duration of labour has been shorter than previously, probably due to the greater use of relaxation, sedation and oxytocin. The figures given below could be considered fairly average today but experience proves that average figures can be misleading.

|  | First Stage | Second Stage | Third Stage | Total |
|---|---|---|---|---|
| **PRIMIGRAVIDA** | 11 hours | $\frac{3}{4}$ hour | $\frac{1}{4}$ hour | 12 hours |
| **MULTIPARA** | $6\frac{1}{2}$ hours | $\frac{1}{4}$ hour | $\frac{1}{4}$ hour | 7 hours |

A considerable number of primigravidae have labours of under 12 hours, a number of multiparae have labours of six to eight hours and in many cases less than six hours. Acceleration of labour by oxytocin i.v. drip has reduced the length of labour to 8 hours in primigravidae.

## THE MECHANISM OF LABOUR

The mechanism of labour is a series of passive movements of the fetus in its passage through the birth canal. Such movements are essential, because the canal is cylindrical, with an inlet and outlet differing in size and shape and a forward curve at its lower end. The fetus is a flexible cylindrical body which, during the process of birth, is made to accommodate itself to the diameters and curve of the pelvic canal. The skilful management of normal delivery is based on a knowledge of the mechanism of labour so it is imperative that these natural movements should be thoroughly understood. The student midwife must be taught the underlying principle of each movement.

Some authorities question the value of teaching the mechanisms of labour (admittedly they are valueless if learned by rote). But when each movement is understood this knowledge enables the midwife to observe the progress of normal and abnormal labour more intelligently. The successful conduct of delivery, whether vertex, breech or face, depends largely on facilitating Nature's method which is mechanism.

## MECHANISM OF VERTEX PRESENTATION

### (*Left Occipito-Anterior Position*)

*The definitions of the terms lie, attitude, presentation, denominator, position and presenting part, used in describing mechanism, are given on page 84.*

**The following movements take place during labour,** as the result of the expulsive action of the uterine and abdominal muscles and diaphragm and the resistance offered by the pelvis, cervix and pelvic floor.

**Flexion of the head**
**Internal rotation of the head**
**Crowning of the head**
**Extension of the head**                *Descent takes*
**Restitution of the head**              *place throughout.*
**Internal rotation of the shoulders**
**External rotation of the head**
**Lateral flexion of the body**

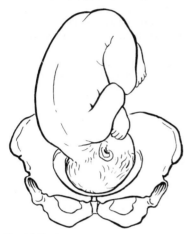

Fig. 15-7   Vertex, right occipito-anterior.        Fig. 15-8   Vertex, left occipito-anterior.

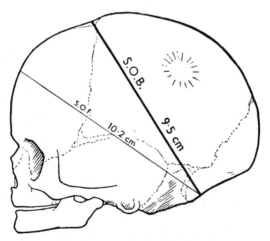

Fig. 15-9   Diagram of fetal skull showing the engaging diameters in a vertex L.O.A. The
S.O.F. diameter lies at the pelvic brim at the onset of labour. With increase of flexion the
S.O.B. diameter engages and passes through the birth canal. The S.O.F. diameter sweeps the
perineum.

### Descent

Descent begins in most primigravid patients two weeks before the onset of labour
when engagement of the head occurs, unless disproportion between head and pelvis

exists. Further descent takes place during the first stage, and is brought about by the action of the uterine contractions. When the head meets resistance, flexion is increased and the dilating cervix allows the flexed head to descend. During the second stage descent is more rapid because the abdominal muscles and diaphragm come into play and the fetus is being actively expelled.

### Flexion of the head

The head is usually flexed at the beginning of labour, with the suboccipito-frontal diameter, 10 cm, lying at the pelvic brim, but when flexion is increased the suboccipito-bregmatic diameter, 9·5 cm, engages. This smaller presenting diameter facilitates descent. Flexion is due to various factors. The fetus *in utero* is already in an attitude of flexion; the uterine contractions will therefore tend to increase the existing attitude.

The result of increased flexion of the head is that the occiput becomes the leading part, and this influences the next movement—that of internal rotation.

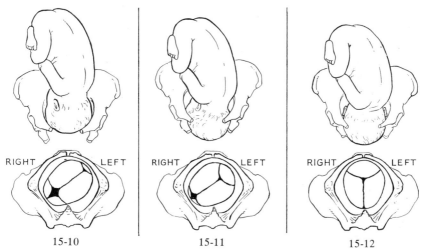

Fig. 15-10   Vertex, left occipito-anterior.   Fig. 15-11   Showing descent with increase in Sutures and fontanelles as seen from below   flexion of the head. Sagittal suture in the prior to flexion of the head.                right oblique of the pelvis.

Fig. 15-12   Showing internal rotation of the head. The occiput lies behind the symphysis pubis, having rotated forwards one-eighth of a circle.

### Internal rotation

Internal rotation is a turning forwards of whatever part of the fetus reaches the anterior, lateral half of the gutter-shaped pelvic floor first. *In an L.O.A.* the occiput rotates forwards. This movement causes the larger diameters of the head, shoulders and buttocks to emerge under the pubic arch in the antero-posterior, which is the largest diameter of the outlet. In an L.O.A. the occiput rotates forwards one-eighth of a circle, from the left ilio-pectineal eminence to the symphysis pubis, where it can escape under the pubic arch and allow the suboccipital region to pivot on the lower border of the symphysis pubis. The factors which bring about internal rotation are: (1) The passive recoil of one lateral half of the pelvic floor. When the leading part reaches the level of the ischial spines it comes in contact with the left half of the pelvic floor. The force of the uterine contractions causes the occiput to stretch the left half of the pelvic floor and push it downwards and outwards; when the contraction passes off the pelvic floor recoils and because it slopes forwards the occiput glides along the left side of the pelvis. If the head is deflexed there is no leading part and the head comes in contact with both halves of the pelvic floor so rotation does not take place. (2) The gutter-shape of the pelvic floor tends to direct the leading part towards the front, where it passes through the weakened area of the pelvic floor and under the pubic arch.

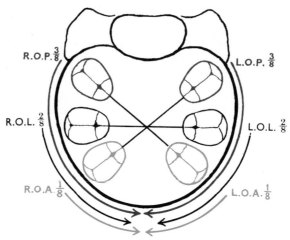

Fig. 15-13 Diagrammatic representation of internal rotation in anterior, lateral and posterior positions of the vertex presentation.

## Crowning of the head

Crowning is the term used when the occipital prominence escapes under the symphysis pubis and the head no longer recedes between uterine contractions. *(A smaller diameter, the suboccipito-bregmatic, 9·5 cm, distends the vulval orifice instead of the larger suboccipito-frontal diameter, 10 cm.)*

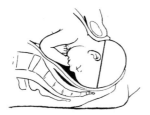

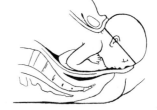

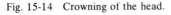

Fig. 15-14   Crowning of the head.          Fig. 15-15   Extension of the head.

## Extension

Extension is a movement by which flexion of the head is undone. The nape of the neck pivots on the lower border of the symphysis pubis while the sinciput, face and chin pass over the thinned-out perineum. Extension results from the action of two forces; the uterine and abdominal muscles exert downward pressure; the pelvic floor and perineum resist this pressure and tend to push the head forwards and upwards through the weak area—the vaginal orifice. *The suboccipito-frontal diameter*, 10 cm, sweeps the perineum.

## Restitution

This is a turning of the head to undo the twist in the neck that took place during internal rotation of the head. In a vertex L.O.A. the occiput restitutes one-eighth of a circle to the left, back to where it was before internal rotation took place. (*This movement reveals whether the position is right or left, and when the midwife knows whether she is delivering an L.O.A. or an R.O.A. she is more likely to manage the birth of the shoulders without causing a perineal laceration.*)

## Internal rotation of the shoulders

This is a movement similar to internal rotation of the head. The shoulders in an L.O.A. are in the left oblique diameter of the pelvic cavity. The anterior shoulder reaches the right side of the pelvic floor and rotates forwards bringing the shoulders into the antero-posterior diameter of the outlet. This should take place with the uterine contraction which occurs after the head has been born.

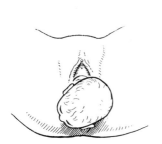

Fig. 15-16   Restitution of the head, occiput turns to left in an L.O.A.

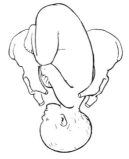

Fig. 15-17   Internal rotation of the shoulders. They are now in the antero-posterior diameter of the outlet. The head has also rotated externally.

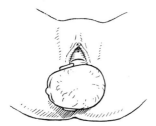

Fig. 15-18   External rotation of the head.

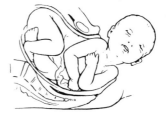

Fig. 15-19   Lateral flexion of the body.

## External rotation of the head

This is a turning of the head which accompanies internal rotation of the shoulders. The occiput turns a further one-eighth of a circle; always in the same direction as in restitution. (*When the head has rotated externally, it indicates that the shoulders are now in the antero-posterior diameter of the pelvic outlet, in readiness for expulsion*).

## Lateral flexion of the body

Lateral flexion is a sideways bending of the spine, which takes place while the body is being expelled, so that it conforms to the curve of the birth canal. The anterior shoulder escapes under the symphysis pubis; the posterior shoulder passes over the perineum, causing a smaller diameter to distend the vaginal orifice than if both shoulders were expelled simultaneously. (*The baby is carried forwards over the symphysis pubis towards the mother's abdomen by the midwife to facilitate lateral flexion.*)

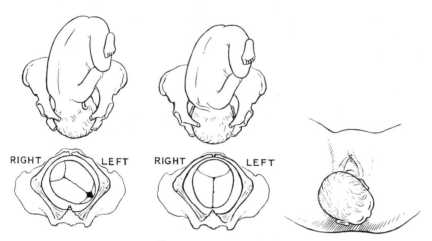

Fig. 15-20 Right occipito-anterior. Head descending. Sagittal suture in the left oblique diameter of the pelvis.

Fig. 15-21 Right occipito-anterior. Occiput has rotated one-eighth of a circle forwards. Sagittal suture in the antero-posterior diameter of the pelvic outlet.

Fig. 15-22 Restitution, occiput turns to the right.

# THE PHYSIOLOGICAL CHANGES DURING LABOUR

## *First and Second Stages*

It is advisable for the midwife to study the physiological changes that occur during labour, to enable her to interpret intelligently such observations as may be made and to appreciate deviations from the normal course.

### DURING THE FIRST STAGE

**Contraction and retraction of uterine muscle.**
**Formation of the upper and lower uterine segments.**
**Development of the retraction ring.**
**Taking up of the cervix. Dilatation of the cervix.**
**Show. Formation of the bag of waters.**
**Rupture of the membranes.**

Uterine contractions are involuntary: they are controlled by the nervous system and by endocrine influence. Palpable contractions rarely last longer than 60 to 70 seconds: if prolonged, the compression of the blood sinuses in the uterine wall interferes with the oxygen supply to the fetus. They usually recur with rhythmic regularity, and the intervals between them gradually diminish from 15 minutes, more or less, at the beginning of the first stage, to two or three minutes at the end of the second stage.

*Fundal dominance.* Each contraction starts in the fundal region and spreads downwards, being stronger and persisting longer in the upper region. The fundus and mid-zone remain hard throughout the period of contraction. On reaching the lower uterine segment the wave of contraction weakens considerably and this permits the cervix to dilate and the strongly contracting fundus to expel the fetus.

*Polarity* is the term used to describe the neuromuscular harmony that prevails between the two poles or segments of the uterus throughout labour. During each uterine contraction these two poles act harmoniously; the upper pole contracting strongly and retracting to expel the fetus, the lower pole contracting slightly and dilating to allow expulsion to take place. If polarity is disorganised the progress of labour is inhibited.

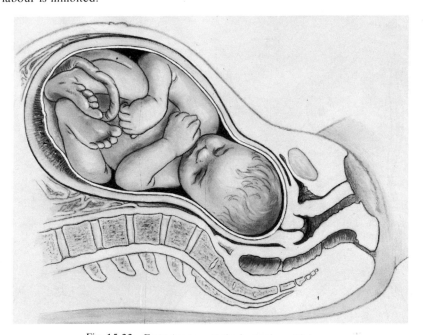

Fig. 15-23   Fetus *in utero* at the beginning of labour.

### Retraction

This is a special faculty of uterine muscle whereby the contraction does not pass off entirely; the muscle fibres retaining some of the contraction instead of becoming completely relaxed. Retraction assists in the progressive expulsion of the fetus; the upper segment of the uterus becomes shorter and thicker and its cavity diminishes.

### Formation of the upper and lower uterine segments

At the end of pregnancy the uterus is divided functionally into two, the upper and the lower uterine segments. The upper segment is the thick muscular contractile part, and the lower segment is the thin distensible area, 7·5 to 10 cm in length, which has developed from the isthmus of the uterus. When labour begins, the retracted longitudinal fibres in the upper segment pull on the lower segment, causing it to stretch: this is aided by the force applied by the descending head or breech.

### Development of the retraction ring

The ridge which forms at the lower border of the thick upper segment where it meets the thin lower segment is known as the retraction, or Bandl's ring. It is present in every labour and is perfectly normal so long as it is not marked enough to be visible above the symphysis pubis. In normal labour there is no need for the lower segment to become unduly distended, because the fetus is gradually being expelled through the dilating cervix. In cases of obstructed labour, where the fetus cannot descend to pass through the cervix, the lower segment must stretch to accommodate it, because the fetus is being pushed out of the shortened upper segment. In such a case the retraction ring would rise and be visible as a depressed ridge running transversely or slightly obliquely across the abdomen above the symphysis pubis. The greater the distension of the lower segment, the higher will the retraction ring rise and the more urgent is the danger of rupture of the uterus.

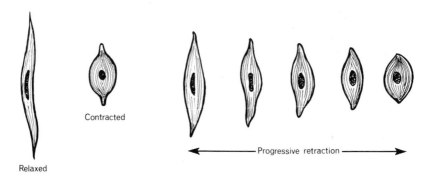

Fig. 15-24 Diagrammatic representation of a uterine muscle fibre, showing how by retraction it retains some of the contraction and becomes shorter and thicker.

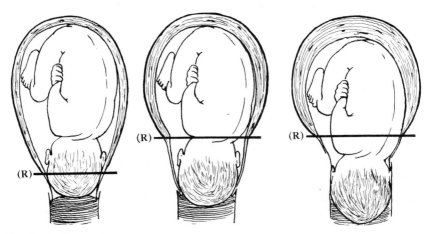

Fig. 15-25 Showing by diagrammatic representation the rising retraction ring (R). As the upper uterine segment contracts and retracts the lower uterine segment has to 'thin out' to accommodate the descending fetus. This continues until the cervix is fully dilated and the fetus can leave the uterus. The retraction ring rises no further, unless labour is obstructed.

*Although the terms 'Bandl's ring' and 'retraction ring' are synonymous,* the term *'Bandl's ring'* is commonly applied to the retraction ring when it becomes visible and 'retraction ring' to the normal invisible one.

### Taking up of the cervix

Some shortening of the cervix has already taken place at the end of pregnancy, but when labour begins, the muscle fibres surrounding the internal os are drawn upwards by the retracted upper segment, and the cervix is shortened as it merges into and becomes part of the lower uterine segment. The cervix is gradually effaced; its canal widens from above to form a funnel, the external os being the narrowed portion. The process could in some measure be likened to the shortening of the neck of a toy balloon when it is inflated. *N.B.* The *'taking up of the cervix'* should not be confused with *'no cervix felt'* on vaginal examination, which denotes complete dilatation of the cervix and signifies the end of the first stage.

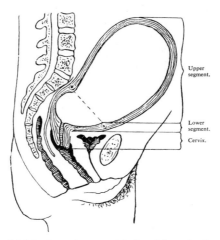

Fig. 15-26    Parturient canal before labour begins.

### Dilatation of the cervix

This causes the enlargement of the external os from a circular opening which would admit a uterine sound to one sufficiently large to permit passage of the fetal head. It is surmised that the upward traction, exerted by the retracted muscle fibres

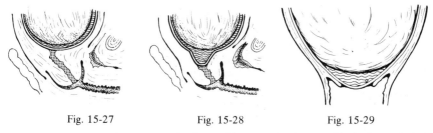

Fig. 15-27              Fig. 15-28              Fig. 15-29

Process of 'taking up' of cervix by which its canal becomes continuous with the lower uterine segment.

in the upper segment, exerts pull on the margin of the weakened area—the cervix—and makes the os enlarge. But without pressure applied from within the uterus, by a well-fitting presenting part, dilatation will not proceed normally. The well-flexed head will, when closely applied to the cervix, aid dilatation.

In the primigravid woman the external os may be closed at the beginning of labour, or it may admit the tip of one finger, and does not dilate until the cervix has been taken up, but the internal os dilates during the process of taking up of the cervix. In the multiparous woman the external os usually admits one finger prior to the onset of labour and the dilatation of the external and internal os proceeds simultaneously with taking up of the cervix.

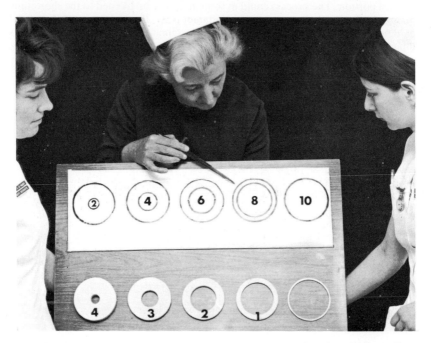

Fig. 15-30   Preparatory teaching of cervical dilatation. Upper—dilatation of os in cm. Lower row—area of thinned out cervix in cm.

*Classroom, Maternity Hospital, Stirling.*

### Show

This is the blood-stained mucoid discharge seen a few hours before, or within a few hours after, labour has started. The mucus is the thick, tenacious substance which formed the cervical plug—the operculum—during pregnancy. The blood comes from the ruptured capillaries of the decidua vera where the chorion has become detached, and from the dilating cervix.

### Formation of the bag of waters

When the lower uterine segment stretches, the chorion becomes detached from it, and the increased intra-uterine pressures causes this loosened part of the sac of fluid to bulge downwards into the dilating internal os, to the depth of 6 mm to 12 mm. The well flexed head fits snugly into the cervix, so that the fluid in front of the head is cut off from the remainder of the amniotic fluid, and is known as the *fore waters*; the remainder is known as the *hind waters*. The purpose of cutting off the fore waters is to prevent the pressure exerted on the hind waters during uterine contractions from being applied to the fore waters, and is Nature's method of keeping the membranes intact during the first stage.

### *General Fluid Pressure*

While the membranes remain intact the pressure of the uterine contractions is exerted on the fluid, and as fluid is not compressible the pressure is equalised throughout the uterus and is known as general fluid pressure. When the membranes rupture and a quantity of fluid escapes, the placenta is compressed between the uterine wall and the fetus during contractions, and the oxygen supply to the fetus is thereby diminished. With intact membranes there is less risk of fetal hypoxia and uterine infection.

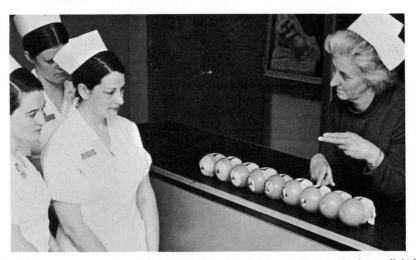

Fig. 15-31   Student midwives being taught dilatation of the cervix 'by touch' prior to clinical experience.

*Classroom, Maternity Hospital, Stirling.*

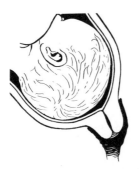

Fig. 15-32   The cervix at the beginning of labour.

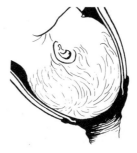

Fig. 15-33   The cervix fully dilated.

#### Rupture of the membranes

The amniotic sac should remain intact until the cervix is fully dilated, but this by no means always happens. The membranes may rupture days before labour begins, or during the first or second stages, and in some instances not until the head is being born. Towards the end of the first stage the bag of membranes receives very little support, because of the extensive dilatation of the cervix. It is also subjected to the increased force of the strong uterine contractions. If, for any reason, there is a badly fitting presenting part, the fore-waters are not cut off effectively and the membranes rupture early, but in some cases this happens for no apparent reason.

## PHYSIOLOGICAL CHANGES DURING THE SECOND STAGE

**The contractions are stronger and more frequent.**
**The abdominal muscles and diaphragm are expulsive in action.**
**The pelvic floor is displaced.**
**The fetus is expelled.**
*The mechanism of labour plays an important role in the second stage of labour.*

The uterus is irritated by being more closely applied to the fetus, when some of the fluid escapes, so its contractile power is intensified. The vagina is being stretched by the fetus and this reflexly stimulates uterine action. The upper uterine segment continues to become short and thick because of the retraction of the muscle fibres: the placental circulation is interfered with to a greater extent than during the first stage. The uterine contractions tend to straighten out the fetal spine and elongate the fetus, so the height of the fundus remains well above the umbilicus although the head is on the pelvic floor.

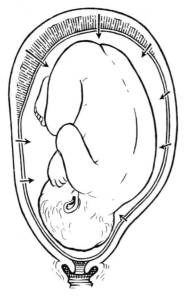
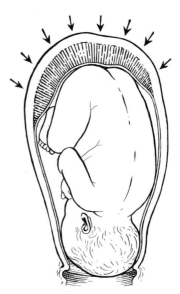

Fig. 15-34 General fluid pressure. The pressure of uterine contractions is exerted on the amniotic fluid and equalised. The placental circulation is only interfered with slightly.

Fig. 15-35 Fetal axis pressure (*aids expulsion of the fetus*). The membranes have ruptured and much of the fluid has drained away. The pressure of the abdominal muscles and diaphragm is exerted on the buttocks and body of the fetus. The placental circulation is interfered with during contractions.

### *Fetal Axis Pressure*

During each contraction the uterus rears forwards and the force of the contraction is transmitted via the long axis of the fetus and directs it through the birth canal. This is known as fetal axis pressure and differs from the general fluid pressure of the first stage.

The contractions of the abdominal muscles and diaphragm now come into play. Their expulsive action, known as *'bearing down'* or *'pushing,'* is largely reflex at first and can be aided by voluntary effort, but when the presenting part reaches the pelvic floor and distends it, this expulsive action becomes involuntary. The secondary powers are of tremendous assistance in overcoming the resistance encountered at the pelvic outlet.

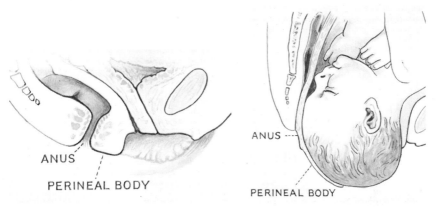

Fig. 15-36 Urethra, bladder, vagina, perineal body and rectum in the non-pregnant state.

Fig. 15-37 Vagina distended, perineal body thinned out, rectum compressed, at the end of the second stage of labour.

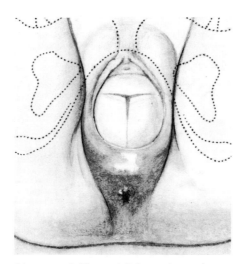

Fig. 15-38 The head is crowned. The occipital prominence has escaped and the sinciput will now sweep the perineum.

## Displacement of the pelvic floor

This occurs when the bladder is drawn up into the abdomen where there is less risk of its being injured by the descending head, and more space is available in the pelvis for the passage of the fetus. The advancing head dilates the vagina and may lacerate the mucosa, causing slight bleeding. The posterior segment of the pelvic floor is pushed downwards in front of the presenting part: the rectum is compressed by the advancing head, and any faecal contents will be expelled. The anus pouts and gradually gapes until the opening is 2·5 cm in diameter, showing the anterior rectal wall. The triangular perineal body is flattened out and instead of being 4 cm by 4 cm it becomes thin and almost transparent with a length of about 10 cm. The thinned out perineum lengthens the posterior wall of the birth canal, causing the vaginal orifice to be directed upwards.

### The fetus is expelled

The head is seen at the vulva, advancing with each contraction and receding between contractions, until crowning takes place: the head is then born by extension. The shoulders and body follow with the next contraction, along with the remainder of the amniotic fluid. The second stage culminates in the birth of the baby.

---

## QUESTIONS FOR REVISION

### *Oral Questions*

What do you understand by normal labour? Name 3 premonitory signs of labour? 3 signs of true labour? Which skull diameters engage in a well flexed head? How would you facilitate lateral flexion of the body during delivery? What do you understand by: polarity, show; bag of membranes?

**Differentiate between:** (*a*) contraction and retraction, (*b*) taking up of the cervix and no cervix felt; (*c*) false and true labour; (*d*) presentation and position; (*e*) restitution and external rotation; (*f*) upper and lower uterine segments; (*g*) retraction ring and Bandl's ring; (*h*) forewaters and hindwaters; (*i*) general fluid pressure and fetal axis pressure; (*j*) abortion and labour.

Describe operculum; crowning; left occipito anterior position; the vertex; bregma.

What are the causes of the onset of labour? How would you recognise that lightening had occurred?

**C.M.B.(Scot.) 30-min. question.** How do you recognise that labour has begun? What changes take place in the uterus during the first stage of labour?

How long does labour usually last in a primigravida, a multigravida? Give length of first, second and third stages.

**C.M.B.(Eng.).** Describe the physiological changes in the uterus throughout labour.

**C.M.B.(Scot.).** What changes take place in the cervix during normal pregnancy? What knowledge can be gained from examination of the cervix (*a*) during pregnancy, (*b*) during labour?

**C.M.B.(Eng.).** Describe briefly the changes which take place in the uterus during the first stage of labour. Give the management of this stage.

**N.Ire.** (*a*) Describe the anatomy of the body of the uterus. (*b*) Describe the changes of its musculature in the three stages of labour.

**N.Ire.** (*a*) Discuss pain relief in labour. (*b*) What are the relevant midwives' rules.

#### MECHANISM OF LABOUR

**Arrange the following movements in correct sequence:**

| | | | | | |
|---|---|---|---|---|---|
| 1. internal rotation of the head | ( ). | 5. crowning of the head | ( ). |
| 2. lateral flexion of the body | ( ). | 6. internal rotation of the shoulders | ( ). |
| 3. flexion of the head | ( ). | 7. extension of the head | ( ). |
| 4. restitution of the head | ( ). | 8. external rotation of the head | ( ). |

### *Practical Application*

Explain how knowledge of the following are useful when delivering the baby: (*a*) external rotation; (*b*) crowning; (*c*) restitution; (*d*) flexion; (*e*) extension of the head. How would you recognise: (*a*) descent; (*b*) flexion of the head during labour. Why should the midwife wait for external rotation of the head before delivering the shoulders?

**Lie** is the relation of the ......................................... to the .............................. of the...............................

**Position** is the relation of the ................................. to the .............................. of the...............................

**Attitude** is the relation of the ................................. to the ...................................................................

*Name the denominators* in the following presentations: Vertex; Beech; Face; Shoulder.

## *C.M.B. Short Questions*

**Eng.** The part played by the pelvic floor in the mechanism of labour. **Eng.** The onset of labour. **Scot.** Effacement of the cervix. **Scot.** Show. **Scot.** Crowning of the fetal head. **Eng.** Spontaneous onset of labour. **Eng.** Cervical dilatation in labour. **Eng.** The advantages of a vertex presentation at delivery. **Scot.** Lower uterine segment. Retraction ring and constriction ring. **Scot.** Entonox apparatus. **Eng.** The use of pethidine in labour. **Eng.** Inhalational analgesics in labour. **Eng.** Nitrous oxide and oxygen analgesia (Entonox). **Eng.** Premature rupture of membranes. **Scot.** Presentation and presenting part.

# 16

# The Management of Normal Labour

*Basic principles. Psychology. Emotional support. Relief of pain and drugs prescribed by midwives. Inhalational analgesia: Entonox. Trichlorethylene. Methoxyflurane. Relief of backache.*

The techniques used in the management of labour are founded on certain basic principles.

### UNDERSTANDING AND MEETING THE WOMAN'S NEEDS: PROVIDING EFFICIENT CARE

A good midwife is essentially a good nurse, and will endeavour to:
**Give comfort; relieve pain;** conserve strength; prevent exhaustion, injury and loss of blood.
**Maintain cleanliness,** antisepsis and asepsis throughout labour.
**Exercise vigilant observation.** This is an integral part of good nursing, and the midwife requires sufficient knowledge and experience to enable her to recognise normal progress and detect deviations from the natural course. The modern midwife is expected to be proficient in supervising maternal and fetal wellbeing when automated devices are employed to induce and accelerate labour and to interpret electronic monitoring of fetal heart rate patterns.

### COPING WITH SUCH EMERGENCIES AS MAY ARISE

Complications should be prevented where possible, recognised early and dealt with promptly and competently until the arrival of the doctor.
These principles are not confined to labour only, for the management of labour begins during the prenatal period by: building up the woman's general health: gaining her confidence, promoting courage and serenity: giving expert supervision and advice: detecting abnormalities which may adversely affect labour.

## THE PSYCHOLOGY OF THE WOMAN IN LABOUR

It has been proved that the emotions of the woman in labour profoundly influence her reaction to discomfort and pain and are a contributory factor in determining the amount of physical and mental exhaustion she will experience. The whole process of childbirth should be handled with sensitivity and compassion.

### The fear of labour

The onset of labour gives rise to various emotions, particularly when it is the first baby. The woman is glad the long waiting period is over and pleased that labour has begun, for she is eagerly looking forward to seeing her infant. These emotions are pleasureable, but they are sometimes counterbalanced by emotions of the opposite type. She may be apprehensive about the process of labour and its possible outcome, and if the thought of the actual birth perturbs her such a state of uncertainty and anxiety culminates in fear. The hospital situation often suggests preparations for a surgical operation rather than a natural event in her life: a more home-like atmosphere should prevail.

### CHILDBIRTH A FAMILY OCCASION

It must never be forgotten that the birth of a baby is an important family affair, and the midwife should give adequate consideration to the relatives, for whom it may be a very trying ordeal. There is no reason why women should be cut off from those who are so deeply concerned. The husband is permitted to remain with his wife, this gives comfort and happiness to both, and she needs the companionship, love and sympathy of those who are dear to her. Patients should always be told of telephone enquiries for them; it is only natural that a woman likes to know her relatives or friends are thinking of her, and it helps to keep up her morale.

When answering telephone calls from relatives during labour, the midwife in charge or her deputy should dictate the reply. It is not sufficient to state that 'Mrs . . . has not had her baby yet'; they should be told something simple and reassuring to allay their natural anxiety, by statements such as—'Had a good sleep during the night.' 'Quite comfortable, not in strong labour yet.' 'Everything is all right.' 'Baby will be here soon: ring again in two hours.' If the woman is not in hard labour and is reasonably comfortable, that information should be conveyed to her relatives.

### The Influence of the Midwife

It has long been known that the personality and attitude of the midwife play an important part in influencing the behaviour of the woman in labour. If the midwife is endowed with a calm, optimistic temperament she is eminently suited from the psychological point of view for the work she is doing. Her approach should always be friendly, and a kindly welcome makes all the difference to an apprehensive patient. The midwife needs sufficient imagination to appreciate what the woman is thinking and suffering, and although labour should be treated as a natural everyday occurrence, the midwife should not in any way belittle the fact that it is a strenuous, uncomfortable process and a momentous experience for the mother.

If the midwife conveys the impression that she is really interested and is doing her utmost to be helpful she will have a soothing influence. The serene way in which the midwife deals with her patients has a reassuring effect; efficiency should always be tempered with mercy. Good human relationships are most essential and the successful midwife has the ability of understanding human nature, adapting her methods of approach to the needs of the different personalities. But the qualities that are acceptable to all women in labour, irrespective of temperament, intelligence, or social status, are *sympathetic understanding* and *patient kindliness*.

Women in labour are sometimes irritable. Some are poorly endowed to endure the discomfort of the first stage of labour, and much tact is needed in handling them. Others are emotionally immature and unable to control their feelings, and in such cases the influence of a calm, patient midwife is invaluable. Although at times firmness must be exercised, this does not necessarily preclude kindness. At all times the midwife should demonstrate the caring attitude. Towards the end of labour the midwife may have to urge the patient to persevere, when her energy and her spirits tend to flag and she becomes disheartened and apprehensive.

### EMOTIONAL SUPPORT

This term is used to embrace the concept of meeting the emotional needs of the woman in labour as a feeling, suffering and probably apprehensive human being. Building up the woman's confidence in the hospital, doctor and midwife, and providing competent physical care during labour, give the woman a feeling of safety that must not be underestimated as a valuable souce of emotional support. But this is not enough. Her emotional requirements must be met in order to prevent labour from becoming a nerve-wracking experience with emotionally traumatising effects. Not only must the midwife desire to give emotional support, she must demonstrate her compassion by words and actions.

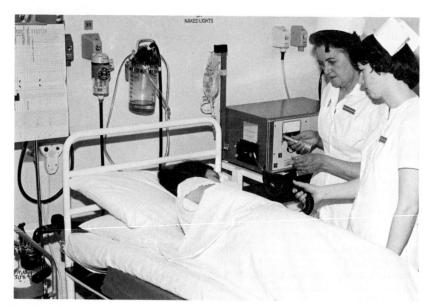

Fig. 16-1   Sister giving emotional support; student midwife observing. Note foam rubber wedge to maintain the lateral position.

*Maternity Hospital, Stirling.*

### Companionship is needed

Loneliness breeds fear. The comforting companionship of the midwife who will listen, explain, encourage and assure, or keep silent as required, is of inestimable value to the woman at this time. When labour is established the midwife should remain in constant attendance. If left for long periods the woman's confidence in her attendants is shattered. The husband, if present, and the woman in labour suffer real anguish in case the baby is born suddenly during the midwife's absence. The companionship the woman in labour needs is the professional presence of the midwife. Husbands are encouraged to stay with their wives; their role being the provision of social companionship and emotional support. This does not absolve the midwife from her responsibility nor is it fair to expect husbands to undertake tasks they are not competent to perform. Their presence is invaluable but is no substitute for the intelligent observation and skilled professional ministrations of the midwife.

### Adequate communication

It is essential for the peace of mind of most women that they be kept informed regarding the progress they are making. Women respond magnificently to a word of praise, and being given reasons or explanations, e.g. prior to vaginal examination the woman is told why this is being done and that if she relaxes, the findings will be more complete: afterwards she is assured that all is well, and that the baby will, or will not, be born soon. If the woman is made aware that she will never be expected to suffer more than she can stand, and that she will be given a sedative when she feels the need of it, she is less likely to clamour for relief too soon or to lose her nerve. Women who scream during labour do so more from fear than from pain, and the midwife should communicate confidence by her calm, competent bearing and kindly actions.

### The Woman's Point of View

The woman desires and needs patient, almost maternal, care and companionship as well as the competent observation and obstetric skill she will undoubtedly receive. Soothing measures, such as rubbing the back, help to alleviate discomfort and the woman interprets this as an expression of solicitude. Some women feel very deeply regarding being permitted to experience what is commonly known as 'natural childbirth' with the profound joy in hearing their baby's first cry. Although the midwife may think it is more humane to administer inhalational analgesia she must respect and comply with the mother's wishes which, in this instance, will have no untoward effect on mother or child.

### A peaceful atmosphere

The atmosphere of the labour ward should be as quiet and tranquil as possible, and it is the midwife in charge who sets the tone. Student midwives may find the urgency of the situation overwhelming at times, but the impulse to rush about must be resisted as this produces an atmosphere of tension which is transmitted to the patients. The woman in labour should never be aware of any doubt or anxiety the student may experience such as inability to hear the fetal heart or that haemorrhage is taking place. Great self-control is needed in maintaining an unperturbed demeanour in the presence of an emergency in which life is endangered and quick action required.

There should be no boisterous urging during the second stage; progress is just as rapid in the absence of excessive exhortation to push. Loud talking and noise create the impression of stress and strain which may leave the memory of terrific turmoil and difficulty when the labour was quite normal and straightforward. No conversation should take place between members of staff in the presence of the woman in labour other than is necessary for the conduct of labour.

*An attitude of reverence should always prevail while in attendance on women during childbirth.*

## RELIEF OF PAIN AND PROMOTION OF COMFORT

Although relief of pain is the dominant reason for the administration of 'sedative' drugs in labour, the promotion of comfort is equally compelling. The woman needs help in coping with apprehension, weariness, tension, and anxiety, therefore tranquillising drugs are as essential as those with analgesic properties. The midwife requires understanding of the principles underlying the administration of the various drugs available, as well as comprehension of the effect of the drugs prescribed by the obstetrician or given on her own authority when practising as a community midwife as sanctioned by The Central Midwives Boards.

### Coping with Pain

Few women experience a painless labour but they can be helped to cope with stress. Women vary in their ability to bear pain depending on temperament: the sensitive 'highly strung' woman may interpret discomfort as acute pain and it is her assessment of pain that should be accepted. Pain exhausts the woman physically and emotionally so it must be relieved by every obstetrically safe means. The midwife by her kindly, confident, bearing and professional proficiency has an assuring beneficient influence.

Drugs are more efficacious when the woman has been educationally conditioned to approach labour with equanimity based on confidence. Midwives should prepare expectant mothers to cope with such stresses as may occur using suggestion and distraction to heighten the pain threshold. Trust in the hospital staff, who will care for her, is a valuable aid. Complete reliance on the psychological method of pain relief is a subordinate feature in the management of labour today: prolonged labour is no longer permitted; it intensifies the perception of pain which becomes more unbearable as the woman's stamina wanes. New drugs and epidural analgesia are now preferred to psychoprophylaxis.

Epidural analgesia is now extensively employed in Britain, providing an almost pain-free labour. The midwife co-operates with the anaesthetist, assessing uterine action in the absence of pain and by her intelligent observation contributing to maternal and fetal welfare.

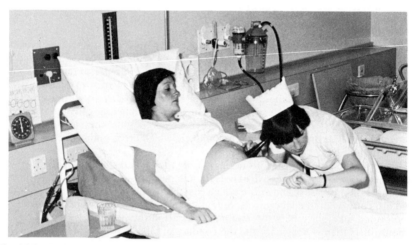

Fig. 16-2 Patient in first stage of labour, comfortable under pethidine. Head 3/5 palpable. Note foam rubber wedge to maintain the propped up position preferred at this hospital.

*Forth Park Maternity Hospital, Kirkcaldy.*

## DRUGS EMPLOYED DURING LABOUR TO PROMOTE COMFORT AND RELIEVE PAIN
### ANALGESICS: SEDATIVES: NARCOTICS: TRANQUILLISERS: HYPNOTICS

It is not possible to classify accurately the action of the above groups of drugs. A small dose of a narcotic would act as a sedative; a large dose of a tranquilliser would be hypnotic. The midwife must know for what reason she is administering a drug, i.e. to allay apprehension; induce sleep; relieve pain: she must also comprehend the main action of the drug she administers.

### ANALGESICS

These drugs are readily definable: they relieve pain without rendering the patient unconscious. Morphine is a most powerful analgesic: being also sedative and hypnotic it calms the woman and provides sleep. Unfortunately it has a profoundly depressant effect on the fetal respiratory centre which limits its usefulness during the phase of labour when pain is most severe.

Pethidine has a somewhat limited analgesic action so drugs such as promethazine (Phenergan), 25 to 50 mg, are given to potentiate this (see p. 263). Pentazocine (Fortral), 30 to 60 mg, is an analgesic drug. Local analgesics such as lignocaine are used to infiltrate the perineum and for pudendal nerve block. Bupivacaine (Marcain) is used for epidural analgesia. Inhalational analgesics such as Entonox, Trilene and Penthrane, when given in the dosage prescribed by the Central Midwives Boards, are analgesic in action.

### SEDATIVES AND TRANQUILLISERS

Sedatives are closely allied to tranquillisers. They do not relieve pain but are useful in early labour to reduce apprehension and induce calmness without producing drowsiness, so they can be administered to patients who are not confined to bed. The phenothiazine derivatives are widely used in obstetrics today: promazine (Sparine) 25 to 50 mg or promethazine (Phenergan) 25 to 50 mg being given with pethidine. Diazepam (Valium) 10 mg is useful to allay tension; larger doses may cause neonatal hypotonia and hypothermia.

**The barbiturates** are sedatives rarely now used in labour, as there is no antidote for the respiratory depression they may produce in the newborn.

#### HYPNOTICS

Chloral hydrate (Welldorm and Trichloryl) tablets are not administered in labour as frequently as in former years since more modern products are now available. Nitrazepam (Mogadon) 10 mg is a most useful drug to induce sleep in non-established labour. Chlormethiazole (Heminevrin) is a sedative and hypnotic mainly prescribed for its anti-convulsant action in severe pre-eclampsia and eclampsia. Because it is not analgesic pethidine may be prescribed with it.

### The Midwife's Role

Inexorably the midwife must adjust to the changing pattern of obstetric nursing care in order to keep pace with modern trends. Acceleration or augmentation by i.v. oxytocin drip has shortened labour but the woman is still given the maximal pain relief consistent with fetal and maternal wellbeing. Drugs are given earlier than previously because when the woman is distraught with pain the effect of the drug is markedly diminished. Many more women have their labours induced and monitored electronically: this demands even more careful supervision of uterine action, additional emotional support and sufficient pain relief.

### SUCCESSFUL SEDATION

*Success and safety depend on:*
1. **The choice of the most appropriate drug** or combination of drugs.
2. **Adequate dosage.** 3. **Proper timing.** 4. **Checking the dose.**

(1) **The choice of drug** will depend primarily on the stage of labour. Tranquillisers and hypnotics are usually indicated in non-established labour: sedatives and analgesics during the latent phase. More powerful analgesics combined with phenothiazines in active labour when pain is dominant, and inhalational analgesics during the second stage. The woman's response to the onset of labour is all important; if apprehensive she needs a tranquilliser: if tired she needs a hypnotic. For discomfort or pain an analgesic and sedative are essential; the modern tendency being to use two drugs, one of which potentiates the action of the other. It goes without saying that fetal safety must always be considered when administering drugs in labour and that the appropriate antagonist, e.g. naloxone (Narcan neonatal) be available to resuscitate the baby.

(2) **Adequate dosage.** It is imperative that the dose of the appropriate drug must

be adequate to produce the desired effect. A woman weighing 80 kg would require a larger dose than one weighing 60 kg. It has been suggested that pethidine should be prescribed as 2 mg per kg body weight (with a limit of 200 mg). If 30 minutes after administration of the drug, relief has not been obtained the doctor ought to be consulted with regard to a supplementary dose. Smaller doses are given later in labour.

(3) **Proper timing** is important. The inexperienced midwife tends to be over-cautious, fearing that early sedation will put the woman 'out of labour'. Oversedation during the latent phase may slow down uterine action but will not stop labour. The timing will be wrong if she gives sedative drugs according to the degree of dilatation of the cervix instead of the degree of discomfort: the interval between doses being too long reduces effective sedation and causes unnecessary suffering. The woman's needs should be anticipated as well as met and this requires judgement. If morphine or diamorphine (heroin) is used, as in posterior vertex presentation, early administration is essential to avoid depression of the fetal respiratory centre at birth.

(4) **The dose must always be checked before being given.** The midwife also has a duty to see that the woman comes to no harm because of her confused state of mind. **Constant vigilance is necessary.**

**The following rule of the Central Midwives Boards must be noted.** 'A practising midwife must not on her own responsibility use any drug, including an analgesic, unless in the course of her obstetric training, whether before or after enrolment she has been thoroughly instructed in its use and is familiar with its dosage and methods of administration or application.' A midwife must observe the requirements of the Misuse of Drugs Amendment Regulations 1974.

#### SEDATIVE DRUGS THAT COMMUNITY MIDWIVES MAY GIVE

**Pentazocine (Fortral),** 30 to 60 mg. **Pethidine,** 100 mg.
**Dichloralphenazone (Welldorm)**
    **tablets,** 0·65 g.         **Promazine (Sparine),** 25 to 50 mg (Eng.)
**Tricloryl tablets,** 0·5 g (dose 1 g).   **Tricloryl syrup,** 5 ml.


### PETHIDINE

#### *(Known Abroad as Dolantin, Demerol)*

Pethidine is rather similar to morphine and atropine in its chemical formula, but is not a derivative of opium, it is habit forming and gives rise to drug addiction of a very severe type. Pethidine 100 mg is about the equivalent of morphine, 10 mg, and comes under the Misuse of Drugs Amendment Regulations 1974, midwives in domiciliary practice being required by law to keep records of the amount issued to and administered by them. Pethidine relieves pain and is sedative; its somewhat limited antispasmodic action relaxes plain muscle, including that of the lower uterine segment. The uterine contractions are not adversely affected. It causes less respiratory depression and vomiting than morphine.

#### *Dosage and Administration of Pethidine*

Community midwives authorised by the Central Midwives Boards to administer pethidine to women in normal labour are required to comply with the Misuse of Drugs Amendment Regulations 1974.

Pethidine, 100 mg, is not considered to be adequate, as an initial dose, by many labour ward sisters: 150 to 200 mg has a deeper and more lasting effect: repeat doses of 100 or 150 mg are given every two, three, or four hours, depending on the needs of the patient. Pethidine is more effective when given by i.m. injection than orally.

Pethilorfan, now rarely used, is not repeated because of the depressant effect of Lorfan on the fetal respiratory centre.

In cases of neonatal asphyxia due to morphine or pethidine excellent results have been obtained by injecting neonatal naloxone (Narcan) into the umbilical vein. Naloxone is a 'Prescription Only Medicine' (POM) which can be administered by midwives (Eng.) under the Prescription Only Order 1978.

The action of pethidine is potentiated by the mono-amine oxidase inhibitors such as Nardil that are sometimes prescribed for mental depression. This combination of drugs may produce coma. Prior to giving pethidine the midwife ought to question the woman regarding drugs she may have been taking.

#### DRUGS GIVEN IN CONJUNCTION WITH PETHIDINE

**Promazine (Sparine),** 25 to 50 mg, may be administered by midwives according to the C.M.B. Eng. (1973). This drug reduces tension; induces a calm state of mind and is useful for the apprehensive woman and in cases of emotional instability. When vomiting is troublesome promazine (Sparine) gives good results; it also potentiates the action of pethidine. Because of its hypotensive action, rapid pulse and a fall in blood pressure may occur if larger doses are given or it is given by the i.v. route and particularly when the patient is dehydrated. Sparine is not administered within 2 hours of giving epidural analgesia.

**Promethazine (Phenergan),** 25 to 50 mg, must be prescribed by the doctor. It is one of the effective and long-acting antihistamines often given with pethidine 150 mg and providing three to four hours of analgesic detachment.

**Pentazocine (Fortral)** is said to be a non-addictive analgesic drug which is not restricted under the Misuse of Drugs Amendment Regulations 1974. In analgesic properties 40 mg is approximately equivalent to 100 mg pethidine. Pentazocine is excreted more rapidly therefore its effect is of shorter duration than that of pethidine; less nausea and vomiting occurs. The drug is available in ampoules of 1 ml (30 mg): and should not be repeated within 3 hours. Two doses are usually sufficient.

Should neonatal respiratory depression occur, and this is rare, neonatal naloxone (Narcan) is administered. Nalorphine (Lethidrone) is not effective.

## OPIUM DERIVATIVES

**Morphine** 15 mg is only given in very early labour; and is not repeated because of its depressant effect on the fetal respiratory centre; this is particularly important should Caesarean section or forceps delivery be anticipated. (If, inadvertently, the baby is born in a state of asphyxia due to the effect of morphine, naloxone (Narcan) 0·01 mg/kg body weight will counteract its depressant action.)

**Papaveretum (Omnopon),** 20 mg, given in conjunction with promethazine (Phenergan) 25 to 50 mg, during early labour has a calming influence on the apprehensive woman as well as being analgesic.

## PSYCHOLOGICAL METHODS OF PAIN RELIEF

Many midwives have, by their sympathetic understanding manner, unknowingly used psychological methods of pain relief. Such techniques can be employed to raise the pain threshold and supplement the pharmacological method.

**The personality of the midwife is of paramount importance** in handling women in labour. If her approach is kindly, her manner reassuring, and she exhibits by word and deed her interest in, and concern for, the woman in labour as an individual, she will provide the emotional support which is so essential at this time. If the woman has been instructed by the midwife during the prenatal period and is sustained emotionally during labour, the maximal analgesic effect of pain relieving drugs is more likely to be achieved.

## INHALATIONAL OBSTETRIC ANALGESIA

Inhalational analgesia is intended for the use of healthy women to relieve the pain of normal labour. The Central Midwives Boards permit midwives to administer under certain conditions laid down by them, the following inhalational analgesics—

**Entonox, premixed nitrous oxide,** 50 per cent, and oxygen, 50 per cent.
**Methoxyflurane** (Penthrane), 0·35 per cent in air.
**Trichloroethylene** (Trilene) 0·35 to 0·5 per cent and air.

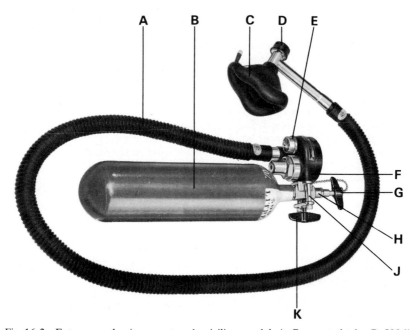

Fig. 16-3   Entonox analgesic apparatus, domiciliary model. A, Corrugated tube. B, 500-litre cylinder (50 per cent nitrous oxide/50 per cent oxygen). C, Face mask. D, Expiratory valve assembly. E, Cylinder pressure gauge. F, Demand regulator. G, Cylinder valve key. H, Non-interchangeable pin-index cylinder valve. J, Cylinder yoke. K, Cylinder yoke key. The new Entonox equipment regulator has been turned 180° so that the outlet faces away from the cylinder as in the hospital model.

*By courtesy of British Oxygen Company Ltd.*

### PREMIXED NITROUS OXIDE AND OXYGEN (Entonox)

The premixed gas and oxygen is a definite advance over gas and air because of increased oxygenation of the fetus. The apparatus consists of a cylinder of premixed gas under pressure (500 litres for domiciliary use: 2,000 litres for hospital use). The cylinder is fitted with a reducing valve that brings the pressure of the gas down to a level safe for inhalation: a pressure gauge provides an indication of the cylinder contents and the demand valve allows the premixed gas to be delivered only on inspiration by the woman inhaling it.

Because premixed gas contains a high percentage of oxygen—50 per cent—and because nitrous oxide is relatively non-cumulative it is safe to prolong its administration over a period of four or even more hours with little risk of fetal hypoxia.

The Central Midwives Boards have approved the Entonox apparatus for use by midwives on their own responsibility provided they have been instructed in its use. Such instruction will include advice on the necessary precautions to be taken against the exposure of the cylinders of premixed gas to cold.

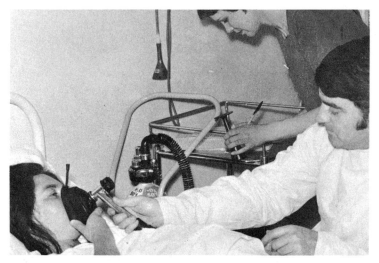

Fig. 16-4   Husband helping to apply the mask.
*Simpson Memorial Maternity Pavilion, Edinburgh.*

### *Cylinders must not be Chilled*

Cylinders of premixed gas must not be exposed to cold, i.e. temperature below freezing, 0°C (32°F). They should be stored at a temperature above 10°C (50°F). If the cylinder is known to have been exposed to a low temperature 0°C (32°F) or shows ice or condensation on its surface, it should be placed in warm water not exceeding 35°C (95°F) for five minutes, avoiding water touching the valve, or placed in the delivery room for at least 2 hours. The cylinder should then be inverted three times to agitate its contents and remix the gases.

*Oil or grease should never be applied to valves or fittings.*

### TRICHLOROETHYLENE B.P. (*Trilene*)

**Trilene** is the trade name of the brand produced by Imperial Chemical (Pharmaceuticals) Ltd. Trichloroethylene in concentrations over 0·5 per cent is an anaesthetic, but midwives are only permitted to use it as an analgesic in concentrations of 0·35 or 0·5 per cent. Two special thermostatically controlled machines have been designed for the use of midwives and approved by the Central Midwives Boards. These are the *Emotril Automatic* and the *Tecota Mark* 6. Both deliver trichloroethylene and air in the following mixtures:

**Minimal or weak concentration,** trichloroethylene, 0·35 per cent.
**Maximal or normal concentration,** trichloroethylene, 0·5 per cent.

A midwife must not on her own responsibility use any other machine or administer trichloroethylene unless she has complied with the requirements of the Central Midwives Boards Rules on the use of trichloroethylene. The machine must be tested every 12 months.

Trichloroethylene is cumulative in effect. For that reason it is not given for prolonged periods, and is usually administered towards the end of the first stage. The fetal heart must be closely observed and a chart kept in graph form. If the woman is **excessively drowsy** the inhalation should be stopped temporarily and the concentration reduced to 0·35 per cent. **Slowing of the maternal pulse or rapid respirations, slowing of the fetal heart to below 120 are indications to cease administration.** It passes the placental barrier and may produce fetal hypoxia and acidosis, when given in conjunction with pethidine within three hours of birth. Trichloroethylene should therefore not be administered until more than two hours after the last dose of pethidine was given.

### METHOXYFLURANE (*Penthrane*)

The Central Midwives Boards (Eng. and Scot.) have approved the use of methoxyflurane B.P. 0·35 per cent in air administered with the approved Cardiff inhaler, by unsupervised midwives. The Cardiff inhaler must be tested when new and tested every 12 months according to British Standards Institution approved specification. Certificates will then be issued by the Boards stating their fitness for use by unsupervised midwives.

Penthrane is administered intermittently to provide analgesia during labour and delivery. The effect of pethidine should have worn off before methoxyflurane (Penthrane) is given. The analgesic effect is good and is usually accompanied by physical and mental relaxation, but the onset of analgesia is slower than with Entonox. Some patients object to the odour. Overdosage is manifest by excessive drowsiness.

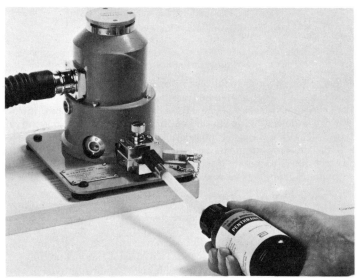

Fig. 16-5   Cardiff inhaler for Penthrane.
*Courtesy of Abbot Laboratories, Queensborough, Kent.*

#### ADMINISTRATION OF INHALATIONAL ANALGESIA

**Entonox**                                             **Penthrane**

To be successful, instruction during the prenatal period is essential, for when feeling nervous on her admission to hospital, distracted with pain or stupefied by drugs the woman cannot comprehend the directions given her. Confidence in herself, and in the safety and efficiency of the apparatus are necessary; she should be shown how to relax and be proficient in using the face-mask. *These points are explained in a talk to mothers-to-be, page 759.*

### Administration during the First Stage

#### (See also p. 759)

The mask is applied closely to the face with the broad end resting on the chin, the narrow end on the bridge of the nose. Nitrous oxide and oxygen has to be inhaled for 15 seconds before having any analgesic effect, and it takes 35 seconds to obtain maximal relief, so inhalation must be started prior to the sensation of pain felt by the woman. Trichloroethylene is slightly more rapid in action. By laying her hand on the fundus the midwife will feel the uterus contracting before the woman experiences pain; inhalation may be started then. The midwife remains in the room, encouraging the woman and helping her to relax between contractions. When administering trichloroethylene the woman must not be left alone in case she extends the period of inhalation, becomes drowsy and rolls over on to her face. The potential dangers of this substance must always be kept in mind and constant vigilance maintained (see p. 266). It should be remembered that the effort of forced inhalation and of repeatedly applying the mask can be very tiring when continued for some time. The mouth becomes parched.

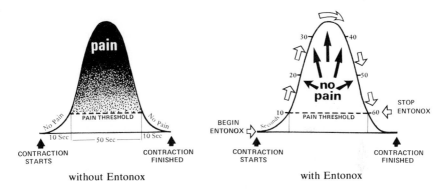

without Entonox          with Entonox

Fig. 16-6    Awareness of pain

### During the Second stage

Inhalation of nitrous oxide and oxygen should be started 40 seconds prior to the uterine contraction: trichloroethylene 30 seconds, in order that as soon as the pain commences the woman can hold her breath and bear down. After doing so she takes one or two breaths of the analgesic gas and pushes again as long as the uterus is in a state of contraction. Timing the contractions is comparatively easy during the second stage as they are recurring at frequent intervals. When the head is crowned an assistant holds the mask snugly in position, and the woman is told to take deliberate breaths to counteract the strong urge to push. During the few moments of the actual birth of the head gas is inhaled continuously.

Rubber masks and corrugated tubing should be thoroughly cleansed with soap and hot water, autoclaved or immersed in activated glutaraldehyde, 2 per cent, (Cidex) for 10 minues otherwise respiratory infections may be spread. Cidex does not attack plastics, rubber or metals.

*Unclean masks have an unpleasant odour.* Irritating antiseptics should not be used, because of the danger of eye and face burns.

## RELIEF OF BACKACHE IN LABOUR

The analgesic drugs that relieve uterine pain do not always have a similar beneficial action on backache. Low back pain may be present from the inception of labour; usually coinciding with the onset of cervical dilatation. The backache persists although it may be less severe during the second stage. The pain is felt in the sacral rather than the lumbar region, sometimes radiating over the buttocks and occasionally down the thighs with a cramp-like sensation.

Occipito-posterior position of the vertex is a well-known cause of backache. The occiput, when posterior, or a very large baby may unduly compress the paracervical ganglia.

### During pregnancy the midwife should——

Advise *re* posture, correct this when faulty, and direct exercises to maintain good muscle tone.

### During labour——

The woman should not be recumbent too soon unless tired. Effective analgesic drugs may be administered. During contractions the woman should be advised to curve her back forwards. She may stand behind a chair on the top of which is placed a pillow on which she rests her arms and head. Squatting, crosslegged, may help some, others find relief by flexing the legs at hip and knee joints.

Back rubbing is one of the most effective means of providing relief employed by midwives and approximately 70 per cent of women obtain some easement from this. With the woman lying on her left side, the midwife, facing the patient's back and head uses her left hand. Power is directed from the shoulder with a relaxed elbow and hand. Deep circular massage is applied mainly over the sacral region. Pressure should be firm but not excessive; the palm being used to a greater extent than the fingers. There should be no friction between the woman's back and the midwife's hand which should adhere to the skin and move the subcutaneous tissues: brisk superficial rubbing is not effective and will only irritate the skin.

---

## QUESTIONS FOR REVISION

### Enlarge on each of the following statements

Childbirth is a family occasion. The midwife should provide emotional support to the woman in labour. Pain exhausts the woman physically and emotionally. The effect of pain-relieving drugs varies in different women. How could you help to relieve backache?

### Oral Questions

Differentiate between: analgesia and anaesthesia; hypnotic and tranquilliser; sedative and narcotic.
How would you prevent or deal with screaming by a woman in labour?
Why is pethidine controlled by the Misuse of Drugs Amendment Regulations?
How would you deal with neonatal asphyxia when pethidine had been administered one hour before delivery? How would you deal with a cylinder of mixed nitrous oxide and oxygen that had been chilled?
Name 3 drugs prescribed by the doctor that are given in conjunction with pethidine?

#### RELIEF OF PAIN

**Gives reasons why and when during labour** you would as a midwife administer each of the following: (1) Entonox; (2) pethidine, 100 mg; (3) Tricloryl tablets 1 g; (4) Trilene, 0·35 per cent; (5) pentazocine (Fortral), 60 mg; (6) promazine (Sparine), 50 mg.

**C.M.B.(Eng.) 30-min. question.** How may a midwife alleviate pain in labour? What regulations must she observe in the use of drugs for this purpose?

**C.M.B.(Scot.) 30-min. question.** Describe the methods available to the midwife to relieve pain in labour.

## PSYCHOLOGY

How would you apply your knowledge of psychology when dealing with the woman in labour? How would you assure and comfort the frightened woman before and during labour. How can you create a 'home-like' atmosphere in a labour ward. What is your attitude to the husband in the labour ward. How can you foster the bonding process during labour. What do you understand by psychological methods of relieving pain?

## *C.M.B. Examination Short Questions*

**Eng.:** Entonox analgesia apparatus. **Eng.:** The use of pethidine in labour. **Eng.:** What are the rules concerning the administration of inhalational analgesia by a midwife? **N. Ireland:** What methods are available to the midwife for the relief of pain in labour. **Scot.:** Entonox analgesia. **N. Ireland:** Pethidine.

# 17
# The Management of Normal Labour (contd.)

*Obstetrical nursing care during the first stage. Cleanliness, antisepsis, asepsis. Admission procedure. Taking the history of labour. Examination of the woman; general and vaginal. Preparation of the woman. Management of labour. Active management, use of the partogram and cervicograph*

Labour should be conducted with the same antiseptic and aseptic precautions that would be employed in a surgical theatre, for the woman must be protected by every available means from infection which may cause ill-health and loss of life.

*The woman is vulnerable to infection for the following reasons:*

Lacerations in her perineum, vulva, vagina and cervix permit organisms to enter.

The large placental site is a raw area through which organisms can readily gain entrance to the blood stream.

The genital tract immediately after labour provides an excellent medium for the growth of organisms.

### The Patient as a Source of Infection

The patient herself can be a source of infection directly and indirectly. She should be free from any focus of infection. The giving of an enema or suppository contributes to the maintenance of a clean field during delivery of the baby. The vulva is swabbed and a shower given after evacuation of the bowels.

The patient's hands should be clean, and she should be instructed not to touch her vulva. All patients who are potentially or actually infected on admission should be isolated and it is a wise precaution when taking the history of the labour to make sure that the woman is not suffering from diarrhoea and has not been in recent contact with an infectious disease.

#### THE MIDWIFE AS A SOURCE OF INFECTION

If the midwife has a cold, sore throat, or other focus of infection, or if she has been nursing a patient suffering from an infectious condition, she should not be in attendance on the woman in labour.

But in our zeal for asepsis we must never underestimate the value of soap and water. Good wholesome cleanliness is the first prerequisite in midwifery and is as important as an impeccable aseptic and antiseptic technique. Throughout labour the midwife should wear a clean dress; during delivery a sterile gown. Her nails should be short and clean; rings and wrist watches should not be worn when hands require to be obstetrically clean. Gloves are worn for vaginal examinations and during delivery.

### Mask Wearing

Unless a mask is worn intelligently, it simply becomes an additional source of infection. The mask should always be worn while 'scrubbing up' to prevent the hands from being contaminated with the spray of saliva while talking. Masks need only be worn when the vulva or sterile equipment is exposed: if worn constantly, the mouth becomes an incubator for organisms.

The mask should never be touched, once it has been applied, because it is infected, and by contaminating the hands infection is spread; nor should one mask be worn for longer than two hours. A mask must never hang around the neck or be carried in the pocket. To do so shows disregard or ignorance of the technique of mask-wearing.

### THE ENVIRONMENT AS A SOURCE OF INFECTION

The risk of cross-infection is very great in hospital because of the large number and close proximity of patients, and on that account special precautions must be taken.

Single labour and delivery rooms are ideal in limiting infection, and should be well aired, as well as being scrupulously clean. Daily dusting should be carried out with clean damp cloths. Thorough washing of the labour ward bed, furniture and floor should follow each delivery.

## ADMISSION OF THE WOMAN IN LABOUR

When the patient arrives in hospital she should be welcomed in a friendly manner and made to feel that she is expected. The midwife notes whether delivery is imminent, and if so, makes immediate preparations to cope with it. While helping the woman to undress, enquiry is made as to whether this is her first baby, and as to the expected date of confinement.

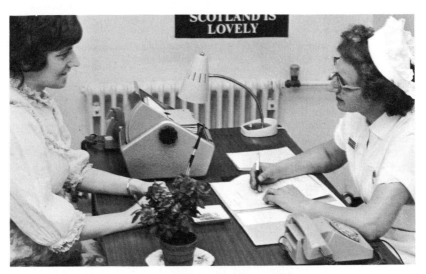

Fig. 17-1   Sister taking history of labour.
*Forth Valley School of Midwifery.*

A decision must be made as to whether the woman is in true labour or not, and this is done by taking a short history of her labour and by examination and observation of the patient. The midwife must also try to decide how far labour has advanced, before giving an enema and carrying out the full admission procedure. If the type of contractions is taken into consideration and how much has been accomplished since the onset of labour, it may be possible to estimate, within limits, whether labour will be long or short. The length of previous labours also gives some idea as to what may be expected, and if the youngest child is under 15 months a more rapid labour can be anticipated.

**The majority of booked patients coming to hospital in labour are normal;** abnormal booked cases are usually admitted for rest and observation previous to the onset of labour.

Relatives ought to be treated with courtesy, and told when to enquire again. The patient's religion and the address of her nearest relative must always be recorded.

## Consent for Operation and Anaesthetic

It is customary and expedient for midwives to request women admitted in labour to sign a permission slip for the obstetrician-in-charge to carry out any treatment or operation which may be considered necessary, including an anaesthetic.

This is a wise precaution. It would even be prudent to include treatment and operative procedures that may be carried out on the fetus and newborn baby. The form should be read to the patient so that she knows the purpose of her signature. The age of consent is now 16 years.

Prior to sterilisation of husband or wife a special consent form must be signed by both: although not legally required, the British Medical Association recommend this.

### TAKING THE HISTORY OF LABOUR

The history of labour is taken under four headings, and the midwife notes whether her own observations coincide with the woman's statements. Questions are asked regarding:

**The uterine contractions.    Rupture of the membranes.**
**Show.    Sleep: rest: food.**

The woman is asked when regular contractions (*pains*) began, how often they are coming and if she has had backache. Discomfort or pain is experienced in the lower abdomen, and when the first stage is more advanced the pain may resemble intestinal colic. Backache may persist throughout labour (see p. 268). The woman's statement regarding the length, strength, severity or expulsive character of the contractions should be corroborated by observation, and a certain amount of discrimination used in assessing the history given, for many women in false labour are under the impression, because they have had occasional pain, that they have been in true labour for one or more days. False labour should never be included in the recorded time of true labour.

### Show

The woman is asked if she has seen any show (*blood and mucus*) and her undergarments examined for staining. Show may appear a few hours before or after the commencement of labour, and the multiparous patient has less than the primigravid one because of her gaping cervix.

### The membranes

The patient may not be sure whether her 'waters' have broken or not; they may have ruptured in the bath or toilet, unknown to her. She should be asked if she has noticed a gush or trickling of water, and the time recorded. Frequency or slight incontinence, may be mistaken for the draining of amniotic fluid. The use of an Amnicator or litmus paper may be helpful, as amniotic fluid is alkaline and urine is commonly acid.

**Sleep: rest: food**

Enquiry should be made as to whether the patient has been deprived of sleep. Many women are kept awake for nights with false, niggling pains and if labour is not being accelerated a hypnotic drug such as nitrazepam (Mogadon) might be prescribed. The patient should be asked if she has had food within 6 hours; if so, this should be recorded.

### OBSTETRIC HISTORY

From her prenatal record, certain important facts regarding previous labours will be noted; but if she is not booked, enquiries will have to be made in regard to them. The weights of her babies delivered spontaneously give a clue to pelvic capacity, particularly if they were 4 kg or over. Previous instrumental delivery, Caesarean section or stillbirth should be reported to the doctor.

The prenatal record will state whether cephalo-pelvic disproportion exists. Her age, if over 30, is significant should this be her first baby or if she has no living children. Any abnormal condition existing during pregnancy will also have been recorded, such as pre-eclampsia, anaemia, diabetes, or cardiac disease. In patients whose Rh factor is negative, antibodies present in her blood should be reported to the doctor at once, so that the paediatrician can be notified and arrangements made for the provision of suitable blood for mother and baby should the need arise.

### EXAMINATION OF THE WOMAN IN LABOUR

**Has labour begun?     Vulval examination.**
**Abdominal examination. Vaginal examination.**
**General examination.**

When labour has really started, little difficulty is experienced in making the diagnosis, but it sometimes takes a number of hours before labour is properly established. At the onset, it is not always easy to decide whether the woman is in false labour or in poorly established true labour.

### *False or True Labour?*

False labour is far more common in multiparous women and is frequently troublesome at night. The contractions tend to be erratic and irregular; they often last longer than one minute and are not usually felt in the back. An enema will generally disperse them, whereas it will stimulate true contractions. No show is present.

If true labour has begun, the midwife may detect on vaginal examination the shortened cervix, and during a contraction the tense bag of waters is felt over the dilating os if the membranes have not already ruptured. The diagnosis is more difficult in the multiparous woman who has a patulous cervix and in whom dilatation of the external os is commonly present during the later weeks of pregnancy, but regular contractions and progressive dilatation of the cervix are the best guides in such cases.

When a woman is near term and has been admitted during the night or from a distance in false labour, it is a good plan to administer a sedative to ensure sleep, e.g. nitrazepam (Mogadon), 5 mg. Labour would likely be induced in the morning.

### ABDOMINAL EXAMINATION

This has been described in detail under inspection, palpation and auscultation on (pp. 131 to 141).

### THE UTERINE CONTRACTIONS

| TRUE LABOUR | FALSE LABOUR |
|---|---|
| Are always present. | Are not always present. |
| Are accompanied by abdominal tightening, discomfort or pain. | Are not always painful. |
| Rarely exceed 60 seconds. | May last three to four minutes. |
| Recur with rhythmic regularity. | Are erratic and irregular. |
| Are often accompanied by backache. | Are not accompanied by backache. |

### THE CERVIX

| TRUE LABOUR | FALSE LABOUR |
|---|---|
| The cervix is shortened. | The cervix is not shortened. |
| The os is dilating progressively. | The os is not dilating. |
| The membranes feel tense during a contraction. | The membranes do not become tense. |
| Show is usually present. | There is no show. |

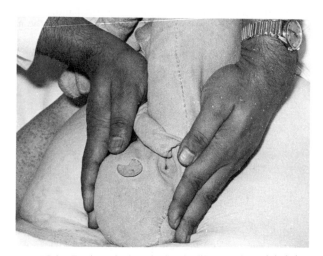

Fig. 17-2   Testing whether the head will enter the pelvic brim.

Labour is said to be established when regular painful contractions occur and the cervix is effaced and 2 cm dilated.

## PREPARATION OF THE WOMAN IN LABOUR

**EVACUATION OF LOWER BOWEL**

*N.B.*—If the woman is suffering from eclampsia or antepartum haemorrhage an enema or suppository is not given.

**It is advisable that the lower bowel is emptied at the beginning of labour.** (Some prefer suppositories, but they are slow in action and do not empty the bowel as effectively as a plain water or disposable enema does so, soiling tends to occur during the second stage.) There is some connection between the nerve supply to the uterus and bowel, so that stimulation of the bowel appears to excite better uterine contractions. This fact should be kept in mind, lest the baby be born during the expulsion of an enema given inadvisedly to a woman in strong labour. Although there would be no risk in giving one to a primigravid woman whose cervix was 6 cm dilated, it would not be wise to give an enema to a multiparous patient at that stage, because in her case the active phase of the first stage is so rapid. When in doubt, it is advisable to make a vaginal examination to ascertain the degree of dilatation of the cervix, but the strength of the uterine contractions and what has been accomplished since the onset of labour should also be taken into consideration.

**An empty rectum allows more room for the descent of the fetus.** If the lower bowel is not emptied, the descending head will cause faeces to be expelled immediately before, and during the birth of the baby. There is less soiling of the sterile field from a firm stool than the fluid from an enema given too late.

### CLEANSING THE VULVA

The traditional procedure of shaving or clipping the pubic hair at the onset of labour has been discontinued at a number of centres. Research has shown that the incidence of sepsis is not increased by so doing.

It would be prudent to cleanse the pubic and vulval area thoroughly using soap and water or Hibiscrub. Swabbing is carried out every four hours during labour for the woman's comfort and always preceding vaginal examination and delivery.

A shower with a mobile handspray is ideal. If not available the woman can kneel in a bath which is one third full. If delivery is imminent, the area from umbilicus to knees can be washed.

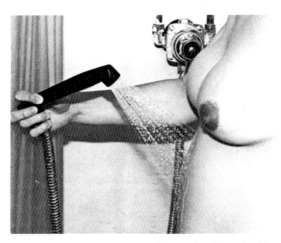

Fig. 17-3 The mobile hand spray. This hand spray is of inestimable value in obstetric practice and particularly during the admission procedure. (This photograph was taken during the post natal period.)

*Royal Maternity Hospital, Glasgow.*

The hair is combed, inspected for pediculi in hospital and subsequently treated if necessary. Long nails harbour organisms and may infect the woman's vulva during labour. No person can handle a baby safely with long sharp nails. It is equally important that *nail-paint, rouge and lip-stick* should be removed during labour, and if the woman is told that her natural colour is the best guide as to how she is faring she will usually co-operate. The use of cosmetics may keep up her morale, but **obstetric precautions must be observed.**

## GENERAL EXAMINATION

**Build and stature. Appearance. Temperature and pulse. Bood pressure. Oedema. Urine analysis.**

Particular attention is paid to the build and stature of the woman, and especially when she is less than 1·6 m in height, or if there is evidence of limp or deformity. Shoes size 3 or less suggest a small pelvis. The doctor should be notified of such cases.

### Appearance

The woman's general appearance will convey an impression of her health and nutrition, and the midwife must be on the alert for conditions that would in any way affect the course of labour. Pallor might be due to anaemia and would be marked in patients admitted because of severe antepartum haemorrhage, but more frequently it is nutritional in origin. Patients with *respiratory infections* should be nursed under barrier precautions because of the danger of infecting others.

If the woman is suffering from a condition that is contagious, e.g. untreated sexually transmitted disease or scabies, she should be seen by the doctor so that isolation and treatment can be carried out. (*Recent or present diarrhoea is significant because of the danger of introducing salmonella gastroenteritis to the unit.*)

### Temperature 4 hourly: pulse every 15 mins.

The temperature is taken and, if elevated, the cause should be sought and the patient isolated or nursed under barrier precautions. The pulse is counted, but not during a uterine contraction, as both pulse and respirations are slightly increased then. Temperature, pulse and respirations do not rise during a normal labour, so any elevation or increase is significant.

### Oedema

Oedema may be due to pre-eclampsia, and if so will be accompanied by raised blood pressure and probably proteinuria. A tight wedding ring or puffiness of the face denotes a marked degree of oedema which is serious. Oedema of the vulva is shown on page 214).

### Urine analysis

Urine is examined for protein, glucose and ketones, the specimen being obtained when the vulva has been swabbed, and before enema and bath, which are likely to cause involuntary micturition. A trace of protein in a voided specimen after the membranes have ruptured has no significance.

The urine is tested for protein and ketones every two hours; some examine every specimen.

### Blood pressure 4 hourly: 2 hourly if 'at risk'

The blood pressure of every woman admitted in labour is taken and if it is over 130/80, the doctor should be notified so that sedatives can be prescribed. The blood pressure rises about 10 mmHg during normal labour, but this is most evident towards the end of the first and during the second stage.

### Vulval examination

If the woman is in strong labour on admission, the vulva may be inspected without actually touching it; and any gaping of the vaginal orifice or anus and bulging of the perineum are suggestive signs of the second stage of labour.

Any bleeding other than a mere show should be reported and the possibility of antepartum haemorrhage considered.

The colour and odour of the amniotic fluid are noted. If the odour is offensive it usually means that the fluid is infected, and this is most likely when the membranes have ruptured early. Green fluid would necessitate listening to the fetal heart, as the presence of meconium early in labour is an ominous sign of fetal distress.

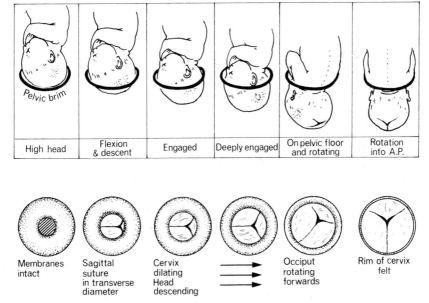

| High head | Flexion & descent | Engaged | Deeply engaged | On pelvic floor and rotating | Rotation into A.P. |

| Membranes intact | Sagittal suture in transverse diameter | Cervix dilating Head descending | | Occiput rotating forwards | Rim of cervix felt |

Fig. 17-4 Diagrammatic representation of head descending through the pelvic brim and findings per vaginam.

**Oedema of the vulva can assume large proportions;** on occasions the labia being the size of the closed fists. This is as a rule due to pre-eclampsia. Reducing the oedema by multiple incisions is recommended by some authorities, but such treatment is seldom necessary as gross oedema of the labia will not appreciably delay the birth of the head but may predispose to labial or perineal laceration. Sores and warts of the vulva are considered under sexually transmitted diseases (p. 220).

# VAGINAL EXAMINATION

A vaginal examination should always be preceded by abdominal examination and made every 4 hours or if at risk 2 hourly. The presentation, position and descent of the fetus can be ascertained by abdominal palpation during the first stage of labour, but there are occasions when it is imperative that a vaginal examination be made. It is the only certain method of determining the degree of dilatation of the cervix, which is one of the criteria by which progress during labour is assessed.

### Indications for Vaginal Examination

Vaginal examinations are now being done more frequently in order to monitor cervical dilatation more accurately in cases of 'high risk' and to diagnose prolongation of the latent phase; e.g. during (a) acceleration of labour and (b) epidural analgesia.

To decide whether the woman is in labour.

When there is doubt regarding the presentation, as may arise in a primigravid patient with rigid abdominal walls.

In an obese patient, to determine whether the head is engaged or not.

Membranes intact?

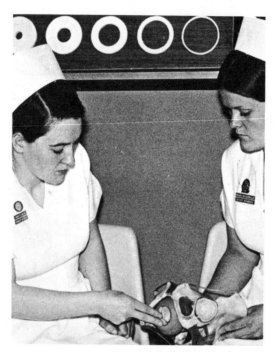

Fig. 17-5   Student midwives learning how to examine the woman vaginally prior to clinical experience in the labour ward.

*Forth Valley School of Midwifery.*

Before giving an enema to a multiparous patient having strong contractions in case she is nearing the second stage.

When in doubt as to whether the second stage has begun, e.g. persistent pushing at end of first stage.

To determine the cause of delay and to report such facts as the level of the presenting part, size of the caput and the degree of moulding to the doctor.

When prolapse of cord is likely to occur:

(a)   After the membranes have ruptured in polyhydramnios.

(b)   After the membranes have ruptured in breech or face presentation.

(c)   After the membranes have ruptured in a multiparous patient when the head is not engaged.

(d)   During labour induced by amniotomy.

In multiple pregnancy if there is doubt regarding the lie of the second twin, or in order to puncture the second bag of membranes when contractions have not recommenced after five minutes.

When some abnormality of the fetus is suspected, e.g. *anencephaly or hydrocephaly.*

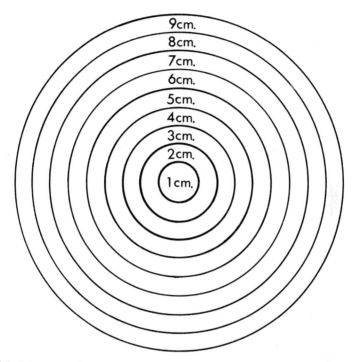

Fig. 17-6 Diagrammatic representation of dilatation of the cervix in centimetres to scale.

### Method of vaginal examination

**Need for asepsis.** The introduction of the fingers into the vagina gives rise to the **danger** of exogenous infection (*introduced from outside the vulva*). The greatest risk lies in the introduction of organisms by the attendant, but intelligent mask-wearing, the conscientious preparation of hands and vulva and wearing of sterile gloves will greatly minimise the risk of sepsis.

The woman should be told what is about to be done, and if she is assured that the procedure will not be painful she is more likely to relax, and the examination will be easier to do and the findings more complete. It is a matter of personal preference whether the midwife examines the patient in the dorsal or left lateral position, but it is generally agreed that the examination can be more comprehensive when the woman lies on her back; when lying on her side, she feels less exposed and less draping is needed. The bladder should be empty.

### Requirements

| | |
|---|---|
| 1 solution bowl. 12 wool balls. | 180 ml Hibitane 1–2000. Hibitane cream. |
| gloves. perineal pad. | 2 paper towels. 1 polythene sheet. |
| 1 sheet steri paper. | 1 polythene bag for soiled swabs. |

The midwife, wearing a mask, prepares her hands and the patient's thighs and vulva prior to swabbing with the left hand. She puts on a gown, and drapes the patient with towels. The first two fingers of the right hand, wearing a disposable plastic glove, are dipped into antiseptic cream and gently inserted into the vagina, while the labia are held apart by the thumb and first finger of the left hand.

Care should be taken not to touch the labia, and the fingers to be introduced are held on a higher level than the vaginal orifice, during their insertion, to avoid contact with the anus. The fingers are directed along the anterior vaginal wall, and should not be withdrawn until the required information has been obtained, for a perfunctory examination will have to be repeated and the risk of infection is in the insertion of the fingers. While turning the hand to explore the vagina, the thumb must not be brought into contact with the anus and then with the vaginal orifice.

### Findings on Vaginal Examination

| | |
|---|---|
| **The condition of the vagina.** | **Presentation.** |
| **The cervix and os.** | **Position.** |
| **The bag of waters.** | **Degree of moulding.** |
| **Level of the presenting part.** | **Abnormalities.** |

The vaginal walls should feel soft and dilatable; when firm and rigid a longer labour can be anticipated. The presence of scar tissue in the lower vagina, following a previous perineal laceration or episiotomy, may, because of lack of elasticity, cause delay during the perineal phase of the second stage of labour, and the perineum is also more liable to rupture. *A cystocele* may be felt in the multiparous woman. A loaded rectum could resemble a tumour, but its putty-like consistency is diagnostic of faeces.

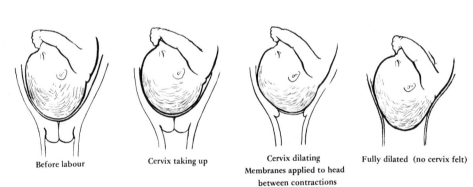

| Before labour | Cervix taking up | Cervix dilating<br>Membranes applied to head<br>between contractions | Fully dilated (no cervix felt) |

Fig. 17-7  The cervix before and during labour.

If the cervix is found to be 2·5 cm long and the os closed, it is usually concluded that labour is not likely to commence for some time, *but some do not accept this*. At the beginning of labour the cervix can be readily felt, although somewhat shortened, but by the time labour is established the cervical canal is completely taken up or effaced and the cervix is often closely applied to the fetal head. A thin, effaced cervix may be difficult to detect, and in primigravid patients it may not lie directly below what is presenting, so the examining fingers should be directed backwards and upwards. If the cervix feels rigid and unyielding, whether it is thick or thin, dilatation is likely to be slow. An oedematous anterior lip of cervix may be present towards the end of the first stage (see p. 402).

**An inexperienced person may mistake the thin cervix** that is taken up and 2 or 3 cm dilated, for one that is fully dilated, but the short contractions and absence of other signs of the second stage should prevent such an error from being made.

### Dilatation of the cervix

This is determined by encircling its circumference with the fingers and forming a mental image of its size. This is described according to the measurement of the diameter of the os in centimetres. Recording dilatation on a cervicograph focuses attention on slow progress.

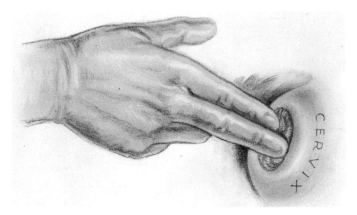

Fig. 17-8   Cervix 4 cm dilated.

**When fully dilated no cervix is felt.** With a 1·5 kg baby full dilatation might be imminent when the diameter of the cervix is 6 cm. It may take longer than three hours for the cervix of the primigravid woman to reach 3 cm dilatation and two hours for the multiparous cervix to reach 4 cm. One cm per hour, after 3 cm has been reached, is the usual rate of cervical dilatation.

**Rim of cervix.** The term is used when the depth of the cervical tissue surrounding the os is 0·5 or 1 cm. This indicates, that, no matter what the measurement of the dilated cervix, the stage of full dilatation is imminent.

An important point to be grasped is that when no cervix is felt it has slipped up over the fetal head, the cervix is fully dilated and the second stage of labour has begun.

### The bag of waters

When the membranes are intact and the amount of forewaters is scanty (6 mm or less in depth) the bag of waters may be difficult to detect on vaginal examination if the membranes lie in close contact with the fetal head. The scalp when covered with mucus has the same smooth slippery feeling that the bag of waters has, but during a uterine contraction the membranes become tense and can then be felt with the hard head lying immediately behind them and fluid between. Usually the forewaters are found by the examining finger to be shaped like a watch-glass but, if the 'fit' between the presenting part and the lower segment is not good, some of the fluid from the hindwaters is forced into the forewaters, causing the membranes to protrude through the cervix like a glove finger. The intra-uterine pressure exerted on these bulging forewaters causes them to rupture early, so they are not often found on examination. Occasionally, in cases where there has been an escape of amniotic fluid and the membranes are believed to have ruptured, the forewaters are found on vaginal examination to be intact. The possible explanation is that there may have been a slight rupture of the hindwaters and when the head was forced into the lower segment by good uterine contractions further escape of fluid was prevented.

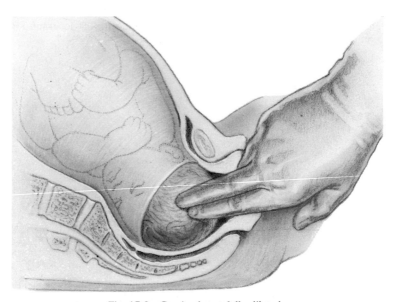

Fig. 17-9   Cervix almost fully dilated.

**Level or station of the presenting part.** If the head is deeply engaged it can be felt low in the pelvic cavity, at the level of the ischial spines. The caput may, however, be below that level. If the head is just engaged it can be touched or tipped, but when the head is above the brim it cannot be reached vaginally.

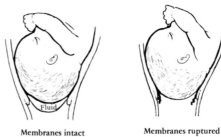

Membranes intact                    Membranes ruptured

Fig. 17-10

**Diagnosis of presentation.** In 96 per cent of cases the vertex presents and is recognised by feeling the hard skull bones, the fontanelles and sutures.

### The diagnosis of position

In the vertex presentation this is determined by recognising which fontanelle lies anteriorly, i.e. the posterior fontanelle in occipito anterior positions, the anterior fontanelle in occipito posterior positions and whether it is to the left or right side of the pelvis.

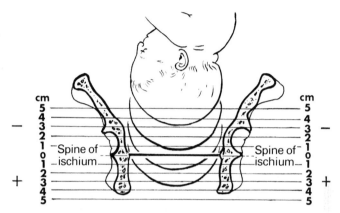

Fig. 17-11 Recording descent of the fetus on abdominal and vaginal examination. The midwife draws a ∪ at the appropriate level in relation to the ischial spines in cm + or −.

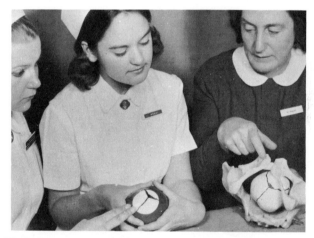

Fig. 17-12 Demonstration of dilatation of cervix and position of the vertex.
Note.—Halves of a series of rubber balls used to denote the dilating cervix.
*Aberdeen Maternity Hospital.*

**The degree of moulding** can be judged by feeling the amount of overlapping of the skull bones, and, when excessive, it suggests that *intracranial injury* is likely to have taken place.

**Abnormalities** such as prolapse or presentation of cord, anencephaly, hydrocephaly and compound presentation can be diagnosed vaginally.

## THE ACTIVE MANAGEMENT OF LABOUR

This modern concept embraces a number of policies and procedures to which midwives must become orientated. The unpredictability of the onset of labour has been eliminated: the negative attitude of watchful expectancy throughout labour which often culminated in a prolonged exhausting experience has been superseded

ANTERIOR

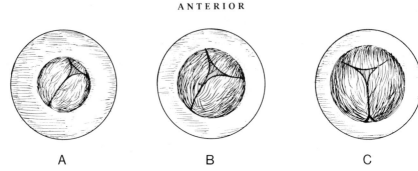

|          A          |          B          |          C          |

Fig. 17-13   Vaginal touch picture of vertex presentation L.O.A.

Post. fontanelle to the left anterior, sagittal suture in the right oblique diameter of pelvis.

Flexion increased.

Posterior fontanelle has rotated one eighth of a circle forward. Sagittal suture in antero-post. diameter of pelvic outlet.

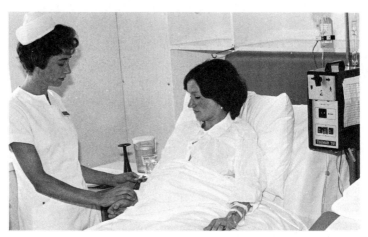

Fig. 17-14   Woman encouraged to sit upright, is receiving Syntocinon i.v. controlled by Tekmar 251.

*Maternity Unit, Southern General Hospital, Glasgow.*

by a planned positive approach. Greater maternal and fetal safety has been achieved by the use of continuous electronic monitoring devices. More frequent use of epidural analgesia, Caesarean section, forceps, episiotomy and controlled cord traction all have a bearing on the active management of labour.

## Induction of labour

The employment of automated i.v. infusion units as well as the gravity drip to dispense oxytocin have proved to be so safe and effective that their use is extended to incorporate additional obstetric as well as social indications to enable the expectant mother to make definitive plans for the onset of labour.

On the day after admission at about 9.00 hours the membranes are punctured and oxytocin administered intravenously: the baby usually being born before nine hours have elapsed.

## THE PARTOGRAM

This provides a graphic method of recording the salient features of labour. Progress can be assessed at a glance because the significant facts are annotated concisely, e.g. the intensity and length of uterine contractions are recorded in three shades of black, the number of contractions in the last 10 minutes of 30 minute periods being depicted.

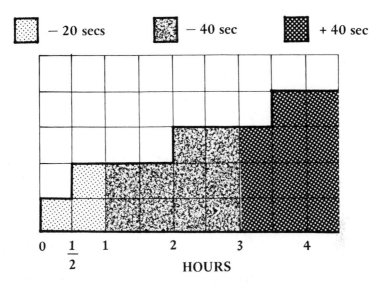

Fig. 17-15   Section of a partogram. Number of contractions in the last 10 minutes of a 30 minute period is recorded in squares. The intensity of the contractions, length and strength is shown in three shades of black.

Half-hourly recording of uterine contractions.

*First half-hour:* In the last 10 minutes of that half-hour there was one contraction lasting less than 20 seconds.

*Third half-hour:* In the last 10 minutes of that half-hour there were 2 contractions lasting over 20 seconds and less than 40 seconds.

*Eighth half-hour:* In the last 10 minutes of that half-hour there were 4 contractions lasting over 40 seconds.

If continuous electronic monitoring is not available the fetal heart rate is recorded by the midwife as on a temperature chart. Descent of the head on abdominal palpation is shown in fifths in relation to the pelvic brim. The station of the head in relation to the ischial spines on vaginal examination is recorded in cm plus or minus. Dilatation of the cervix is depicted on a cervicograph (see Fig. 17-17).

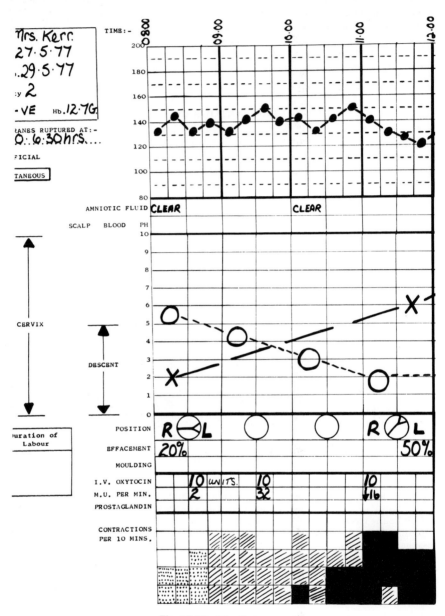

Fig. 17-16 The Partogram.

Most hospitals develop a partogram to suit their own requirements. There is no standard partogram.

*Other facts recorded are*

**maternal and fetal condition;
blood pressure; temperature: pulse;
fluid balance; urine analysis;
drugs administered including i.v. oxytocin;
epidural and inhalational analgesia.**

Such documentation requires diligent observation of the patient; the visual display of progress providing an early warning system which facilitates recognition of deviation from normal and alerts the labour ward staff to the need for medical assistance. The results are:—more careful accurate observation; greater safety for mother and child and improved management of labour; fewer prolonged labours and instrumental deliveries; higher Apgar scores in the newborn and a lower perinatal mortality rate. The graphic type of recording requires less time than writing a descriptive assessment of procedures and progress.

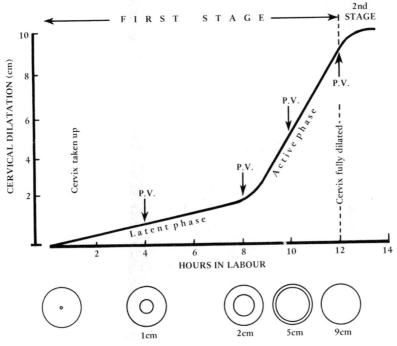

Fig. 17-17 Diagrammatic representation of Cervicograph. Dilatation of the cervix is recorded by an **X** every 2 or 4 hours.

### THE LATENT AND ACTIVE PHASES OF THE FIRST STAGE

The period from the onset of labour to 3 cm cervical dilatation is known as the latent phase. Progress during the latent phase is slow and may last for 6 hours in a primigravida. The active phase extends from 3 cm dilatation until the end of the first stage and should proceed at not less than 1 cm per hour in primigravidae and 1·5 cm in multiparae.

### THE CERVICOGRAPH

The cervicograph (see Fig. 17-17) is used as a guide line to plot dilatation of the cervix in centimetres against time in hours. Zero time is taken as the hour of admission in labour (in preference to the spontaneous onset which is often in doubt), or the time of induction (usually by amniotomy and oxytocin drip).

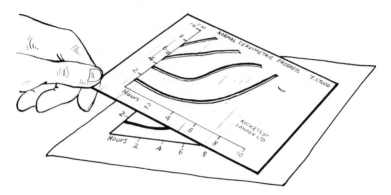

Fig. 17–18    Studd's Stencil

The stencil is used to draw one of four curves according to the dilatation of the cervix in cm on admission in labour or at the time of induction. (See cervicograph Fig. 17-17.)

Acrylic stencils (Studds) are available from Rocket of London Ltd to provide a normal cervicometric progress curve for cases admitted with cervical dilatation of 2, 4, 6, or 8 cm. If the patient's cervical dilatation curve extends 2 hours to the right of the stencil curve, labour is considered to be prolonged, so the doctor may decide to accelerate it by giving a Syntocinon i.v. drip.

**Acceleration of labour**

If the cervicograph shows that dilatation of the cervix is too slow, labour may be accelerated. An assessment is made to exclude any contraindication to vaginal delivery and if none is evident the membranes are punctured and an i.v. automated or gravity drip started at 0·5 units Syntocinon in 540 ml 5 per cent glucose. Increase to one unit in 30 minutes and gradually up to 2·5 units if the maternal and fetal conditions warrant this. The fetal heart should be monitored assiduously in such cases, preferably electronically.

A vaginal examination is made every 2 hours. Tranquillisers are given as necessary but a vaginal examination should be made prior to administering any analgesic type of drug, e.g. pethidine. The Syntocinon drip is continued until 1 hour after completion of the third stage and then reduced gradually. Caution should be observed in stimulating the uterus of the multiparous woman.

---

### QUESTIONS FOR REVISION

What do you understand by: established labour, active management of labour, acceleration of labour, the latent phase of labour? What are the uses of the partogram? What does intelligent mask wearing imply?

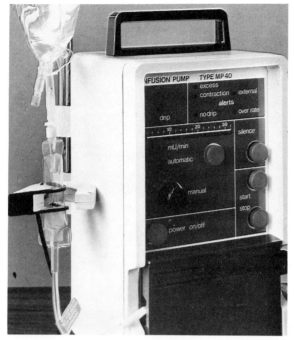

Fig. 17-19 Pye Dynamics type MP40 Infusion Pump, which administers a progressively increasing dose of oxytocin. Warning alerts are sounded if certain undesirable conditions are detected. It can be controlled manually and is intended to be used in conjunction with a standard fetal monitor.

### ADMISSION OF THE WOMAN IN LABOUR

How would you approach and receive the woman in labour?

What do you ask re. contractions, show, membranes, sleep, food?

Under what circumstances should a vaginal examination not be made by the midwife?

Give reasons why the woman in labour should be given an enema. When should an enema not be given?

**C.M.B.(Scot.).** How is the onset of true labour recognised? What are the indications that labour is progressing normally in the first, second and third stages.

**C.M.B.(Eng.).** Describe in detail the admission procedure for a patient in labour.

**C.M.B. (Eng.).** Describe the records kept in the first stage of labour, and the reasons for the recordings.

### CLINICAL APPLICATION

**Give examples** as to how domestic cleanliness can prevent infection in the labour ward. In what way is the history of labour significant? How would a woman, admitted in false labour, be dealt with?

**State whether labour is true or false** in the following circumstances:

**Contractions** (a) Painful ......; (b) lasting 2 minutes ......; (c) erratic ......; **on vaginal examination** (a) cervix is shortened ......; (b) os not dilating ......; (c) membranes tense ......; (d) no show ......

How do you give emotional support to the woman in labour?

**Discuss** (a) bath *versus* mobile hand spray; (b) shaving *versus* non-shaving; (c) water enema *versus* suppository.

**Differentiate between** (a) urine and amniotic fluid; (b) the vulva of a primigravid and a multiparous woman; (c) thin cervix 2 cm dilated and one that is fully dilated; (d) an L.O.A. and an R.O.P. vaginally; (e) intact and ruptured membranes P.V.

What are the advantages in using a partogram to record the progress of labour?

How often do you (a) take and record: the blood pressure; temperature; pulse. (b) examine the urine and for which substances. (c) examine the abdomen. (d) make a vaginal examination?

What do you understand by palpating the fetal head relative to the pelvic brim in fifths?

What is Studd's cervicometric stencil?

**C.M.B.(Eng.) 30-min. question.** Give the reasons for the measures which are adopted to avoid infection in a maternity unit.

**(N. Ireland) 30-min. question.** What are the indications for vaginal examination during labour? Indicate how the findings might influence the conduct of labour.

**(N. Ireland) 30-min. question.** An unbooked multiparous patient is admitted in early labour. What would make you think the labour should proceed normally?

**C.M.B.(Eng.).** List the indications for vaginal examination of a patient between the beginning of pregnancy and the end of the puerperium.

**N. Ire.** Describe the anatomy of the vagina. Discuss the indications for making a vaginal examination in pregnancy and labour.

## C.M.B. Short Questions

**Eng.** Indications for vaginal examination. **Eng.** Measures to prevent infection during labour.

**Eng.** Assessment of progress during the first stage of labour.

**Eng.** Urinary catheterisation in labour.

**N.Ire.** How may the condition of the fetus and mother be assessed during labour?

What can you learn from making a vaginal examination during labour?

What do you mean by the latent and the active stages of labour?

# 18
# The Management of Normal Labour (contd.)

*Obstetrical nursing care in the first stage. Diet. Attention to bladder. Observation.*
*Fetal condition. Fetal distress. F.H. monitoring. Maternal condition.*

The management of labour has been modified to a considerable extent during recent years: prolonged labour no longer being permitted. Syntocinon i.v. is given by electronic automated units: biochemical control maintained. 'High risk' maternal and fetal cases are monitored by cardiotocograph. These procedures demand technical skill and meticulous supervision by the midwife.

### Posture in labour
No hard and fast rule can be laid down regarding the posture to be adopted by the woman in labour. If she is tired she should relax and rest. In the upright position the antero-posterior diameter of the brim enlarges slightly. Bending the back and drawing in the abdominal muscles will facilitate engagement of the head: a similar advantage being obtained by sitting in a low chair or in bed leaning forwards during uterine contractions. Some encourage the woman to sit upright in bed until labour is established and sedation is required.

**The lateral position is now recommended** because vena caval compression occurs during the first stage in some women and the supine hypotensive syndrome ensues when they lie on their backs (see p. 125). Kidney function is facilitated when the woman lies on either side. The foam rubber wedge is useful to maintain the lateral position.

When the intensity of the contractions gives rise to suffering, the woman should of course be in bed in order that analgesics may be given to relieve the pain.

## DIET DURING LABOUR

This subject presents great difficulties; the nutritional and biochemical requirements of the woman and the grave risk of anaesthetic deaths must be given due consideration. In many centres food is withheld when labour is established (cervix 3 cm dilated) and glucose, 5 per cent, is given intravenously. Deprivation of glucose leads to ketosis which produces vomiting, extreme exhaustion and a predisposition to shock, so the urine is examined for ketones every 2 hours or each specimen. When ketones are present an intravenous drip of 5 or 10 per cent glucose is set up, but many women in labour are given i.v. glucose when food is withheld.

*During early labour* tea and a digestive biscuit; strained non-greasy soups; fruit jellies; cornflour pudding; ice-cream is served in some centres.

Pain and nervous tension inhibit appetite and retard the absorption of food which may be vomited after 8-12 hours.

But even when no food has been partaken for hours during labour, inhalation by the unconscious woman of the acid gastric juice may produce bronchospasm, cyanosis, pulmonary oedema and, in some cases, death may ensue. To counteract the acidity of the gastric contents most obstetricians prescribe Aludrox or magnesium trisilicate, 15 ml two hourly throughout labour.

**Prolonged labour can present serious problems** for midwives in some developing countries. If food is withheld for many hours until the woman is profoundly dehydrated and suffering from ketosis she is a very grave risk when operative measures under general anaesthesia are undertaken. A glucose drip i.v. 5 or 10 per cent, should be given.

Dehydration must be avoided so the woman in labour should receive about 75 ml of fluid per hour. Some give weak tea or water. Copious aerated fruit juices may cause nausea, vomiting and dehydration as well as gaseous distension of the stomach and intestine. A fluid balance chart should be kept; vomitus being subtracted from intake.

### Possible anaesthetic difficulties

The question as to whether a general anaesthetic will be necessary should be kept in mind, and the woman ought not to be given food or oral fluids within three hours of delivery. Many obstetricians are using pudendal nerve block and perineal infiltration in preference to a general anaesthetic for forceps delivery.

A plastic oesophageal tube No. 18 F.G. should be passed if the woman has had food before a general anaesthetic is administered, the woman being propped up or on her side but not supine during the procedure.

### Biochemical Control and Electrolyte Replacement

Ketonuria indicates the presence of ketosis due to deficient carbohydrate intake, interfering with the metabolic breakdown of fats: dehydration aggravates the situation (hot climate or overheated labour wards cause fluid loss). Potassium becomes depleted. Fluid is administered i.v., e.g. 5 or 10 per cent glucose; potassium being added in severe cases.

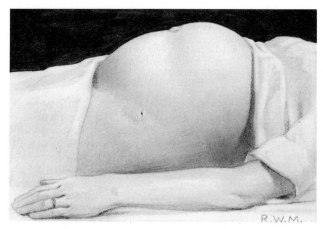

Fig. 18-1   Distended bladder during labour.

### ATTENTION TO THE BLADDER

It is the duty of the midwife to see that the woman empties her bladder (every two hours) throughout labour, every specimen being tested for ketones and protein. A bladder containing 90 to 120 ml of urine will be seen and felt, well above the symphysis pubis during labour, and it will have a soft fluctuating consistency. When overdistended, it forms a smooth round tense swelling and above its upper margin a very definite depression is evident. This dip may be mistaken for Bandl's ring (see p. 247).

**A full bladder may prevent the head from entering the brim,** and this is most frequently seen in the multiparous woman. It may retard descent of the fetus, so in all cases of delay the bladder should be palpated and percussed. It will cause much unnecessary pain during labour, and by interfering with the tone of the bladder may predispose to retention of urine after delivery.

Poor uterine contractions are often associated with a full bladder, and in such cases an improvement in uterine action is usually apparent as soon as the bladder is emptied. When minor cephalo-pelvic disproportion exists, the bladder may be nipped between the fetal skull and pelvis, but this is most likely to happen when the bladder is not emptied regularly. The bruised area may slough during the puerperium giving rise to a vesico-vaginal fistula.

## RETENTION OF URINE

*This occurs during labour, for the following reasons:*

The bladder may lack tone, especially when hypotonic uterine action is present.

Using the bedpan is an uncomfortable procedure for the cumbersome woman in labour. (It should be placed on a low stool beside the bed, or better still, in a sanichair, which gives firm support to her arms and buttocks and allows better relaxation of the pelvic floor muscles.)

Inability to void during the latter part of the first stage is usually due to pressure of the fetal head on the neck of the bladder, and in such circumstances posture and suggestion are of no value. If the woman has not passed urine for six hours, the bladder is visibly distended and the woman unable to void, a catheter ought to be passed. Medical permission should first be obtained.

### Catheterisation

Plastic disposable catheters are used. If difficulty is encountered while introducing the catheter, the sterile gloved forefinger of the left hand should be inserted into the vagina and placed along its anterior wall. The tip of the catheter can then be felt, and if it is directed parallel with the finger in the vagina, the catheter will enter the bladder without injury to the urethra. If the catheter is obstructed by the fetal head, upward pressure on the head by the finger in the vagina will permit passage of the catheter.

In all cases where medical aid is summoned during labour, the patient should be encouraged to empty her bladder. Many obstetricians are reluctant to pass a catheter unless the bladder is distended and the woman unable to void. Others consider that damage to the bladder can be more dangerous than urinary tract infection and that catheterisation should be performed prior to vaginal operative manipulations during labour.

### Attention to the bowel

An enema should never be given at the end of the first stage, because during its expulsion it is usual for the action of the uterus to be intensified, and further descent of the fetal head may prevent the complete return of the fluid, so that with each subsequent contraction there will be spluttering of liquid faeces.

**It is not commendable to permit patients to use 'the toilet' throughout labour.** They are unable to differentiate between the desire to defaecate and the similar sensation preceding expulsion of the baby's head. When a bedpan is used and the midwife empties it, the amount of urine can be measured and any abnormal vaginal discharge noted.

### Rest and sleep

The need for adequate rest and sleep during early labour cannot be overemphasised; for discomfort, pain and anxiety are each exhausting and the woman in labour may experience all three.

The usual nursing procedures to induce sleep should be employed:

The bladder is emptied; a nourishing drink given; the bed ought to be comfortable; the room darkened; an effort is made to ensure quietness.

In early labour if the woman is assured that 'all is well,' given a suitable analgesic and tucked up in a kindly manner, she will almost certainly relax and sleep.

### Comfort and assistance

The midwife can add greatly to the comfort of the woman in labour by attending to her personal toilet. She should wash the patient's face and hands and help to dress her hair. The buttocks and thighs should be washed and the vulva swabbed four-hourly for the woman's comfort, even by those who do not consider it to have any antiseptic value. Clean clothing is most refreshing. Soiled bed linen is unhygienic as well as uncomfortable, and when amniotic fluid is draining freely, pads can be placed beneath the buttocks.

Cramp in the leg may be very distressing, and one way of obtaining quick relief is to extend the leg and dorsiflex the foot. (The toes of the straightened leg are brought towards the knee.) Backache (see p. 268).

Bearing down should be forbidden during the first stage of labour, because, when the cervix is not fully dilated, the woman pushes her uterus downwards and puts such great strain on the transverse cervical ligaments and the para-cervical tissue, that subsequent uterine prolapse is likely. Premature pushing causes the cervix to be compressed between the fetal head and the pubic bone, making the anterior lip of cervix become oedematous and hard, thereby increasing the pain and delaying labour. The increased intra-uterine pressure may cause premature rupture of the membranes as well as fetal distress. The patient who bears down too soon must be asked to stop, turned on her side and shown how to refrain by breathing deliberately, accentuating inspiration rather than expiration during contractions. If inhalational analgesia is administered, the woman can co-operate more readily.

## OBSERVATION OF THE WOMAN IN LABOUR

This is an integral part of good obstetrical nursing care, and, although the majority of labours are normal, the midwife must never lower the high standard of conscientious observation needed for the safety of the two lives in her care.

*Observation can be considered under the following headings:*

| | |
|---|---|
| Uterine action. | Discharge from the vagina. |
| Dilatation of the cervix. | The fetal condition. |
| Descent of the presenting part. | The maternal condition. |
| Complications. | |

The frequency, length and strength of the contractions should be noted. The strength of a contraction cannot be judged by the reaction of the woman, but always by laying the hand on the uterus and noting the degree of hardness during the contraction and by timing its length. Some women appear to experience great pain and yet the contractions may be neither long nor strong and very little is accomplished; other women appear to suffer very little, yet good progress is made.

When a uterine contraction begins, it is painless for a number of seconds and painless again at the end, so the midwife is aware of the approach of a contraction before the patient feels it, and this knowledge can be utilised when giving inhalational analgesia. The uterus should always relax between contractions. Should the contractions be unduly long or very strong and rapid, concern would be felt in case fetal hypoxia develops.

### Dilatation of the cervix

Until the cervix begins to dilate, the woman is not considered to be in true labour but when it is 3 cm dilated with regular contractions at about 10 minute intervals labour is said to be established. The progress of labour is usually assessed by the degree of dilatation of the cervix and this can be recorded on a cervicograph which demonstrates whether progressive dilatation is taking place when a vaginal assessment is recorded every 2 or 4 hours (see also Fig. 17-17).

In cases where the doctor wishes to be present for the delivery it is usual to call him when the cervix is fully dilated in a primigravida and when 7 cm in a multiparous woman, but other factors, such as the strength and frequency of the contractions and the rate of advance, must be taken into consideration when predicting the probable time of delivery.

### Descent of the presenting part

During the first stage this can be noted almost entirely by abdominal palpation but when doubt exists a vaginal examination is made. In the primigravid woman the fetal head is commonly engaged before labour begins and its continued descent can be followed by abdominal palpation. Should the head be above the brim in a primigravida, close watch must be kept by frequent palpation to find out whether with good contractions the head enters the brim.

When the head is engaged the biparietal diameter has passed through the pelvic brim, the occipital prominence can only be felt with difficulty from above. The sinciput may still be palpable above the brim because of the increased flexion of the head until the occiput reaches the pelvic floor and rotates forwards.

In a multiparous patient the head may not descend appreciably until labour is well established and sometimes not until the membranes rupture. A full bladder may prevent descent.

The descent of the presenting part can also be detected from below by vaginal examination and in cases where there is excessive moulding and a large caput, a misleading impression of advance may be gained, as it is possible for a caput to be showing inside the vulva while the head is actually above the ischial spines and the cervix not fully dilated.

Some record descent on a graph in which the ischial spines are zero. The station of the head is depicted by a curved line on the cm scale plus or minus the spines (see p. 283).

### Discharge from the vagina

Show is the blood stained mucus seen early in labour. Towards the end of the first stage a trickle of blood may appear, due to the slight laceration of the cervix which usually takes place when it is dilated to its maximum.

Amniotic fluid may be seen trickling from the vagina after the membranes have ruptured, but if doubt exists as to whether it is urine or liquor, its alkaline reaction, obtained by the use of litmus paper, will help to settle the question. The presence of meconium in the liquor suggests fetal distress, except during the second stage in cases of breech presentation. If the fluid looks milky or contains white specks, this is only due to vernix caseosa and has no significance. Golden liquor is seen in some cases when the fetus is suffering from Rh haemolytic disease.

#### Early Rupture of the Membranes

If the membranes have been ruptured for 24 hours or more, which is frowned on today, the amniotic fluid may become infected and will have an offensive odour. This is dangerous, because the fetus may inhale some of the fluid, with resultant pneumonia. The doctor should be notifed; an endocervical or high vaginal swab is taken; an antibiotic, such as ampicillin, 500 mg followed by 250 mg, 6 hourly or cephaloridine is usually prescribed.

## ELECTRONIC MONITORING DURING LABOUR

Expectant mothers should be orientated to appreciate and accept the use of electronic monitoring equipment before being subjected to it during labour. They ought to be told that constant supervision of the fetal heart can only be attained by an electronic monitor and that fewer mentally retarded babies are now born, because of the detection by monitors of conditions that are harmful to the baby during labour. The woman should also be aware that the monitor is recording her uterine contractions, a valuable safety measure.

**As a suffering human being,** the woman should receive more rather than less care when her condition is being monitored. Midwives must be careful that the woman does not get the impression that more attention is being paid to the equipment than to her.

### THE PURPOSE OF ELECTRONIC MONITORING

**(1) for the early diagnosis of fetal distress,** identification of the cause, and if possible rectification or alleviation of the hypoxia before cerebral damage has been inflicted or fetal death supervenes.

**(2) Recording the uterine contractions on the same strip as the fetal heart rate pattern** is invaluable to detect the effect of the contractions on the fetal heart, as in induction or acceleration of labour by Syntocinon when the contractions may be too frequent, long or strong.

**(3) During epidural analgesia,** the woman experiences no pain so the uterine contractions are visually recorded.

**The midwife must**

(a) **Understand the significance** of what is being recorded.
(b) **Interpret the findings** in relation to the clinical situation.
(c) **Be alert in reporting adverse signals to the doctor.**

### Recording Uterine Activity

**The internal method** of recording uterine contractions—tocography—is the more reliable and the most commonly employed. An open ended Teflon catheter filled with fluid is introduced through the cervix into the amniotic cavity and changes in the amniotic fluid pressure are transmitted through the catheter and detected by a sensitive pressure transducer which converts them into electrical signals that are displayed on the strip-chart. Each contraction is depicted as an upward deflection. Uterine tonus is not successfully depicted so the fingers by indenting the uterus abdominally can assess tonus.

**The external method** utilises a pressure transducer placed on the midline of the abdomen at about fundal level. The abdominal belt interferes with palpation, is uncomfortable and easily displaced. To avoid skin irritation it should be moved every hour.

### Recording the fetal heart rate pattern

**The internal or direct method of cardiography** is carried out most successfully by an ECG electrode (spiral) attached to the fetal scalp; avoiding fontanelles. The buttock can be used in breech presentation. The cervix should be at least one cm dilated, membranes ruptured.

**The external method** whereby a microphone is placed on the maternal abdomen over the site of maximal fetal heart intensity has the same disadvantages as in external tocography.

## Phonocardiography

Fetal heart sounds are detected by a transducer that contains a sensitive contact microphone which is placed on the maternal abdomen. The sounds are amplified but relatively noise-free surroundings are necessary.

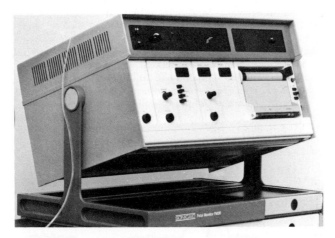

Fig. 18-2    Sonicaid FM3R. The various modules record fetal heart rate pattern: fetal ECG from scalp electrode: an ultrasound module displays the fetal heart rate pattern on the oscilloscope to aid transducer placement. (Cabinet with 3 drawers on which the FM3R is positioned at bedside level is not shown.)

*By courtesy of Sonicaid Ltd., Bognor Regis, West Sussex.*

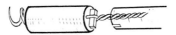

Fig. 18-3    Showing detail of the spiral electrode.

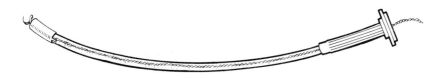

Fig. 18-4    Introducer for spiral electrode. Attached to the fetal scalp, not over a fontanelle, when cervix is more than 1 cm dilated. Impulse directed by electric lead to a fetal heart monitor where the impulse is displayed on the strip chart.

## THE FETAL CONDITION

The fetal heart rate pattern is the best indication as to how the fetus is faring during labour. Undue frequency, length and intensity of uterine contractions can have an adverse effect on the fetal heart because they diminish uterine and placental blood flow; thus reducing the supply of oxygen to the fetus. The traditional, intermittent, method of auscultation by using Pinard's fetal stethoscope gives very limited information regarding the fetal heart status and does not provide early warning signs of fetal hypoxia, so it has been replaced in many centres by continuous fetal heart rate monitoring equipment.

**Interpreting the recorded signals requires a degree of expertise and judgment;** the record on the strip-chart must be co-ordinated with and interpreted in relation to the clinical progress of labour. The midwife still applies her traditional facility for observation of the woman's general condition, uterine action, fetal wellbeing, descent and cervical dilatation. A new terminology has been introduced so the midwife must extend her vocabulary and gain some understanding of the signals displayed on the strip chart.

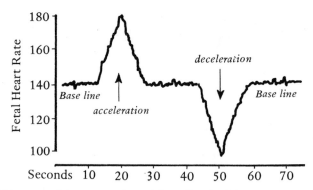

Fig. 18-5   Diagrammatic representation of base line fetal heart rate pattern showing acceleration and deceleration.

### Baseline fetal heart rate

This is the FH pattern between uterine contractions ranging normally from 120 to 160 beats per minute. When above 160 the term 'baseline tachycardia' is used; when below 120 it is 'baseline bradycardia'. Both should be considered as reflections of fetal hypoxia and should not be disregarded.

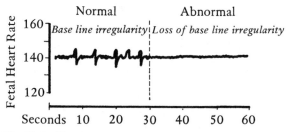

Fig. 18-6   Showing normal and abnormal base line variability.

**Baseline variability** (formerly known as 'beat to beat variation')

In normal circumstances there is a difference of more than 5 beats, and more than 2 such oscillatory shifts in 30 seconds. Loss of such variation reflects loss of adaptive ability of the circulatory system or depression of the cardiac reflex centre in the brain.

### Type 1 Dips (early deceleration)

The fetal heart slows by approximately 30 beats per minute, the lowest point of deceleration coincides with the acme of the uterine contraction and returns to base line at the end of the contraction. It is thought to be due to pressure on the fetal head by bony or soft tissues e.g. the pelvis or cervix. It is not seriously significant but should not be ignored.

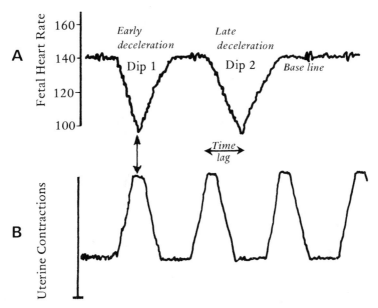

Fig. 18-7  Showing relationship between uterine contractions and fetal heart rate, early sounds

*Aberdeen Maternity Hospital.*

### Type 2 Dips (late deceleration)

**The fetal heart rate slows by about 40–50 beats per minute:** the lowest point being reached after the uterine contraction has ceased; this is known as time lag and the greater the lag the more serious is the situation: the bigger the dip the greater the danger. Type 2 dips persist into the resting phase of uterine activity and are an ominous fetal heart rate pattern usually associated with utero-placental insufficiency and demanding urgent treatment. A vaginal examination is made to rule out prolapse of cord. If treatment by rectifying vena-caval occlusion, discontinuing oxytocin, giving i.v. fluids and intermittent hyperoxic therapy are of no avail, operative delivery is considered.

### The ultrasonic fetal heart detector

This FH monitor which has a low intensity beam is also used, the Doppler principle being employed. The Doptone, Sonicaid and Hewlett Packard monitors are in common use.

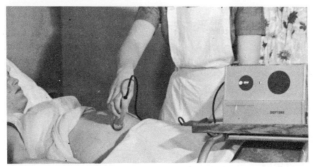

Fig. 18-8    The Doptone ultrasonic fetal heart monitor used to clarify fetal heart sounds.
*Aberdeen Maternity Hospital.*

**Fetal telemetry is now employed** during the first stage of labour in some centres. A portable battery-operated transmitter (Hewlett Packard) is carried about by the ambulant woman. The scalp electrode transmits the fetal ECG through a radio transmitter to the 8030A cardiotocograph where it is recorded on the strip-chart.

### When modern electronic equipment is not available

The fetal heart rate should be carefully assessed at the beginning of labour so that the average rate for each particular fetus is known; the normal rate being 120 to 160 beats per minute. Volume and rhythm should also be noted. When labour is established the fetal heart is auscultated every 15 minutes, during and after the uterine contraction.

### High risk conditions

These may involve the placenta; cord; hypertonic uterine action; maternal diseases; drugs; anaesthetics.

(1) **Severe pre-eclampsia, diabetes, antepartum** haemorrhage, multiple pregnancy, the older primigravida.

(2) **Rh haemolytic disease, uterine growth retardation,** preterm labour, small for date babies, low daily fetal movement-count.

(3) **Oxytocin induction or acceleration of labour** with or without puncture of membranes.

(4) **Epidural analgesia if undue hypotension occurs.**

(5) **Prolapse of cord.**

### FETAL DISTRESS

**In cases where fetal distress is suspected or anticipated,** as in severe pre-eclampsia, auscultation during every uterine contraction should be carried out; also towards the end of the first stage when the woman is in strong labour and particularly so when the membranes are no longer intact. The fetal heart rate should always be checked when the membranes rupture because of the risk of prolapsed cord, especially when there is a malpresentation or when there is polyhydramnios and in parous patients because the head may not be engaged at that time. During labour, induced by amniotomy, prolapse of cord is a fairly frequent occurrence.

**Hypoxia is the commonest cause of fetal distress.** Oxygen lack can cause stillbirth; in less severe cases the baby is born in a state of asphyxia with a low Apgar score. When the brain cells are deprived of oxygen they are damaged and mental retardation and spastic paralysis may result.

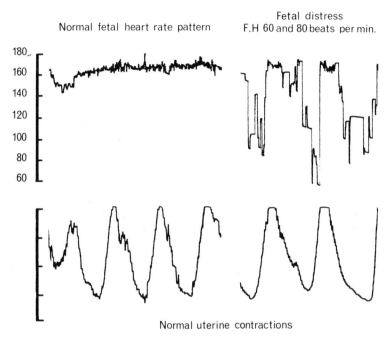

Fig. 18-9   Sonicaid tracing of fetal heart rate pattern and uterine action.
*Aberdeen Maternity Hospital.*

### Signs of fetal distress

**An increase of over 20 beats** is an early sign of mild oxygen lack; a rate of over 160 beats per minute should cause concern.

**A slow fetal heart is significant** and a rate of below 120 or a decrease of 20 beats usually indicates oxygen lack. The rate may become progressively slower and when under 110 gives rise to anxiety; under 100 puts the fetus into the danger zone. Rates as slow as 80 can occur. When the FH takes progressively longer to recover its normal rate after each uterine contraction or a slow beat persists for over 15 seconds after the contraction has ceased, the outlook is serious. (See also early and late decelerations, p. 299).

**The passage of meconium** may not be significant without other signs of fetal distress and in breech presentation during the second stage due to compression of the abdomen. Slight green staining of the amniotic fluid may be the result of previous distress from which the fetus has recovered. Some obstetricians prefer to puncture the membranes early in labour to detect the presence of meconium.

### Management of fetal distress by the Midwife

**Medical aid is obtained.** If an oxytocin drip is being administered it should be stopped: i.v. fluids being continued. The woman is turned on her side to rectify any vena caval occlusion. Maternal oxygen lack, as may be present in cardiac failure, severe APH or eclampsia may be treated by giving oxygen at interrupted periods. During the second stage, delivery may be expedited by making an episiotomy. Preparations should be made for fetal blood sampling; delivery, by forceps under pudendal nerve block or by Caesarean section should be anticipated.

The paediatrician should be notified and equipment for resuscitation of the infant made available.

### SALING METHOD OF DETECTING FETAL HYPOXIA

When the fetus is hypoxic the pH of its blood falls and this is a guide to the oxygenation of the fetus. The normal level is around 7·35: below 7 the brain cells will perish. Fetal distress is always accompanied by respiratory and metabolic acidosis with a lowering of the pH of the blood.

**Fetal blood sampling** is now mainly used to confirm variations in the fetal heart rate pattern. It is also done when fetal distress is anticipated as in placental dysfunction, Rh immunisation and in breech presentation during the period of cord compression.

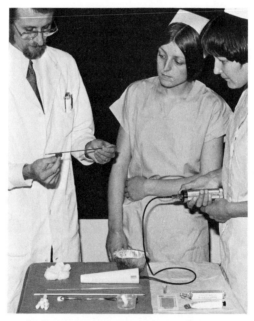

Fig. 18-10   Fetal blood sampling. Non sterile set up for clinical instruction. Fibre optic light. The obstetrician is running a magnet along the capillary tube to move the iron filing and mix heparin and blood.

*Queen Mother's Hospital, Glasgow.*

### Procedure

The vulva is cleansed, amnioscope inserted, fetal scalp dried, sprayed with ethyl chloride to produce hyperaemia, smeared with silicone grease. A small incision is made with a 4 mm blade and 0·5 ml of blood sucked into heparinised capillary polythene tubing. An iron filing is added to the blood, the tube sealed with wax (See Fig. 18-10).

**The pH of the blood is assessed by the Astrup micro apparatus:** serial tests being made in suspicious cases, i.e. pH under 7·25. Termination of labour is considered when the pH is 7·2 or less.

## ACTIVE TREATMENT OF FETAL DISTRESS

### Administration of oxygen

When the mother has a deficiency of oxygen in her blood as occurs in eclampsia, cardiac failure, or in collapse due to severe antepartum haemorrhage, oxygen should be administered. The woman is turned on to her side.

### Caesarean section

During the first stage of labour Caesarean section should be anticipated and the necessary preparations made.

### Episiotomy

Should marked fetal distress occur because the head is held up by a rigid perineum, and there is no possibility of getting the doctor in time, a midwife would make an episiotomy under local analgesia.

### Application of forceps

This will often ensure a live baby, but, when forceps are applied under general anaesthesia in cases of established fetal distress, the baby is liable to be born in a state of severe asphyxia. Pudendal nerve block or epidural analgesia is preferred.

The paediatrician should be notified in order that he may be present to resuscitate the baby.

# THE MATERNAL CONDITION

The woman's general condition should be under constant surveillance. It is not good obstetric practice to allow signs of distress to become manifest. Such a state should be anticipated, ketonuria being an early sign.

During normal labour there is rarely any need for anxiety regarding the woman's general condition. If given light sieved food early in labour to maintain her strength, analgesic drugs for the relief of pain and to ensure adequate rest and sleep, the average woman remains in good physical condition throughout labour. Pulse and temperature are useful guides as to how she is standing up to labour, and on that account both should be taken on admission and at **four-hourly intervals** throughout the first stage. The pulse is taken every one or two hours when in strong labour and should be reported when over 100. Blood pressure should be estimated four-hourly, some do so two-hourly. A fluid balance chart is kept. Every specimen of urine should be examined for protein and ketones.

### Emotional distress

The woman may exhibit a certain amount of psychological fatigue. She is more discouraged than exhausted, and the student midwife must learn to differentiate between such a condition and ketoacidosis, which is commonly known as maternal distress. The emotionally tired woman shows no physical signs of exhaustion, such as rising pulse and temperature. She is disheartened because she may feel that very little progress is being made. Many women in this state say '*they cannot stand it any longer*', but that is no real indication of maternal distress. Much encouragement is needed to tide them over this difficult period, and drugs such as pethidine are invaluable. In such cases, as soon as labour is over the woman recovers quickly, she is interested in her baby and ready for food.

Ketoacidosis is serious, and does not arise in good midwifery practice, nor does it happen like a *'bolt from the blue'*, for it is usually associated with delayed labour, the cause of which the midwife should have diagnosed earlier. The condition may occur when dehydration has been allowed to develop and the woman has lost much sleep. This is unlikely to occur today: an effort being made to accelerate retarded labour.

### Early Signs of Ketoacidosis

Ketonuria and dehydration are present.

A rising pulse rate is significant and when over 100 constitutes a definite warning.

Temperature over 37·2°C (99°F).

For later signs see p. 403.

**Treatment includes giving 10 per cent glucose, i.v. and sedatives.**

## COMPLICATIONS DURING THE FIRST STAGE

Conditions present during pregnancy such as eclampsia or antepartum haemorrhage may persist during labour, but the commonest complications during the first stage are due to factors which give rise to delay, e.g.

Contracted pelvis: rigid cervix: Big baby: malpresentation: malposition.

Such complications should be prevented when possible, recognised early and medical aid summoned. (*They are considered elsewhere under their respective headings*.) Emergencies must, however, be dealt with proficiently by the midwife until the arrival of the doctor.

---

## QUESTIONS FOR REVISION

### OBSTETRICAL NURSING CARE IN NORMAL LABOUR

### Oral Questions

What is the new terminology for 'loss of beat to beat variation'?
How can the history of labour influence your management?
Why is Aludrox or magnesium trisilicate given during labour?
What can you learn from abdominal examination during the admission of a woman in labour?
What can you learn from inspecting the vulva during labour?
What are the signs that labour is established?
How can you avoid vena caval compression?
How do you record the station of the descending fetal head?
What do you understand by a 'high-risk' fetus? What is the purpose of fetal scalp blood sampling?
**Write short notes on:** (*a*) attention to the bladder in labour; (*b*) attention to the bowel in labour; (*c*) comfort and assistance in labour; (*d*) early rupture of the membranes; (*e*) findings on vaginal examination in labour; (*f*) intelligent mask wearing; (*g*) established labour; (*h*) acceleration of labour; (*i*) uterine tonus.
**Differentiate between:** (*a*) physical and emotional distress; (*b*) the cervix of a primigravid and a multiparous woman; (*c*) true and false labour; (*d*) latent and active phase of labour. (*e*) Fetal heart rate pattern early dip: late dip. (*f*) Base line acceleration. (*g*) Base line deceleration.
**What could be done** for the following conditions: Backache, cramp in the leg, premature bearing down?
Give five signs of fetal distress. Give five signs of ketoacidosis.
When no electronic FH monitors are available, how often should the midwife auscultate the fetal heart during labour?
What are the causes of fetal distress? What is fetal scalp blood sampling? Why is it done?
What preparations should be anticipated as necessary treatment for fetal distress.
State what changes may occur in the fetal heart: rate, rhythm, regularity.
Why are uterine contractions and FH signals recorded on the same strip chart?
Name 5 conditions that create a 'high risk' for the fetus. What is the purpose of the Astrup apparatus.

## C.M.B.QUESTIONS

**C.M.B.(Eng.) 30-min. question.** Describe the anatomy and relations of the bladder. Why is it important to keep the bladder as empty as possible during labour?

**C.M.B.(Eng.) 30-min. question.** A primigravida is in early labour, the membranes rupture and the liquor is meconium-stained. What may the cause of this be, and what should the midwife do?

**C.M.B.(Eng.) 30-min. question.** What are the signs of fetal distress during labour? Give the causes of this condition and describe how you would deal with it.

**C.M.B.(Eng.) 30-min. question.** Describe the methods available for assessing the state of the fetus during pregnancy and labour.

**C.M.B.(Eng.) 30-min. question.** Describe the care a midwife should give to the patient in the first stage of normal labour. What signs would indicate that the labour was becoming abnormal?

**C.M.B.(Scot.).** What factors predispose to intra-uterine hypoxia? What are the signs of this condition? What action should be taken by the midwife when this condition is suspected?

## *C.M.B. Short Questions*

**Eng.:** Ketosis in labour. **Eng.:** What factors are taken into account when assessing the progress of labour? **Eng.:** Monitoring the fetal heart during labour. **Eng.:** Premature rupture of the membranes. **Eng.:** Clinical signs of fetal distress. **Scot.:** Accelerated labour. **Eng.:** Causes of retention of urine during labour. **N. Ire.:** Acetone in the urine during labour. **Eng.:** Signs that labour is progressing normally. **Eng.:** Fetal heart recordings during labour. **Eng.:** Signs of maternal distress in labour. *Eng.:* Fetal distress.

## ELECTRONIC MONITORING

Explain how this benefits the parturient woman and her fetus. How will you avoid the impression that the machine gets more attention than the patient? How does it aid the diagnosis of hypoxia? Define: baseline fetal heart rate; baseline variability; baseline deceleration; Dip 1; Dip 2, or early and late. What is a spiral scalp electrode? Why is electronic monitoring useful in epidural analgesia?

# 19
# The Management of Normal Labour (Second Stage)

*Signs. Observation. Fetal condition. Maternal condition. Methods of delivery. Prophylactic use of Syntometrine. Precipitate labour. Prevention of perineal laceration. Immediate care of the baby. Apgar scoring. Attention to the umbilical cord. Means of identification. Bonding.*

During the second stage of labour mother and fetus require unremitting supervision, for both are subject to trauma and other dangers which do not arise during the first stage. The midwife must now remain in constant attendance; indeed, the woman in her own home should not be left from the time the cervix is 6 cm dilated.

**C.M.B.(Scot.) Rule. (Eng.) Code of Practice.** *When in charge of a case of labour, a practising midwife must not leave the patient without giving an address by which she can be found without delay. After the beginning of the second stage she must stay with the patient until the expulsion of the placenta and membranes, and as long as may be necessary (Scotland, at least one hour).*

### SIGNS OF THE SECOND STAGE

The transition from the first to the second stage is not always clearly defined clinically. There is only one positive sign, which involves making a vaginal examination, and it is neither desirable nor necessary to make repeated vaginal examinations for this purpose. There are a number of probable signs and an aggregation of these can be accepted with a fair degree of reliance, but no one probable sign is infallible.

### POSITIVE SIGN

#### *No Cervix felt on Vaginal Examination*

#### PROBABLE SIGNS

| | |
|---|---|
| **Expulsive uterine contractions.** | **Tenseness between coccyx and anus.** |
| **Trickling of blood.** | **Vulva gaping.** |
| **Rupture of membranes.** | **Presenting part appearing.** |
| **Anus pouting and gaping.** | **Bulging of perineum.** |

**The expulsive type of contraction** is fairly diagnostic, but when the head is deeply engaged, the rectum loaded or the occiput posterior, the woman may have a strong inclination to bear down during the latter part of the first stage.

**A trickle of blood** may come from slight lacerations of the cervix when it is stretched to nearly full dilatation, but with a large head the cervix may sustain slight laceration before then. There may, of course, be no bleeding although the cervix is fully dilated. Later, when the head descends into the vagina, lacerations of the vaginal mucosa may cause slight bleeding.

**Rupture of the membranes** may occur before labour begins or at any time up until the birth of the head: a most uncertain sign.

**Pouting and gaping of the anus occurs** when the head has reached the pelvic floor, but this may take place during the last phase of the first stage if the head is engaged deeply in a multipara with a lax pelvic floor. When the anus gapes and faeces are expelled the cervix is usually fully dilated. If a woman in labour, particularly a multiparous patient, asks urgently for a bed-pan because she thinks her bowels are about to move, the student midwife should first look at the vulva: the head will probably be showing.

306

**Tenseness between anus and coccyx** is a very useful test that can be made by pressing the middle finger deeply between the anus and coccyx. Before the head is low enough to be felt, there is a tenseness of the tissues that is probably due to the pressure exerted by the descending head on the rectum and pelvic floor. When the head descends further, its hard consistency can be recognised by this method.

**Gaping of the vulva** is a more valuable sign in the primigravida, for the vulva of the multiparous woman will gape if she resorts to premature bearing down.

**The presenting part appearing** is usually accepted as being an almost positive sign, and in the majority of instances it is so; but in the case of a footling breech presentation, the cervix would not necessarily be fully dilated although a foot appeared at the vulva. On rare occasions, when there is excessive moulding of the head, a large caput may be visible inside the vagina during a contraction, although the head may be above the ischial spines and the cervix only 6 cm dilated.

**Bulging of the perineum** is one of the good later signs and usually means that delivery is imminent.

### DURATION OF THE SECOND STAGE

The second stage is relatively short, but its length is vitally important, for, if unduly prolonged, it is fraught with danger to mother and child. For that reason it is essential that the midwife should recognise its onset. A primigravid patient may be half an hour or more in the second stage before the presenting part appears at the vulva so the commencement of the second stage should not be calculated from the time of the appearance of the head.

Most obstetricians deprecate a prolonged second stage and would prefer that the midwife made an episiotomy. In some hospitals the application of forceps is considered when the head is seen and not advancing satisfactorily in 30 minutes. Time may be a convenient means of assessment for the novice, but with greater knowledge and additional experience the midwife develops judgment and will take the strength and frequency of the contractions and the condition of mother and fetus into consideration. Many multiparous patients have a second stage of 15 minutes or less, but it would probably be safer to allow a primigravida, who always has a strong uterine wall, to go one hour, than to permit a woman who has had more than four children to go much longer than half an hour.

It is expedient to divide the second stage into two phases:

**The stage of descent** lasts for only a few moments in the majority of multiparous women, the head descending to the perineum almost immediately after full dilatation of the cervix. In a primigravida the head is usually showing within 30 minutes, and if it does not appear then, a vaginal examination should be made to determine the cause of delay.

**The perineal phase.** From the time that the head appears it is generally agreed that it should be born within three-quarters of an hour. Some authorities believe that half an hour is sufficient, but the strength and rate of the contractions and the maternal and fetal conditions have also to be considered. Advance should take place with each contraction and some obstetricians wish to be summoned if no advance occurs with good contractions during a period of 15 minutes.

## OBSERVATION

### THE FETAL CONDITION

The fetal heart is listened to assiduously, for the risk of hypoxia and intracranial injury is infinitely greater during the second stage. The fetal heart should be auscultated during and after every contraction. If fetal distress is anticipated or suspected, the FH should be auscultated before, during and after each contraction if an electronic or ultrasonic monitor is not available.

The point of maximal intensity of the fetal heart moves downwards and towards the midline of the mother's abdomen as the second stage advances, and when the head is on the perineum the fetal stethoscope should be placed just above the symphysis pubis.

## THE MATERNAL CONDITION

This must be noted, and the pulse taken every 10 minutes, or more often if the second stage is prolonged. Uterine action requires particular attention; the strength and frequency of the contractions and whether the uterus is relaxed between them must be closely watched. Although tonic contractions rarely occur and Bandl's ring is seldom seen, such possibilities must always be kept in mind, particularly in the multiparous woman, for the possibility of rupture of the uterus is much more likely during the second stage.

For signs of ketoacidosis see page 403.

**Advance of the presenting part** should proceed steadily even if slowly, and this can be seen from below. But only because of the delay that may occur before vulval signs of advance are manifest, should it be necessary to resort to vaginal examination.

## GENERAL CARE AND ASSISTANCE

Because of the danger of inhaling vomited fluid under general anaesthesia, nothing more than a mere sip should be taken during the second stage of labour. When inhaling analgesic gas, the mouth becomes very dry: the woman is warm, perspiring and thirsty when pushing, especially in a hot climate and will appreciate having her face and hands sponged with cool water.

### THE BLADDER

A full bladder should be recognised and emptied at the end of the first or the beginning of the second stage. If the woman is unable to void at this time, the fetal head is no doubt compressing the urethra or the neck of the bladder. Catheterisation will be necessary if the woman has not passed urine for six hours and the bladder is visibly distended. On no account should a woman be permitted to enter the third stage with a full bladder, for this may interfere with the process of separation and expulsion of the placenta. Because a distended bladder can inhibit good uterine contractions during and after the third stage, postpartum haemorrhage is likely to ensue, a catastrophe every midwife will endeavour to prevent.

### *Puncture of Membranes*

The membranes should have ruptured by the end of the first stage, their function is finished and they are only a hindrance during the second stage. The descent of the fetus will be retarded if it is still contained within the intact sac of fluid, which is attached to the uterus by the placenta. The membranes should be punctured, when tense during a contraction, by using a pair of artery forceps. Should the intact membranes appear at the vulva they ought to be punctured at once. The baby's head will then appear and be born with the next contraction or within a few minutes. If the membranes are not punctured there will be more delay and the baby's head may be born covered with amnion (a caul or cap) which must be removed from the face immediately to allow the infant to breathe.

## POSITION OF THE PATIENT

Some prefer patients to be propped up on three pillows or 2 foam rubber wedges.

### In the dorsal position

The woman can push more effectively. She can rest and relax between contractions and will often doze for short periods.

Observation of her abdomen can be more easily carried out, and at this stage intensive vigilance is necessary. The fetal heart can be listened to more readily and more frequently. The woman's face is in full view the whole time. A close check can be kept on her general condition, and early signs of distress detected.

Patients with cardiac disease and cases of multiple pregnancy are more comfortable in the dorsal position. If signs of vena caval occlusion are manifest the woman should be turned on to her side but this is not so likely when the head is deep in the pelvic cavity.

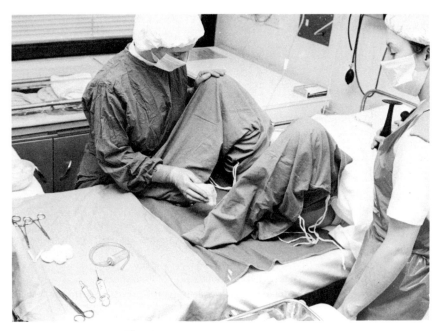

Fig. 19-1 Conducting normal delivery.
*Aberdeen Maternity Hospital.*

### When to bear down

The woman may be told to 'push' when the presenting part appears at the vulva; to do so before then incurs the risk of the cervix not being fully dilated. The natural urge to 'bear down' is experienced by the woman when the presenting part reaches the pelvic floor, so then would seem to be the proper time for her to be encouraged to do so. If she is told to 'push' as soon as the cervix is fully dilated and the head has not descended to the pelvic floor, she fritters away her energy and will have no strength left to push properly when the need arises to overcome the resistance of the perineum.

*(Some authorities do not approve of encouraging the woman to make any expulsive effort and do not find undue prolongation of the second stage because of this.)*

### How to 'bear down'

At the onset of each contraction the woman flexes her knees and places her feet flat on the bed. Her back is curved, chin on chest and knees wide apart. To allow the baby to escape more easily she relaxes her pelvic floor area while pushing. In some hospitals two midwives help the woman to raise her flexed legs while she grasps her thighs under the knees. This procedure is more tiring than placing the feet on the bed.

When about to push the woman takes a deep breath, holds it, closes her lips and glottis and 'bears down': (a long, sustained push is more efficacious than a series of short ones). Between contractions her legs should be flat so that she can relax and rest.

The woman must not cry out or make any sound, because much of the expulsive force will be wasted. The woman should not be permitted to push between contractions, or she will overstretch the transverse cervical ligaments and predispose to uterine prolapse.

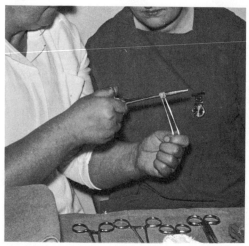

Fig. 19-2    Non-sterile demonstration on normal delivery: pre-packed tray: student midwife being shown rubber band for cord ligation.

| LINEN AND DRESSINGS | INSTRUMENTS |
|---|---|
| 1 gown. 2 draping sheets. 2 dressing towels. | 2 Mayo forceps. |
| 10 wool swabs. 1 baby wrap. | 1 Mayo scissors (15 cm). |
| 1 polypropylene receiver for placenta. | 1 Mayo scissors (20 cm). |
| 1 hand lotion and 1 swabbing bowl. | 1 Spencer Wells forceps to apply cord rubber band. |

| LOWER SHELF | DRUG TRAY |
|---|---|
| Pre-packed gloves and hand towel, catheter, mucus extractors, cord ligatures, syringes, needles, baby identification bands, jug to measure blood loss. | Syntometrine, ergometrine, Syntocinon, Lignocaine 1 per cent, and 0·5 per cent. |

#### REQUIREMENTS FOR RESUSCITATION OF INFANT

Laryngoscope, mechanical suction, endotracheal tubes naloxone (Narcan neonatal)
*Simpson Memorial Maternity Pavilion, Edinburgh.*

Encouragement should be given, and a word of commendation after each effort is opportune, for praise is a good stimulus to continued endeavour. As a rule, women complain less of pain at this stage, no doubt because they are taking an active part in the proceedings and are conscious that progress is being made and that labour is nearly over.

About one hour prior to the expected time of delivery and before the head is showing the woman ought to be encouraged to empty her bladder. If she fails to do so and the bladder is distended catheterisation is indicated.

The pubic region, thighs and buttocks should be washed with soap and water, using a sterile perineal pad. A clean short gown is put on.

The room, baby's cot and cellular cotton blanket must be warm, identification bracelet prepared: delivery pack, basins and floor bucket are placed in position. Hypodermic tray is in readiness for immediate use.

### When to 'Scrub Up'

It is not possible to state the exact time at which the midwife should start scrubbing her hands in readiness for delivery: it depends on the rate of advance and whether the woman is a multipara or primigravida. In the multiparous woman who is progressing rapidly, towards the end of the first stage would be appropriate. In the primigravida, a reasonable time would be when a diameter of about 5 cm of head is showing at the vulva during contractions. Experience is the best teacher. The midwife should not be 'scrubbed up' too soon, or she is liable to become contaminated and the woman may disarrange the sterile drapes.

### Method

The midwife, with clean hands, puts on a plastic apron, clean cap and mask; prepares hand and swabbing lotions; opens packs; places the patient in the correct position for swabbing and delivery. Hands and arms are scrubbed with a soft brush in running water for five minutes. It is a good plan to swab the vulva with the scrubbed hands before wearing gloves in order to avoid contaminating them. Sterile forceps can be used for this purpose and also to apply antiseptic cream. The only areas which should be considered sterile are: the equipment on the trolley; swabbing lotion; the inner surface of the vulva and the baby's head. Drapes and gown soon become contaminated when in contact with the patient and the bed, and should be touched with the gloved hands as little as possible.

## METHODS OF DELIVERING THE BABY

The technique used in delivering the baby varies in different countries and different hospitals, but the basic principles are the same; in all cases an endeavour is made to deliver an uninjured child with minimal trauma to the mother. Where doctors and trained midwives are in attendance and when analgesics and anaesthetics are administered the dorsal or left lateral position is employed but a squatting attitude is the one adopted by primitive tribes.

### DELIVERY IN THE DORSAL POSITION

The woman lies on her back with knees flexed and widely separated. Some place a firm pad under the woman's buttocks thereby facilitating delivery of the head and shoulders. The midwife stands on the right side of the bed, facing towards the woman's feet. She places the palm of her left hand on the advancing head, with fingers pointing to the sinciput and may alter her grip as in the left lateral position (p. 312), so that the parietal eminences are grasped, to assist in completing extension of the head.

### Advantages of the dorsal position

It is less tiring for the woman than the left lateral position in which the right leg has to be held up by an assistant or the patient herself. When a midwife is delivering a woman alone, it is easier for both; there is less opportunity or temptation to interfere prematurely with the natural process of extension of the head, and so perineal trauma is minimised.

One particular advantage in using the dorsal position is that the woman does not have to be turned on her side previous to crowning, nor on to her back again for the conduct of the third stage.

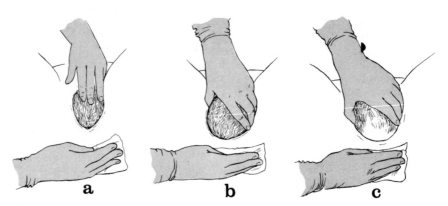

Fig. 19-3    Delivering the head. (*a*) Controlling the crowned head. (*b*) Grip altered to extend the head. (*c*) Widest diameter distending perineum.

#### DELIVERY IN THE LEFT LATERAL POSITION

The woman lies on her left side, buttocks at the edge of the bed and legs slightly flexed. When the head is almost ready for crowning the midwife stands behind the woman's buttocks, facing her feet, and an assistant on the right or left side of the bed raises the right leg sufficiently to take its weight off the midwife's hand. By passing her left arm over the patient's abdomen the midwife brings her hand between the thighs and down to the vulva where the fingers rest lightly on the baby's head, poised in readiness to retard any sudden expulsive movement.

### Advantages of the left lateral position

More assistance can be given in aiding extension of the head in cases where the woman is anaesthetised. It is claimed by some that fewer perineal lacerations occur. When difficulty is encountered with the shoulders of a large baby, the necessary manipulation is more easily carried out.

#### DELIVERY OF THE HEAD

The majority of midwives agree that not until the occipital prominence is free (*the head crowned*) should active extension be permitted to take place. When the stage of crowning approaches, the woman is asked to stop pushing; she continues to inhale whatever analgesic gas is being administered. During and after crowning the fingers are spread equally over the vertex (to avoid depressing one of the skull bones) with their tips pointing towards the bregma, in order to restrain any sudden expulsive effort. The sinciput is allowed to glide slowly over the perineum at the end of a contraction and during this time the woman is inhaling analgesic gas with

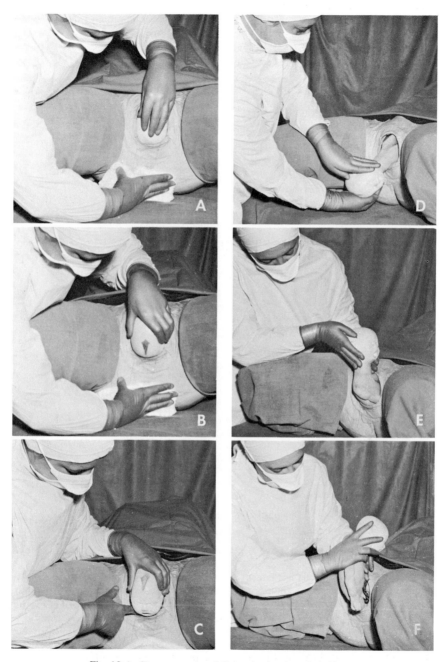

Fig. 19-4   Demonstrating delivery in the dorsal position.
*Simpson Memorial Maternity Pavilion, Edinburgh.*

deliberate breaths to avoid pushing. A certain amount of restraint may have to be applied to the baby's head during the height of this contraction, and such pressure should be evenly distributed to avoid intracranial injury.

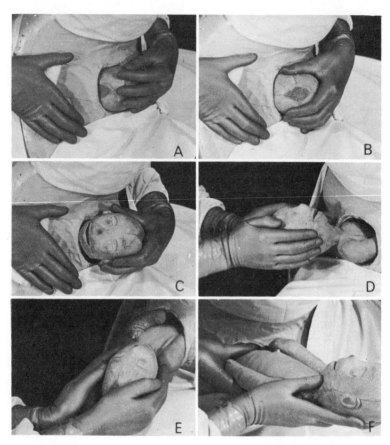

Fig. 19-5  Demonstrating delivery in left lateral position.
*Simpson Memorial Maternity Pavilion, Edinburgh.*

Those who deliver in the left lateral position usually aid extension of the head. A pad held in the palm of the right hand is placed over the anus and when crowning has taken place the midwife exerts steady foward pressure with the heel of her right hand on the area between anus and coccyx, while with her left hand she retards any sudden expulsive movement. A few midwives draw the perineum down over the baby's face after the prominent part of the sinciput has escaped. Such a manoeuvre is probably traditional rather than necessary and if the thumb and middle fingers are placed on the outer lateral borders of the perineum and brought slightly towards the midline, tension on the perineum is diminished while it is being wiped down over the face. The chin is freed, if necessary, by slipping the index finger under the side of the jaw and sweeping it below the chin and out at the other side.

### *Attention to the Cord around the Neck*

In about 30 per cent of cases the umbilical cord is looped round the baby's neck usually once but sometimes two or three times. Unwinding these loops seldom cause difficulty, but the novice tends to be over-anxious and is inclined to premature clamping and cutting of the cord, when it is not necessary. In a case at the Simpson Maternity Pavilion a 107 cm cord, looped five times around the neck, was slipped over the head without clamping.

The fingers of the clean hand (*not the hand that was used to hold the pad over the anus*) should be inserted into the vagina to feel if the umbilical cord is around the baby's neck. The finger tips should be placed down the baby's back to shoulder level and drawn up towards the neck, where they will find the coil of cord which should be gently taken over the baby's head. Strong traction must not be used in case a thin cord should break, but if the cord will not come over the head two Mayo forceps should be applied and the cord cut between them. *This should never be done without due cause*, as the baby's oxygen supply is now cut off, and if there is delay in the delivery of the shoulders, or if the baby is hypoxic, his chances of survival are reduced.

Should the shoulders appear before there is time to deal with the loop of cord, an attempt should be made to slip it over the anterior shoulder and to deliver the baby through the loop. Cord manipulation may induce spasm of the umbilical vessels and cause hypoxia but the baby usually recovers quickly from the short period of oxygen deprivation at this stage of labour.

### DELIVERY OF THE SHOULDERS AND BODY

While waiting for the shoulders to rotate internally, an opportunity is provided to wipe any mucus from the mouth and nostrils with a gauze swab.

**a**

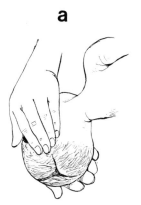

**b**

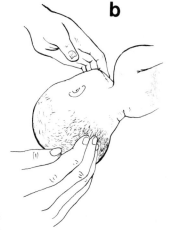

Fig. 19-6 Delivery of the shoulders. Demonstrating how downward traction is applied after shoulders have rotated into the antero-posterior diameter of the outlet (lateral view).

Fig. 19-7 Some prefer to grasp the head by the mentum and occiput (lateral view).

In a natural birth the shoulders are born during the contraction following the birth of the head. This contraction causes the anterior shoulder to rotate forwards so that the shoulders are in the antero-posterior diameter of the outlet. This will be evident by seeing external rotation of the head. The tendency to hurry this phase of the delivery should be resisted. The baby's face will certainly look reddish blue, but such congestion is a necessary stimulus to respiration. Many experienced midwives practice slow delivery of the body and do not drag the baby out. If, however, the blue colour becomes dark the uterus ought to be stimulated to contract by massaging it, and applying fundal pressure, or asking the woman to push to expel the baby.

Syntometrine, 1 ml, is given when the anterior shoulder appears, remembering the danger should there be a second fetus *in utero*. If the baby is large this is the ideal time to give Syntometrine.

To facilitate expulsion of the anterior shoulder the head may be gently depressed towards the anus but no attempt made to get the anterior arm out. If the anterior arm comes of its own accord it is not likely to be harmed, but if it is deliberately brought down under the pubic arch the risk of fracturing the humerus is intensified. The important point is that traction exerted should be minimal and ought not to make the neck twist or bend sideways because of the risk of injury to the brachial plexus, causing paralysis of the baby's upper arm. (Erb's paralysis.) When the anterior shoulder is free, the head is guided in an upward direction towards the mother's abdomen so that the posterior shoulder can escape over the perineum. This should take place slowly and smoothly; the contraction of the uterus being sufficient to accomplish the expulsion of the body.

As soon as the baby is born the midwife looks at the clock, which should be at the correct time, so that the exact moment of birth can be recorded on the birth certificate. The airway is cleared (see also p. 319). The normal baby breathes and cries within a few seconds of birth.

The baby may be held upside down for a few seconds to drain fluid from the respiratory passages.

### Delay with the Shoulders

The conscious woman can be asked to bear down or an assistant, if present, may apply fundal pressure. Delay at this stage is usually due to incomplete internal rotation of the shoulders, so a finger is hooked into the anterior axilla to exert forward rotation followed by downward traction, but care must be exercised. (See shoulder dystocia, p. 651.)

#### ATTENTION TO THE EYES

Each eyelid should be wiped with separate swabs of dry, sterilised cotton wool to remove secretions containing organisms from the birth-canal. *Some authorities do not approve of wiping the eyelids.* The midwife's hands should be clean when dealing with the eyes, and dipping them into weak antiseptic solution is not an efficient method of cleansing them. Wool swabs if used should be the size of a golf ball, so that antiseptic lotion and organisms from badly fitting or contaminated gloves will not come in contact with the baby's eyes.

#### PERINEAL LACERATIONS

Perineal lacerations cannot always be avoided, but the extent of the damage can often be minimised by skilful manipulation. The various methods of delivery have been devised with the intention of giving maximal control during the expulsion of the infant. The midwife ought to know which measurements of the skull are involved in the various presentations and whether, by assisting flexion or extension of the baby's head, the smallest possible diameters can be made to distend the vulval orifice. Certain conditions other than faulty management by the midwife predispose to perineal lacerations and they are usually due to disproportion between the fetal head and the outlet of the birth canal.

*The principles of management are:*

That the smallest possible diameters of head and shoulders should be permitted to emerge and distend the vulval orifice.

That the actual birth of the head should take place slowly and without expulsive force.

### CAUSES OF A THIRD DEGREE TEAR

**A large baby; vertex face to pubes; face presentation; the aftercoming head in a breech presentation.**

**A rigid perineum,** and particularly when scar tissue from a previous laceration or episiotomy is present.

**The android type of pelvis** causes the head to be forced backwards on to the perineum.

## Signs that the Perineum is liable to Tear

A perineum that resists the pressure of the descending head and is not stretching.

A long perineum, particularly if it lacks elasticity or is oedematous.

Trickling of blood from the vagina when the head is on the perineum is usually due to laceration of the vaginal mucosa on the inner surface of the perineum, which tears as a rule before the perineal skin.

When the perineum has a bluish appearance in the midline, which later becomes white, shiny and transparent.

If the fourchette begins to tear before the head is crowned, an extensive laceration can be anticipated. On rare occasions a perineal laceration may start in the centre of the perineum, the so-called 'button-hole' or central tear.

### MEANS OF LESSENING THE RISK OF PERINEAL LACERATION

**Obtaining the woman's co-operation.** She should have been told, prior to, or at the beginning of labour what she is expected to do. When distracted with pain or stupefied by analgesic drugs, the woman is incapable of comprehending instruction. The woman who is frightened is liable to become hysterical and unmanageable: the midwife prevents this. The only satisfactory method of inhibiting the desire to push, which is involuntary and overwhelmingly strong when the head is distending the perineum, is for the woman to take deliberate breaths through her mouth without accentuating expiration. It is imperative that, from the time of crowning, the woman should only push when instructed to do so. Uterine contraction alone is sufficient at this stage, and while the head is actually being born the woman must desist from any expulsive effort.

**Having control of the advancing head.** The woman may push, cough or move suddenly, and the midwife must always anticipate such a possibility by having her finger tips on or near the head, poised ready to restrain it.

**Getting small diameters to distend the vaginal orifice.** By maintaining flexion and controlling too rapid extension of the head in vertex presentations.

**Preventing 'active' extension before crowning.** The sinciput should not be permitted to glide over the perineum, until the occipital prominence, and, if possible, the parietal eminences have been born.

**Keeping the hands off the perineum.** Supporting, or what is commonly called 'guarding,' the perineum will not prevent lacerations. Any pressure applied by the fingers thins the perineum still further or causes bruising which favours tearing.

**Delivering the head at the end of or between contractions.** If the head is born during a uterine contraction, too much force is exerted by the primary and probably by the secondary powers. The perineum is more tense then and will rupture more readily.

**Allowing the woman to 'breathe the head out'.** This midwife's phrase lucidly explains a manoeuvre whereby the actual extension of the head takes place with a slow gliding movement. During this time the woman breathes in a deliberate way to avoid pushing while the sinciput and face emerge from under the perineum.

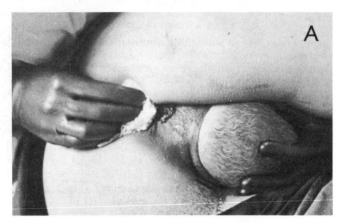

Fig. 19-8   Head ready for active extension.

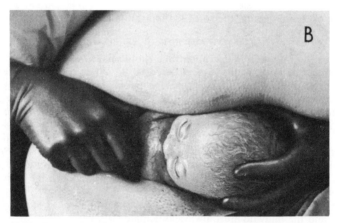

Fig. 19-9   The head is allowed to extend slowly to prevent perineal laceration.
*Simpson Memorial Maternity Pavilion, Edinburgh.*

**Taking care in delivering shoulders and body.** If the shoulders are dragged or pushed out before they have rotated internally, they will rotate while passing through the vulva and the strain on the perineum is liable to result in a perineal tear. Not all lacerations of the perineum occur during the birth of the head. Very often a slight nick is extended into a gash during the birth of the shoulders. The occurrence of restitution is not an indication to deliver the shoulders. External rotation of the head must take place as this signifies that the shoulders have rotated into the antero-posterior diameter. By permitting the anterior shoulder to escape first a smaller diameter emerges, and when the baby is carried upwards over the mother's abdomen its weight is taken off the perineum. As the baby is being born its arms should be grasped alongside the body. If the midwife grasps the body under the arms their outward thrust puts additional strain on the perineum.

## PRECIPITATE LABOUR

Precipitate labour is one in which the fetus is expelled after three or four painful uterine contractions. The condition is rare, and the term should not be applied when early signs of labour have been overlooked. It is probable that the woman has had a painless first stage and that the cervix and vagina are unusually soft and dilatable.

The risks are greatest when the birth occurs in some inconvenient place, such as the 'toilet' or the street. The baby may suffer from intracranial injury or cephalhaematoma, due to rapid expulsion; he might fall to the ground and be injured; the cord may rupture, but bleeding does not occur to the same extent as when the cord has been cut. The mother may sustain a perineal laceration; inversion of the uterus, due to cord traction, is not likely to occur, because the uterus will be contracting strongly. When a woman has had one precipitate labour, she should be admitted to hospital prior to her next confinement to avoid such consequences as those mentioned above.

## IMMEDIATE CARE OF THE BABY

### Clearing the air passages

This is an urgent duty that must be performed without delay, for, if the baby inhales into its bronchi the mucus and amniotic fluid which may be present in the pharynx, atelectasis or pneumonia may ensue. If the baby cries immediately there should be no need to use any means of clearing the airway, but the trachea of the asphyxiated baby is often blocked with thick mucus which may be tinged with blood from the vagina, or meconium that has been passed by the distressed fetus. It is imperative that this material be removed without delay. Some hold the baby upside down, with the head slightly extended for a few seconds before laying him on the bed, to allow any fluid in the trachea to drain out; this should not be done if the infant is shocked. To avoid letting the baby slip, the forefinger of the hand grasping the ankles should be placed between them.

**Resuscitation Equipment**

| | |
|---|---|
| Baby Laryngoscope, McIntosh. | Neonatal naloxone (Narcan) |
| Warne endotracheal tubes F.G. 10, 12, 14. | Konakion 1 mg. |
| Suction tubes F.G. 6. | 10 ml amps. Sodium bicarbonate 8·4 per cent. |
| Beelee catheter FG14 | 10 ml amps. Calcium Gluconate 10 per cent. |
| Mucus extractors. | 10 ml amps. Sodium chloride 0·9 per cent |
| Paediatric i.v. Administration Set. | 20 ml amps. Glucose 10 per cent. |

Selection of syringes 1 ml and 20 ml.

The infant cannot breathe if the airway is plugged with mucus, and if inhaled into the lungs its tenacious consistency prevents the alveoli from becoming inflated and its irritant propensity is likely to cause pneumonia. Thick mucus will not drain out when the infant is held upside down.

### The Use of Suction

Various mechanical devices for applying suction are employed, e.g. electric apparatus, rubber mucus extractors with a plastic trap or most commonly disposable extractors. All must be used with gentleness and due caution.

The tubing must be fine with a lumen of 2 or 3 mm and the end bevelled like a rectal tube. In an emergency, a rubber catheter, No. 12 F.G., a gauze swab, or the finger can be used to remove mucus. In using a mucus extractor it should be directed over the dorsum of the tongue into the pharynx, not more than 5 cm of tubing being inside the baby's lower gum. Undue prodding with the sucker, too often and too far may cause laryngeal spasm and respiratory arrest.

A word of warning is necessary in regard to the excessive use of suction, for if continued after the airway is clear, the baby is deprived of oxygen. Inexperienced midwives can produce shock by this means. The mucus extractor is a life-saving device when used judiciously.

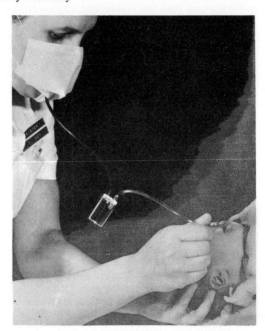

Fig. 19-10   Using disposable mucus extractor.
*Aberdeen Maternity Hospital.*

## APGAR SCORING

This is a means of standardising the method of evaluating and recording the condition of the baby, in numerical terms at one minute after birth and if necessary at 5 minutes.

Five vital signs are each given a score of 0, 1 or 2 points, i.e. colour, respiratory effort, heart beat, muscle tone, reflex response. Heart beat is the most important observation.

| Signs | Score | | |
|---|---|---|---|
| | 0 | 1 | 2 |
| **Colour** | blue pale | body pink limbs blue | completely pink |
| **Respiratory effort** | absent | slow, irregular weak cry | strong cry |
| **Heart beat** | absent | slow, less than 100 | over 100 |
| **Muscle tone** | limp | some flexion of limbs | active movement |
| **Response to flicking foot** | absent | facial grimace | crying |

Severe 0—2      Moderate 3—4      Mild 5—7      No asphyxia 8—10

*The paediatrician is notified if the score is 3 or under at 1 minute.*

### FIVE MINUTE SCORE

The score at 5 minutes gives a more accurate prediction regarding survival: a low score at 5 minutes being more serious than a low score at one minute.

*The paediatrician is notified if the score is 6 or under at 5 minutes.*

### Gastric suction

In some hospitals mucus is extracted from every baby's stomach. This procedure is believed to reduce the incidence of vomiting and mucus gastritis.

## MEANS OF IDENTIFICATION

Before cutting the cord, whatever means of identification is used should be applied to the infant. The system of checking the name and verifying the sex should be foolproof. It entails grave responsibility, and the danger of mixing babies in hospital must constantly be kept in mind. The mother should be shown the identification wrist tape and the sex of the baby in the labour ward.

### The different methods are:

Wrist name tape, some apply one on each wrist. (*These should be checked daily and a record kept of this.*)

A string of lettered china beads that are clamped with a lead seal around the neck or wrist before the umbilical cord is cut.

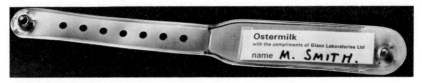

Fig. 19-11    Identification bracelet. The holes allow the bracelet to be tightened as necessary.

*Courtesy of Glaxo Laboratories Ltd.*

Footprints are a positive means of identification if they are clear enough to make the fine ridge detail on the baby's skin legible. A high standard of legibility is not readily attained by finger-print experts much less the nursing staff in a busy labour ward. Footprints must always be read by a finger-print expert so they are not as useful as beads and name-tapes for the daily routine identification of babies in maternity hospitals.

### EXAMINATION OF THE BABY

Particular attention is paid to the baby's respirations and colour: a vigorous cry usually denotes satisfactory respiratory effort. The presence of pallor or cyanosis is noted, the baby treated if necessary and closely observed for improvement. Muscle tone should be good. Serious illness or gross malformation is readily detected (*medical aid is summoned*); a detailed examination is carried out later, usually prior to bathing. More than a cursory glance at the genital organs is needed before recording the sex of the infant. When doubt exists expert investigations are made.

### The Need for Warmth

While the baby is being attended to, he must not be allowed to become chilled. The thermal centre does not function well at birth, and the baby loses much heat by evaporation from his wet skin (see neonatal hypothermia, p. 543). The room in which the baby is born should be 21·1°C (70°F); the baby should be dried and received into a warm sterile towel and two warm cellular cotton blankets, one of which is wrapped over his head. The baby can lose a lot of heat from his exposed wet head which is one quarter of the area of the baby. Labour ward cots should be heated, mattress and blankets warm. Plastic cots with lids or portable incubators can be used when transferring babies from the labour ward through cold corridors to the postnatal ward.

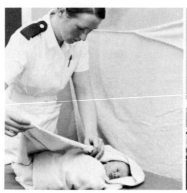

Fig. 19-12   Turkish towelling baby wrap and head cover 90 cm square. The triangular piece (hood) is flat to facilitate laundering.

*Aberdeen Maternity Hospital.*

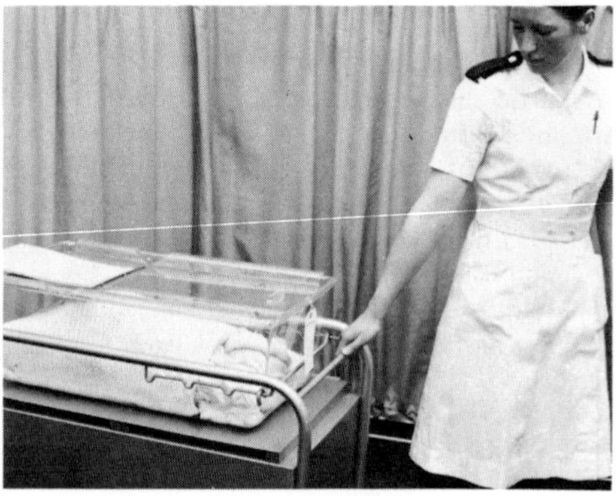

Fig. 19-13   Plastic cot with cover to transport baby to postnatal ward or nursery.

*Aberdeen Maternity Hospital.*

**Hot-water bottles are potentially dangerous** in a busy unit, where inexperienced staff may use water that is too hot or neglect to apply adequate covering to the bottles. The newborn baby's skin is extremely sensitive and will blister very readily. If as is the practice in some hospitals, the baby is wrapped in a 90 cm cotton cellular blanket with a sterile towel it can wriggle until it comes in contact with the hot-water bottle. Blankets should be adequate in size to envelop the baby properly and so avoid exposure due to limb movements. Electric blankets are not without risk.

#### ATTENTION TO THE UMBILICAL CORD

There are differences of opinion as to whether to tie the cord immediately or to wait for pulsation in the cord vessels to cease. It has been stated that the infant obtains 40 to 60 ml of extra blood from the placenta if the cord is not tied until pulsations cease. Others believe that the baby obtains the full complement of placental blood within 30 seconds of birth. By tying the cord at once, excessive exposure and chilling of the wet infant is avoided: this also prevents over transfusion which raises the baby's normal blood pressure.

### Tying and cutting the cord

Plastic clamps, rubber bands, linen or tape ligatures are applied to the umbilical cord to act as a haemostat to the umbilical blood vessels. A ligature that is too fine, even although strong, might sever the cord, so traction on the ligature should be exerted slowly, without jerking, and the knot should be of the reef or other variety that will not slip. If the mother is Rh immunised or diabetic or if the baby weighs less than 2 kg umbilical catheterisation may be necessary. In such cases the cord should be ligated not closer than 4 cm from the umbilicus.

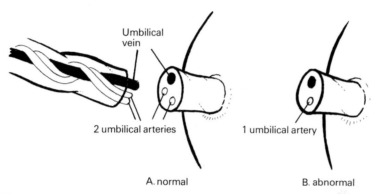

Fig. 19-14   Examination of severed cord. There should be two arteries, if there is only one a congenital abnormality may be present.

The first ligature may be placed about 2·5 cm from the umbilicus. Another ligature is applied 5 cm on the outer side of the first one as a precautionary measure in case the placenta *in utero* is being shared by another baby, a monozygotic twin.

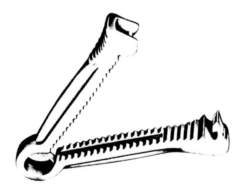

Fig. 19-15   Hollister umbilical cord clamp.
*Obtainable from C. F. Thackray Ltd., Park Street, Leeds.*

The scissors used to cut the cord should be blunt-pointed and sterile, and those previously used for episiotomy are no longer sterile. While cutting the cord it should be placed in the palm of the hand and the points of the scissors directed into the partly closed fist to avoid injuring the kicking infant. *Some spray the cord with Polybactrin before and after cutting. The cut end of the cord is examined; the absence of one artery occurs in 1–200 babies and suggests the presence of congenital abnormalities.* 21 cases of one artery were detected during one year at the Simpson Memorial Maternity Pavilion, Edinburgh.

When the baby goes to the ward a second ligature is applied, after bathing, about 2·5 cm from the umbilicus.

**Disposable plastic cord clamps** are applied about one centimetre from the umbilical skin and closed by finger pressure. The cord is cut 1 cm beyond the clamp to prevent it from slipping off the cut end of the cord. The clamp should be removed after 24 hours, but some prefer to leave it until the third day. Plastic clamps are effective but expensive.

**Rubber bands,** 3·5 cm long by 2 mm wide, are wound four times round an average size cord: they are considered to be more efficient than tape which may allow leakage: rubber bands may cut through a thick cord.

Rubber bands provide continued pressure as the cord shrinks.

**Pieces of compression tubing** (*not ordinary rubber tubing*) 4 mm wide are most effective. Umbilical cord-tape 15 cm long is threaded through the lumen of the tubing and knotted.

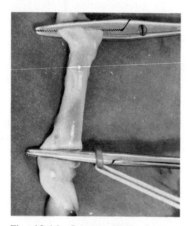

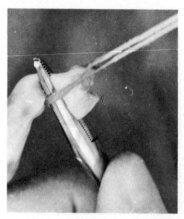

Fig. 19-16 Spencer Wells forceps, with latex tubing, applied 5 cm from umbilicus.

Fig. 19-17 After cutting the umbilical cord between the two Spencer Wells forceps, the tape is used to pull the latex band on to the stump of cord.

*Bellshill Maternity Hospital, Lanarkshire.*

**Method.** Through the lumen of the tube a pair of sterile 18 cm Spencer Wells forceps is passed to just beyond the joint. With these forceps the cord is clamped 5 cm from the umbilicus; another pair of forceps is applied 2·5 cm from the first pair on the placental side of the cord. The cord is cut between the two pairs of forceps. The umbilical cord tape is used to draw the latex tubing off the Spencer Wells forceps, on to the cord stump; the tubing is positioned 2·5 cm from the skin edge. Forceps and tape are then removed. The tubing is more easily applied when wet.

### Cord haemorrhage

The midwife must look repeatedly at the cord during the first six hours to make sure there is no bleeding. There is less bleeding when rubber bands are applied. Fatal haemorrhage can occur, for the loss of 30 ml of blood to the newborn is equivalent to the loss of 600 ml to an adult. Artery forceps should be sterilised pending the doctor's arrival and applied if medical aid is not available.

### CARE OF THE EYES

No longer is the routine instillation of silver nitrate or argyrol in the eyes of the newborn advocated. It is believed that silver nitrate, 1 per cent, produces a mild chemical burn which lowers the resistance of the conjunctiva to organisms and may predispose to conjunctivitis neonatorum. With the increase in gonorrhoea, vigilant observation is necessary; smear and culture of any discharge should be sent for examination.

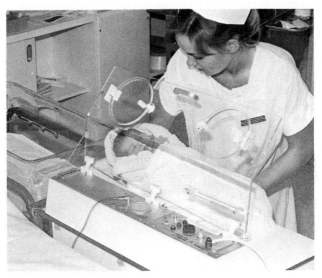

Fig. 19-18    All babies in this hospital are transferred to postnatal ward or nursery in a heated incubator.

*Maternity Unit, Southern General Hospital, Glasgow.*

## Rest after the Trauma of Birth

The baby should be placed in a warmed cot and allowed to recover from the strenuous experience of birth. Routine lowering of babies' heads is not now advocated.

The baby's colour should be noted. Any mucus ought to be removed from the nose and mouth.

There should be no routine time, such as one hour after birth, for giving the first bath: the correct time is when the baby is pink, warm and vigorous. Bathing is not an essential procedure and should be postponed for 12 hours to prevent hypothermia. A clear airway and warmth are the baby's immediate needs.

### Telephone Inquiries

Student midwives should be meticulously careful when receiving inquiries and giving information over the telephone regarding the birth of a baby, for much dissatisfaction is caused to relatives when erroneous statements are made. The name should be clearly identified and repeated, for more than one patient may have the same surname. The use of the words 'boy' and 'girl' are less likely to be confused than 'male' and 'female'.

The Sister will always confirm name and sex from the chart, and will answer the call herself if the baby is stillborn.

## MOTHER AND BABY

Some authorities think the mother should see and touch her infant immediately he is born, and before the umbilical cord is severed, believing that the emotional stimulus will cause the uterus to contract strongly. The wishes of the mother should be ascertained and respected. The interaction of mother and baby during the hours immediately following birth is believed to establish an emotional bond. Any routine that separates mother and baby may interfere with the bonding process. In hospital, women are shown their babies in the labour ward, including sex and identification bracelet, before they are taken to the nursery.

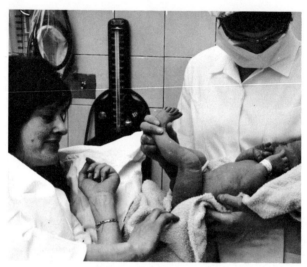

Fig. 19-19　Mother being shown baby's sex and identification bracelet before leaving the labour ward.

*Aberdeen Maternity Hospital.*

Midwives should remember that they are accustomed to the appearance of newborn babies, but an inexperienced mother seeing her own infant for the first time, unwashed, may experience a feeling of disappointment that she may later regret ever having entertained towards her child. The first glimpse of her baby is a momentous occasion and should be treated with due regard to its importance. The main thing is that the mother's feelings are considered and everything done to foster her appreciation of the beauty and sanctity of motherhood.

## BONDING OF MOTHER AND BABY

**Bonding** is the establishment of a loving relationship between the mother and her child. Most women experience a surge of affection, the maternal instinct, for their newborn babies. At this time the woman feels relief, thankfulness and joy but the tender protective feeling of love for her baby transcends all other emotions. In many women the bonding process is initiated during pregnancy: much depends on their sensitivity and temperament: it is a revealing indication of their attitude to love, marriage, motherhood and to the type of person they are. Nature has created this response as a stimulus to the provision of tender loving care for the helpless infant. By caressing, cuddling, gentle handling and a soothing tone of voice one would expect the babe to feel loved and secure. The loving mother strives to give suitable food, warmth and comfort, and with such devoted care the child thrives physically and emotionally.

**Bonding would seem to be a basic attribute.** Adults and children alike, respond in a kindly protective manner towards babies and young animals. Ferocious wild beasts treat their offspring with loving, devoted care.

**In some women the response is weak** or delayed. When the bond is tenuous such procedures as separating mother and baby for neonatal intensive care may accentuate the lack of maternal affection and in such cases a greater incidence of baby battering has been found to occur.

MIDWIVES SHOULD DO ALL IN THEIR POWER TO FACILITATE THE BONDING PROCESS

**By exhibiting kindly qualities** in her attitude to motherhood and baby care, the midwife may motivate the expectant mother to comprehend and foster any dormant maternal feelings.

**By administering sedatives during labour,** the association of pain with the baby may be avoided: the provision of caring, companionship and friendly communication during labour gives an opportunity to further the loving mother and child relationship.

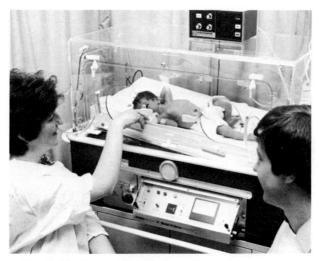

Fig. 19-20   Parents visiting baby in the special care nursery.
*Aberdeen Maternity Hospital.*

**By encouraging fathers to be present** to give emotional support during labour, the marriage and family bond is strengthened.

**By ascertaining and complying with** (if possible) **the mother's wishes regarding the bonding process:** (a) she may wish to be conscious to hear the baby's first cry (she could be assured that the first cry she hears is as compelling as his first cry, as would occur after forceps delivery or Caesarean section); (b) some wish to grasp the baby's hand as he is being born; (c) a few may wish to suckle their baby at the breast, usually if they intend to breast feed; (d) skin to skin contact by laying the baby on the mother's abdomen is desired by some mothers. But the baby should be considered too: he needs rest and warmth and the exposure may chill him and cause hypothermia. The 'high risk' baby should be laid below the level of the placenta *in utero* to receive the blood he needs and will get (unless the cord has been severed). Traction on the cord must be avoided.

**By allowing the mother to cuddle her wrapped baby** as soon as possible: the midwife handling the infant tenderly; the husband being present if available.

**By practising rooming in,** the mother's love is strengthened by the continuous close association with her baby. The family triad is furthered when baby, mother and father are together at visiting time. When the baby needs intensive care, the mother should visit and caress him at least three times every day; the father visiting when possible.

### Dealing with the Crying Baby

The persistently crying baby can have a devastating effect on the delayed bonding process. Community midwives and Health Visitors have a responsibility to make provision and take action in regard to the crying baby. No mother should have to endure more than one night disturbed by her crying child. A 24-hour service, whereby advice can be given by telephone or personal call, should be inaugurated. Crying babies are particularly liable to be subjected to non-accidental violence and mothers need counsel on the prevention of battering.

---

## QUESTIONS FOR REVISION
### MANAGEMENT OF SECOND STAGE OF LABOUR

#### Oral Questions

Name 6 probable signs of the second stage. How do you know when the cervix is fully dilated? How often do you auscultate the fetal heart during the second stage? Why is the fetus in greater danger during the second stage?

How would you deal with the following: (*a*) membranes at the vulva intact; (*b*) cord around the baby's neck; (*c*) delay with the shoulders; (*d*) Apgar score of 5 at 5 minutes; (*e*) bleeding from the umbilical cord.

Write short notes on: (*a*) the bladder during the second stage; (*b*) teaching the mother how to bear down; (*c*) avoiding perineal laceration.

What assistance can the midwife give to a woman during the second stage of labour? State the length of time you would consider as safe for the second stage. What are your duties when it is unduly prolonged?

What is a precipitate labour?

What precautions do you take when using the mucus extractor?

How can the midwife foster the bonding process during labour?

**(N. Ire.) question.** Describe in detail your treatment of the umbilical cord at birth and subsequently. What possible complications may arise and how would you avoid them?

**C.M.B.(Eng.) question.** What indications would lead you to send for a doctor during the second stage of labour?

**C.M.B.(Scot.) question.** Discuss the causes of delay in the second stage of labour. Enumerate the procedures which may be adopted to effect delivery.

**(N. Ire.) 30-min. question.** Describe the Apgar score system. What measures would you take to resuscitate a baby who does not breathe after normal delivery?

**Scot. C.M.B.** Describe the appearance of a baby who has an Apgar score of 2 one minute after birth. What are the immediate and long term dangers?

**Scot. C.M.B.** Define the second stage of labour. How do you recognise that the patient is in this stage? What may be (*a*) the causes and (*b*) the signs of delay?

**N. Ire.** (*a*) How would you recognise that the second stage of labour has begun? (*b*) Describe the management of the second stage of labour.

**N. Ire. 30-min. question.** Describe the vagina and perineum. Explain how injuries to these structures may be minimised during labour.

#### C.M.B. Short Questions

**Scot.:** Second stage of labour. **Eng.:** Observations during the second stage. **Eng.:** Signs of full dilatation of the cervix. **Eng.:** Causes of delay in the second stage. **Eng.:** Causes of perineal laceration. **Eng.:** Apgar scoring. **Eng.:** Treatment of the umbilical cord at birth. **Eng.:** Initial examination which the midwife makes of the baby. **Eng.:** Identification of the newborn. **Eng.:** Maternal distress in labour. **Eng.:** Describe the methods available for monitoring the fetus during pregnancy and labour. **Eng.:** Prevention of perineal lacerations in labour. **Eng.:** Ketosis in labour. **Scot.:** What is 'Bonding'? **Eng.:** Partogram. **Scot.:** Describe late deceleration of the fetal heart. **Eng.:** Syntometrine. **Eng.:** Fetal monitoring in labour. **Eng.:** The establishment of mother/child bonding.

# 20
# The Third Stage of Labour

*Physiology. Control of bleeding. Management. Observation. Controlled cord traction. Traditional method of placental expulsion. Examination of the placenta. Retained membranes. Fourth stage of labour. Recording.*

## PHYSIOLOGICAL CHANGES

The third stage is that of the separation and expulsion of the placenta and membranes which lasts from the birth of the baby until the placenta is expelled. The usual length is 5 to 15 minutes, but any period up to one hour may be considered normal.

*The administration of oxytocic drugs with the anterior shoulder or birth of the head shortens the third stage and most authorities are of the opinion that 30 minutes should now be considered the limit of normal.*

### MECHANISM OF PLACENTAL SEPARATION

Separation of the placenta is brought about by the contraction and retraction of the uterine muscle, which thicken the wall and reduce the capacity of the upper uterine segment so that the area of the placental site is diminished.

**A**
**B**

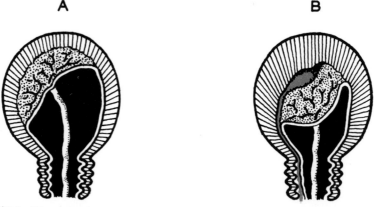

Fig. 20-1  Diagrammatic representation of placental separation. A, Uterine wall partly contracted but not sufficient to cause separation of placenta. B, Further contractions and retraction thicken uterine wall, reduce the size of the area of the placental site, and cause the placenta to become detached. *Note*—The thin lower uterine segment has collapsed like a concertina following the birth of the baby.

The placenta has no power of contraction, but it does become thicker and more compact when its cotyledons are crowded more closely together. Before the end of the second stage the area of the placental site is somewhat diminished, and it is surmised that it must be reduced by half before placental separation begins. There is a marked reduction in the size of the placental site during the contraction that expels the baby's body; after the birth of the baby further contractions and

330

retraction of the uterine muscle continue the process of separation: the more powerful the contractions the sooner will the placenta be detached, probably within five minutes.

Separation usually begins in the centre of the placenta, but may begin at the lower edge, and at the level of the deep spongy layer of the decidua, but if the ovum has embedded too deeply separation will not readily take place. The process has been likened to the detachment of postage stamps at the perforations between them. At the area of separation the blood sinuses are torn across, causing 30 to 60 ml of blood to collect between the maternal surface of the placenta and the decidua basalis—the retroplacental clot or haematoma. Subsequent uterine contractions completely detach the uterus from the placenta which is then forced out of the upper segment into the lower uterine segment or the vagina. The lower segment, which had collapsed like a concertina as the baby was born becomes distended with the placenta. The empty upper uterine segment contracts effectively, forming a hard round mass, that is pushed upwards and perched on top of the placenta which is now lying in the lower uterine segment. The membranes do not separate as readily as the placenta, for they tend to wrinkle, thus accommodating themselves to the diminished area of the uterus. The traction of the descending placenta slowly peels them off the decidua, but the membrane attached to the area round the cervix may remain adherent until the placenta is actually being expelled outside the vulva.

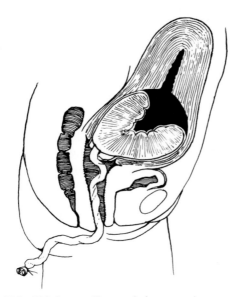

Fig. 20-2   Third stage. Placenta in lower uterine segment.

## CONTROL OF BLEEDING

If Nature did not make some provision whereby bleeding from the large uterine blood vessels could be controlled, the woman would bleed to death in a matter of minutes. The contraction and retraction of the uterine muscle fibres that bring about separation of the placenta also act as **'living ligatures'** by compressing the blood vessels and controlling the bleeding. Clotting of blood plays little part during this phase, but a few hours later, when the uterine contractions are less vigorous, bleeding is prevented by the blood clot which has formed in the sinuses. Recent research has shown a transitory activation of the coagulation and fibrinolytic mechanism in the placental site circulation during and immediately following placental separation. This beneficial clotting occurs in the uterine blood vessels and sinuses at the placental site.

*N.B.—The presence of clots in the uterine cavity would inhibit sustained retraction and predispose to haemorrhage.*

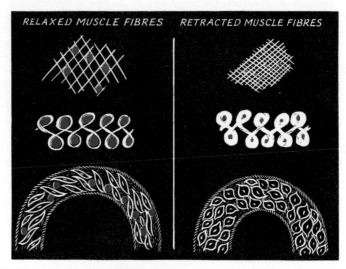

Fig. 20-3  Diagrammatic representation of the action of the uterine muscle fibres in the control of postpartum bleeding from the placental site.

### Nature's Method of Expulsion of the Placenta

Nature has two methods of expelling the placenta, which have been described by Schultze and Matthews Duncan. These methods are not under the control of the attendant.

The Schultze method is said to be the more common. The placenta slips down into the vagina through the hole in the amniotic sac; the fetal surface appears at the vulva with the membranes trailing behind like an inverted umbrella as they are peeled off the uterine wall. The maternal surface of the placenta is not seen, and any blood clot is inside the inverted sac.

The Matthews Duncan method. The placenta slides down sideways and comes through the vulva with the lateral border first, like a button through a buttonhole. The maternal surface is seen, and the blood escapes as it is not inside the sac. There is more likelihood of ragged membranes with the Matthews Duncan method, as they are not peeled off as completely as in the Schultze method.

## MANAGEMENT OF THE THIRD STAGE OF LABOUR

Good management of the third stage begins during the prenatal period, for the woman should be brought into labour in excellent physical condition, so that the uterus will have the power to contract and retract, and in order that normal blood loss will not produce collapse. Such management should continue during the first and second stages of labour, when the midwife prevents conditions arising that would exhaust the woman and seeks medical assistance for the treatment of complications that interfere with good uterine action. Many experienced midwives believe that slow delivery of the baby's body lessens the incidence of postpartum haemorrhage.

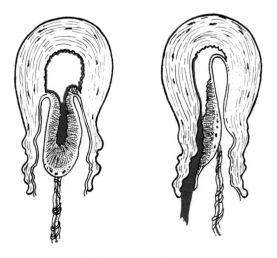

Expulsion of the placenta.

Fig. 20-4   The Schultze method.   Fig.   20-5   The   Matthews   Duncan method.

**The administration of oxytocic drugs,** e.g. Syntometrine 1 ml with the birth of the anterior shoulder shortens the third stage, reduces blood loss and the incidence of haemorrhage.

### ASEPSIS AND ANTISEPSIS

The need for asepsis is greater now than in the preceding stages of labour, for the mother's resistance, both general and local, is diminished. Laceration and bruising devitalise the tissues of the vulva and vagina, and render them prone to invasion by organisms. In the raw placental site and the alkaline lochia, organisms find an ideal nidus in which to flourish. An aseptic technique must be rigorously observed.

## POSITION OF THE PATIENT
*The dorsal position has numerous advantages:*

The uterus can be observed better. It is more comfortable for the woman. Cord traction can be applied more effectively.

The uterus remains in the midline. Her face is in full view. To detect perineal laceration the woman who has been delivered in the left lateral position can have her perineum examined before she is turned on to her back, and if two wool swabs are used to separate the labia, the perineum and posterior vaginal wall can be inspected quite easily. The hands should, of course, be scrubbed and the vulva gently swabbed to remove blood. Medical assistance ought to be obtained to suture all lacerations other than a mere nick.

The need for warmth at this time should be appreciated, for the woman has undergone strenuous physical exercise which has made her perspire, and she has lost much heat from her body in the baby and amniotic fluid. If exposed, an attack of shivering is likely to occur, which is not a true rigor, but often alarms the woman and can be prevented by the avoidance of chilling. The room should be warm and any soiled wet linen removed from under the patient.

### GENERAL CONDITION

In the majority of cases, the woman's general condition is good; she may feel rather tired, but not ill. In the case of twins, or after the birth of a very large baby, the woman may feel limp, although not actually shocked, because of the great reduction in abdominal pressure. But after a long, exhausting labour, a difficult delivery, or when there has been much bruising or laceration of the birth canal, the woman may suffer from shock. A pulse rate over 90 and rising, with pallor, is a very serious sign caused by haemorrhage, shock or cardiac failure. The blood pressure is taken and the systolic should be over 110 mm Hg.

## OBSERVATION

### (1) The pulse is the best guide to the loss of blood.

The midwife should keep her fingers on the pulse throughout the third stage. During this time the pulse is slightly slower than normal, probably because additional blood has entered the circulation from the contracted uterus. If the pulse is rising and particularly when it reaches 90, the possibility of haemorrhage must be considered. The skin should feel warm and dry; the systolic blood pressure over 110 mm Hg. Action should be taken by the midwife to control excessive bleeding even though the amount is not sufficient to be classified as post-partum haemorrhage.

### (2) Guarding the uterus. (rarely done when controlled cord traction is used).

This term is used to describe the traditional method of observing the uterus by abdominal palpation while waiting for separation and descent of the placenta. The hand is kept perfectly still; kneading and squeezing the uterus disturbs the clotting of blood which should be taking place in the sinuses at the placental site.

### (3) Consistency of the uterus

After the birth of the baby the uterus has the consistency of a firm tennis ball: the upper border being about 2·5 cm below the level of the umbilicus. In shape the uterus is broader laterally than anteroposteriorly. Every two or three minutes, when a contraction occurs the uterus will feel more like a cricket ball for about 30 seconds: but the student midwife must not expect this cricket ball consistency to be constantly maintained. Between contractions the firm distinct outline of the uterus should be clearly defined; it should not be soft and flabby. A firmly contracted uterine muscle will prevent haemorrhage.

### (4) Size of the uterus

If after the birth of the baby the fundus is more than 2·5 cm above the umbilicus, four causes must be considered.

(a) **There is another baby** *in utero*. Palpate for fetal parts, listen for a fetal heart.

(b) **The placenta is unduly large.** This would be present in multiple pregnancy and if the Rh baby suffered from hydrops fetalis.

(c) **Blood clot is present.** When the uterus is atonic it cannot control bleeding and may not expel the blood so it clots *in utero*. The pulse will be rapid, no blood may be visible. The clots must be expressed.

(d) **A full bladder.** This would only occur if the woman had not been under competent supervision.

### (5) Amount of blood loss

To detect blood loss the vulva is constantly exposed. There may be, in the uterus, more than 300 ml of blood before any escapes. Pallor is a late sign. Quickening of the pulse may not take place until one minute or more after the onset of bleeding. Clots may form within the uterus and no bleeding is obvious.

**Post-partum haemorrhage is an ever present risk** during the third stage of labour. This danger has been reduced since the administration of Syntometrine has been employed during the birth of the anterior shoulder but preventive measures must still be utilised and diligent observation practised during the third stage of labour. The average amount of blood lost during and immediately after the third stage is approximately 120 to 240 ml but as there is usually some amniotic fluid in the blood, such an amount is not serious. Blood is a very precious fluid and midwives should endeavour to conduct the third stage with minimal blood loss. All blood should be measured including clots from the placental surface; the amount spilt on bed linen assessed.

## EXPULSION OF THE PLACENTA

The expulsion of the placenta was probably intended by Nature to be accomplished in the squatting attitude as adopted for defaecation, but when the woman lies in the dorsal position, help is usually required to express it. The woman lies with knees flexed and well separated: she is told that the procedure will be uncomfortable but not painful.

### Three Methods are Described

**(1) Controlled cord traction**

**(2) Using fundal pressure**

**(3) Bearing down by the woman**

**(1) Controlled Cord Traction** is the method most commonly employed in Britain; having superseded the traditional method of 'using fundal pressure'. Delivering the placenta by controlled cord traction following the administration of Syntometrine 1 ml intramuscularly at the time of the appearance of the anterior shoulder or after the birth of the head, provides a safe and successful means of reducing blood loss and shortening the third stage of labour. By this regime normal blood loss has been diminished by 30 to 60 ml; the incidence of postpartum haemorrhage lowered from 7 to 3 per cent. Successful results depend upon understanding the pharmacological action of Syntometrine; timing the procedure properly; being alert to the possibility of twins *in utero*.

Syntometrine 1 ml consists of 5 units of oxytocin (Syntocinon) and 0·5 mg ergometrine maleate B.P. When administered intramuscularly the Syntocinon acts within 2½ minutes and the ergometrine within 6 to 7 minutes. Ergometrine tends to cause spasm of the lower uterine segment so the placenta should be delivered before the ergometrine acts; (when ergometrine is given intravenously its rapid action within 1 to 2 minutes may cause trapping of the placenta as well as hypertensive episodes).

When Syntometrine is given intramuscularly hypertensive episodes are slight, transient and less frequent than with ergometrine given intravenously. Preeclamptic patients and those with essential hypertension are given Syntocinon, 5 units, in preference to Syntometrine or ergometrine. Syntometrine does not cause hypertensive episodes in normotensive women.

### Timing the Administration of Syntometrine

Giving Syntometrine when the anterior shoulder appears has certain advantages; the length of time between administration of the drug and delivery of the placenta can be accurately controlled. If given with crowning of the head Syntometrine may be administered too soon, for the act of crowning is not always properly understood or recognised; the placenta is not then delivered within 4 minutes and is liable to be trapped. Some administer Syntometrine when the head is born, others think that shoulder dystocia is less likely to occur if it is given when the anterior shoulder appears.

*Syntometrine must not be used after the expiry date,* **i.e. nine months after manufacture.**

### SYNTOMETRINE 1ml
**(Syntocinon 5 units and ergometrine 0·5mg)**

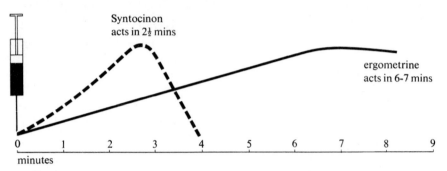

Fig. 20-6   Showing the rapid action of Syntocinon in comparison with ergometrine.
*Courtesy of Sandoz Products Ltd.*

### *Timing of Controlled Cord Traction*

The placenta should be extracted with the first uterine contraction after the birth of the baby usually between 2 to 4 minutes. (Some do not wait for this, but attending to the baby occupies two or three minutes.)

### *Method of Controlled Cord Traction*

Apply Mayo's artery forceps to the cord near the vulva. This provides a better hold for traction and reinforces the sensation of placental descent to a greater degree than when the cord is wound around the fingers. Wait for a strong uterine contraction, usually about 2–4 minutes after delivery.

Place the left hand on the lower abdomen, the palmar surface bracing back the upper uterine segment, the fingers stretching the lower uterine segment upwards towards the umbilicus to prevent inversion of uterus. Traction on the umbilical cord should begin gently, and be continued steadily, without jerking to avoid breaking the cord. Should the uterus relax, traction is stopped temporarily. The hand on the abdomen can, with practice, detect that the uterus is not being pulled downwards as would occur if the placenta were still adherent to it. If after 20 to 30 seconds of traction the placenta does not descend, the attempt should be abandoned for one or two minutes when it can again be resumed. The direction of pull should first be downwards then outwards as the placenta descends and upwards when it appears at the vulva, followng the axis of the birth canal. The safety of the procedure, in avoiding inversion of the uterus, lies in bracing back the uterus while cord traction is applied. Fundal pressure and cord traction must never be combined as this would be very liable to cause inversion of the uterus.

## BREAKING OF THE CORD

Cord traction should not be applied when the fetus is macerated, or if the baby is preterm: in both instances the tensile strength of the cord is much reduced. Fundal pressure would be preferable if the woman cannot expel the placenta by her expulsive effort. If the cord should snap, the sterile gloved hand is introduced into the vagina and the placenta grasped and extracted.

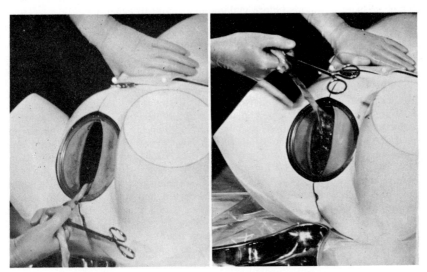

Fig. 20-7                                           Fig. 20-8

Classroom demonstration of controlled cord traction. *Note left hand bracing back the uterus.*
*Aberdeen Maternity Hospital.*

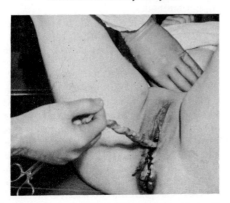

Fig. 20-9    Controlled cord traction. The left hand braces the contracted uterus upwards.
*Simpson Memorial Maternity Pavilion, Edinburgh.*

### Brandt-Andrews manoeuvre

Brandt, during 1930, and Andrew, during 1940, modified Aristotle's method of delivering the placenta by cord traction. They recommended applying tension, but not traction, to the umbilical cord with one hand; the other hand on the abdomen pushing the uterus upwards off the placenta, which in most cases was partially, if not completely separated. Controlled cord traction, a refinement of this method, is usually preferred.

## PLACENTAL SEPARATION AND DESCENT

When using method (2) Fundal pressure or method (3) Bearing down by the woman, it is essential that the placenta has separated and is lying in the lower uterine segment or vagina before making an attempt to expel it.

### Signs of Placental Separation and Descent

No one sign is absolute but a collection of signs is usually accepted as being reliable.

**(a) The fundus is globular** instead of having a broad flattened contour. It feels hard because when empty the uterus contracts better. The fundus rises to the level of the umbilicus because it is perched on top of the placenta now lying in the lower uterine segment. The uterus is also nearer the surface. Because it is no longer restrained by lying within the brim of the pelvis, it is mobile: only the thumb and middle finger are used when testing mobility and great gentleness exercised.

**(b) The cord lengthens at the vulva.** Slight traction on the cord is made to straighten out any kinks. Fundal pressure is then applied—the uterus being firm—and when the pressure is released, the cord outside the vulva will not recede if the placenta has separated and descended. It will recede if separation is not complete.

**(c) A gush of blood 30-60 ml usually appears when** the placenta starts to separate but does not indicate that separation is complete. As long as no separation takes place no bleeding can occur.

### (2) Using the Fundus as a Piston

Although this method is seldom employed in Britain today, midwives in developing countries may not use Syntometrine nor controlled cord traction so they will employ this traditional method.

The placenta must be separated and lying in the lower uterine segment or vagina.

The firmly contracted fundus is used as a piston to push the placenta out, in the same way that the piston is used to push fluid out of the barrel of a syringe.

### Method

The woman is asked to open her mouth and to breathe through it slowly and quietly, for the abdominal muscles must be relaxed. The midwife stands on the woman's right and uses her left hand to grasp the fundus, during a contraction, with her fingers behind the uterus and her thumb on the anterior surface (using only one hand). Pressure is applied with the palm of the hand in the axis of the pelvic inlet, then in a downward and backward direction. The causes of failure are usually due to pushing in the wrong direction, so that the placenta is jammed against the pubic bones. A full bladder makes the procedure very difficult indeed.

The right hand receives the placenta at the vulva, but when it is almost completely expelled both hands should be used, as the placenta is too big and slippery for a midwife to hold with one hand. The membranes usually slip out with the placenta, but if not, they may be still attached to the decidua in the area of the lower uterine segment near the cervix.

#### ADHERENT MEMBRANES

In an attempt to detach adherent membranes the placenta can be turned round to make a complete circle which will twist the membranes into a rope and strengthen them. The usual method employed is to apply a pair of artery forceps to the membranes and to exert gentle traction in an up and down, sideways and circular manner, in an endeavour to coax the membranes out.

### (3) The woman's bearing down effort (rarely used)

When the placenta has separated and descended and the uterus is contracted she is instructed to hold her breath and bear down as she did for the birth of the baby. Some multiparous women have lax abdominal muscles which cannot be effectively used in bearing down. The midwife could assist in such cases by laying both her hands, palms downwards, across the woman's abdomen below the umbilicus to provide a brace against which the woman can push.

The primigravida often has a rigid pelvic floor, and assistance may be required to overcome its resistance, unless an episiotomy has been made, or an extensive perineal laceration is present. If the woman fails to expel the placenta by pushing, assistance must be given.

### SUMMARY OF FUNDAL HEIGHTS DURING THIRD STAGE

| | | |
|---|---|---|
| A, **At the beginning of third stage** | 2·5 cm below | 15 cm above |
| B, **Placenta in lower segment** (separated) | 1·5 cm above | 19 cm above |
| C, **End of third stage** (placenta expelled) | 4 cm below | 14 cm above |
| | **The umbilicus** | **The symphysis pubis** |

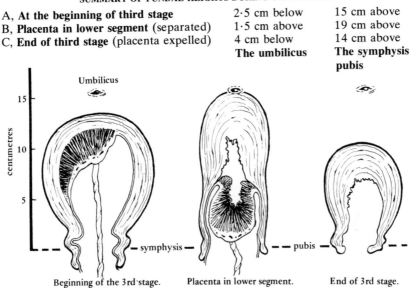

Fig. 20-10   Fundal height relative to the umbilicus and symphysis pubis.

## EXAMINATION OF THE PLACENTA

Management of the third stage is not complete until the placenta has been examined to make sure that no part of it has been retained, and this must be done in a careful systematic manner. It is advisable to examine the membranes first, as they are apt to become torn while inspecting the maternal surface of the placenta.

### Inspection of the membranes

The amount of chorion should be sufficient to have contained the fetus and amniotic fluid and, if not complete, an effort must be made to assess the amount of membrane that is missing.

The amnion ought to be peeled from the chorion right up to the umbilical cord, for it is not possible to determine that the chorion is complete until the amnion has been detached from it. When the membranes are stained with meconium it is possible that the baby may have inhaled meconium-stained amniotic fluid and develop pulmonary complications.

### Blood Vessels in the Membrane may denote a Succenturiate Lobe

Blood vessels in the membrane should be traced from source to destination. They may run from the main placenta to a succenturiate lobe situated in the membrane, and when such a lobe is present (*visibly*) there is no cause for concern, but if the lobe has been retained, the vessels will be seen running to the hole in the membrane where the lobe had been. There will, of course, be a large hole in the membrane through which the baby has come, and there may be a hole due to the retention of a piece of membrane; but in neither instance will there be any blood vessels going to these holes. The vessels may run to a velamentous insertion of cord, or they may return to the placenta again—the so-called aberrant vessels which are of no significance.

### Incomplete Membranes

The state of the membranes must be recorded on the chart, eg. 'complete', 'half retained', and if the membranes are torn but appear to be complete the term 'ragged membranes' is used. When the membranes are incomplete, the midwife in remote areas may give one of the ergot preparations, b.i.d. for two or three days; and inspect all lochial discharge until the membrane is passed. The danger of haemorrhage must be kept in mind and the doctor summoned if the membrane is not passed within 48 hours, if the lochia are persistently red, or if postpartum or puerperal haemorrhage occurs.

### Inspection of the maternal and fetal surfaces

Blood clot should be removed from the maternal surface and placed in the jug used for measuring blood loss. The placenta should be dark bluish-red in colour and of firm consistency. An unhealthy placenta is soft and mushy, and when hydrops fetalis is present the placenta is large, pale and oedematous, with water oozing from it. (Other abnormalities are considered on page 46.)

All the cotyledons should be present, and, if the placenta is laid flat, they will fit together if the placenta is intact. The placenta is inspected for infarcts, which are whitish areas usually about 2·5 cm or more in diameter. The position of the insertion of the cord is noted, its length measured and the presence of 1 or 2 arteries established. The placenta is weighed, and pertinent facts regarding it are recorded on the chart. The examination of the placenta is a most important duty, and because of the grave danger of a cotyledon (*or a succenturiate lobe*) being left behind, the Central Midwives Board for Scotland rules state that the placenta and membranes must be examined before they are destroyed. If the placenta is normal and the doctor has not requested that it should be kept for his inspection, it is disposed of by burning if possible.

### Dangers of retained Lobe of Placenta

Serious postpartum or puerperal haemorrhage may occur when a lobe of placenta is left behind and no steps are taken to promote its expulsion. Retained placental tissue is more dangerous than retained membrane, because it is deeply embedded and when it sloughs off may open up large uterine vessels. This haemorrhage may occur after the woman has been discharged, and can be fatal. To avoid such a catastrophe the obstetrician will detect retained products by a sonar scan, explore the uterus under a general anaesthetic in the operating theatre and remove the lobe. Blood should be available for transfusion.

In domiciliary practice medical assistance must be obtained when the placenta is not complete; it is likely that the woman will be transferred to hospital. If the retained piece of placenta is very small, ergometrine, 0·5 mg, or other ergot preparation will be ordered and given b.i.d. Continued red lochial discharge is a warning sign, which should be reported at once and preparations made for exploration of the uterus.

## THE FOURTH STAGE OF LABOUR

The first hour after expulsion of the placenta is sometimes designated the fourth stage of labour, in order to stress the fact that vigilance is still necessary in case haemorrhage should occur. The empty uterus should now be firmly contracted. If an oxytocic drug has not already been given the midwife should now administer an ergot preparation, such as ergometrine, 0·5 mg, or Syntometrine, 1 ml. Any blood clot present should be expelled while the uterus is in a state of contraction by gently squeezing and cautiously pressing the uterus in a downward and backward direction with due regard to the danger of predisposing to uterine prolapse. Routine massage of the uterus at this period, when it is contracting satisfactorily, is to be deprecated.

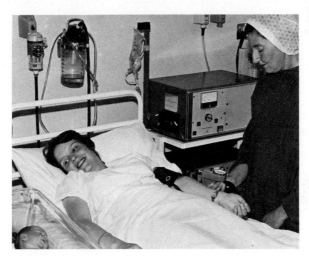

Fig. 20-11  Midwife taking the blood pressure with an electronic sphygmomanometer. No stethoscope required. Radiant maternal bonding is obvious.

*Maternity Hospital, Stirling.*

### Nursing care

The vulva is swabbed and a sterile pad placed in position, buttocks dried and any wet linen removed, so that the woman will be warm and comfortable. A sterile towel is laid over the lower abdomen and thighs and the woman covered with warm cellular cotton blankets. The midwife remains at the bedside, noting the woman's pulse and colour. At frequent intervals she palpates the uterus to make sure it is not filling up with blood, and looks at the pad to ensure that the blood loss is not excessive. The pulse rate should be between 60 and 70, but if it is over 90 investigation and continued supervision are necessary. The temperature is taken, and may be subnormal because of loss of body heat, but occasionally it is 37·2°C

(99°F), due to reaction following a difficult labour.

**The blood pressure** is taken during the first half hour after delivery; the systolic pressure should be above 110 mm Hg, but, if less, and especially if accompanied by a pulse of over 100, it is usually due to collapse from haemorrhage or shock. If the blood pressure is higher or lower than anticipated it is taken every half hour.

The woman is encouraged to pass urine before being left in her home or transferred to the postnatal ward in hospital, but if she has emptied her bladder prior to delivery she may have no desire to urinate. Vulval swabbing is repeated, and a large perineal pad placed on the vulva.

She will appreciate a cup of tea and toast, and there is no reason why she should not have a light meal if she desires it.

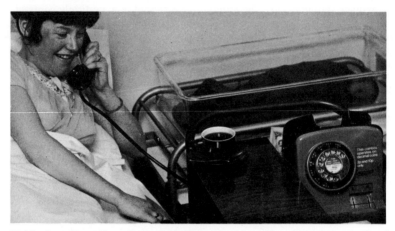

Fig. 20-12   Portable trolley telephone. Newly delivered mother talking to her husband.
*Simpson Memorial Maternity Pavilion, Edinburgh.*

Rest and sleep should be encouraged. After seeing her husband, the room should be darkened and quietness assured. Even although the mother may feel elated and not inclined for sleep, it is sound practice to give a sedative at this time.

C.M.B.(Scot.) Rule. *The midwife must not leave her patient until at least one hour after the birth of the placenta. And only then if:*

**Vaginal blood loss normal.          Pulse below 90.          Fundus firm.**
**Systolic blood pressure** 110 mm/Hg or over          **Baby's condition good.**

The more common reasons for obtaining medical assistance during the third stage are: haemorrhage, adherent and retained placenta. These and the other complications are discussed on page 423.

### RECORD KEEPING

It is the duty of the midwife, to record her observations during labour. The best aids to good record keeping are:

(1) A plan of work that ensures the carrying out of every essential treatment and examination at stated times throughout labour; (2) Suitable charts such as the partogram that are designed for the recording of all necessary observations and treatment at specific intervals. Such charts serve as a reminder for making observations and giving treatments and help the midwife to organise the nursing care of the woman in labour.

There are differences of opinion as to which observations are absolutely necessary and how frequently they should be made. The midwife in charge uses her discretion, allowing the woman to rest and sleep when necessary.

### Prompt Recording should be the Rule

The filling up of charts, long after the findings were made, is most unreliable. If facts are recorded at once, the progress of labour can be assessed by any member of the staff, in the absence of the person who made the examination. Charts should, if possible, be completed as soon as labour is over, so that they can be sent to the post natal ward along with the patient. The sister will, of course, make her own observations of mother and baby as soon as they are admitted to her ward; but she should be given certain information regarding the type of delivery and what the condition of mother and baby has been during the first postpartum hour. The postnatal ward sister will note the following facts, which should have been recorded so that any necessary precautions and treatment can be instituted.

**Delivery:** Spontaneous; accelerated; malpresentation; forceps; Caesarean.

**Anaesthetic:** General; epidural; local.

**Blood loss:** Amount.

**Placenta and membranes:** Complete; incomplete.

**Perineum:** Laceration; episiotomy; number of non-absorbable sutures.

**Drugs given to mother:** e.g. Oxytocic preparations; sedatives.

**Baby:** Preterm. Light for date. Condition at birth. Apgar score. Rh haemolytic disease? Drugs given, e.g. Konakion (vitamin $K_1$); naloxone (Narcan).

Legibility is essential and the dosage of drugs given ought to be clearly printed. *Abbreviations* should be avoided, except for those which are universally employed, such as, L.O.A., P.V.

### Accuracy is imperative

The chart should present a clear, concise, reliable record so that when reviewing the case at the end of labour, or prior to a subsequent delivery, the pertinent facts are available. Records are sometimes utilised for statistical purposes and for obstetrical research, so facts and figures must be correct. They are kept for a number of years in case of litigation.

The legal aspect of record keeping is also important during labour. The date and hour of birth, sex of the child, and whether alive or stillborn, are required for the registration and the notification of births. The length and weight at birth might be needed as evidence of the period of gestation in cases when the paternity of the child is under question.

---

## QUESTIONS FOR REVISION
### THE THIRD STAGE OF LABOUR

#### Oral Questions

**What observations does the midwife make during the third stage?** Why is it important to take the pulse during the third stage? How could you help a woman to expel her placenta? When should you not apply cord traction? What would you do if the cord broke? What is the normal amount of blood loss?

The patient's condition should be satisfactory when left one hour after the placenta has been expelled. Explain what you mean by **'satisfactory'** under three headings. How can the midwife endeavour to prevent postpartum haemorrhage? What is meant by 'living ligatures'? If the uterus is unduly large what are the four possible causes? Why is it important to make sure a second twin is not *in utero* prior to giving Syntometrine? Why is the timing of administration of Syntometrine important? Why does giving ergometrine i.v. cause trapping of the placenta? Why is Syntometrine not given in cases of pre-eclampsia? How would you examine the placenta?

Describe the mechanism of placental separation and natures method of preventing haemorrhage.

**Give 5 pertinent facts re:** (a) prevention of excessive blood loss; (b) blood pressure after delivery; (c) retained lobe of placenta; (d) nursing care during the fourth stage.

**Differentiate between:** (a) the Schultze and Matthews Duncan method; (b) Brandt-Andrews method and controlled cord traction; (c) adherent and retained placenta; (d) Syntometrine and Syntocinon.

Why is it important that the bladder is not overdistended during the third stage? How would you deal with (a) adherent membranes; (b) a retained lobe of placenta?

Explain what is meant by "using the fundus as a piston" "guarding the uterus" "hypertensive episodes" "cricket ball consistency".

Describe the nursing care during the fourth stage of labour. How do you carry out "controlled cord traction" what are the benefits of this procedure.

**C.M.B.(Scot.) 30-min. question.** Describe briefly how you would examine the placenta, and state what complications may occur if the placenta or membranes are found to be deficient.

**(N.Ire.) 30-min. question.** Discuss the conduct of the third stage of labour in a patient with a history of postpartum haemorrhage at an earlier confinement.

**(N.Ire.) 30-min. question.** Describe the placenta at term. Why is it important to make a careful examination of it immediately the third stage is completed?

**(N.Ire.) 30-min. question.** Describe the mechanism of placental separation and expulsion. Give the management of the normal third stage of labour.

**C.M.B.(Eng.) 30-min. question.** Describe the management of the third stage of labour. What complications may arise?

**C.M.B.(Scot.) 30-min. question.** Describe the physiology and management of the normal third stage of labour.

## C.M.B. Short Questions

**Eng.:** Signs of separation and descent of the placenta. **Eng.:** Management of the third stage of labour. **N. Ire.:** Syntometrine. **Eng.:** Examination of the placenta and membranes. **N. Ire.:** Signs of complete placental separation and descent. **Eng.:** Control of bleeding in the third stage. **N. Ire.:** Use of oxytocic drugs in the third stage. **Eng.:** Physiology of the third stage. **N. Ire.:** Controlled cord traction. **N. Ire.:** Retained placenta. **Eng.:** Manual removal of placenta. **Eng.:** Principles of management of the third stage of labour.

# 21

<table>
<tr>
<td>

## Occipito-posterior
## Positions of the Vertex
*Diagnosis. Mechanism. Management. Deep transverse arrest. Unreduced occipito-posterior*

</td>
<td>

## Multiple Pregnancy
*Types. Diagnosis. Effect on pregnancy and labour. Management. Complications*

</td>
</tr>
</table>

## Postmaturity

---

## RIGHT OCCIPITO–POSTERIOR POSITION

Although the vertex is a normal presentation, the course of labour can border on the abnormal when the occiput occupies a posterior instead of an anterior part of the pelvis.

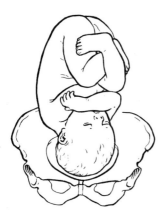 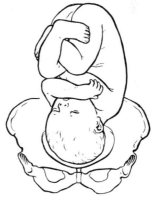

Fig. 21-1   Right occipito-posterior.        Fig. 21-2   Left occipito-posterior.
Vertex presentation.

### DIAGNOSIS (Right Occipito-posterior)

#### ABDOMINAL EXAMINATION

**On inspection** there is a saucer-shaped depression at or immediately below the umbilicus, because when the back is not in front, there is a 'dip' between the upper and lower poles of the fetus. The high head with the depression above it looks rather like a full bladder.

**On palpation the head is high:** the commonest cause of a high head in a primigravida during the later weeks of pregnancy is posterior position. This is because the large engaging diameter O.F. 11·5 cm will not enter the brim until labour begins and flexion takes place.

**The head feels unduly large,** this is due to the larger circumference of the deflexed head.

**The occiput and sinciput are on the same level.**

345

**The back is difficult to palpate** because it is placed well out on the right side. The anterior shoulder will be 7 to 10 cm from the midline, and because the head is high, the shoulder will be about 12 cm above the symphysis pubis.

**Limbs are felt on both sides of the midline** whereas in anterior positions they are only felt on one side.

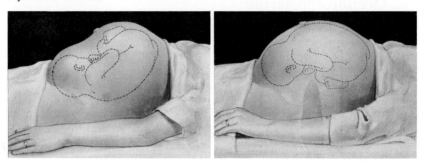

Fig. 21-3   Posterior.                    Fig. 21-4   Anterior.

Comparison of abdominal contour in posterior and anterior positions of vertex presentation.

**On auscultation** the fetal heart beat will be located in the right flank, somewhat muffled as the muscles there are thick. It may also be heard in the midline near the umbilicus or slightly to the left, because when the back is not well flexed the fetal heart is heard through the fetal chest which is thrown forwards.

### DIAGNOSIS DURING LABOUR

Posterior position should be suspected where there is no disproportion and a vertex presentation is held up at the brim in spite of good uterine action.

The vaginal findings will depend on the degree of flexion of the head, and locating the anterior fontanelle to the left anterior is diagnostic of an R.O.P. The sagittal suture will be in the right oblique diameter of the pelvis.

**ANTERIOR**

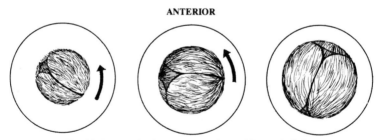

Fig. 21-5   Touch picture per vaginam. Vertex L.O.P.

| Anterior fontanelle felt in right anterior. Sagittal suture in the left oblique diameter of the pelvis. | Anterior fontanelle felt in the right lateral. Sagittal suture in the transverse diameter of the pelvis. | With increased flexion the posterior fontanelle is felt in the left anterior. Sagittal suture in the right oblique diameter of the L.O.A. It is now an L.O.A. |

During the second stage of labour a vaginal examination is often necessary because of delay. The large caput may make identification of sutures and fontanelles difficult and in such cases the doctor usually inserts his hand so that an accurate diagnosis and assessment of the situation can be made.

*Mechanism of Right Occipito-posterior Position*

The lie is longitudinal.
The attitude is that of flexion.
The presentation is the vertex.
The position is the R.O.P.

The denominator is the occiput.
The presenting part is the middle
or anterior area of the left
parietal bone.

The occipito-frontal diameter, 11·5 cm lies in the right oblique diameter of the pelvic brim. The occiput points to the right sacro-iliac joint, the sinciput to the left ilio-pectineal eminence.

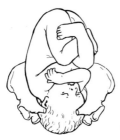

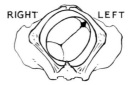

Fig. 21-6   Head descending with increase in flexion.

Fig. 21-7   Sagittal suture in the right oblique diameter of the pelvis.

Right occipito-posterior.

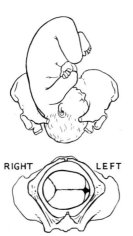

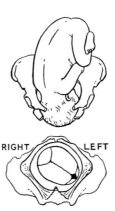

Fig. 21-8   The occiput and the shoulders have rotated one-eighth of a circle forwards. The sagittal suture is in the transverse diameters of the pelvis.

Fig. 21-9   The occiput and shoulders have rotated two-eighths of a circle forwards, now being similar to an R.O.A. The sagittal suture is in the left oblique diameter of the pelvis.

**Flexion.** Descent takes place with increasing flexion. The occiput becomes the leading part.

**Internal rotation of the head.** The occiput reaches the pelvic floor first and rotates three-eighths of a circle forwards along the right side of the pelvis. The shoulders turn two-eighths of a circle with the head from the left to the right oblique. (*This is not internal rotation of the shoulders as they have not yet reached the pelvic floor.*)

**Crowning.** The occiput escapes under the symphysis pubis and the head is crowned.

**Extension.** Sinciput, face and chin sweep the perineum and the head is born by a movement of extension.

**Restitution** takes place and the occiput turns one-eighth of a circle to the right and the head rights itself with the shoulders.

**Internal rotation of the shoulders.** The shoulders enter in the right oblique of the pelvis, the anterior shoulder reaches the pelvic floor first and rotates one-eighth of a circle forwards, along the left side of the pelvis.

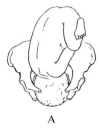

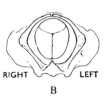

RIGHT            LEFT

A                                B

Fig. 21-10

A, Occiput has rotated three eighths of a    B, The sagittal suture is in the antero-
circle forwards. Note twist in neck.              posterior diameter of the pelvic outlet.

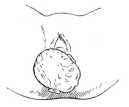

Fig. 21-11    Restitution. The occiput turns one-eighth of a circle to the right.

**External rotation of head.** The occiput turns a further one-eighth of a circle to the right.

**Lateral flexion.** The anterior shoulder escapes under the symphysis pubis, the posterior shoulder sweeps the perineum and the body is born by a movement of lateral flexion.

### *The Probable Course of Labour*

**Long internal rotation** of the head commonly takes place. Good uterine contractions produce flexion and descent of the head so that in 90 per cent of cases the occiput rotates forwards three-eighths as described above.

**Short internal rotation** of the head takes place in 10 per cent of posterior positions because flexion of the head does not occur; the sinciput reaches the pelvic floor first rotates forwards and the baby is born face to pubes.

**Deep transverse arrest of** the head occurs in the pelvis which has projecting ischial spines that inhibit forward rotation of the head.

**Labour may be prolonged** because larger diameters of the skull present, and the suboccipito-frontal diameter 10 cm instead of the suboccipito-bregmatic diameter 9·5 cm will have to pass through the pelvis. The cervix will have to dilate to a greater extent to allow passage of the larger circumference of the head. The anterior lip of cervix may be nipped between the head and the pubic bone. Weak uterine contractions are sometimes associated with occipito-posterior positions, because the deflexed head does not fit snugly into the lower uterine segment and stimulate the cervical nerve endings. The deflexed head does not dilate the cervix effectively.

$$\frac{5}{5} \qquad\qquad \frac{4}{5} \qquad\qquad \frac{3}{5}$$

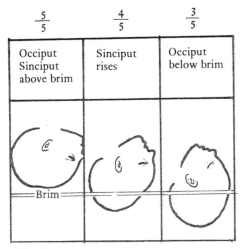

Fig. 21-12    Showing high head, slow descent.

**The necessity for interference is greater. Epidural analgesia** may be used for backache. Rotation of the head may have to be assisted manually or by forceps; application of forceps is frequently required because of delay in the second stage, or on account of fetal or maternal distress.

**The fetal mortality and morbidity rates are higher** because of intracranial injury and hypoxia.

### Summary of Clinical Features

The head descends slowly, even when there are good contractions.

The uterine contractions are sometimes weak. Dilatation of the cervix is retarded.

The membranes usually rupture early. Backache is frequently complained of.

Difficulty in micturition is common.

The urge to bear down at the end of the first stage is especially great, probably because the occiput is pressing on the rectum.

### Nursing care

Although only 10 per cent of these patients will have a prolonged or difficult labour, such a possibility should be anticipated in every case so that further complications can be averted. Additional nursing care, including observation of the maternal and fetal conditions will be necessary.

## DEEP TRANSVERSE ARREST

The head is arrested deep in the pelvic cavity, with the sagittal suture in the transverse diameter of the pelvis. Arrest may be due to weak contractions: it is sometimes associated with the type of pelvis with a straight sacrum, or with one that is narrowed at the bispinous diameter of the outlet, and the occiput is prevented from rotating forwards.

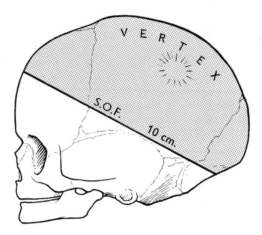

Fig. 21-13    The suboccipito-frontal diameter of the skull passes through the birth canal in posterior vertex positions.

### Diagnosis

Deep transverse arrest would be suspected when, after half an hour (or less) of second stage contractions, the head is not visible at the vulva. On vaginal examination the sagittal suture will be felt in the transverse with a fontanelle at either end. The head will be at the level of the ischial spines, although the caput may be below this.

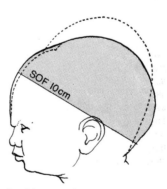

Fig. 21-14    Moulding of the head in an occipito-posterior position of the vertex. Shown by dotted line.

### *Treatment*

Medical assistance should be obtained, and pending the doctor's arrival the woman could be given an inhalational analgesic. Perineal infiltration or pudendal nerve block should be anticipated and preparations made for catheterisation, episiotomy, forceps delivery, the reception of a hypoxic baby and perineal suturing.

The doctor will attempt to increase flexion by pushing up the sinciput and with his whole hand in the vagina will rotate the head. Obstetricians frequently rotate the head with Kielland's forceps.

## PERSISTENT OCCIPITO-POSTERIOR

When the occiput fails to rotate forward in an R.O.P., it is known as a persistent or right unreduced occipito-posterior R.U.O.P. The sinciput reaches the pelvic floor first and rotates forward so the occiput goes into the hollow of the sacrum. The baby is born face to pubes.

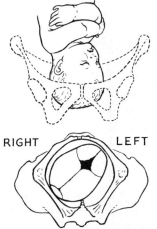

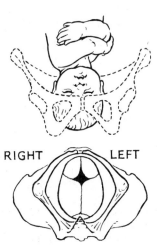

Fig. 21-15  R.U.O.P.—Head in right oblique diameter of pelvis.

Fig.  21-16  R.U.O.P.—Head  in  antero-
posterior diameter of pelvis.

### CAUSES

Deficient flexion of the head and spine. In posterior positions the fetus tends to adopt the military attitude and the occipito-frontal diameter, 11·5 cm, presents in the right oblique diameter of the pelvic brim. The wide biparietal diameter 9·5 cm is liable to be caught in the sacro-cotyloid dimension 9 cm. (*If the head becomes flexed, the parietal eminences are brought forwards and clear the sacro-cotyloid dimension*.) Descent of the occiput is retarded, the sinciput becomes the leading part, reaches the pelvic floor first and rotates forwards.

If the head is small in relation to the pelvis, it need not flex before descent can take place and in that case the sinciput might reach the pelvic floor first and rotate forwards.

### DIAGNOSIS OF PERSISTENT OCCIPITO-POSTERIOR POSITION

During labour the head is slow to engage, and the usual degree of flexion does not take place. The fetal heart may be heard clearly in the midline at about umbilical level, because the chest of the fetus is in close proximity to the abdominal wall. Delay in the second stage should arouse suspicion and a vaginal examination would reveal the anterior fontanelle behind the symphysis pubis. Sometimes the fontanelle is obliterated by a large caput and in that case the doctor will feel for the pinna of the ear which if directed towards the sacrum will determine that the occiput is posterior.

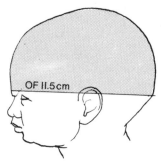

Fig. 21-17    Diameter engaging when head is deflexed. Occipito-frontal 11·5 cm.

Excessive bulging of the perineum and gaping of the anus are sometimes evident because the broad biparietal diameter instead of the bitemporal is distending the perineum. In this case the head will be showing and the anterior fontanelle can be felt just below the symphysis pubis. The baby is born face to pubes.

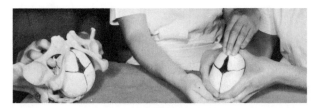

Fig. 21-18    Holding sinciput back until occiput sweeps the perineum.

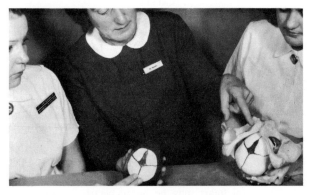

Fig. 21-19    Allowing the sinciput to emerge from under the pubic arch by a slight movement of extension (note half of rubber ball as cervix).

*Aberdeen Maternity Hospital.*

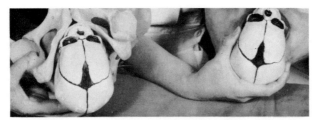

Fig. 21-20   Face born from under symphysis pubis.
*Photographed at Aberdeen Maternity Hospital.*

ANTERIOR

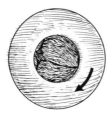 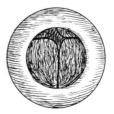

Fig. 21-21   Vaginal touch picture unreduced left occipito-posterior.

Anterior fontanelle to the right anterior: sagittal suture in the left oblique of the pelvis.

Anterior fontanelle in front behind symphysis pubis.

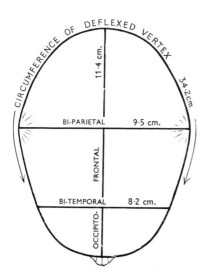 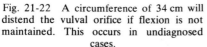 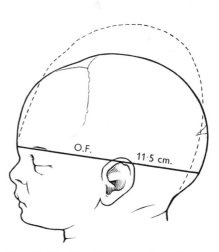

Fig. 21-22   A circumference of 34 cm will distend the vulval orifice if flexion is not maintained. This occurs in undiagnosed cases.

Fig. 21-23   Moulding in vertex, face to pubes, shown by dotted line. Note the 'sugar loaf' head.

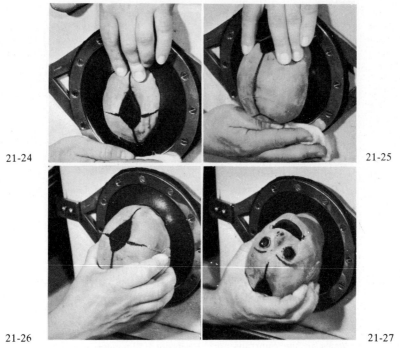

21-24                                                                                     21-25

21-26                                                                                     21-27

Demonstrating delivery of vertex face to pubes in the dorsal position.
Fig. 21-24   Holding the sinciput back until the occiput sweeps the perineum.
Fig. 21-25   The occiput is born by a movement of flexion.
Fig. 21-26   Grasping the head to bring the face down from under the symphysis pubis.
Fig. 21-27   The movement is now one of extension.
*Aberdeen Maternity Hospital.*

### Management

An episiotomy will facilitate delivery and avoid serious perineal trauma. The midwife will maintain flexion by holding the sinciput back under the symphysis pubis so that the area anterior to the bregma will be the point which pivots under the symphysis pubis. After the occiput comes over the perineum, the midwife grasps the vertex and brings the face down from under the symphysis pubis.

### UNDIAGNOSED FACE TO PUBES ON DELIVERY

The forehead is seen slipping down under the symphysis pubis, the head pivots on the glabella and the occipito-frontal diameter distends the vulval orifice. Because the biparietal diameter is also stretching the perineum, a third-degree tear is likely.

The moulding of the head in these babies is typical, with the caput on the anterior part of the parietal bone, giving what is known as the '*sugar-loaf*' head. Because the vault of the skull is raised, intracranial injury and haemorrhage may occur so vitamin $K_1$ should be administered to the baby at birth.

# Multiple Pregnancy

When there is more than one fetus *in utero* the term 'plural' or 'multiple' pregnancy is applied. Twins occur approximately once in about every 90 pregnancies, and the tendency is manifest in certain families. Triplets occur once in about every 9,000 pregnancies, quadruplets once in 700,000 but quintuplets are very rare indeed. In recent years sextuplets and septuplets have been conceived due to stimulation of the ovaries, by drugs given in cases of infertility to promote ovulation; many have aborted, a few have been born viable.

### MONOZYGOTIC (UNIOVULAR)

Monozygotic or single ovum twins are known as identical twins because their physical and mental characteristics are so similar. They develop from one ovum which has been fertilised by one spermatozoon and are always of the same sex. They are definitely uniovular if they share one placenta and one chorion; a few have two chorions. There is a connection between the circulation of blood in the two babies. Finger and palm prints are identical in monozygotic twins.

Errors in development are more likely in monozygotic twins, so abnormal fetuses are more common; conjoined twins, usually known as Siamese, are uniovular in type. The perinatal mortality rate is higher than in dizygotic twins.

### DIZYGOTIC (BINOVULAR)

Dizygotic or double ovum twins, which are three times more common than uniovular twins, develop from the fertilisation of two ova and two spermatozoa. The babies may or may not be of the same sex and their physical and mental characteristics can be as different as in any two members of one family. Dizygotic twin bearing is hereditary either through the mother or father, but probably mainly *via* the mother. They each have a separate placenta and chorion, but, although the placentae may fuse, the fetal circulations do not mix. The differentiation between monozygotic and dizygotic twins at birth is not always easy, because some monozygotic twins have two chorions.

If the babies are of different sexes or have two separate placentae, they are definitely dizygotic. But sometimes the two zygotes embed close to each other so that the placentae fuse and appear to the naked eye to be one single placenta. In that case, if the sex of the babies is the same, the diagnosis is made by examination of the membranes of the fetal sac, and in dizygotic twins two chorions are present.

| MONOZYGOTIC OR Uniovular | DIZYGOTIC OR Binovular |
|---|---|
| One ovum. | Two ova. |
| One spermatozoon. | Two spermatozoa. |
| One placenta. | Two placentae (*may fuse*). |
| One chorion (*a few have two*). | Two chorions. |
| Two amnions. | Two amnions. |
| One sex. | One or two sexes. |

Very occasionally one fetus may die and be retained *in utero* until term when it will be expelled with the placenta as a flattened paper-like fetus—a fetus papyraceous.

Although twin babies are as a rule small and often preterm, ranging from 2,260 g to 2,720 g, normal weights are not uncommon; the author having seen twins weighing 4,060 g and 3,960 g; 4,340 g and 4,300 g.

## DIAGNOSIS OF TWINS

The diagnosis of twins is not always easy in primigravid women with firm abdominal walls, or in obese women, and experienced doctors and midwives may not always detect them. The period of gestation is also difficult to assess.

**DIZYGOTIC OR BINOVULAR**

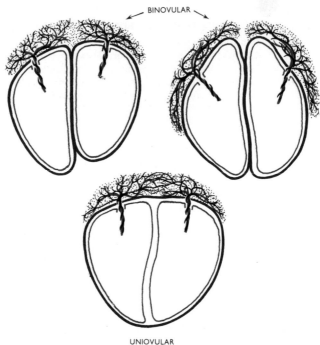

BINOVULAR

UNIOVULAR

**MONOZYGOTIC OR UNIOVULAR**

Fig. 21-28  Twin placentae. Dizygotic twins have two placentae which may fuse, and two chorions. Monozygotic twins have one placenta; if they have one chorion they are definitely uniovular, but some have two chorions.

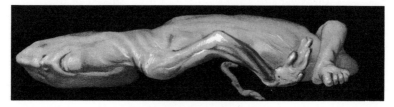

Fig. 21-29  Fetus papyraceous.

An ultrasonic scan will demonstrate two heads at 15 weeks: two gestational sacs have been seen at eight weeks. X-rays may be used after the 30th week.

Twins may first be diagnosed by finding the uterus large and the fundus well above the umbilicus after the birth of the first baby.

### On inspection

Suspicion is aroused when the uterus is unduly large for the period of gestation after the 20th week. The uterus looks round or broad and fetal movement may be seen over a wide area, but this is not diagnostic. At term, a woman of average build has an abdominal girth of about 100 cm. The possibility of polyhydramnios must be considered, and it can be present in conjunction with or independent of twins, but palpation should help to clinch the diagnosis.

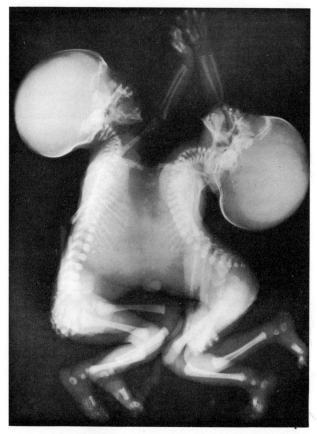

Fig. 21-30   X-ray of conjoined twins delivered by Caesarean section at onset of labour at 35th week of pregnancy. (Note extension of heads and spines.)
*Simpson Memorial Maternity Pavilion, Edinburgh.*

### On palpation

Finding two heads is diagnostic. When one head lies in the fundus and one in the lower pole, they are more readily palpated; but in 40 per cent of cases both fetuses present by the vertex, and the second head may be palpated in the iliac fossa. If one fetus lies in front of the other, it may not be easy to detect two heads or two backs. Should the fetal head seem small in comparison with the size of the uterus this rather suggests the presence of two fetuses. Excessive fetal parts might make one surmise that twins were present.

**Auscultation**

Hearing two fetal hearts is not a reliable method of diagnosis because with a large, vigorous fetus, the fetal heart can sometimes be heard over a wide area.

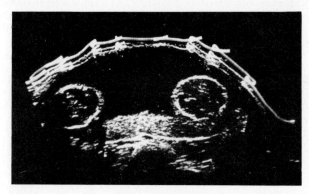

Fig. 21-31    Ultrasonogram. Twins at 21½ weeks gestation demonstrated by both heads seen in oblique section. Note placenta (speckled area situated posteriorly near the bottom of the picture).

*Courtesy of Queen Mother's Hospital, Glasgow.*

### THE EFFECT OF TWINS ON PREGNANCY

**Pre-eclampsia** is more common than in single pregnancies.

**Polyhydramnios** frequently occurs with twins and adds to the woman's discomfort. Acute polyhydramnios is invariably associated with uniovular twins: the usual outcome being abortion.

**Anaemia** develops because of the increased fetal demands for iron: the incidence of megaloblastic anaemia is increased and may be suspected by a sudden fall in haemoglobin.

**The minor disorders** and general discomforts of pregnancy are more pronounced: morning sickness, nausea and heartburn are more persistent.

**Pressure symptoms due** to the weight and size of the uterus may be troublesome. (*a*) The tendency to oedema of the ankles and varicose veins is increased because of pressure on the veins returning blood from the lower limbs. (*b*) Dyspnoea and indigestion are more marked: backache is common.

### *Management of Pregnancy*

As soon as twins are diagnosed a close check should be kept on the mother's haemoglobin and advice given regarding foods rich in iron. Ferrous preparations are usually prescribed and vitamin supplements are essential. Most obstetricians give a preparation of folic acid e.g. Ferfolic contains 30 mg Fe and five mg folic acid, one three times daily. The woman should drink at least 1,200 ml of milk daily to prevent her calcium reserves from being depleted. Her protein intake must be adequate.

In order to detect pre-eclampsia which is three times more common in multiple pregnancy, the woman is seen weekly from the time twins are diagnosed about the 20th week.

To relieve the discomfort of a heavy uterus, a good supporting maternity belt will be appreciated. A 'roll-on' worn at night in the later weeks gives abdominal support, and extra pillows are needed for sleep, as the woman feels more comfortable when propped up. When lying on her side a small pillow tucked under her abdomen will ease any dragging sensation. Vague pains due to overstretched muscles and ligaments, as well as the excessive fetal movements, tend to disturb sleep and in some cases a mild sedative is necessary. Adequate rest is essential during the last 12 weeks to increase uterine blood flow.

The woman may be admitted to hospital from the 30th to the 36th week to avoid preterm labour by providing rest, and to improve her nutrition. She should not be permitted to go beyond term but many go into labour prior to then.

## THE EFFECT OF TWINS ON LABOUR

Although multiple pregnancy may not be regarded as abnormal in itself, many complications that endanger fetal and maternal life do arise (see p. 361). Labour is often preterm: the babies tend to be light for date even when at term, so their blood glucose levels should be assessed (see p. 534).

The perinatal mortality rate is about 8 per cent, as against less than 1·7 per cent in single births. The mortality rate of the second twin is twice that of the first, and this may be due to reduction in the placental circulation and partial separation of placenta following the birth of the first twin. Malpresentation is more common.

For these reasons hospitalisation for delivery is advocated.

### The Management of Labour

Heavy sedation should be avoided. Some authorities use epidural analgesia. If delay occurs due to hypotonic uterine action an oxytocin drip may be given after puncture of the membranes and kept running until one hour after both babies and placentae are delivered.

Preparations should be made for the reception of two immature babies, who may show signs of asphyxia or intracranial injury. Additional swabs, cord clamps, ligatures, scissors, mucus extractors and baby blankets should be set out. Wrist name tapes marked 1 and 2. Two incubators or cots should be in readiness.

The room ought to be warm and extra cotton blankets should be available for the slight degree of shock that often follows delivery because of marked reduction in abdominal pressure. Syntometrine 1 ml should be drawn up in readiness to be given as soon as the anterior shoulder of the second twin is born, or during the third stage if haemorrhage occurs. It is a wise precaution to have 600 ml of cross-matched blood available if the haemoglobin is below 9 g/dl.

### Active Treatment

The woman may be more comfortable in the dorsal position with additional pillows. A lateral tilt on a foam rubber wedge is popular.

Perineal infiltration or pudendal nerve block is commonly employed and an episiotomy is made *in an endeavour to lower the high perinatal mortality rate.*

The airway of the first baby is cleared. The cord should be ligatured in two places, for although the placental end of the cord is tied or clamped at every delivery, it is because of the possibility of undiagnosed monozygotic twins that this is done. The first baby, after being marked No. 1, is laid in a warm cot and the midwife keeps her *'ear and eye on it'.*

The abdomen is palpated without delay to ensure that the lie of the second twin is longitudinal. Presentation and position are diagnosed, but are of less importance: the fetal heart is listened to. The midwife stands by. She will closely observe the uterus, probably keeping her hand lightly on it to detect uterine contractions. The fetal heart should be checked frequently.

With three or four good contractions and the woman pushing effectively the second baby ought to be born. But if, when 5 minutes have elapsed, contractions have not recommenced, the midwife should scrub up and after making sure that the head or the breech is presenting she should puncture the bag of membranes and massage the uterus to stimulate uterine action. The second baby should be born within 15 minutes after the first baby. (Doctors in hospital frequently deliver the second baby within a few minutes.)

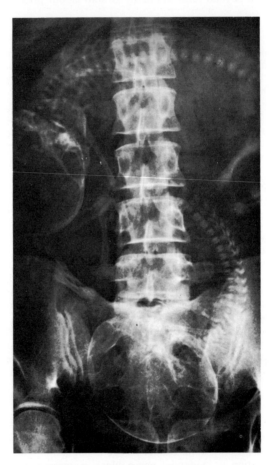

Fig. 21-32   Twins. One is presenting by the vertex; the other is lying transversely in the fundus.

*Simpson Memorial Maternity Pavilion, Edinburgh*

Ergometrine, 0·5 mg or Syntometrine, 1 ml, should be given intramuscularly as soon as both placentae are born to prevent postpartum haemorrhage. If Syntometrine is given inadvertently after the birth of the first baby, the second baby must be expelled immediately by fundal pressure. Midwives must always remember the possibility of an undiagnosed twin when they administer Syntometrine during the actual birth of a baby. The woman should not be left until at least two hours after the birth of the placentae and to ensure sleep a sedative is given.

**Transverse lie of the second twin**

If, after the birth of the first baby, the second baby is found to be presenting by the shoulder, the midwife should send for the doctor, but she must act pending his arrival because of the risk that the second bag of membranes will rupture and the arm prolapse. The midwife ought to attempt external version between contractions: this should not be unduly difficult, if the membranes are intact (see pp. 609, 649). The doctor will probably perform internal version for transverse lie of the second twin and do a breech extraction. In very remote areas, with no medical help available, the midwife should do likewise if external version has not been successful.

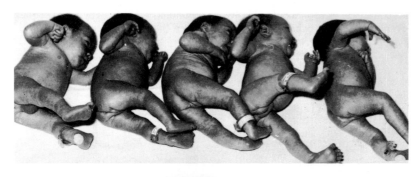

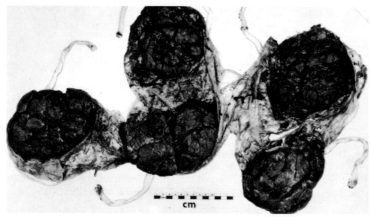

Fig. 21-33    Quintuplets born 1972. Weights: 1,470 g; 1,250 g; 1,490 g; 1,596 g; 1,250 g; Placentae 1,780 g.

Fig. 21-34    All discharged alive at 67 days. Mother's abdominal girth at 34 weeks = 125 cm.

*Maternity Unit, Bangour Hospital, Broxburn, West Lothian.*

**Delay in the birth of the second twin**

Should contractions not recommence within 20 minutes after having punctured the membranes medical assistance must be sought. Cases are known in which two or three days have elapsed between the births of the first and second babies: this should not be permitted to occur.

*The disadvantages of such delay are:*

The fetus *in utero* may die of anoxia should the placenta separate.

The risk of sepsis is increased when the cord is lying outside the vulva.

The cervix closes to a certain extent and will have to dilate again.

Having ensured that the lie is longitudinal, the doctor will probably puncture the membranes, and give an oxytocin drip, then when the uterus begins to contract he may apply forceps or use the Malmström vacuum extractor.

**The expulsion of a placenta or bleeding** before the birth of the second twin gives warning that the placenta still *in utero* may also be separating and causing hypoxia of the unborn twin; in which case, the midwife should massage the uterus and expel the second twin as soon as possible by using fundal pressure. (The usual sequence of events is for both babies to be born and then the placentae.)

**Postpartum haemorrhage** (see p. 423).

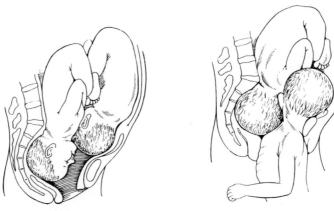

Fig. 21-35                    Fig. 21-36
Two varieties of locked twins.

**Locked twins** are very rare indeed, and the most serious variety occurs when the first fetus is presenting by the breech and the head of the second fetus which is presenting by the vertex gets in front of the aftercoming head of the first baby. The heads become impacted and decapitation of the head of the first baby is usually necessary.

### Management of the Puerperium

Involution of the uterus may be slow; afterpains are more troublesome. The care of the babies is a most urgent problem, as the number of twin babies who die is alarmingly high, the smaller one may be light for date (see p. 534). The mother will need help and advice in regard to feeding, and should not be discharged from hospital until the babies are gaining weight satisfactorily.

## POSTMATURITY

**After the 41st week of pregnancy postmaturity is assumed.** Recent recommendations to allow pregnancy to continue until the 42nd week are now being reconsidered: the high death rate of postmature babies being associated with conditions that cause placental dysfunction, e.g. pre-eclampsia. Postmaturity and pre-eclampsia, a combination that is particularly lethal to the fetus during labour ought to be avoided.

**Older primigravidae** and others with a poor obstetric history are not usually permitted to go beyond 40 weeks. Unfortunately conclusive evidence of postmaturity is not always available when the decision has to be made whether the woman has gone beyond the calculated date of confinement.

The date of her last menstrual period may be in doubt and 'post pill' amenorrhoea is conducive to this.

On abdominal palpation at term the amount of amniotic fluid seems scanty and more so after term.

## MANAGEMENT

### Induction of labour

**To ripen the cervix,** Prostaglandin $E_2$ gel may be introduced into the extra amniotic space or posterior vaginal fornix: a further dose may be needed to induce labour.

**The fetus being at risk is monitored carefully during labour.** Because of the hard head, moulding does not occur successfully and delivery by forceps may be necessary.

### THE POSTMATURE BABY

There are no absolute criteria of postmaturity. Hard skull bones, small fontanelles and narrow sutures are suggestive, but not conclusive. Excessive weight is not decisive: babies at term may weigh 4·5 kg. The baby's skin is loose, due to loss of subcutaneous fat. and may be dry, cracked and desquamating, nails long; but these are sometimes seen in babies who are not postmature. The placenta gives no reliable clue.

---

## QUESTIONS FOR REVISION
### OCCIPITO-POSTERIOR POSITION OF THE VERTEX

#### Oral Questions

Why does a high head occur in posterior positions of the vertex? How would you diagnose posterior position on (a) inspection; (b) palpation; (c) auscultation.

Describe on vaginal examination: R.O.P.; deep transverse arrest.

What is the probable course of labour?

Describe head moulding in face to pubes. How would you diagnose face to pubes when the head is on the perineum?

Why is the perineum liable to be lacerated?

Describe how you deliver the head face to pubes.

Describe (a) diagnosis of R.O.P. during labour; (b) clinical features of labour in R.O.P.; (c) management of deep transverse arrest.

**C.M.B.(Scot.) 30-min. question.** What do you understand by the term 'persistent occipito-posterior'? How would you recognise that delay in labour was due to this cause?

**C.M.B.(Eng.) 30-min. question.** How may the posterior position of the occiput affect the course and outcome of labour?

**C.M.B.Eng.** Labour is commencing with the fetal occiput in the posterior of the mother's pelvis. Discuss the possible outcomes of this labour.

#### C.M.B. Short Questions

**Eng.:** Occipito-posterior positions in labour. **Scot.:** Deep transverse arrest of the head. **N.Ire.:** Diagnosis of occipito-posterior position. **Eng.:** Recognition of deep transverse arrest of the fetal head. **N.Ire.:** Possible effects of occipito-posterior in labour. **Scot.:** Delivery of the head face to pubes.

### MULTIPLE PREGNANCY

## *Oral Questions*

Why is it advisable for twins to be born in hospital? What procedures, normally outside her province, might a midwife have to perform during delivery of twins?

Give another name for: (*a*) conjoined twins; (*b*) monozygotic twins; (*c*) fetus papyraceous. Why does the woman pregnant with twins become anaemic? Why is folic acid always prescribed? What advice could you give to relieve pressure symptoms? How would a midwife diagnose multiple pregnancy? What is the danger of giving Syntometrine in a twin labour? How would you do external version for the second twin? The smaller of twin babies may be light for date, what will the midwife be required to do in such a case?

Differentiate between: (*a*) uniovular and binovular twins; (*b*) twins and polyhydramnios; (*c*) multiple pregnancy and multiparity.

For what complications would you require medical assistance?

Describe (*a*) the effect of twins on pregnancy; (*b*) nutrition of the pregnant woman with twins; (*c*) the effect of twins on labour; (*d*) the management of labour in twins; (*e*) delay in the birth of the second twin.

**N.Ire. 30-min. question.** What features would make you suspect that a patient had a multiple pregnancy? In what way is such a patient at increased risk during the antenatal period?

**C.M.B.(Scot.) 30-min. question.** Describe the management of labour in a patient with multiple pregnancy.

**C.M.B.(Eng.) 30-min. question.** What would make you suspect a multiple pregnancy? Discuss the antenatal complications and the management of a twin pregnancy.

**N.Ire.** (*a*) How may a twin pregnancy be recognised? (*b*) Describe the management of a multiparous patient with a twin pregnancy during the last trimester.

## POSTMATURITY

Why is the woman with pre-eclampsia not permitted to go beyond term?
Describe the nursing care in postmature labour.
Why is the fetus at high risk?

# 22
# Malpresentations

*Breech: diagnosis, management, extended legs, arms, head. Face: diagnosis, management. Brow. Shoulder. Unstable lie*

## BREECH PRESENTATION

In breech or pelvic presentation, the fetus lies with its buttocks in the lower pole of the uterus. Breech presentation occurs in 2·5 to 3 per cent of cases after the 34th week of pregnancy. During mid-term the frequency is higher because the greater ratio of amniotic fluid facilitates spontaneous version of the fetus.

### VARIETIES

**Complete breech**

The fetal attitude is one of complete flexion, thighs and legs both flexed.

**Incomplete breech**

Breech with extended legs (frank breech). The legs are extended on the abdomen, thighs flexed.

Footling presentation (*rare*). One or both feet present because neither thighs nor legs are fully flexed.

Knee presentation (*rarer still*). Thighs are extended, one or both legs are flexed.

**Positions**

There are six positions, the denominator being the sacrum.

| | | | |
|---|---|---|---|
| Right sacro-posterior | R.S.P. | Left sacro-posterior | L.S.P. |
| Right sacro-lateral | R.S.L. | Left sacro-lateral | L.S.L. |
| Right sacro-anterior | R.S.A. | Left sacro-anterior | L.S.A. |

**Causes**

In the majority of cases there is no obvious reason why the fetus presents by the breech at term, for the ovoid shape of the uterine cavity and greater breadth in the fundus is conducive to cephalic presentation:

| | | |
|---|---|---|
| **Preterm labour** | **Polyhydramnios** | **Extended legs** |
| **Multiple pregnancy** | **Hydrocephaly** | |

Extended legs occur in over 80 per cent of cases, commonly in primigravid women with high uterine muscle tone, and this inhibits the free turning of the fetus which usually occurs at mid-term.

In polyhydramnios the cavity of the uterus may be round because of excessive amniotic fluid but the breech is readily diagnosed on the X-ray performed in such cases and easily rectified by external version.

The fetal head may be proportionately large as in hydrocephaly or to some extent in the preterm baby and can be more readily accommodated in the fundus.

## PRENATAL DIAGNOSIS

This may not be easy in the primigravid woman who has firm abdominal muscles. The figures of undiagnosed breech presentation range from 10 to 15 per cent.

### ABDOMINAL EXAMINATION

**Inspection**

The abdominal contour of the complete breech is not different from that of the vertex presentation.

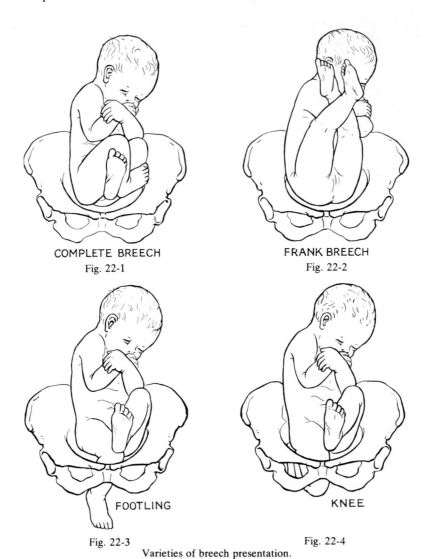

| | |
|---|---|
| COMPLETE BREECH | FRANK BREECH |
| Fig. 22-1 | Fig. 22-2 |
| FOOTLING | KNEE |
| Fig. 22-3 | Fig. 22-4 |

Varieties of breech presentation.

**Palpation**

At the pelvic brim a large, soft, indefinite mass is felt.

In the fundus, at one or other side, a round, hard mass may be detected, and by ballotting this mass with one or both hands it can be made to move independently of the back (nodding of the head). To identify the head, the fetal back is grasped between the palms of both hands and an attempt made to ballotte with the fingers what is thought to be the head. If the breech is anterior and the fetus well flexed it may be difficult to locate the head. If doubt exists, the combined grip is useful (p. 138).

### Auscultation

The fetal heart is heard at or above the level of the umbilicus in a complete breech, because the presenting part does not usually engage until labour begins. The fetal heart is further from the buttocks than from the head; when the legs are extended the breech engages so the fetal heart is heard at a lower level.

## PRENATAL MANAGEMENT

If the midwife suspects or detects a breech presentation on or after the 32nd week she should arrange for her patient to see a doctor or attend a prenatal clinic.

X-rays may be employed because of doubt in diagnosis and in cases of failed version.

### *The following points are noted on X-ray:*

The size and shape of the pelvis.       Whether the legs are extended.
Size of the fetus.                      Fetal abnormalities, e.g. hydrocephaly.

**Ultrasonography** may be used, the head being located in the fundus.

### *External Version*

External version may be attempted (if no contraindications exist) for two reasons:

1. Cephalo-pelvic disproportion cannot be detected unless the head is at the pelvic brim. 2. To avoid the dangers to the fetus of breech delivery.

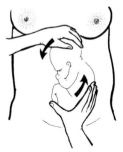 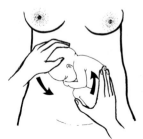 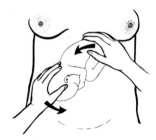

Fig. 22-5  Right hand lifts breech out of pelvis. Left hand makes head follow the nose. Flexion of head and back maintained throughout.

Fig. 22-6  Flexion is continued. Left hand brings head downwards. Right hand pushes breech upwards.

Fig.    22-7  Pressure   is exerted on head and breech simultaneously until head is lying at the pelvic brim.

External version of breech to vertex.

Spontaneous cephalic version may take place up to the 34th week (*rarely later*). The risks of external version are rupture of membranes and placental separation due to traction on the cord, but these are less frequent than the actual dangers of breech delivery. The doctor is likely to decide against external version if there is hypertension, Rh−ve patient, antepartum haemorrhage or if a Caesarean section has previously been performed.

The optimal time for performing version is between the 32nd and 36th weeks: but some authorities do so earlier. If external version fails a careful assessment of the pelvis is made. Extended legs and scanty amniotic fluid are the main causes of failed version.

If the fetus is hydrocephalic, breech presentation is an advantage, as it may be possible after the buttocks are born to drain off the cerebrospinal fluid *via* the spinal canal.

### MECHANISM OF LABOUR

**Left sacro-anterior, L.S.A.**

**Lie,** longitudinal.  
**Attitude,** Complete flexion.  
**Presentation,** breech.  
**Position,** left sacro-anterior.  
**Denominator,** sacrum.  
**Presenting part,** anterior buttock.

The bitrochanteric diameter, 10 cm, enters in the left oblique diameter of the pelvic brim. The sacrum points to the left ilio-pectineal eminence.

**Descent** takes place with increasing compaction, due to increased flexion of limbs.

**Internal rotation of the buttocks.** The anterior buttock reaches the pelvic floor first and rotates one-eighth of a circle forwards along the right side of the pelvis. The bitrochanteric diameter is now in the antero-posterior diameter of the outlet.

**Lateral flexion of the body.** The anterior buttock escapes under the symphysis pubis, the posterior buttock sweeps the perineum and the buttocks are born by a movement of lateral flexion.

**Restitution of the buttocks.** The anterior buttock turns slightly to the patient's right side.

**Internal rotation of the shoulders.** The shoulders enter in the same oblique of the brim as the buttocks—the left oblique. The anterior shoulder rotates forwards one-eighth of a circle along the right side of the pelvis and escapes under the symphysis pubis, the posterior shoulder sweeps the perineum and the shoulders are born.

**Internal rotation of the head.** The head enters in the transverse diameter of the pelvic brim. The occiput rotates forwards along the left side, and the sub-occipital region (*nape of the neck*) impinges on the under surface of the symphysis pubis.

**External rotation of the body.** The body turns so that the back is uppermost, a movement which accompanies internal rotation of the head.

**Birth of the head.** The chin, face and sinciput sweep the perineum and the head is born in a flexed attitude.

### DANGERS TO THE BABY

The dangers to the baby are very great indeed and except in the hands of experts the perinatal mortality rate is 10 per cent. Some induce labour at 38 weeks if the fetus is large because big babies are especially vulnerable.

**Preterm birth,** particularly if the baby weighs under 1·8 kg, intensifies all the other dangers and 50 per cent of breech stillbirths are preterm. The skull bones are soft and the brain is easily damaged. The relatively large head may be 'held up' by a cervix which has allowed extended legs to pass, causing dangerous delay and hypoxia. (*The complete breech dilates the cervix to a greater extent.*)

**Intracranial haemorrhage** is due to the rapid compression of the aftercoming head which has not had the opportunity of slow moulding as when the vertex presents. Fetal blood is forced upwards into the intracranial venous sinuses and the hypoxia, frequently present, causes venous congestion.

The severe compression of the head coming through the cervix and vulva and its sudden release if extracted quickly (like a cork out of a bottle) also produce intracranial trauma. To avoid the latter an episiotomy is made.

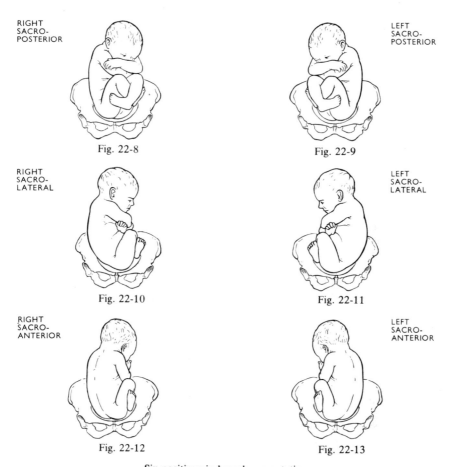

RIGHT SACRO-POSTERIOR

Fig. 22-8

LEFT SACRO-POSTERIOR

Fig. 22-9

RIGHT SACRO-LATERAL

Fig. 22-10

LEFT SACRO-LATERAL

Fig. 22-11

RIGHT SACRO-ANTERIOR

Fig. 22-12

LEFT SACRO-ANTERIOR

Fig. 22-13

Six positions in breech presentation.

### Hypoxia may be due to the following causes:

#### (A) *Interference with the Utero-placental Circulation*

By the application of fundal pressure (*inadvisedly*).
When the placenta separates while the head is still in the vagina.
By marked retraction of the placental site before birth of the head.

#### (B) *Interference with the Cord Circulation*

**Cord compression.** This is inevitable with a large baby and when the legs are extended, because the cord becomes nipped when the fetal shoulders and head pass through the pelvic brim and through the cervix. (The head enters the brim when the baby presenting by the breech is born as far as the umbilicus.) The cord is severely compressed also when the hard head is passing through the vulval ring.

**Prolapse of cord** occurs because the complete breech is a badly fitting presenting part and also because the umbilicus is so near the buttocks.

### (C) *Premature Inspiration*

If the oxygen supply is diminished because of the preceding causes, the fetus will be stimulated to breathe and will inhale fluid or mucus which may prevent expansion of the lungs at birth and may cause pneumonia.

### (D) *Injuries*

The fetus is usually injured because of rough or wrong handling. Patience and gentleness are needed but when interference becomes imperative the midwife must know how to avoid injuries such as:

Fractures of humerus or clavicle when dealing with extended arms.
Damage to the brachial plexus by twisting the neck, causing Erb's paralysis.
Ruptured liver, produced by grasping the abdomen.
Damage to adrenals by grasping the baby's body at kidney level.
Crushing the spinal cord or fracturing the neck by bending the body backwards over the symphysis pubis while delivering the head.

## MANAGEMENT OF LABOUR

Because of the risks to the fetus, multiparae as well as primigravidae should be delivered in hospital where expert assistance is available. The woman should not be allowed to go beyond her date, labour is induced, sometimes at 38 weeks. Caesarean section is frequently performed for breech presentation per se as well as for complications such as infertility, older primigravida, bad obstetric history, contracted pelvis, fetal distress.

Epidural analgesia is now employed more frequently; advantages being that the urge to push prematurely is inhibited and the incidence of fetal and maternal acidosis is reduced. The woman can push on command: necessary manipulative measures are facilitated.

### *The Principles of Treatment are:*

Intelligent observation.
The avoidance of unnecessary interference.
Prompt action, carried out with manual dexterity when assistance is needed.
The avoidance of fetal injury and hypoxia.

### THE FIRST STAGE OF LABOUR

Labour is conducted as in vertex presentation, including sedation. An enema should be given, and if the breech is engaged the woman ought to be allowed up unless bed rest is necessary for electronic monitoring or the administration of i.v. oxytocin to accelerate the retarded latent phase of labour. The passage of meconium during the first stage may be a sign of fetal distress but is likely to be due to compression of the fetal abdomen.

### VAGINAL EXAMINATION

A vaginal examination is always made in breech presentation, immediately after the membranes rupture, for the following reasons:

To find out whether the cord has prolapsed.

To ascertain whether the breech is complete or incomplete.
To determine the dilatation of the cervix.
To assess the station of the breech.

### Findings

**Prolapse of cord** is probably the cardinal indication for making the vaginal examination and is a serious complication.

**Complete breech.** A high, soft, irregular mass presents, with feet lying alongside the buttocks: sacrum and coccyx are recognisable. The anal sphincter will grip the examining finger. (Meconium on the examining finger is diagnostic of breech presentation.)

**Incomplete breech.** If the legs are extended, no feet are felt. The external genitalia are very evident. In a footling presentation doubt may arise as to whether the prolapsed limb is a hand or a foot. Toes are all the same length; they are shorter than fingers and the great toe cannot be abducted. The foot is at right angles to the leg and the os calcis (heel bone) has no equivalent on the hand.

**Dilatation of the cervix.** This ought to be carefully assessed, because it is important that the midwife should be aware when the first stage is completed.

**The station** of the breech may be high during the latent phase; descent being more rapid during the active phase.

### Monitoring the Fetal Condition

The fetal heart rate should be auscultated before, during and for 15 seconds after each contraction during the active phase of the first stage. In a number of centres continuous electronic monitoring of the fetal heart rate pattern is carried out as soon as labour is established: an electrode being attached to the fetal buttock. If the tracing indicates hypoxia, fetal blood sampling is done. Some take blood samples at the end of the first stage when cord compression by the cervix is maximal, and again when the umbilicus appears at the vulva because the contracting empty fundus diminishes the placental site area and reduces the oxygen supply to the fetus.

### The Avoidance of Premature Pushing

No pushing should occur until the buttocks are bulging at the vulva. If the buttocks are forced through an imperfectly dilated cervix, the birth of the head may be delayed at the critical moment after the shoulders are born. In a footling presentation the cervix may be only 5 cm when the foot appears at the vulva. (It is possible that with extended legs the cervix may not be fully dilated although the buttocks are visible on separating the labia.)

The head of the preterm baby, being proportionately large, is liable to be held up by the cervix which has not been sufficiently dilated by the smaller buttock mass.

**A vaginal examination should always be made to ensure that the cervix is fully dilated before allowing the woman to push.**

### THE SECOND STAGE

**An assisted breech.** The legs and trunk are born by the natural forces, assistance being given for the birth of the shoulders and head.

**A breech extraction.** A manipulative delivery under inhalational or epidural analgesia by the doctor.

## MANAGEMENT

When the buttocks are bulging at the vulva, the woman should be lying on her back, with two pillows under her head, and encouraged to bear down. The temptation to assist, by using fundal pressure, must be resisted in case the placental circulation is impeded, oxygen supply reduced and the fetus stimulated to breathe *in utero*. Using traction is much more liable to cause extension of arms and head than the mother's expulsive efforts so she must be encouraged to push.

ANTERIOR

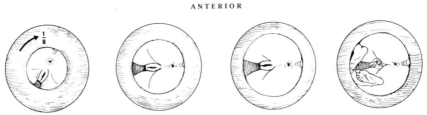

Figs. 22-14–22-17　Vaginal touch pictures of breech presentation L.S.A.

Fig. 22-14　Left sacro-anterior position. Anal sphincter grips examining finger.

Fig. 22-15　Anterior buttock has rotated forwards one-eighth of a circle. Bitrochanteric diameter in antero-posterior diameter of pelvis.

Fig. 22-16　No feet felt. Legs extended.

Fig. 22-17　Feet felt. Complete breech presentation.

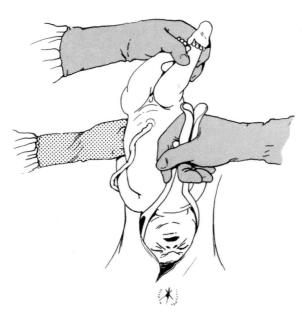

Fig. 22-18　Application of forceps to the aftercoming head.

The room and the cot should be warm, resuscitation equipment ready to treat a hypoxic infant, vitamin $K_1$ available. The bladder should be empty so that suprapubic pressure will be effective and bladder injury avoided.

Syringes, a local analgesic, requirements for local analgesia, scissors and suturing requirements ought to be set out for a large episiotomy.

Forceps for the aftercoming head should always be in readiness, for, if required, there must be no delay. This is a routine procedure in many centres, to give adequate control of the head.

Some give epidural analgesia: good pelvic floor relaxation being advantageous.

The paediatrician is present in a number of hospitals to take charge of the baby.

### BIRTH OF THE BABY

With the patient's buttocks at the edge of the bed it is possible to allow the baby to hang and to apply suprapubic pressure to the head if required. The midwife would be justified in making an episiotomy, e.g. a primigravid woman, or a multipara with a small or very large baby. (It is essential that a doctor or senior midwife, who is competent and thoroughly experienced in breech deliveries, should be 'scrubbed up' in readiness to assist the novice should the need arise.) The administration of Syntometrine is delayed until the baby is born.

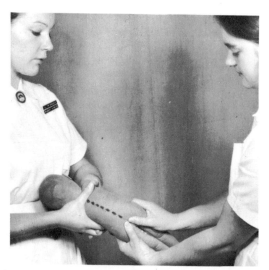

Fig. 22-19 Student midwives practising delivery of breech. Grasping iliac crests: thumbs on sacrum to avoid compression of adrenals: using downward traction to deliver the anterior shoulder.

*Aberdeen Maternity Hospital classroom.*

The buttocks should be expelled by the unaided, bearing-down efforts of the mother and it is therefore an advantage to have a conscious patient so that she can co-operate.

**'Hands off the breech'** is a good motto at this stage for the midwife, who should exhort the woman to push. The buttocks curve upwards, the feet become disengaged at the vulva, and with the same contraction the baby is born as far as the umbilicus. *Doctors in hospital tend to do an 'episiotomy and assisted breech delivery'; some give a pudendal nerve block.* Fetal blood sampling to detect hypoxia is sometimes carried out when the baby is born as far as the umbilicus.

A loop of cord is pulled down, mainly to avoid traction on the umbilicus. The cord should be handled gently to avoid inducing spasm of the cord vessels; traction on the umbilicus occurs if the cord is not pulled down and this will also induce spasm. If the cord is being nipped under the pubic arch it should be moved down to the perineum. Feel if the elbows are on the chest: they usually are. Wait for the next contraction but do not delay too long; keep the dangers of hypoxia in mind.

### DELIVERY OF THE SHOULDERS

The weight of the buttocks will bring the shoulders down on to the pelvic floor, where they will rotate into the antero-posterior diameter of the outlet.

The midwife can assist the expulsion of the shoulders by using downward traction while the uterus is contracting and the woman pushing. The baby should be grasped by the iliac crests (*with thumbs on the sacrum and not high enough to compress the adrenals*). A small towel may be wrapped round the baby's hips as they are slippery to hold but this must not be allowed to interfere with the necessary manipulation.

When the anterior shoulder escapes, the buttocks are elevated to allow the posterior shoulder and arm to pass over the perineum. The back must not be turned uppermost until the shoulders have been born, in order that the head will descend through the transverse diameter of the pelvis. If the back is turned up before the shoulders are born, the head will enter the antero-posterior diameter of the brim and become extended; the shoulders may then become impacted at the outlet and the extended head may cause difficulty.

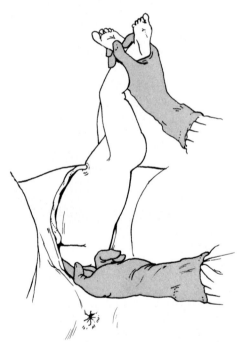

Fig. 22-20  Delivery of the posterior shoulder.

### DELIVERY OF THE HEAD

#### The Burns Marshall Method

As soon as the shoulders are born, the infant is allowed to hang by its own weight, which brings the head down to the pelvic floor on which the occiput rotates forwards. If this does not take place two fingers should be placed on the malar

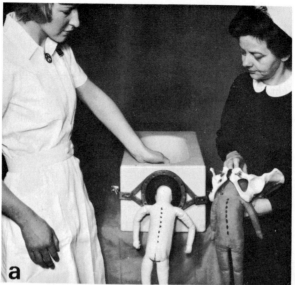
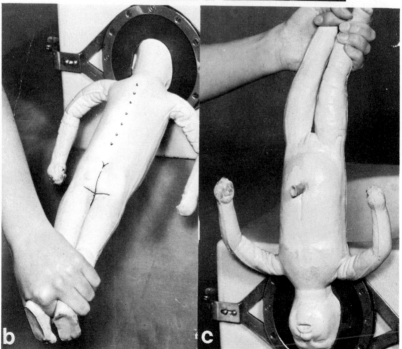

Fig. 22-21 The Burns Marshall method of delivery.

a, Baby hangs for one or two minutes until the hairline appears.
b, Baby grasped by the feet and held on the    c, Mouth and nose are free. The vault of the
stretch.                                                          head is delivered slowly.

*Aberdeen Maternity Hospital.*

bones and the head rotated. The back is now uppermost. The baby can be allowed to hang for one or two minutes. Gradually the neck elongates, the hair-line appears and the suboccipital region can be felt.

The baby is grasped by the feet and held on the stretch; sufficient traction being applied to prevent the baby's neck from bending backwards and being fractured. The suboccipital region, and not the neck, should pivot under the apex of the pubic arch, or the spinal cord may be crushed. The feet are taken up through an arc of 180 degrees until the mouth and nose are free at the vulva. The baby is now being held upside down and any mucus or amniotic fluid can drain from the lungs and trachea. Mechanical suction or mucus extractors may be used. The nose and mouth are wiped with gauze swabs. If the airway is clear the baby will breathe because lungs, trachea, nose and mouth are free. Two or three minutes should elapse to allow the vault of the head to be expelled, and this is best accomplished when the mother takes deliberate regular breaths—**'breathing the head out'.** Supra-pubic pressure may be required to aid expulsion of the head.

# BREECH WITH EXTENDED LEGS

The frank breech occurs in about 80 per cent of breech presentations and is commonly found in primigravid women, probably because firm uterine walls and strong abdominal muscles predispose to a more rigid attitude of the fetus.

**On inspection**

The uterus looks long and narrow.

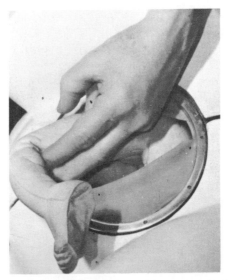

Fig. 22-22 Classroom demonstration of assisting delivery of extended legs at the vulval orifice. Pressure on popliteal space. Splinting and abduction of femur. Flexion of knee joint. Extraction of foot.

*Aberdeen Maternity Hospital.*

**On palpation**

The frank breech forms a snug, firm mass that may engage before labour begins and may easily be mistaken for the head. If the breech does not engage, the straight spine may cause the head to be pushed under the costal margin where it is not readily palpated. (The woman complains of pain in that region when she is sitting.) The nodding movement of the head is not manifest if the head is caught between the feet; the knobbly feet and knees are not palpable. Failed external version is suggestive of extended legs.

### On auscultation

The fetal heart will be heard below the umbilicus when the frank breech is engaged, and this adds to the likelihood of the diagnosis of vertex, L.O.A., head engaged—instead of breech, L.S.A.

### Per vaginam

If, after the cervix is 5 cm dilated, no feet can be felt, the legs are extended. The buttocks are firm to the touch, round and smooth because the presenting mass is more compact. The external genitalia are more evident.

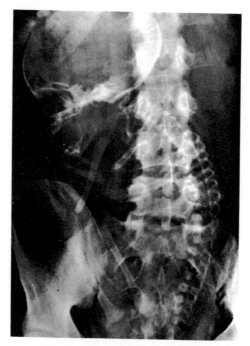

Fig. 22-23   X-ray of frank breech.
*Simpson Memorial Maternity Pavilion, Edinburgh.*

### *Management of Extended Legs*

The frank breech is a better fitting presenting part than the complete breech, so it descends more rapidly during the first stage. The cervix dilates more quickly and the risk of cord compression is greater but prolapse of cord is less likely. Delay may occur at the outlet because the legs splint the body and impede lateral flexion of the spine. An episiotomy is made.

The baby can be born with its legs extended, but assistance is usually required. When the popliteal fossae appear at the vulva, pressure on the fossa of the most accessible leg combined with abduction of the thigh will flex the knee and aid extraction of the foot which should be swept over the baby's abdomen.

The knee is a hinge joint that bends only in one direction so traction must not be exerted on the anterior surface of the knee. Severe injury to the knee joint can occur from doing so.

# EXTENDED ARMS

Extended arms are diagnosed when the elbows are not felt on the chest after the umbilicus is born or if there is no advance then, with good contractions. In the absence of medical aid the midwife must act promptly or the baby may be hypoxic: she must know what to do and how to do it; unless the manipulation is carried out competently, fracture or paralysis of the arms may result.

The Løvset manoeuvre is successful in the bringing down of extended arms.

## THE LØVSET MANOEUVRE

This manoeuvre is a combination of rotation and downward traction, that can be used successfully whether the arms are extended, flexed, or round the nape of the neck. It makes delivery of inaccessible extended arms possible, and is efficacious in cases when, because of a large baby, there is no room in the vagina for manipulation in bringing arms down. The direction of rotation must always bring the back uppermost. The arms are delivered from under the pubic arch.

A, When the umbilicus is born and the shoulders are in the antero-posterior diameter, downward traction is applied until the axilla is visible, the midwife grasping the baby by the iliac crests with thumbs on the sacrum.

B, The body is rotated half a circle, 180 degrees (when starting rotation the back must be turned uppermost in order that the shoulders may enter the transverse of the pelvic brim). Downward traction must be maintained throughout the manoeuvre or it will not succeed. Rotation is in an anticlockwise direction in an L.S.A.

C, The arm that was posterior is now anterior, ready for delivery.

D, The arm now anterior is delivered from under the pubic arch. The first two fingers of the left-hand splint the humerus to avoid breaking it and the elbow is drawn downwards.

E, The posterior arm must now be made anterior so the body is rotated half a circle in a clockwise direction: still using downward traction.

F, The back is uppermost during the half-circle rotation started in E.

G, Downward traction makes the anterior arm accessible.

H, Using the right hand, the humerus is splinted and drawn downwards if it is not delivered without aid.

## EXTENDED HEAD

If, when the body has been allowed to hang, the neck and hair-line are not visible, it is probable that the head is extended.

### MAURICEAU-SMELLIE-VEIT MANOEUVRE

This method should only be used when forceps are not available. Traction on the shoulders may cause Erb's paralysis.

A moderate degree of suprapubic pressure is used in a downward, backward

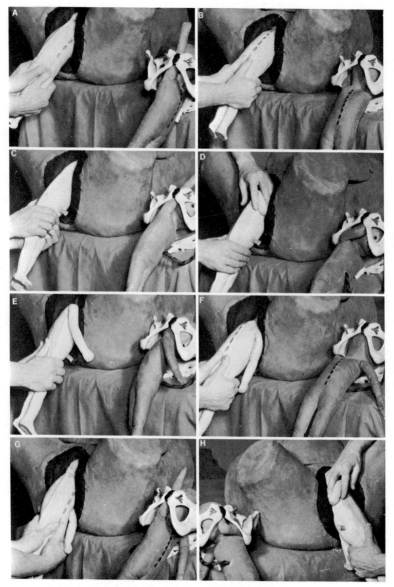

Fig. 22-24   The Løvset manoeuvre, L.S.A.
*Photographed at Aberdeen Maternity Hospital.*

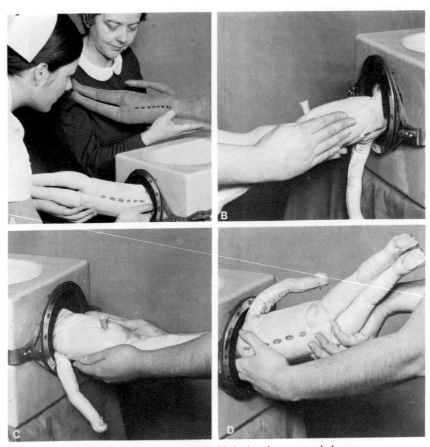

Fig. 22-25  Classical method of bringing down extended arms.

A, Midwife's left hand supports the buttocks. Posterior arm brought down first, using hand corresponding to the baby's back. Index and middle fingers splint the humerus to avoid fracturing it. Baby's forearm is flexed over his face like a 'cat washing its face'. The elbow is brought down, wrist grasped and the hand brought out.

B, The hands splint the body while rotating it in the same direction as the hand that is out is pointing (otherwise the arm in the vagina will be displaced behind the baby's neck in the nuchal position, a serious complication which can be avoided or rectified by the Løvset manoeuvre).

C, Rotation is continued until the arm in the vagina is in the hollow of the sacrum, i.e. posterior.

D, Midwife's right hand supports the buttocks and with her left hand the posterior arm is brought down as in (A).

*Photographed at Aberdeen Maternity Hospital.*

direction to increase flexion and descent of the head. (To avoid injury to the bladder, while using suprapubic pressure, the bladder is always emptied during preparation for delivery of breech presentation.)

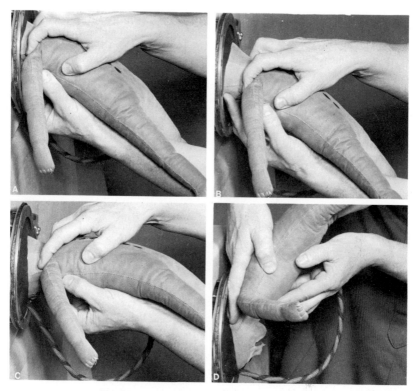

Fig. 22-26   Mauriceau-Smellie-Veit manoeuvre.

A, Baby astride left arm with palm supporting chest. First and third fingers of left hand on malar bones to flex head. (Some place the middle finger in the mouth (well back) to aid flexion.) First two fingers of right hand hooked over shoulders, pull in a downward direction. Traction on the shoulders must not be excessive.

B, Controlled traction is exerted in a downward direction as the head descends in the curved birth canal.

C, Traction continued in an outward direction until suboccipital area appears. If upward traction is carried out too soon fracture of the neck could be inflicted.

D, Traction exerted in an upward direction to expedite birth of the head. Nose and mouth are free so the air-way is cleared. The vault is delivered slowly.

*Photographed at Aberdeen Maternity Hospital.*

### Causes and Treatment of Delay in Breech Presentation

**Delay in the first stage is rare** and may be caused by impaction due to a large baby or a small pelvis or to weak contractions. Medical aid is necessary. Caesarean section would no doubt be performed.

**Delay during the second stage** is usually caused by extended legs and in such a case the midwife should not interfere until the buttocks are bulging at the outlet. If the doctor is not available and fetal distress is manifest, a medio-lateral episiotomy ought to be made then steady traction should be used with two fingers in the groins, pulling mainly in the posterior groin, in an outward upward direction, to aid lateral flexion.

**Delay in the birth of the head** may occur because the head of a preterm baby is large in proportion to the breech and is held up by the insufficiently dilated cervix.

If the midwife is unable to extract the head and the baby is making gasping movements, she should mop the vaginal wall in contact with the baby's face and by inserting two fingers make a channel through which air can reach the baby.

If the head is arrested high in the pelvic cavity disproportion may exist; suprapubic pressure may help but the application of forceps will likely be necessary. Should the baby be small the possibility of a hydrocephalic head must be considered.

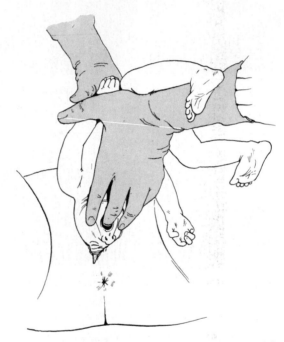

Fig. 22-27   Extraction of the head by Mauriceau-Smellie-Veit grip.

### Posterior Rotation of the Occiput

This malrotation of the head is rare and is usually the result of mismanagement, for the back should not be turned upwards until the shoulders are born.

To deliver the head, face to pubes, the chin and face are permitted to escape under the symphysis pubis as far as the root of the nose; the occiput then sweeps the perineum. The application of forceps may be necessary.

*All breech babies should be admitted to the special care unit for the first few days: vitamin K₁ is administered.*

## FACE PRESENTATION

When the attitude of the head is one of complete extension, with the occiput in contact with the spine, the face will present at the pelvic brim.

The frequency is about 1 in 500 cases and the majority develop from vertex to face after the onset of labour, i.e. secondary face presentation. When the face presents before labour, the term 'primary face presentation' is used, and the anencephalic fetus is the main example.

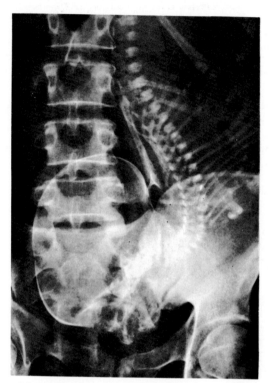

Fig. 22-28   X-ray of face presentation. Left-mento-posterior. Note extension of the spine.

## POSITIONS

*There are six positions in face presentation: denominator the mentum*

| | | |
|---|---|---|
| **Right mento-posterior R.M.P.** | **Left mento-posterior** | **L.M.P.** |
| **Right mento-lateral   R.M.L.** | **Left mento-lateral** | **L.M.L.** |
| **Right mento-anterior  R.M.A.** | **Left mento-anterior** | **L.M.A.** |

## CAUSES

### Anterior uterine obliquity

This is the commonest maternal cause. When the fetus presents as a posterior vertex in a multiparous patient the pendulous abdomen causes the fetal buttocks to lean forwards and the force of the uterine contractions is exerted in a line directed to the chin rather than to the occiput, causing the head to extend.

### Contracted pelvis

In the flat pelvis, the head enters in the transverse of the brim and the parietal eminences may be held up in the obstetrical conjugate, the head becomes extended and face presentation develops. Or, if the head in the posterior position (vertex presenting) remains deflexed, the parietal eminences may be caught in the sacrocotyloid dimension, the occiput does not descend, the head becomes extended, and face presentation results.

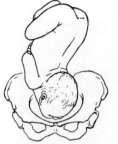
Fig. 22-29   Right mento-posterior.

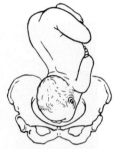
Fig. 22-30   Left mento-posterior.

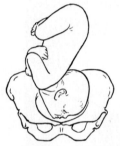
Fig. 22-31   Right mento-lateral.

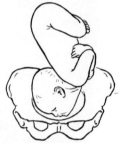
Fig. 22-32   Left mento-lateral.

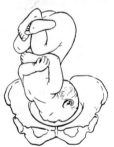
Fig. 22-33   Right mento-anterior.

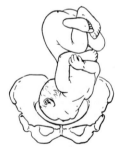
Fig. 22-34   Left mento-anterior.

Six positions of face presentation.

### Polyhydramnios

If the vertex is presenting and the membranes rupture spontaneously, the head may extend with the rush of fluid as it sinks into the lower uterine segment.

### Anencephaly

This is a common fetal cause because the vertex is absent, and if the head lies in the lower pole of the uterus when labour starts the face enters the pelvic brim.

### DIAGNOSIS

**On inspection.** There is nothing diagnostic.

**On palpation.** Face presentation may not be detected. (If the doll is placed in the pelvis as a right mento-posterior, the prominent occiput may be seen in the left anterior quadrant of the pelvis with a furrow between the occiput and the extended back, but in practice the prominent occiput may be mistaken for the sinciput and an erroneous diagnosis of vertex (R.O.A.) made.) In mento-anterior positions the limbs are readily palpated being in close proximity to the abdominal wall.

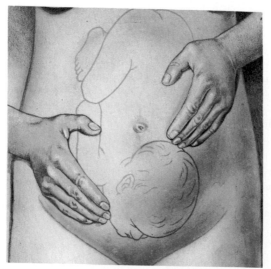

Fig. 22-35   Palpation of head in face presentation. Right mento-posterior.

ANTERIOR

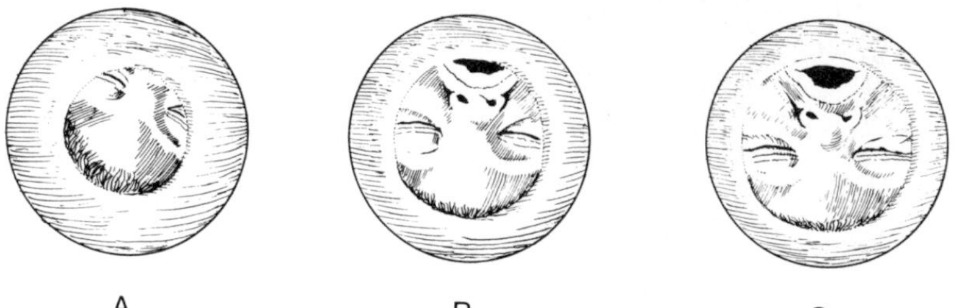

| A | B | C |

Fig. 22-36   Vaginal touch picture—left mento-anterior.

A, Mentum points to left anterior. Orbital ridges in left oblique diameter of pelvis.

B, With increased extension of the head the mouth (gums are diagnostic) can be felt.

C, Face has rotated one-eighth of a circle forward. Mentum now anterior and will eventually escape under the pubic arch.

**Auscultation.** When the chin is anterior the fetal heart is heard distinctly because the fetal chest is in contact with the mother's abdominal wall. When the chin is posterior the fetal heart is not easily heard because the fetal thorax is in contact with the mother's spine.

**Vaginal examination.** The presenting part is high, soft and irregular. A malpresentation is suspected when the smooth, hard vertex is not felt and sutures and fontanelles are absent.

Gums are diagnostic. Confusion between mouth and anus could arise, but the mouth is open, whereas the anus grips the examining finger and stains it with meconium. Lips and labia majora might be confused.

To determine position the chin should be located and, if it is posterior, the midwife should decide whether it is lower than the sinciput; if so, it will rotate forwards. In an R.M.A. the orbital ridge will be in the right oblique diameter of the pelvic brim or cavity.

Care must be taken to neither injure nor infect the eyes with the examining finger.

### MECHANISM OF LABOUR

The mechanism is fundamentally similar to that in a vertex presentation, except that, instead of an increase in flexion, there is increased extension, and the chin, instead of the occiput, becomes the leading part and rotates forwards. The head is born by flexion instead of extension.

### *Left Mento-anterior*

**Lie,** longitudinal.                         **Position,** L.M.A.
**Attitude,** extension of head and      **Denominator,** mentum.
                                    back
**Presentation,** face.                    **Presenting part,** left malar bone.

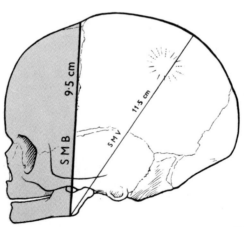

Fig. 22-37 Engaging diameters. The submento-bregmatic diameter, 9·5 cm, presents at the brim and appears at the vulva. The submento-vertical diameter, 11·5 cm, sweeps the perineum.

**Descent** takes place with increasing extension. **Internal rotation** occurs when the chin reaches the pelvic floor and rotates forwards one-eighth of a circle. The chin escapes under the symphysis pubis. **Flexion** takes place when the sinciput, vertex and occiput sweep the perineum; the head is born. **Restitution** occurs when the chin turns one-eighth of a circle to the patient's left. The shoulders enter in the left oblique and the anterior shoulder rotates one-eighth of a circle forwards along the right side of the pelvis, accompanied by external rotation of the head. (The shoulders are born as in a vertex presentation.)

## PROGNOSIS AND COURSE OF LABOUR

If the chin is anterior, less difficulty is encountered; if posterior and the head is well extended and contractions are effective, the chin will rotate forwards and the face will be born as in the anterior position.

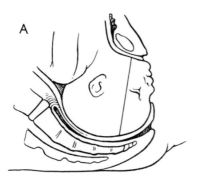 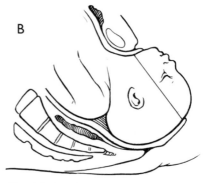

Fig. 22-38   Mechanism of birth of head in mento-anterior position.

A, Submento-bregmatic diameter at outlet, chin escapes under symphysis pubis.

B, Head is born by movement of flexion; the submento-vertical diameter will sweep the perineum.

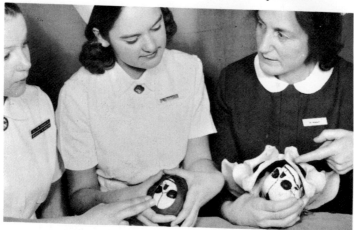

Fig. 22-39   Delivery of face presentation in dorsal position. Tutor demonstrates with doll: hands used as vulva, left mento-anterior. Keeping sinciput back until chin is delivered.

*Aberdeen Maternity Hospital.*

### *Delay in Labour is common for the following reasons:*

The face is a badly fitting presenting part which does not stimulate good uterine contractions and is a poor cervical dilator. The face bones do not mould. The face is shallow and to enable the chin to reach the pelvic floor the shoulders must also enter the pelvic cavity. There is misdirected force, because the fetal axis pressure is directed to the chin, and the head is almost at right angles to the spine.

Internal rotation may be arrested when the chin is posterior and the face becomes impacted when persistent mento-posterior occurs.

*The cord may prolapse.*
*Perineal laceration occurs* because the submento-vertical diameter, 11·5 cm, sweeps the perineum, which is also distended by the biparietal diameter.

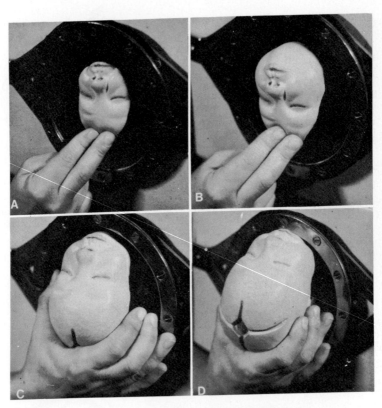

Fig. 22-40   Delivery of face presentation.
A, Holding back sinciput to increase extension of the head until the chin is born.
B, Chin is born, the head can now be flexed by the mother 'breathing the head out'.
C, Bringing the occiput over the perineum.
D, Flexion completed—head born.
*Aberdeen Maternity Hospital classroom.*

## MANAGEMENT OF LABOUR

The midwife must notify the doctor, but in 75 per cent of cases the babies are born spontaneously. A vaginal examination is made when the membranes rupture, to find out whether the cord has prolapsed; taking care neither to infect nor injure the eyes.

The fetal heart requires careful observation, an electronic monitor being advantageous. In mento-posterior cases the midwife must observe closely that the chin is the lowest point and that rotation and descent are taking place. If the head remains high in spite of good contractions, Caesarean section should be anticipated.

## DELIVERY OF THE BABY

The important point is to get the chin out before the head flexes, so, when the face appears at the vulva, extension should be maintained by holding back the sinciput to permit the chin to escape under the symphysis pubis before the occiput is allowed to sweep the perineum. In this way the submento-vertical diameter, 11·5 cm, distends the vaginal orifice instead of the mento-vertical diameter, 13·5 cm. An episiotomy and delivery by forceps may be necessary. The baby should be cot-nursed and kept quiet for a few days. Head retraction persists for some days; the face is congested and bruised, the eyelids and lips are oedematous. The babies stand labour remarkably well, however, considering the stretching to which the blood vessels and nerves in the neck are subjected. If the blue discoloration and the disfiguring oedema are excessive the mother should be assured before she is permitted to see her baby. Some wait until the bruising has subsided.

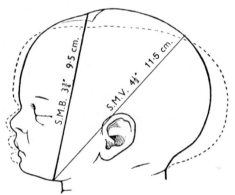

Fig. 22-41   Typical moulding in a face presentation, shown by dotted line.

### PERSISTENT MENTO-POSTERIOR

In this case the head is incompletely extended and the sinciput reaches the pelvic floor first and rotates forwards one-eighth of a circle: the chin goes into the hollow of the sacrum. There is no further mechanism: the face becomes impacted because the head and neck are completely extended and cannot negotiate the posterior wall of the pelvis. (Whatever lies in the hollow of the sacrum must sweep the perineum to be born.) In a persistent mento-posterior that is not possible because the fully extended neck lies in the hollow of the sacrum and the head cannot extend further.

### *Management*

The midwife must get medical aid at once and anticipate Caesarean section or pudendal block, episiotomy, forceps delivery and an asphyxiated baby. The doctor may attempt to increase extension of the head by pushing up the sinciput; he will then manually rotate the head and apply forceps.

In a neglected case when the face is impacted and the baby dead, craniotomy through the orbit will be necessary.

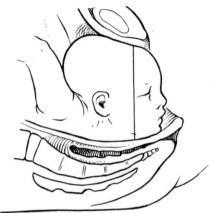

Fig. 22-42   Persistent mento-posterior position. Head cannot extend further to sweep the perineum, so the face becomes impacted.

## BROW PRESENTATION

The fetus presents by the brow when the area of the skull bounded by the orbital ridges and the anterior fontanelle lies at the brim of the pelvis. The attitude of the head is midway between that of a vertex and a face presentation; in fact, during the process of a vertex developing into a face presentation, the brow will present temporarily, and in 1 in 1,000 cases brow presentation will persist.

The maternal causes are similar to those of face presentation (see p. 383).

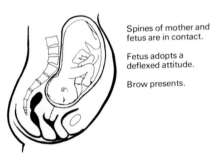

Spines of mother and fetus are in contact.

Fetus adopts a deflexed attitude.

Brow presents.

Fig. 22-43   Brow presentation.

It is not necessary to consider the positions in brow presentation because only on rare occasions is any mechanism of labour possible. Commonly, the head attempts to enter the pelvis with the mento-vertical diameter 13·5 cm in the transverse diameter of the brim.

### DIAGNOSIS

Brow presentation may be suspected when the head seems to be unduly large but is not usually detected until labour begins.

**On abdominal examination** the head is high, seems to be unduly big, and in spite of good uterine contractions does not enter the pelvic brim.

**On vaginal examination** the presenting part cannot be reached, but as labour proceeds the anterior fontanelle may be felt at one side of the pelvis and the orbital ridges at the other; neither vertex nor face can be felt.

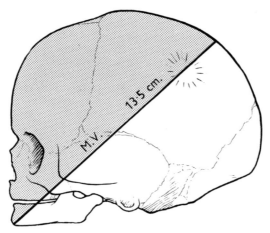

Fig. 22-44   Brow presentation. The mento-vertical diameter, 13·5 cm, lies at the pelvic brim.

### Management

It is possible that with a large pelvis in a multiparous woman, a small baby could be born with the aid of forceps. The brow reaches the pelvic floor, rotates forwards and is born by a mechanism rather similar to that of a vertex face to pubes. The midwife should never anticipate such a favourable outcome, as the majority of brow presentations give rise to obstructed labour.

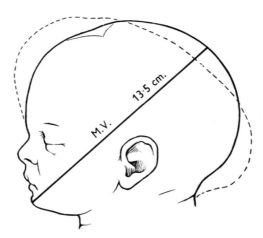

Fig. 22-45   Typical moulding in a brow presentation shown by dotted line.

When the back is anterior and the condition is diagnosed early, before the membranes rupture, the doctor may, by combined abdominal and vaginal manipulation, attempt to increase flexion of the head and convert the brow into a vertex. Caesarean section is usually resorted to. When the back is posterior, the doctor may attempt to increase extension and convert the brow into a face presentation, because an anterior face might be more favourable than a posterior vertex, but Caesarean section is often necessary.

The moulding of the head is typical, with a large caput on the brow.

In cases of neglected brow presentation when the head is wedged into the pelvic brim, or when labour has been in progress for some time and the uterus is moulded round the fetus, it may be necessary to perform craniotomy to avoid rupture of the uterus. The midwife must always view brow presentation with concern and immediately send for medical assistance. The doctor will transfer the patient to a specialist obstetric unit without delay.

# SHOULDER PRESENTATION

When the fetus lies with its long axis across the long axis of the uterus (*transverse lie*) the shoulder is most likely to present. Occasionally the lie is oblique, but this does not persist, as the uterine contractions during labour make it longitudinal or transverse.

Shoulder presentation occurs in 1 in 250 cases near term and the incidence is five times greater in multiparae than in primigravidae.

*Two positions are commonly described*

### Dorso-anterior
The fetal back is in front, conforming to the mother's abdominal wall: the acromion process (*and, of course, the head*) could be to the right or the left.

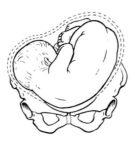
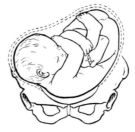

Fig. 22-46  Shoulder presentation, dorso-anterior.

Fig. 22-47  Shoulder presentation, dorso-posterior.

### Dorso-posterior
The fetal back is behind, directed towards the mother's spine, the acromion process and head are to the left or right.

### CAUSES
Any condition that increases the mobility of the fetus *in utero* or which prevents the head from entering the brim will produce any malpresentation, including shoulder.

### MATERNAL

**Anterior obliquity of the uterus.** When the abdominal muscles are lax, the uterus leans forwards and the fetus does not maintain the longitudinal lie.

**Preterm.** Because the amount of amniotic fluid is relatively greater, the fetus is more mobile.

**Multiparity.** If the uterine walls have been frequently stretched, due to repeated childbearing, the snug ovoid shape of the uterus is absent.

**Polyhydramnios.** Because the uterus is globular, the fetus can move freely in the excess fluid.

**Bicornuate uterus.** When the septum extends part way down into the uterine cavity, the fetal head may be in one horn, the breech in the other: **external version fails.**

**Contracted pelvis**
**Placenta praevia** ⎫ may rarely prevent the head from entering the
**Fibroid tumours** (low) ⎭ pelvic brim.

### FETAL

**Twins,** especially the second twin.

**Macerated fetus.** Lack of muscle tone causes the fetus to slump down into the lower pole of the uterus.

## DIAGNOSIS

Every qualified midwife should be competent to diagnose shoulder presentation during pregnancy and early labour; (traditional birth attendants should also be taught this). It is reprehensible when the condition is not recognised until labour is well advanced. The results can be disastrous, i.e. obstructed labour, rupture of uterus, maternal and fetal death.

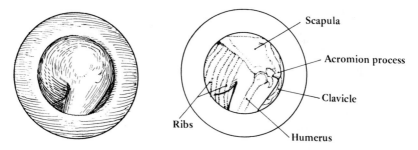

Fig. 22-48A and B    Shoulder presentation. Vaginal touch picture of findings: ribs; edge of scapula, humerus and clavicle.

### *During Pregnancy*

**Inspection.** The fundus is low, sometimes being higher at one side than the other; the uterus is wide.

**Palpation.** On pelvic and fundal palpation, neither head nor breech is felt. The mobile head is located in the iliac fossa, the breech on the opposite side, slightly higher.

**Auscultation.** The fetal heart is heard below the umbilicus but this is not diagnostic.

### During Labour

When the membranes have ruptured the irregular outline of the uterus is more marked. If the uterus is contracting strongly and becomes moulded round the fetus, palpation is very difficult; the pelvis is no longer empty, the shoulder being wedged into it.

**Per vaginam**

Early in labour the presenting part is so high that it is beyond the reach of the midwife's fingers and this should immediately arouse suspicion. The membranes have usually ruptured because of the badly fitting presenting part.

Later, the shoulder is felt as a soft irregular mass and if the fetus is small the ribs may be palpated; their gridiron conformation being diagnostic. When the shoulder enters the brim, prolapse of an arm is liable to occur.

### A hand can be differentiated from a foot as follows:

**The elbow** feels sharper than the knee.     **The thumb** can be abducted.
**The fingers** are longer than the toes     **The palm** is shorter than the sole.
    and are of unequal length.         **No os calcis** can be felt.
       **The hand** is not at right angles to the arm.

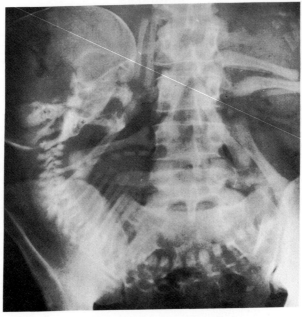

Fig. 22-49   X-ray of transverse lie.

### There is no Mechanism for a Shoulder Presentation

The rare processes by which a macerated, preterm fetus may be expelled in a doubled-up manner are only of academic interest to midwives. These are: Spontaneous evolution. Spontaneous expulsion (see Glossary). The likelihood of the lie becoming longitudinal by the occurrence of spontaneous version or spontaneous rectification at the beginning of labour, is so remote that the midwife should never even entertain the idea of such a possibility.

**In all cases of transverse lie the midwife must get medical assistance.**

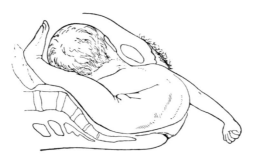

Fig. 22-50    Spontaneous evolution.

### *Treatment*

The main treatment is prophylactic and where adequate prenatal care is practised a shoulder presentation ought to be diagnosed, the cause investigated, and the condition rectified or appropriate treatment arranged for prior to labour. Contracted pelvis in the primigravid woman and the possibility of placenta praevia will be considered; in both instances Caesarean section would be performed at term.

External version is performed when the lie is transverse after the 32nd week of pregnancy. If unsuccessful or if the lie is again transverse when seen within a few days the woman is admitted to hospital where a full investigation is made to determine the cause.

At the beginning of labour if the membranes are intact, the doctor may do external cephalic version, followed by puncture of membranes; close supervision is essential to ensure that the longitudinal lie is maintained.

Caesarean section is the method of choice (*a*) when attempts to correct shoulder presentation have failed; (*b*) when the membranes are ruptured; (*c*) if the cord prolapses; (*d*) if labour has been in progress for some hours.

**Prolapse of cord is a possible complication,** so a vaginal examination is made immediately the membranes rupture. Caesarean section is a recognised method of treating prolapse of cord as well as of shoulder presentation.

## NEGLECTED SHOULDER PRESENTATION

In this condition, the shoulder becomes impacted. It is forced down and wedged into the pelvic brim; the membranes will have ruptured and if the arm has prolapsed it becomes swollen and blue. The uterus goes into a state of tonic contraction, the over-stretched lower segment is tender to touch, the fetal heart fails and all the maternal signs of obstructed labour are manifest. The outcome is that of obstructed labour, with rupture of uterus and stillbirth.

### *Treatment*

A general anaesthetic is given immediately, to stop the contractions, in an endeavour to avert uterine rupture, and preparations made for Caesarean section.

Internal version is dangerous and may rupture the uterus. Some obstetricians consider the risk of uterine rupture to be so great that they perform a Caesarean section even if the fetus is dead.

In remote areas it may be necessary to decapitate the fetus: evisceration may be needed if the neck is not accessible.

With adequate prenatal care and competent supervision during labour, impacted shoulder presentation should never occur. The midwife must always treat shoulder presentation during labour as a dangerous emergency which demands immediate action by the doctor.

# UNSTABLE LIE

This term is applied when after the 36th week of pregnancy the lie, which should at this time be stable as longitudinal, is found to vary (breech, vertex, or shoulder presenting), from one examination to another.

### Causes

Any condition in late pregnancy that increases the mobility of the fetus *in utero*, e.g. lax uterine muscles as in multiparity, polyhydramnios.

## MANAGEMENT OF UNSTABLE LIE

1. The woman is admitted to hospital at the 37th–38th week of pregnancy and remains there until she is delivered to avoid the unsupervised onset of labour with a transverse lie and to receive the essential expert supervision necessary prior to and throughout the labour. Ultrasonography is used to rule out placenta praevia.

2. Further attempts to correct the abnormal presentation by external version are made. If unsuccessful Caesarean section is considered.

3. Some authorities puncture the membranes at the 38th week, having first corrected the transverse lie, to ensure that the woman goes into labour with the vertex presenting: others do so when labour starts. A number of obstetricians do not approve of puncturing the membranes because of the risk of prolapse of cord.

4. An intravenous oxytocin drip is usually given after version; extreme caution being exercised if the woman is a grande multipara.

5. Vigilant supervision is mandatory throughout labour to ensure that the longitudinal lie is maintained: a meticulous abdominal examination being made at the onset of labour, and repeated at frequent intervals. The fetal heart must be auscultated more frequently than is usual and monitored electronically, because of possible prolapse of cord.

6. The bladder should be emptied every two hours (the rectum having been evacuated at the onset of labour) to facilitate preservation of the longitudinal lie.

## COMPOUND OR COMPLEX PRESENTATION

When a hand, or occasionally, a foot, lies alongside the head, the presentation is said to be compound. This tends to occur with a small fetus or roomy pelvis and seldom is difficulty encountered except in cases where it is associated with a flat pelvis. On rare occasions, head, hand and foot are felt in the vagina; a serious situation which usually occurs with a dead fetus. If diagnosed during the first stage of labour, medical aid must be sought. An attempt could be made to push the arm upwards over the baby's face.

If during the second stage the midwife sees a hand presenting alongside the vertex she could try to hold the hand back, directing it over the face. The author saw a case in which both feet were showing at the vulva with the head (*following external version in a frank breech*); the feet were held back, and with no delay the baby was delivered spontaneously.

MALPRESENTATION

### Breech presentation

Fill in the following facts.—The percentage of breech presentations at term .......... The perinatal mortality rate .......... Main cause of fetal death ..........

How would you diagnose a frank breech on inspection—palpation—auscultation—vaginal examination. Give three maternal and three fetal causes of breech presentation.

Give two reasons why external version should be performed during pregnancy.

Describe the following procedures: (a) Burns-Marshall method; (b) Løvset manoeuvre; (c) Mauriceau-Smellie-Veit manoeuvre.

How would you differentiate P.V. between: (a) complete and frank breech; (b) knee and elbow; (c) hand and foot. Differentiate between assisted breech and breech extraction.

Why is it advisable that breech presentations should be delivered in hospital? Give two reasons why the cord is liable to prolapse.

What is meant by the nuchal position?

Explain how the following are produced: hypoxia; intracranial injury; rupture of liver; fracture of humerus; fracture of neck; Erb's paralysis.

Why should the following procedures be avoided? (a) fundal pressure; (b) traction on the breech; (c) turning the back up prior to birth of the shoulders; (d) pulling the head out quickly.

The following colloquial terms are useful reminders—explain them. 'Hands off the breech', 'like a cat washing its face', 'not like a cork out of a bottle', 'breathing the head out'.

Why must the midwife be able to deliver 'the breech baby' competently although delivery in hospital is modern policy.

How would you deal with extended legs, extended arms, extended head?

**C.M.B.(Scot.) 30-min. question.** Describe the management of a breech delivery where the legs are extended.

**C.M.B.(Eng.) 30-min. question.** How is a breech presentation diagnosed? Discuss the investigations which would be made and what treatment would be carried out during the antenatal period.

**C.M.B.(Scot.) 30-min. question.** What is the mechanism of labour in a breech presentation? Describe the complications which may arise during labour.

**C.M.B.(Eng.).** List the causes of breech presentation. Describe the management of the second stage of a breech labour.

## Oral Questions

Why is it important to make a vaginal examination when the membranes rupture? When might an L.O.A. and an L.S.A. be confused on abdominal examination? Why is intracranial injury more likely to occur in breech than vertex presentation? Why is it important that the bladder is empty prior to delivery? When is Syntometrine given in breech delivery? Why is it essential that the cervix is fully dilated before the woman is allowed to 'push'? Why is vitamin $K_1$ administered to the baby? Give reasons for delay in the first stage, second stage, during expulsion of the head.

### Face presentation

Give three maternal and three fetal causes of face presentation. In making a vaginal examination, what is the diagnostic landmark? Why must you avoid the eyes?

## Explain

(a) **The management of labour in face presentation:** (b) **persistent mento-posterior.**

**Why labour is long?** Which diameters of the skull (a) engage; (b) appear at the vulva; (c) sweep the perineum?

**C.M.B.(Eng.) 30-min. question.** How would you diagnose a face presentation during labour? Briefly describe the conduct of labour in such a case.

**C.M.B.(Scot.) 30-min. question.** Describe the course of labour in a face presentation and indicate briefly the treatment of any difficulties which may arise.

## Oral Questions

How would you differentiate P.V. between lips and labia; mouth and anus; vertex and face? How would you assist in getting the chin born first? Why do the face bones not mould? Why is the cord liable to prolapse? In a posterior face what finding P.V. would indicate that the chin will rotate forward?

### Brow presentation

How would you (a) suspect a brow presentation, on abdominal examination; (b) diagnose it on vaginal examination? What would you do in such circumstances? What treatment might be carried out?

Why could brow presentation obstruct labour? Describe the shape of the moulded head. What would the treatment be in a case of neglected brow presentation?

**Shoulder presentation**

Give three fetal and three maternal causes of shoulder presentation and explain why they produce a transverse lie. Place the doll in the dorso-anterior position and explain what the findings would be on abdominal examination.

What would you do if the shoulder was presenting in the following circumstances? In the overseas service, with the doctor ten hours' journey distant: (a) woman at beginning of labour; (b) cervix (6 cm); (c) shoulder impacted.

Why is it imperative that transverse lie is diagnosed prior to the onset of labour?

## Describe

(a) **The outcome** of an undiagnosed shoulder presentation. (b) **Unstable lie.**

(c) **The dangers of internal version** during labour for shoulder presentation.

condition and what are the dangers to mother and baby?

Why is shoulder presentation more common in multigravid women?

Why is it dangerous to perform version when labour has been established for some time?

Differentiate between elbow and knee; fingers and toes; palm and sole, on vaginal examination.

Define unstable lie. Why is delivery in an obstetric unit imperative? What details should the midwife observe during labour?

**C.M.B.(Scot.) question.** What are the complications and dangers of transverse lie at full term? How may they be avoided? In what type of patient are you likely to find a transverse lie?

**C.M.B.(Scot.) 30-min. question.** Describe the cause, diagnosis and management of transverse lie.

**C.M.B.(N. Ireland) 30-min. question.** What is meant by unstable lie? What are the causes of this

# 23
# Disordered Uterine Action: Prolonged Labour

*Hypotonic, inco-ordinate, constriction ring, cervical dystocia. Contracted pelvis. Trial labour. Obstructed labour*

Disordered uterine action rarely gives rise to difficulty in centres where the active management of labour is practised. Some believe that all forms of disordered uterine action respond favourably to amniotomy and i.v. infusion of oxytocin.

Many theories have been propounded regarding the causation of disordered uterine action, but none provides a satisfactory solution. The condition may be manifest as hypotonic uterine action and inco-ordinate uterine action.

## (1) HYPOTONIC UTERINE ACTION

This term is usually applied when uterine contractions are weak and dilatation of the cervix is slow. Early signs are manifest by using the cervicograph, the latent phase of labour being retarded. Efficiency of uterine action is reflected in the rate of cervical dilatation.

### *Treatment*

The membranes are punctured.

A low dosage Syntocinon i.v. infusion is started, 0·5 units in 540 ml glucose, 5 per cent, at 1 ml per minute: increased to 1 unit in 30 minutes and gradually up to 2·5 units if maternal and fetal conditions are satisfactory. The drip is continued until one hour after completion of the third stage then gradually reduced. Sedatives are prescribed as required. Cervical dilatation is recorded on a cervicograph.

Biochemical control and electrolyte replacement are instituted. Maternal and fetal conditions are monitored by electronic means: fetal blood sampling being done when the fetal heart rate pattern deviates from normal. Nursing care is similar to that for normal labour.

### *Operative measures*

Caesarean section is now performed earlier in cases where cervical dilatation is persistently slow. Epidural analgesia is preferred by some. Forceps delivery under pudendal nerve block may be necessary to avoid fetal hypoxia during the second stage.

## (2) INCO-ORDINATE UTERINE ACTION

This state of dysfunction is manifest when the progress of labour is very slow in spite of frequent painful contractions. The two poles of the uterus do not function rhythmically: the cervix dilates slowly and feels tight and unyielding.

## (3) HYPERTONIC UTERINE ACTION

The condition known as hypertonic uterine action in which the tone of the uterus is high during and between contractions, with severe backache is dealt with by the administration of epidural analgesia and i.v. low dosage oxytocin. All cases of uterine dysfunction, i.e. inco-ordinate, hypotonic and hypertonic, respond favourably to low dosage oxytocin (see above).

*Treatment of Hypertonic Uterine Action*

**Exclusion of cephalo-pelvic disproportion.**
**Trial of oxytocin**

Syntocinon, 0·5 units, in 540 ml of glucose, 5 per cent, is administered intravenously starting with one ml per minute. The drip method is used if an automated titration unit is not available.

Constant supervision with the fingers palpating uterine tonus is mandatory: the fetal condition being monitored by an electronic unit if possible.

Effective pain relief is obtained by epidural analgesia or other pain relieving drugs, e.g. pethidine which may be added to the 'drip'.

Urine analysis, fluid balance, and nursing care are similar to that in normal labour (p. 276). A cervicographic record is kept.

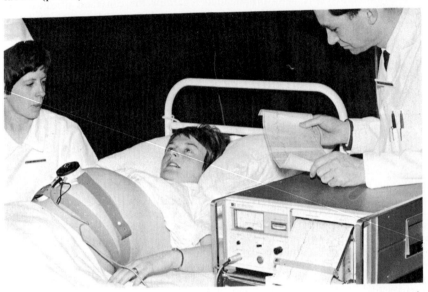

Fig. 23-1 The Hewlett-Packard cardiotocograph system. This apparatus simultaneously measures and records uterine activity and fetal heart frequency. The outputs of the transducers are fed to two distinct channels in the cardiotocograph, where they are processed to give a direct reading of fetal heart frequency and relative uterine activity. These readings are indicated by meters on the front panel of the instrument and simultaneously by the recorder.

*Simpson Memorial Maternity Pavilion, Edinburgh.*

In remote areas, patients may be admitted to hospital having been 24 hours in labour with a hypertonic uterus.

Dehydration and ketoacidosis must be combated and electrolyte control instituted: the intravenous route being utilised, oral fluids discontinued.

Heavy sedation is achieved, then when the patient (and uterus) is rested a trial of oxytocin is begun cautiously.

An endocervical swab is taken and a bacterial culture made. If the membranes have been ruptured for 24 hours some give ampicillin, 500 mg, followed by 250 mg six hourly until the bacteriological report is received.

Caesarean section may be carried out if dilatation of the cervix is slow.

Nursing care is similar to what is now routine in normal labour (p. 256).

## EFFECT ON THE WOMAN AND FETUS

**Ketoacidosis**

This metabolic disturbance gives rise to signs formerly known as those of maternal distress. It is due to deficient intake of carbohydrates interfering with the metabolic breakdown of fats. Ketone bodies appear in the urine, dehydration and lack of food accentuate the condition. This in turn contributes to uterine dysfunction and if neglected the maternal and fetal conditions deteriorate. Electrolytes—particularly potassium—are depleted.

Hypertonic uterine action is extremely dangerous for the fetus even when the membranes are intact. Ketoacidosis adds to the hazards. The fetus is deprived of oxygen because the utero-placental circulation is diminished by the hypertonic state of the uterus. Some recommend epidural analgesia because it is beneficial for the fetus. Fetal hypoxia is a constant threat that becomes more serious in ratio to the length of time the membranes have been ruptured and labour has lasted. Neonatal pneumonia is common in cases when the membranes have been ruptured for 24 hours. The fetal mortality rate is doubled after 36 hours.

## CONSTRICTION RING DYSTOCIA

This localised spasm of a ring of muscle fibres, a condition occurring in about 1 in 1,000 labours, is due to disorganised uterine action. It may occur in the upper or lower segment, commonly near the junction of both, and usually embraces a narrow part of the fetus, e.g. the neck. The constriction ring may form during the first or second stage and when present during the third stage is known as an hour-glass contraction.

**Causes**

The spasm may arise in such circumstances as: when the uterus is hypertonic: when the membranes rupture early and the uterus becomes irritated by being moulded round the fetus: following intra-uterine manipulation, e.g. internal version.

**Signs**

There is no advance of the presenting part. The upper segment feels tender to touch. The constriction ring is diagnosed vaginally, while investigating delay or during operative delivery. It must not be confused with Bandl's retraction ring.

### Treatment

Papaveretum or pethidine may be prescribed. It may be necessary to achieve immediate relaxation of the constriction ring in order to deliver the placenta, and the inhalation of 1 ampoule of amyl nitrite, or the administration of 10 ml of a 20 per cent solution of magnesium sulphate intravenously, is sometimes successful in relieving the spasm. A general anaesthetic may be necessary.

## CERVICAL DYSTOCIA

**Rigid cervix**

In this rare condition the cervix dilates very slowly although the uterine action is normal. The condition occurs mainly in primigravidae; the first stage of labour is prolonged and painful, backache is severe and persistent. On vaginal examination the cervix feels thin, tight and unyielding, but may become thick and oedematous later.

## Treatment

The treatment is as for hypertonic uterine action: Caesarean section being performed in most cases.

*N.B.*—Cervical rigidity may occasionally be due to other causes, e.g. scarring from previous injury or infection.

### Oedematous anterior lip of cervix

In cases of disproportion when the cervix is nipped between the fetal head and the brim of the pelvis a lip of cervix becomes swollen and oedematous; it does not stretch well and gives rise to delay and much suffering. Oedema of the cervix may also be caused by the woman bearing down during the first stage. The oedematous anterior lip is felt on vaginal examination as a firm ridge, sometimes as thick as a finger. On occasions, when the condition is not recognised and treated, the glistening cervix may be seen at the vulva between the occiput and the lower border of the symphysis pubis.

## Treatment

The woman is told to breathe rhythmically with her mouth open, throat relaxed, without accentuating expiration during contractions, in order to refrain from pushing; a midwife should be in constant attendance to ensure this. Turning the woman on her side and elevating the foot of the bed may help to take the pressure of the fetal head off the cervix. Inhalational analgesia may be helpful, but in persistent cases an attempt is made between contractions to push the cervix up over the head. This must be done very gradually to avoid lacerations.

### Annular detachment of cervix

This occurs in rare instances due to prolonged pressure of a large head on a rigid cervix producing an ischaemic area which inhibits dilatation: bearing down during the first stage may be conducive to this. The necrosed ring of cervix becomes detached and expelled. Medical aid must be obtained.

# PROLONGED LABOUR

Labour is said to be prolonged when it exceeds 24 hours; false labour should not be included. But delay can be inferred prior to then, if with good contractions, the presenting part remains high or descends slowly, and when dilatation of the cervix is retarded.

This situation is not permitted to occur or persist in modern obstetric practice. Many conditions likely to prolong labour can be diagnosed during pregnancy, e.g. contracted pelvis, large baby, occipito-posterior position. Major degrees of disproportion are dealt with by Caesarean section.

A long second stage has been proved harmful to the fetus: hypoxia and acidosis both being present in such cases (see p. 307).

## Admission to Hospital

The patient should be admitted to hospital if the first stage is still in progress after 12 hours and there is no likelihood of the early completion of labour.

The woman needs constant supervision, and unless good nursing care is provided ketosis develops; her condition begins to deteriorate after about 24 hours, and when 36 hours have elapsed the danger zone is reached.

**History of labour,** including records, is obtained from doctor or midwife: length, type and frequency of contractions; when membranes ruptured? This is significant because after 24 hours the risk of puerperal sepsis and neonatal pneumonia is very great: pyrexia of 37·5°C or over during labour is an absolute indication for the administration of antibiotics. An endocervical or high vaginal swab is taken.

**Enquiry re:** analgesic drugs given; food and fluid taken; vomiting; evacuation of bowel and bladder.

**Examination of woman:** general appearance—distressed, exhausted, dehydrated; temperature and pulse—an increase in either would be significant; urine analysis—concentrated urine suggests fluid imbalance and dehydration. Ketostix reagent strips will detect ketoacidosis which must be rectified at once.

**Abdominal examination:** uterine tonus—strength, length and frequency of contractions; presentation, position, engagement, size of fetus, disproportion, fetal heart rate.

**Vaginal examination:** dilatation and consistency of cervix, membranes ruptured, level of presenting part, presentation, position, moulding and caput formation.

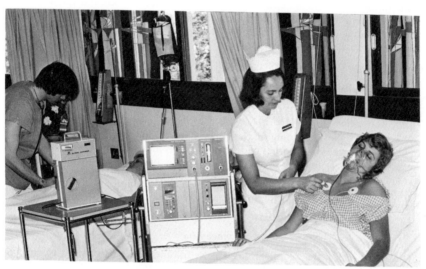

Fig. 23-2   Intensive care labour ward unit.
*Bellshill Maternity Hospital, Lanarkshire.*

### Early signs of ketoacidosis

Pulse over 90, temperature over 37·2°C. The woman is apathetic and feels weak. Ketones are present in the urine.

### Late signs of ketoacidosis

**Anxious expression.** The woman has a drawn, anxious expression with a degree of circumoral pallor; her nose and mouth look pinched, and with an imploring glance she appeals for help. The woman looks and feels ill.

Beads of perspiration are seen on the upper lip. Signs of dehydration are evident, e.g. dry lips, parched tongue, concentrated urine. Marked restlessness. Between uterine contractions she does not relax; she is distracted and restless. Vomiting when persistent, with dark-coloured vomitus welling up into the mouth, is an ominous sign.

## DANGERS OF A PROLONGED SECOND STAGE

### To the fetus

During the perineal phase the fetal head is being exposed to great pressure; it is being forced downwards by the contracting uterus and resisted by the pelvic floor, and the excessive moulding may give rise to intracranial injury and hypoxia. The placenta is compressed between the retracted thickened wall of the upper uterine segment and the buttocks of the fetus, and because much of the amniotic fluid will have drained away, interference with the placental circulation occurs, resulting in fetal hypoxia. A prolonged second stage causes fetal metabolic acidosis (*Signs of fetal distress must be watched for.*) (See p. 301.)

If the head does not appear after half an hour of good contractions, a vaginal examination should be made to find the cause of the delay; excessive moulding or a large caput would indicate that the fetal head is being exposed to undue stress. When the head is showing at the vulva and good uterine contractions do not overcome the resistance of the perineum within half an hour, or if no advance is made during that time, an episiotomy and forceps delivery are indicated.

The last hour of labour may do more damage to mother and baby than the whole of the preceding hours, and, if the midwife delays too long in sending for the doctor, the infant's chances of survival are poor.

### To the uterus

If the presenting part does not advance with good contractions, the lower uterine segment may be stretched to such an extent that it ruptures—a serious accident.

### To the pelvic floor

When the head is pounding on the pelvic floor for longer than three-quarters of an hour, the perineum becomes oedematous and is more likely to tear; in addition, the pelvic floor is unduly stretched and uterine prolapse, cystocele and stress incontinence are liable to ensue. The urethra being persistently compressed by the fetal head becomes bruised and this may give rise to retention of urine during the puerperium.

#### *Management*

The first need is the rectification of dehydration, ketoacidosis and electrolyte imbalance by i.v. glucose, 10 per cent, and Ringer's lactate solution. This is imperative prior to a general anaesthetic and to operative procedures. Caesarean section may be performed during the first stage for disproportion, fetal distress, disordered uterine action. During the second stage episiotomy, forceps or ventouse vacuum extraction may be necessary. The baby may require resuscitation.

Assiduous supervision of the fetal condition is necessary and if electronic equipment for constant monitoring is not available auscultation during and following uterine contractions should be carried out.

**Nursing care** is as prescribed for normal labour (p. 284).

## CONTRACTED PELVIS

A pelvis is contracted when one or more diameters are less than the minimal normal range by over 1 cm, thereby making the delivery of an average-sized baby by the natural route difficult or impossible. Undiagnosed, contracted pelvis will give rise to prolonged, difficult and possibly obstructed labour, which may result in injury or death of mother and child. The recognition of signs which indicate possible contraction of the pelvis is one of the fundamental duties of a midwife.

*Diagnosis*

**Contracted pelvis** is more commonly seen in women whose height is less than 1·5 metres. The more gross deformities may be due to diseases such as rickets, and tuberculosis of spine or hip. Diminutive height, if due to disease such as rickets, is more serious than when occurring in the small woman with fine bones. A limp, waddling gait, bony deformity of the hips or spine, and any sign of rickets, will arouse suspicion of serious pelvic malformation. A medical history of injury or disease of spine or pelvis is significant.

### Obstetrical history

If the patient gives a history of difficult labour, forceps delivery, Caesarean section, or stillbirth, the cause must be sifted. A woman who has given birth spontaneously to a 3·6 kg baby is likely to have an adequate pelvis, but subsequent babies may give rise to difficulty if over that weight.

### Examination of the pregnant woman

Every woman must be examined for cephalo-pelvic disproportion at the 37th week, even when her pelvis is of normal shape and dimensions; when a high head or malpresentation is found, further investigation is essential. Pelvimetry by the use of X-rays is resorted to after the 32nd week, if clinical signs of contraction are manifest. Digital exploration of the pelvic canal will reveal pelvic size and shape (p. 127). A pendulous abdomen in a primigravid woman near term usually indicates pelvic contraction or spinal deformity which diminishes the accommodation between the ribs and pelvis and so causes the uterus to become anteverted.

Medical assistance must be obtained by the midwife when she suspects pelvic contraction or cephalo-pelvic disproportion. The obstetrician will decide whether trial labour or Caesarean section is indicated, depending on the degree of disproportion; admission to hospital at term will be arranged.

## THE JUSTO MINOR PELVIS

This pelvis has been likened to a gynaecoid pelvis in miniature. All the pelvic measurements are diminished but are in correct proportion. These women are petite, usually under 1·5 m in height, with small hands and feet, shoes size 3 or less, but occasionally the justo minor pelvis may be present in a woman of normal stature.

The difficulty encountered will depend on the degree of cephalo-pelvic disproportion, and will persist throughout the first and second stages. The mechanism proceeds in the usual way, but there will be exaggerated flexion of the head. If vaginal delivery is possible, a trial labour is carried out. Caesarean section may be necessary, but fortunately these women often have small babies.

# THE FOUR BASIC TYPES OF PELVIS

**Female pelves have been classified into four basic types,** each being designated according to the shape of the brim. Gross abnormalities, due to developmental errors and accidents, as well as deformities brought about by diseases such as rickets and tuberculosis of the spine or hip, may be superimposed on any of the four basic types.

## (1) GYNAECOID

**This, the true female pelvis, is normal in size and shape.** (It has been described under the normal pelvis—p. 22.)

### (2) THE ANDROID PELVIS

This pelvis has a heart-shaped brim, and because the cavity is deep and the outlet narrow it has been likened to a funnel. Marked contraction of the intertuberischial and the bispinous diameters is the oustanding characteristic. The subpubic angle and the sacro-sciatic notches are found to be acute on vaginal examination; the ischial spines prominent. Because of the depth of the cavity the diagonal conjugate may be greater than 12 cm, giving a misleading impression regarding the adequacy of the obstetrical conjugate.

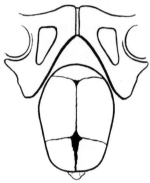
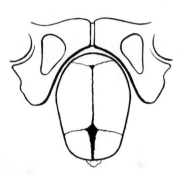

Fig. 23-3  Outlet of android pelvis. The head does not fit into the acute pubic arch and is forced backwards on the perineum.

Fig. 23-4  Outlet of gynaecoid pelvis. The head fits snugly into the pubic arch.

**Effect on labour**

Posterior positions of the vertex are more common, because the biparietal diameter is more easily accommodated in the posterior segment of the heart-shaped brim. Deep transverse arrest of the head sometimes occurs.

The head is forced back into the posterior segment of the outlet, because it cannot be accommodated in the acute pubic arch; much bruising or laceration of the pelvic floor and perineum results.

The fetus does not stand up well to the stress and delay which may occur during the second stage. An episiotomy and forceps delivery are usually necessary.

### (3) THE ANTHROPOID PELVIS

In this pelvis the brim is oval, with the transverse diameter less than the antero-posterior. The head may engage with the occiput anterior: if it engages with the occiput posterior the baby is born face to pubes.

### (4) THE PLATYPELLOID OR SIMPLE FLAT PELVIS

The brim is kidney-shaped, with a diminished antero-posterior diameter and an enlarged transverse. The antero-posterior diameters of the cavity and outlet are also reduced, the whole sacrum being displaced forwards. This simple flat pelvis is said to be due to a subclinical form of rickets.

The effect on labour is similar to that in the rachitic flat pelvis, but the difficulty persists throughout labour, as the antero-posterior diameters of the brim, cavity and outlet are all diminished.

### THE RACHITIC FLAT PELVIS

This deformed pelvis is due to rickets in early childhood, and is rarely encountered in pronounced form because of the facilities now provided for child health. The condition may be seen in immigrant mothers and babies. Clinical signs of rickets may be evident, such as bow legs and deformities of the spine which, in conjunction with defective growth of bone, tend to diminish stature.

The only diameter diminished in the rachitic flat pelvis is the obstetrical conjugate. The sacro-cotyloid dimension is also reduced. All the other diameters are increased. The brim is kidney-shaped because the sacral promontory projects so far forwards. The sacrum lacks the normal curve, and in some cases is straight, with the coccyx bending acutely forwards. The ischial tuberosities are farther apart, so the pubic arch may be greater than a right angle: the outlet is therefore capacious.

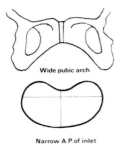

Wide pubic arch

Narrow A.P. of inlet

Wide A.P. of outlet

Fig. 23-5   Rachitic flat pelvis.

Note wide pubic arch.
Note kidney-shaped brim.

The lateral view shows the diminished antero-posterior diameter of the brim and the increased antero-posterior diameter of the outlet.

### *Effect of Flat Pelvis on Labour*

Caesarean section will be necessary if the degree of contraction is severe. In minor or moderate degrees a trial labour may be carried out (see p. 408). Many hours will elapse before the head passes through the pelvic brim, but when this is accomplished the remainder of the labour will be unusually rapid in the rachitic pelvis.

Face presentation, prolapse of cord and fetal distress are complications to be anticipated during labour.

### MECHANISM OF LABOUR

**The fetal head enters in the transverse diameter of the brim,** and both fontanelles remain on the same level. The head negotiates the pelvic brim in the following manner.

**Anterior asynclitism or Naegele's obliquity.**—This is a lateral tilting of the head. The anterior parietal bone moves slowly down behind the symphysis pubis until the parietal eminence has passed through the brim. The movement is then reversed, the head tilting in the opposite direction until the posterior parietal bone is pushed past the promontory. Flexion, internal rotation and extension then take place in the usual way.

**Posterior asynclitism or Litzmann's obliquity** is similar to anterior asynclitism, but the movements are reversed. The posterior parietal bone enters first and is driven past the promontory of the sacrum; then the anterior parietal bone passes down behind the symphysis pubis. This mechanism is less common and occurs in the more severe degrees of flat pelvis.

### RARE PELVIC DEFORMITIES

#### OSTEOMALACIC OR MALACOSTEON PELVIS

This extreme deformity is due to the disease, osteomalacia, which is found in certain localities but is rarely seen in Britain or America. It occurs in multigravidae and is due to gross deficiency of minerals and vitamins in the diet. All the bones of the skeleton soften and the sides of the pelvic canal are squashed together until the brim becomes a mere Y-shaped slit.

**Naegele's pelvis has only one wing** to the sacrum probably due to maldevelopment or disease of the sacro-iliac joint with ankylosis during infancy. The brim is obliquely contracted.

**Robert's pelvis** is one in which there are no wings to the sacrum and the brim consists of a narrow opening.

**Spinal deformities.** When kyphosis (forward angulation) or scoliosis (lateral curvature) is evident, or any limp or deformity is present, the midwife must refer the woman to a doctor. Such marked deformities are readily diagnosed, but greater vigilance is needed in detecting the lesser degrees of pelvic contraction or cephalo-pelvic disproportion.

# TRIAL OF LABOUR

**Some authorities question the need for trial of labour:** they consider that every normal labour is a trial labour. But when a minor or moderate degree of cephalo-pelvic disproportion exists, labour is not normal and should be conducted with the same degree of expert supervision accorded to other abnormal conditions in labour. Admittedly skilled midwives are needed for normal labour but for trial labour expert staff (usually more senior) are invaluable because they are highly proficient, and have the priceless faculty of interpreting clinical observations and applying knowledge and practical experience judiciously. Conducting a trial of labour is a searching test of the clinical judgment of those in charge. The use of a partogram is commendable but does not replace the wisdom and competence of the professionally accomplished obstetrician or midwife.

### THE OUTCOME

**The outcome of a trial of labour depends on:**

**The effectiveness of the uterine contractions.**
**The degree of moulding of the fetal head.**
**The give of the pelvic joints.**

These factors are not predictable until labour is established, so judgment is withheld, as to whether Caesarean section will be necessary, until the amount of progress made over a period of hours has been assessed.

It is not a trial of how much the woman or her fetus can endure and is not permitted to continue until signs of fetal or maternal exhaustion are exhibited. The outcome should be a live mother and child who have sustained a minimal amount of trauma.

### *Management*

The woman, usually a primigravida, is allowed to go to term, because the spontaneous onset of labour is more likely to result in efficient uterine action; the mature fetus is better equipped to withstand the stress of labour.

Labour is conducted in a specialist obstetric unit, where constant supervision, expert care and provision for operative procedures are available. Progress is recorded on a partogram. Sedation should be adequate.

Opinions differ regarding the length of trial labour. So many factors have to be considered that *'time in hours'* can be a treacherous criterion on which to make the decision. Some authorities consider that, on weighing up the situation after four hours of established labour, they can predict whether a safe vaginal delivery is possible. Delaying the decision until the cervix is fully dilated is precarious. If the cervix dilates slowly with good contractions or if the contractions are poor the outlook is gloomy. The decision rests with the obstetrician.

## THE MIDWIFE'S DUTIES

### *Careful Abdominal Examination on Admission*

The presentation will be the vertex; the position should be diagnosed, L.O.A. being most favourable.

The head will not be engaged, but its level in relation to the pelvic brim should be assessed. This can be checked by vaginal examination.

The degree of flexion of the head and the amount of overlap at the brim is noted.

The fetal heart rate is carefully monitored or recorded in graph form.

### *Vigilant Observation*

*The midwife remains in constant attendance—observing, recording, and maintaining the woman's morale.*

**Uterine action.** The time of the onset of contractions, their frequency, length and strength should be recorded. A monitoring device is constantly employed.

**Fetal condition.** The fetal heart rate should be taken every 5 to 15 minutes and recorded in graph form or monitored electronically.

**Early signs of fetal distress are watched for,** because of the excessive moulding necessary to allow the head to engage. Fetal scalp blood sampling may be done.

**Progress.** The midwife should assess what is accomplished in a given time, i.e. every two hours, taking into consideration the type of uterine contractions, cervical dilatation and fetal descent.

**The maternal condition** needs close supervision. Biochemical control and electrolyte balance are maintained.

Routine nursing care is similar to that which is given for normal labour (p. 291).

### On abdominal examination

Increase of flexion and descent of the head in fifths should be noted.

### On vaginal examination

Level of the head and degree of flexion: dilatation of the cervix; consistency of cervix; membranes intact or ruptured; excessive moulding; a large caput.

### Conditions to be reported to the doctor

Rupture of membranes, colour of amniotic fluid, time of occurrence. Number of hours in labour.

Unsatisfactory advance when contractions are good, e.g. head still high after six hours in labour.

Early signs of fetal distress and maternal ketosis.

Change of vertex presentation to brow or face.

# OBSTRUCTED LABOUR

Obstructed labour is present when there is no advance of the presenting part in spite of strong uterine contractions and is due to some fault in the passages or passenger (but not in the powers) producing an impassable barrier. Obstruction should not occur, as the cause should have been detected during pregnancy or early in labour.

Obstruction usually occurs at the pelvic inlet but can take place at the outlet, as in cases of android pelvis and when undiagnosed deep transverse arrest of the head occurs.

## CAUSES

**Contracted pelvis,** cephalo-pelvic disproportion.

**Malpresentation.** Shoulder. Brow. Face. (*persistent mento-posterior*).

**Large fetus.** When the fetus is over 4·5 kg and the pelvis average in size, there will be delay and difficulty, but actual obstruction is more likely with a fetus weighing over 5·5 kg.

**Fetal abnormalities:** hydrocephaly being most common, conjoined twins are rare.

**Fibroid tumours** rarely give rise to obstruction unless situated in the lower pole of the uterus; bony tumours are rarer still.

### EARLY SIGNS

The presenting part does not enter the pelvic brim in spite of good contractions. It should be remembered that a full bladder and a large bag of membranes may prevent the head from engaging.

The cervix dilates slowly and hangs loosely like 'an empty sleeve' because the presenting part cannot descend and become applied to it.

The membranes tend to rupture early.

### LATER SIGNS

These would only occur in remote areas where competent obstetric supervision was not available.

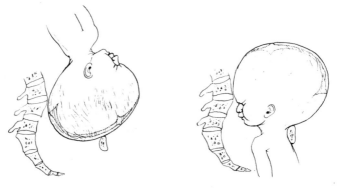

Fig. 23-6   Hydrocephalus.

Fore-coming head.                          After-coming head.

The uterus becomes moulded round the fetus and does not relax properly between contractions. The presenting part becomes wedged and immovable when it descends partly into the pelvis. The cranial bones overlap excessively and a large caput forms.

Uterine exhaustion; contractions may cease for a period to recommence with renewed vigour, usually in primigravid women. Bandl's ring may occasionally be seen abdominally, rising nearer the umbilicus as the lower uterine segment becomes progressively thinner and longer.

Evidence of maternal ketoacidosis and fetal distress are usually manifest.

## DANGERS

### Maternal

Rupture of the uterus, due to excessive thinning of the lower uterine segment.

Death of the mother. In neglected cases the woman may die from exhaustion, undelivered, or from shock following urgent operative delivery especially when ketosis and dehydration have not been combated. She may die from rupture of the uterus. (Sepsis and haemorrhage can usually be dealt with by modern methods.)

Vesico-vaginal fistula may occur, due to bruising of the bladder, or to injury during a difficult instrumental delivery.

### Fetal

Stillbirth. Neonatal death, asphyxia, intracranial haemorrhage, pneumonia.

### *Treatment of Obstructed Labour*

### During pregnancy (prophylaxis)

Recognition of, and reporting to the doctor, conditions which would give rise to obstruction. Examination of every woman at the 37th week by a doctor, to exclude cephalo-pelvic disproportion.

External version for shoulder presentation. Making arrangements in cases of hydrocephaly for admission to hospital, where craniotomy will be done during labour when the cervix is 5 cm dilated.

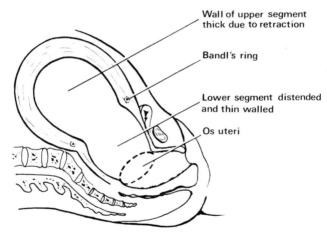

Wall of upper segment thick due to retraction

Bandl's ring

Lower segment distended and thin walled

Os uteri

Fig. 23-7 Representation of excessive thinning of the lower uterine segment, which is liable to rupture.

### During labour

Lower segment Caesarean section is performed if conditions are present which would cause obstruction or if early signs of obstruction are manifest. It is the duty of the midwife to recognise these and summon medical assistance.

Intravenous glucose, 5 or 10 per cent, is given prior to, and during operative delivery. Preparations are made to treat a shocked mother and baby. Blood should be at hand. Embryotomy may be necessary in neglected cases.

## TONIC CONTRACTION AND RETRACTION

This serious condition arising during the uterine effort to overcome an obstruction should not be permitted to occur: the contractions occurring more frequently and more strongly, until one long contraction is maintained. Retraction is extreme and the upper segment becomes hard and excessively thick: the lower uterine segment is abnormally thin, tender to touch, and may rupture, particularly in multiparous patients. Bandl's ring may be seen abdominally. The fetus dies of anoxia, due to the constant contractions diminishing its supply of oxygen.

### Treatment of Tonic Contractions

Medical assistance must be summoned urgently.

A general anaesthetic is needed to damp down uterine activity and prevent rupture. The uterus is emptied without delay and Caesarean section is usually performed but if not practicable embryotomy may be necessary. Such a state of affairs should not arise; the midwife ought to have diagnosed the condition causing obstructed labour and obtained medical assistance prior to the onset of tonic contractions.

---

## QUESTIONS FOR REVISION
### PROLONGED LABOUR

Give six signs of maternal ketosis. Mention the dangers of a prolonged second stage, under the following headings (a) the fetus; (b) the uterus; (c) the pelvic floor.

### Oral Questions

For what reasons are the following done? pH of fetal blood estimated; intravenous fluid administered? Which urine tests are made?

Differentiate between: fetal tachycardia and bradycardia; ketonuria and proteinuria.

Why is biochemical control necessary during prolonged labour?

Why is an endocervical swab taken when the membranes have been ruptured for 24 hours?

Define: dystocia; annular detachment of cervix; hypertonic uterine action; prolonged labour; tonic contractions; uterine dysfunction; constriction ring; cervical dystocia.

**C.M.B.(Scot.) 30-min. question.** What are the causes of delay in the first stage of labour? Describe the management of a patient with delay in the first stage.

**N. Ire. 30-min. question.** What are the causes of delay in the second stage of labour? What are your duties in such a case?

### CONTRACTED PELVIS

### Rearrange correctly:

| Description | Term | | |
|---|---|---|---|
| 1. Funnel shaped pelvis | Justo minor | ( | ) |
| 2. Small pelvis | Gynaecoid | ( | ) |
| 3. Narrow transverse diameters | Platypelloid | ( | ) |
| 4. Round brim | Anthropoid | ( | ) |
| 5. All antero-posterior diameters diminished | Android | ( | ) |
| 6. Y shaped brim | Roberts | ( | ) |
| 7. One ala to sacrum | Malacosteon | ( | ) |

What would make you suspect contracted pelvis: (a) from the medical and obstetrical histories; (b) from the woman's appearance.

Why is rickets seen in some immigrant expectant mothers. What are the 4 basic types of pelvis?

**C.M.B.(Scot.) 30-min. question.** (a) What is a contracted pelvis? (b) what would lead you to suspect this deformity? (c) what effects might it have on the course of the patient's pregnancy and labour?

What are the features of the four main types of pelvis. How may divergence from normal shape and size affect the course of labour?

How would you (a) prevent and (b) deal with an oedematous lip of cervix.

What are the (a) early and (b) late signs of ketoacidosis. What could the midwife do to prevent this.

## TRIAL LABOUR

**Define Trial Labour.** On what three unpredictable factors does the outcome depend? Describe the abdominal examination you would carry out at the beginning of labour. What observations would you make and record during labour? What would you report to the doctor?

**N.Ire. 30-min. question.** What are the important points in the nursing of a case of 'trial labour'?

**C.M.B.(Scot.) 30-min. question.** Describe the management of a patient during a trial labour.

**C.M.B.(Scot.) 30-min. question.** Describe the main characteristics of the following types of pelvis (*a*) justo minor, (*b*) simple flat, (*c*) rachitic flat. Discuss the care of a patient having a trial labour.

## OBSTRUCTED LABOUR

Define: obstructed labour; cephalo-pelvic disproportion. What weight of fetus is liable to obstruct labour.

What is meant by vesico-vaginal fistula. Why may it occur during obstructed labour?

**C.M.B.(Scot.) 30-min. question.** What are the causes of obstructed labour? How can these be prevented by proper antenatal care? What are the early signs of obstructed labour?

## *C.M.B. Short Questions*

Constriction ring and retraction ring; gynaecoid pelvis; tonic contraction; cervical dystocia; Bandl's ring; oedematous anterior lip of cervix; cervicograph; ketoacidosis.

# 24
# Obstetrical Emergencies

*Rupture of uterus. Prolapse of cord. Amniotic fluid embolism. Acute inversion of uterus*

## RUPTURE OF THE UTERUS

This is one of the most serious accidents in obstetrics, occurring in approximately 1 in 3,000 cases, commonly in multiparous patients.

*The four main causes are:*

**Weak Caesarean section scar.       Obstructed labour.**
**Trauma during operative manipulation per vaginam.**
**The unwise use of oxytocic drugs.**

### 1. DUE TO WEAK CAESAREAN SECTION SCAR

*Factors causing a weakened scar are:*

When the wound did not heal by first intention.
If another pregnancy occurs within six months.
Overdistension as in subsequent twins or polyhydramnios.

The scar may rupture during the last four weeks of pregnancy but more commonly during the first stage of labour, and as the signs are not as dramatic as in obstructed labour, the term 'silent rupture' is applied. During late pregnancy the woman may experience intermittent pain in her right side, not necessarily severe, which may persist over a period of four or five days. Pain is due to irritation of the peritoneum by the trickling of blood from the uterine scar which is 'giving way'.

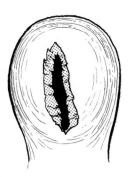
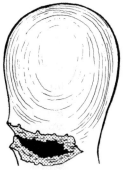

Rupture through a                     Tranverse rupture
classical Caesarean scar              of lower segment

Fig. 24-1

**During labour** severe constant abdominal pain accompanied by vomiting, even when the pulse is below 100, is a significant sign of scar rupture. Shock comes on slowly in some cases, and abruptly in others depending on the degree of rupture and the amount of internal haemorrhage. Vaginal bleeding may occur.

414

*Management*

All labours subsequent to Caesarean section should be conducted in hospital because of the danger of scar rupture; the author having seen a case of ruptured scar prior to which the woman had one spontaneous and one forceps delivery subsequent to a classical Caesarean section for placenta praevia. These patients should be under the care of an obstetrician, who will admit them to hospital for the last two weeks of pregnancy. (Oxytocin is rarely given to induce labour in such cases and if so beginning with low dosage: constant monitoring is mandatory.)

Impending scar rupture may not be detected under epidural analgesia.

The midwife's responsibility is heavy, and she must pay close attention to the following points. (*a*) Abdominal palpation should be reduced to a minimum and performed with great gentleness.

(*b*) **The following features should be reported to the doctor:**

Slight or no advance, with good contractions during first stage.

| | |
|---|---|
| Increasing tenderness over the scar. | A rising pulse rate. |
| Constant pain in the abdomen. | Vaginal bleeding. |
| Insufficient advance during second stage. | Signs of shock. |

## 2. DUE TO OBSTRUCTED LABOUR

The uterus ruptures because of excessive thinning of the lower uterine segment, and in view of the possibility of this catastrophe midwives must know the causes of obstructed labour and detect them during pregnancy (p. 410). Recognition of the signs of obstructed labour is equally important, but such a state of affairs does not arise in the practice of a competent midwife; she detects the conditions causing obstruction and seeks medical assistance. The patient is usually a grande multipara whose uterus is liable to have much fibrous tissue that does not stretch well. Rupture has, to the author's knowledge occurred when the woman had been one hour in the second stage and less than 12 hours in labour. It occurs more commonly during the second stage.

*Warning Signs*

**General and abdominal signs of obstructed labour are manifest,** such as a rising pulse rate, tonic contractions and Bandl's ring.

**The lower segment is exquisitely tender. Vaginal bleeding is an ominous sign.**

### ACTUAL RUPTURE

**Excruciating pain occurs, uterine contractions cease:** the woman may feel that 'something has given way', but not in all cases.

She feels faint and rapidly becomes profoundly shocked. The uterus may be felt as a separate mass. Cessation of the fetal heart beat occurs. The fetus, now in the peritoneal cavity, can be palpated beneath the abdominal wall. Any abdominal or shoulder pain experienced is due to the presence of blood or of the uterine contents in the peritoneal cavity. These signs will be less pronounced when uterine rupture is not extensive; shock comes on more slowly.

*Treatment of Ruptured Uterus*

**On district.** The 'Flying Squad' is summoned and the woman treated for shock (see p. 433). Blood transfusion will be given if necessary and a sedative administered prior to transferring the patient to hospital as quickly as possible.

**In hospital.** The woman is laid flat. Treatment for shock is given. Preparations are made for blood transfusion and for hysterectomy (the rent *may be* sutured in scar rupture and in *other* cases where the tear is not irregular).

The prognosis is less good in cases of obstructed labour, the maternal mortality rate being 50 to 60 per cent. The fetal mortality rate is almost 100 per cent in cases of complete rupture.

### 3. DUE TO TRAUMA DURING DYSTOCIA

**Internal version for shoulder presentation** may cause rupture.

When labour has proceeded for some time with a shoulder presentation, the thinned lower uterine segment is unduly stretched, therefore any internal manipulation to rectify the lie carries a grave risk. The woman exhibits signs of shock during or after the procedure: Caesarean section is usually preferred.

**Extraction of the after-coming head of the hydrocephalic baby** may cause a severe cervical tear which extends upwards into the body of the uterus. On district the treatment is to give ergometrine, 0·5 mg intramuscularly, and summon the 'Flying Squad'. A pack will be inserted, a sedative given and the patient transferred to hospital for hysterectomy.

**During a destructive operation** injury to the uterus may (rarely) occur. In such cases the baby is extracted vaginally; the signs are similar to those of incomplete rupture.

### 4. DUE TO THE UNWISE USE OF OXYTOCIC DRUGS

When given intramuscularly (inadvisedly) to induce labour, rupture of the uterus may occur: signs of rupture may not be manifest for a number of hours after its administration. Buccal Pitocin has been associated with uterine rupture. Oxytocin is never administered by a midwife during the first stage of labour, except under written instructions from a doctor. Oxytocin is equally dangerous during the second stage should obstruction to advance of the fetus be present. (*Intravenous drip is a safer method of administration.*)

### INCOMPLETE RUPTURE

In this condition the myometrium and endometrium are ruptured, the perimetrium remains intact and the baby is born vaginally. The diagnosis is made during the third stage of labour, when signs of shock develop. Whenever shock during the third stage is more severe than the type of delivery or blood loss warrants, or if the woman does not recover from shock when given the necessary treatment, the possibility of incomplete rupture of the uterus should be considered.

### Treatment

This is the same as for complete rupture. (In remote areas the rent and vagina may be packed with gauze to control bleeding and the woman transferred to hospital for hysterectomy.)

## PRESENTATION AND PROLAPSE OF CORD

**Presentation of cord** is the term applied when the umbilical cord lies in front of the presenting part and the membranes are intact.

**Prolapse of cord** is the term applied when the cord lies in front of the presenting part and the membranes are ruptured.

**Occult prolapse of cord** is the term used when the cord lies alongside, but not in front of, the presenting part.

### CAUSES

Any condition in which the presenting part does not fit accurately into the lower uterine segment will permit the umbilical cord to slip down in front of the presenting part. Multiparity is a contributory factor because the head may not be engaged when the membranes rupture. Anterior obliquity and malpresentations are both more common in multiparae.

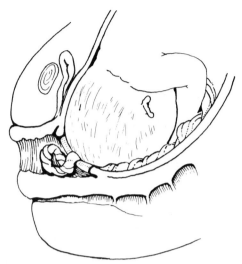

Fig. 24-2    Prolapse of cord.

### MALPRESENTATIONS

**Complete breech presentation** is a common cause, as the umbilicus is so near the buttocks. The prognosis is fairly good, because the presenting part is soft and does not compress the cord as the head would.

**Shoulder presentation.** If in remote areas it is not possible to perform Caesarean section internal version is done and this also succeeds in replacing the prolapsed cord, but the manipulation increases the risk of stillbirth and is not recommended.

Face and brow presentations are less common causes.

### POLYHYDRAMNIOS

The cord is liable to be swept down in the rush of fluid if the membranes rupture spontaneously: some puncture the membranes at the beginning of labour with due precautions (see p. 180) to prevent this. Polyhydramnios and malpresentation occur in twins and both cause the cord to prolapse.

### HIGH HEAD

If the membranes rupture spontaneously with the fetal head high, the cord may prolapse. This tends to occur in multiparous patients because the head may not be engaged when the membranes rupture.

**Puncture of membranes:** because the incidence of cord prolapse is increased when labour is induced by puncture of membranes this should only be undertaken in a hospital where Caesarean section can be performed without delay. Close supervision of the fetal heart is essential.

## CORD PRESENTATION

Presentation of cord is rarely encountered, because the conditions causing the cord to present tend to produce early rupture of the membranes. It can only be diagnosed by feeling the cord inside the intact fore-waters.

The midwife should feel if the cord is pulsating, and then withdraw her fingers because of the danger of puncturing the membranes. If pulsating, the doctor should be sent for urgently, and the woman placed in the exaggerated Sims' left lateral position. Using the Trendelenburg position or having the foot of the bed raised 50 cm is less tiring for the woman, but less effective. Preparations are made to deal with prolapse of cord, which is certain to take place within a short time. The theatre should be set up quickly for Caesarean section.

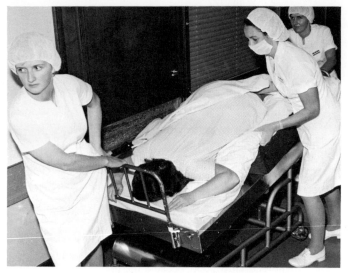

Fig. 24-3   Patient being transported from labour ward to theatre. Midwife elevating the fetal head PV to take pressure off the cord.

*Bellshill Maternity Hospital, Lanarkshire.*

## PROLAPSE OF CORD

The cord may be felt in the vagina, or be seen lying outside the vulva. Early diagnosis and prompt treatment may save the baby's life, so the midwife must always be on the alert for the possibility of this complication.

The fetal heart should be auscultated when the membranes rupture, during every labour, but if conditions liable to cause prolapse of cord exist, a vaginal examination should be made as soon as the membranes rupture. Suspicion of prolapsed cord will be aroused when fetal distress occurs for no apparent reason. Any disturbance in the fetal heart rate, particularly slowing, especially during the first stage, is significant; a vaginal examination will verify the diagnosis; presentation of the fetus and dilatation of the cervix are noted.

### Management

**During the first stage.** Caesarean section is performed if the fetus is alive. Attempts to replace the cord inside the uterus either fail or the cord prolapses again, and valuable time is wasted.

If the cord is outside the vulva it should, after being cleansed with a warm antiseptic solution, be placed in the vagina to keep it clean and warm. Chilling and rough handling of the cord will produce spasm of the umbilical blood vessels and this will further impede the supply of oxygen to the fetus.

**During the second stage.** Episiotomy, application of forceps or breech extraction as indicated.

The risks to the fetus are hypoxia and stillbirth. Head presentations are most serious: complete breech most favourable, and 10 minutes is the maximal time the fetus can be expected to survive cord compression, but the length of time depends on the degree of compression.

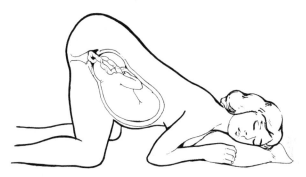

Fig. 24-4   Patient in the knee elbow position. Thighs must be straight. The fetus gravitates towards the fundus and pressure on the cord is relieved. Not so useful during transportation.

### To Relieve Pressure on the Cord

The woman is placed in the exaggerated Sims' left lateral position and two foam rubber wedges are inserted under her buttocks to elevate them still further. This causes the fetus to gravitate towards the diaphragm and takes the pressure off the cord. The presenting part is elevated manually by the sterile gloved fingers in the vagina. The procedure is less tiring when maintained for a long period if the woman lies in Sims' position as described above. Elevation of the presenting part should be continued (1) from the time prolapse of cord is diagnosed, (2) during the journey to hospital by ambulance, (3) while being transported in hospital from labour ward to operating theatre.

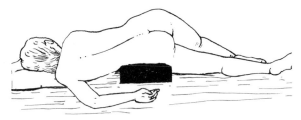

Fig. 24-5   Woman in the exaggerated Sim's left lateral position. Two large foam rubber wedges or pillows give additional elevation of buttocks.

A patient with prolapse of cord was admitted to the Simpson Maternity Pavilion after a three-hour journey by ambulance, during which pressure on the cord was reduced by the adoption of Sims' position and manual elevation of the fetal head vaginally. A live baby was born by Caesarean section. At Bellshill Maternity Hospital, Lanarkshire, five babies during one year were born alive under similar circumstances.

## AMNIOTIC FLUID EMBOLISM

This catastrophe with a maternal mortality rate over 80 per cent usually occurs near the end of the first stage of a labour that is apparently normal but characterised by rapid, strong tumultuous contractions, the membranes having ruptured. The administration of oxytocin may be a predisposing factor. It tends to occur in women over 35 years of age and may result in sudden death. Amniotic fluid (which is high in thromboplastin) is forced into the maternal circulation via the utero-placental site and this gives rise to blood coagulation disorders, e.g. hypofibrinogenaemia.

### SIGNS AND SYMPTOMS

**Respiratory distress of sudden onset.**  **Severe dyspnoea.**  **Hypotension.**
**Cyanosis: Pulmonary oedema.**  **Sudden collapse.**  **Tachycardia.**

### *Treatment*

Oxygen is administered.

A general anaesthetic may be necessary to damp down the tetanic uterine contractions. An anaesthetist will cope with the cardio-respiratory emergency. Aminophylline is administered slowly to reduce bronchial spasm.

Blood transfusion will be given slowly: fresh (not stored) blood being preferred to fibrinogen or plasma to combat the hypofibrinogenaemia which is invariably present. The transfusion is monitored by central venous pressure measurement to maintain adequate blood volume and avoid cardiac failure.

Delivery by forceps.

Torrential uncontrollable postpartum haemorrhage will occur if the clotting defect is not rectified and the uterus is atonic.

# ACUTE INVERSION OF THE UTERUS

Inversion means that the uterus is turned inside out, and is a serious complication of the third stage. In acute cases the inner surface of the fundus appears at the vaginal orifice.

The frequency of this condition is said to be about 1 in 100,000 deliveries, and it is only by being aware of and avoiding the causes that it does not occur more often.

### CAUSES

Forcibly attempting to expel the placenta by using fundal pressure when the uterus is atonic.

Combining fundal expression and cord traction to deliver the placenta.

*Precipitate labour is an unlikely cause as the uterus is contracting strongly.*

### SIGNS AND SYMPTOMS

The uterus may be seen outside the vulva. The fundus is not palpable abdominally.

Shock is an outstanding sign and is probably due to traction and compression of the ovaries, Fallopian tubes and broad ligaments (Fig. 24-6).

Bleeding will be present unless the placenta is completely adherent to the uterine wall.

Pain is usually severe.

In less acute cases the fundus is partially inverted and may or may not pass through the cervical os; it is neither visible at the vulva, nor can it be palpated abdominally.

### Treatment on District

The inverted uterus should be replaced immediately or as soon as possible.

The midwife sends urgently for medical assistance ('Flying Squad'), and if the uterus is outside the vulva it should be wrapped in a towel wrung out of warm Hibitane solution. Raising the foot of the bed will partly relieve the traction on the ovaries: to alleviate pain the midwife may give an injection of pethidine, 100 mg. The doctor may attempt to replace the uterus without removing the placenta, and this is less difficult if done at once.

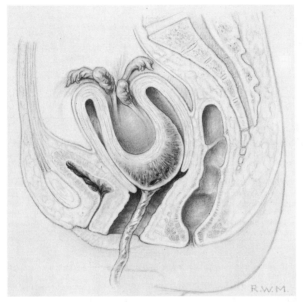

Fig. 24-6   Acute inversion of the uterus. Note traction on ovaries and Fallopian tubes which gives rise to shock.

**In remote areas**

The midwife attempts to replace the inverted uterus under inhalational analgesia. With the fingers of the hand in the vagina, pressure is applied on the area near the cervix, and gradually the corpus is replaced. The fundus goes back last by pressure with the palm of the hand. Abdominally slight counter pressure is applied to prevent the uterus from being pushed up too far. If the midwife fails to replace the uterus she should insert it into the vagina and then introduce a gauze pack or a recorded number of perineal pads to maintain it in position. Raising the foot of the bed 50 cm will relieve traction on the ovaries.

### Treatment in Hospital

**Controlling haemorrhage.** In doing so it may be necessary to strip off the remainder of the placenta and apply hot towels to the uterus.

**Replacing the uterus.** Delay increases the difficulty of replacement. The part which came down last goes back first, e.g. the lower segment first, fundus last.

The hydrostatic pressure method of replacement has been used with success in a series of cases. The vagina is douched with Hibitane solution. The solution is then changed to sodium chloride, and the vaginal orifice blocked by the forearm or hand. No douche nozzle is used, and to create the necessary pressure the douche-can may have to be raised above the usual level for douching. The pressure exerted by the fluid distends the vagina and reduces the inverted uterus.

**Combating the shock.** The degree of shock does not improve until the uterus is replaced, but when shock is profound following delay or a long ambulance journey resuscitative measures should be instituted prior to replacement. Immediate blood transfusion is essential; Ringer's lactate may be used until blood is available.

**Preventing subsequent inversion.** Ergometrine, 0·5 mg, or Syntometrine 1 ml is given after replacement.

### The Midwife prepares the equipment for

Blood transfusion. Catheterisation. Anaesthesia. Cleansing of the parts. Douching with large volume of sodium chloride solution.

---

## QUESTIONS FOR REVISION
### RUPTURE OF THE UTERUS

#### Oral Questions

Give 4 main causes of uterine rupture. Give 4 signs of actual rupture.

Give examples of trauma that might cause uterine rupture: (1) how a midwife could try to prevent rupture of the uterus; (2) care of a woman during labour who has had a previous Caesarean section; (3) obstructed labour as a cause of rupture.

What is meant by: silent rupture; the unwise use of oxytocic drugs; grande multipara?

Give 3 reasons why a Caesarean scar is likely to rupture. When does this occur? What are the warning signs? Which malpresentations, if not diagnosed, might cause rupture? State the signs of impending rupture due to obstruction. What is meant by incomplete rupture? How and when is it diagnosed?

**C.M.B.(Scot.) 30-min. question.** What factors predispose to and what are the imminent signs of rupture of the uterus? **Eng.:** Management of labour in a woman with a uterine scar.

#### Acute inversion of the uterus

Give two ways in which an incompetent midwife might cause inversion: how would the condition be treated on the district? What is the reason for raising the foot of the bed? What preparations would the midwife make for such a case in hospital? Why is precipitate labour unlikely to cause inversion? What is meant by the hydrostatic method of replacement?

**C.M.B.(Scot.) 5-min. question.** Acute inversion of the uterus.

#### Amniotic fluid embolism

During what stage of labour does amniotic embolism occur? Give 4 signs. Mention 4 procedures you could anticipate being carried out by the doctor. Name 3 substances that may be administered intravenously. If the woman survives the immediate episode what further danger exists?

#### PROLAPSE OF CORD

Differentiate between: presentation and prolapse of cord; treatment during first and second stages of labour.

Explain why cord prolapse occurs in polyhydramnios and what a midwife could do to avert or recognise this.

Give (a) causes of prolapse of cord; (b) treatment of prolapse of cord when the cervix is 4 cm dilated.

Describe how you would relieve pressure on a prolapsed cord during a long ambulance journey.

How would you prevent prolapse of the cord during transport from labour ward to theatre.

**C.M.B.(Scot.) 30-min. question.** Define prolapse of the cord. Describe the predisposing factors and management of such a case.

**N. Ire.** What conditions predispose to prolapse of the umbilical cord? You are attending a patient during labour and the cord prolapses. Describe your management pending the arrival of a doctor.

**N. Ire.** (a) Describe the structure and the functions of the umbilical cord. (b) Briefly discuss the abnormalities of the cord which may occur. (c) What action should be taken by the midwife if the cord prolapses?

**C.M.B.(Eng.).** Differentiate between cord presentation and cord prolapse. On which factors does the management of these complications depend and why?

# 25
# Complications of the Third Stage of Labour

*Postpartum haemorrhage (atonic; traumatic). Adherent placenta. Retained placenta. Vulval haematoma. Collapse and shock. Blood transfusion. Central venous pressure*

## POSTPARTUM HAEMORRHAGE

This is one of the most serious complications in obstetrics, and the woman's life depends on the midwife's prompt, intelligent action, for what might become an alarming haemorrhage can often be checked or kept under control by good management.

**Definition.** Postpartum haemorrhage is severe bleeding during the third stage of labour, or within 24 hours after the expulsion of the placenta. Haemorrhage occurring after 24 hours and within six weeks of delivery is known as puerperal haemorrhage. This is considered under complications of the puerperium (p. 478).

### Sending for Medical Aid

The amount of blood-loss which constitutes haemorrhage cannot be gauged entirely in millilitres. Medical aid should be obtained when over 500 ml is lost, even with no systemic signs, or if the loss of under 500 ml is accompanied by deterioration in the woman's general condition. It is the effect of blood-loss rather than the amount of blood lost that matters. In cases of anaemia, whether nutritional or due to antepartum haemorrhage, the loss of under 300 ml of blood might be serious.

The average blood-loss during a normal third stage is 120 to 240 ml, and when a woman loses more than 300 ml the midwife should take action to control the bleeding, but need not send for medical assistance if the woman's general condition is satisfactory and the loss is less than 500 ml. (*In some hospitals the resident doctor is summoned for a blood-loss of 300 ml*). All blood should be saved until bleeding is under control. A fall in Hb postpartum 2 to 3 g/dl is presumptive evidence of postpartum haemorrhage if the Hb had been done shortly prior to delivery.

### ATONIC HAEMORRHAGE

**Atonic** is the more common type and is always from the placental site. As the name implies, it is due to lack of tone in the uterine muscle and any condition that interferes with uterine contraction and retraction will predispose to it.

### Causes

**Mismanagement of the third stage. Atonic uterus. Antepartum haemorrhage. Fibroids. Blood coagulation disorders are an additional hazard.**

#### Mismanagement of the third stage

This is probably the most common cause of postpartum haemorrhage and one which is under the control of the person conducting the labour. If the woman is permitted to come into the third stage of labour with a full bladder, this inhibits proper placental separation, and as a result haemorrhage is liable to follow. It is reprehensible to have to pass a catheter when postpartum haemorrhage occurs; the need should not exist; the bladder should have been emptied at the end of the first stage.

Massaging, kneading, squeezing and pushing, over-stimulate the uterus and cause irregular contractions and partial separation of the placenta. Such contractions are inadequate to control the bleeding from the separated areas. Too much massage may prevent clot formation in the blood sinuses of the placental site.

**The grande multipara** may have a lax uterus.

**Narcosis and anaesthesia.** If large doses of sedative drugs are administered and when deep general anaesthesia is necessary the uterus becomes sluggish.

**Rapid expulsion of a large baby.** It may be that the muscle fibres in the upper segment do not have time to retract properly during rapid expulsion of the baby. Midwives should not pull the baby out.

**Twins.** The overdistended uterus may not contract well and the large placental site provides a more extensive bleeding area.

### Antepartum haemorrhage

In cases of placental abruption, blood percolates amongst the muscle fibres and inhibits their contractility. In placenta praevia the muscle fibres in the lower uterine segment do not furnish the 'living ligature' action as do those in the upper segment.

### Subendometrial fibroids

When situated in the placental site area fibroids may interfere with the uterine muscle action that closes the blood sinuses.

### Blood coagulation disorders

If in the presence of this condition the uterus is atonic, torrential and uncontrollable haemorrhage will occur.

*Retained products* cause bleeding: the uterus cannot retract completely until it is empty; blood clot in the cavity of the uterus interferes with uterine action, and a partially separated placenta has the same effect. When a piece of placenta is left adhering to the uterine wall, it inhibits the effective closure of the surrounding blood sinuses. Later it may slough off, giving rise to serious puerperal haemorrhage.

#### SIGNS OF POSTPARTUM HAEMORRHAGE

| Bleeding. | Boggy uterus. | Pallor (*a later sign*). |
|-----------|---------------|--------------------------|
| Big uterus. | Pulse rapid. | Collapse (*see* p. 431). |

### Bleeding

In atonic haemorrhage the bleeding does not as a rule begin until a few minutes after the birth of the baby, and there is no difficulty in making the diagnosis when blood is seen pouring from the vagina. It tends to come in gushes, because the inert uterus fills up with blood and the large clots which collect in the uterus or vagina are expelled when a contraction occurs.

### Big uterus

When the fundus rises above the level of the umbilicus or feels large the cause must be investigated (p. 334). On rare occasions the fundus has been known to reach the xiphisternum, because the inert uterus was filled with clot and no blood was escaping from the vagina. This could only happen when there was **ignorance or gross negligence** on the part of the person in charge of the case.

### Boggy uterus

A uterus distended with blood lacks the firm consistency of the well contracted empty uterus. In severe cases the uterus may be so soft and flabby that it is impossible to detect its outline.

**Pulse rapid**

When the pulse rate rises to 90 beats per minute it is abnormally rapid, but the midwife should realise that one or more minutes may elapse before the pulse increases, even when 500 ml of blood has been lost.

**Pallor**

This is usually noticed in the face, and is a later sign; a striking feature often indicating collapse (p. 431).

### PROPHYLAXIS

**Treatment of anaemia** during pregnancy so that the woman is not exsanguinated by average blood loss. This is particularly applicable in the African countries.

**The following women should be delivered in hospital.** Women who have a history of postpartum haemorrhage or adherent placentae as they are liable to have a recurrence.

The grande multipara (*more than five confinements*) is particularly likely to bleed.

Those who have had antepartum haemorrhage.

The woman with fibroid tumours.

**Good management of the second stage of labour**

The bladder should be emptied at the end of the first stage.

Slow delivery of the baby's body during a contraction.

**Good management of the third stage of labour** (See p. 332, also Mismanagement, p. 423).

The practice of giving Syntometrine and using controlled cord traction has reduced the incidence of postpartum haemorrhage from 7 to 3 per cent.

**Anticipation of blood coagulation disorders**

This condition may exist in cases of placental abruption, prolonged retention of a dead fetus, or amniotic fluid embolism, and if the uterus is atonic, may cause torrential haemorrhage.

**The use of oxytocic drugs**

Intramuscular injection of Syntometrine, 1 ml, is given by most British doctors and midwives as soon as the anterior shoulder is born.

Oxytocin drip.—This would be set up as a prophylactic measure in cases when postpartum haemorrhage is anticipated and when the uterine contractions are weak: it is kept running for one hour after completion of the third stage.

### *The Principles of Treatment*

**Stop the bleeding.   Replace fluid lost.   Treat circulatory failure (shock).**

### ACTIVE TREATMENT (*prior to expulsion of placenta*)

**To stop the bleeding** the uterus must be stimulated to contract, and this can best be accomplished when it is empty, so blood clot and placenta must be expelled.

**Massage and knead the uterus until it contracts**

Then squeeze out the blood clots. Remove the placenta by controlled cord traction.

### Send for the doctor or the 'Flying Squad'

But never leave the patient while doing so. Send a responsible person, if available, and make it clear that the doctor is urgently needed. If the blood group and Rh factor are known, notify this to the 'Flying Squad'. Instruct the person to give the name and address clearly, and, if remote, directions for finding the house or flat. Valuable time will be saved at night having a lighted window to attract attention; in multistoried blocks of flats some person should be strategically placed to direct the 'team'.

### Administration of oxytocic drugs

If the placenta cannot be expelled because it is not completely separated, the midwife should give Syntometrine, 1 ml, which consists of **ergometrine, 0·5 mg, and oxytocin (Syntocinon), 5 units.** Given intramuscularly Syntocinon acts in $2\frac{1}{2}$ minutes, ergometrine acts in 6 to 7 minutes. Syntometrine may be given intravenously unless the patient is of doubtful cardiac status.

The left hand is kept on the fundus, and when the contraction induced by the Syntometrine occurs the midwife should deliver the placenta by controlled cord traction. If the placenta does not separate completely, she should not meddle any further; the Syntometrine already given ought to control the bleeding; but if not and the loss is profuse a second dose may be administered in ten minutes. If haemorrhage continues and medical assistance cannot be obtained in time, manual removal of the placenta will have to be performed by the midwife.

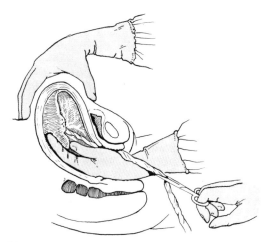

Fig. 25-1    Manual removal of placenta. Fingers separating the placenta.

### Manual removal of the placenta

This formidable procedure should not be undertaken by the midwife except in a grave emergency, for when done without a general anaesthetic the risk of shock is intensified. But when the need arises, the procedure should be carried out before the patient is exsanguinated. When serious postpartum haemorrhage occurs in hospital, manual removal of placenta is carried out under general anaesthesia without delay, usually within one minute following the intravenous injection of ergometrine, 0·5 mg.

*Method*

The patient is placed in the lithotomy position. An assistant cleanses the vulva quickly with a suitable disinfectant, and smears the labia with obstetric cream. The midwife makes her hands as aseptic as possible in the very short time at her disposal, e.g. she washes them quickly, draws on a sterile gauntlet glove (if available) and smears her gloved hand with Hibitane cream.

The left hand holds the umbilical cord taut while the right hand, with the thumb in the palm, shaped like a cone, is inserted into the vagina and follows the cord up to the placenta. On finding the separated area the ulnar border of the extended fingers is insinuated between placenta and decidua, the palm facing the placenta: with a sideways slicing movement the placenta is gently detached.

Throughout the separation procedure the left hand steadies the uterus abdominally. When the placenta is completely separated the left hand rubs up a contraction and expels the hand with the placenta within its grasp.

## TREATMENT OF ATONIC POSTPARTUM HAEMORRHAGE
*(after the placenta is expelled)*

**The uterus should be massaged until it contracts.** Blood clots are then expelled. **Medical aid or the 'Flying Squad' is summoned Oxytocic drugs are given Syntometrine, 1 ml, given intramuscularly acts in two and a half minutes.**

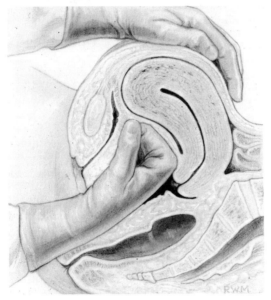

Fig. 25-2   Internal bimanual compression of the placental site. The left hand is on the abdomen.

**Ergometrine, 0·5 mg, given intramuscularly acts in seven minutes.** The doctor may give ergometrine intravenously; by this route it acts in 45 seconds, dose 0·5 mg, but may cause the placenta to be trapped. Midwives may use the intravenous route but if inexperienced in the technique of intravenous injection they will waste valuable time in attempting to inject the vein of a collapsed patient, so they should give i.m. Syntometrine.

If bleeding continues, an oxytocin intravenous drip is given; i.e. glucose (5 per cent) 540 ml, with 10 units Syntocinon at 40 drops per minute.

The midwife should not discard any blood until the haemorrhage is under control, and the amount of blood lost should always be measured and recorded. (For treatment of collapse due to haemorrhage, see p. 431.)

### Bimanual compression of the placental site

This method is useful in controlling severe haemorrhage until oxytocic drugs take effect. The patient is in the dorsal position. An assistant, if available, cleanses the vulva. The right hand is made as aseptic as possible in the manner described for manual removal of placenta and inserted into the vagina like a cone; the hand is closed and the flat part of the closed fist is placed into the anterior vaginal fornix and against the anterior uterine wall. The right elbow rests on the bed between the woman's thighs. The left hand is placed down behind the uterus abdominally, with the fingers directed towards the cervix. The uterus is brought forwards and with the palm of the left hand it is pressed on to the fist in the vagina. In this way the placental site is compressed between the two hands.

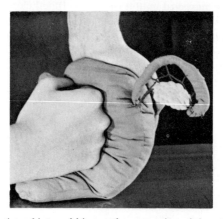

Fig. 25-3  Demonstration of internal bimanual compression of the uterus. Model of uterus used at Aberdeen Maternity Hospital for student midwives. *Note.*—Ovaries are not being compressed.

Bimanual compression must be maintained until the uterus contracts and retracts, even although the bleeding is controlled by pressure. Packing the uterus is a useless procedure which will not control atonic haemorrhage.

## TRAUMATIC POSTPARTUM HAEMORRHAGE

Traumatic haemorrhage is usually due to lacerations of the cervix or upper vagina. (Bleeding from a lacerated perineum is readily controlled, but when from the region of the clitoris the flow may be profuse and necessitate the insertion of sutures. The midwife should apply pressure with a sterile pad in an endeavour to control bleeding.)

### Causes

Traumatic haemorrhage can take place during the spontaneous delivery of a large baby, or when a large diameter presents as in face to pubes, or during extraction of the after-coming head in a breech presentation, but is more commonly associated with a difficult instrumental delivery.

**SIGNS**

Bleeding starts immediately after the baby is born.

The flow of blood is continuous, often a heavy trickle, although it may collect and form clots in the vagina, especially when the woman is lying on a sagging bed.

The uterus is in good tone and may be firmly contracted.

### *Treatment*

The only satisfactory treatment is suturing of the lacerations, so medical aid should be obtained. The requirements for suturing are outlined on page 615. The woman is anaesthetised and the vagina swabbed as dry as possible. For visual inspection a Sims-Ferguson's speculum and a good light are essential. The anterior and posterior lips of the cervix are grasped with sponge-holding forceps, as teneculae are liable to tear the soft cervix. The bleeding points are tied, and the lacerated edges sutured with catgut.

#### Treatment in remote areas by the midwife

Only in very remote areas will the midwife have to cope with traumatic haemorrhage alone, and in such circumstances she may have to resort to packing the vagina in order to compress the bleeding vessels. Such packing will not control bleeding from an atonic uterus.

Clots should be swabbed out of the vagina and the bladder emptied.

If a sterile gauze pack is not available sterile perineal pads smeared with obstetric cream may be used. If no speculum is available, the woman is placed in Sims' left lateral position and, while using the first and second fingers of her left hand as a perineal retractor, the midwife should pack the vagina snugly and then apply a perineal pad which is held firmly in position by being attached to a T-binder. The recorded number of pads are removed in six hours.

## VULVAL HAEMATOMA

Vulval haematoma is a condition which may give rise to a form of traumatic haemorrhage. It is caused by rupture of the subcutaneous veins of the vagina which produces an effusion of blood into the connective tissue of the vulva and vaginal wall. A small haematoma may be associated with the repair of a medio-lateral episiotomy or perineal laceration. It may be a few hours after labour before signs are manifest. The woman complains of discomfort and pain in the perineum and/or labia; the labia majora may be distended to such a degree that the skin is glistening; the haematoma may bulge into the vagina.

### *Treatment*

Without delay and under a general anaesthetic an incision is made into the haematoma by the doctor, the blood clot removed and the bleeding vessels tied or the tissues sutured. Otherwise the wound is firmly packed with gauze wrung out of hot sodium chloride solution. In a case seen by the author 450 ml of blood clot was removed. Blood transfusion may be required.

## ADHERENT PLACENTA

The placenta is said to be adherent if, 30 minutes after the birth of the baby, there are no signs that it has left the upper uterine segment. The most likely cause is that the uterus is not contracting and retracting strongly enough to diminish the area of the placental site sufficiently to separate it from the placenta. A full bladder may predispose to weak uterine action.

### Placenta accreta

Very rarely the placenta is morbidly adherent, because there is no spongy layer of decidua and the chorionic villi are embedded into the uterine muscle. The treatment is hysterectomy, but it occurs so seldom that the midwife need not anticipate such an unlikely event.

### *Treatment of Adherent Placenta* (*See manual removal*, p. 426)

The midwife should seek medical assistance, the 'Flying Squad'. When the doctor is not immediately available, the midwife should give the woman a sedative and remain with her until medical assistance can be obtained. If there is no separation of the placenta there will be no bleeding and on no account should the midwife attempt to detach the adherent placenta or she will cause partial separation and haemorrhage, as well as shock.

Most authorities consider that the woman must not be transferred to hospital with the placenta *in situ* lest partial separation and profuse haemorrhage occur *en route*. The 'Flying Squad' will remove the placenta and give a blood transfusion if necessary. In hospital practice manual removal of the placenta will be performed even in the absence of bleeding, in 30 minutes, under a general anaesthetic. Ergometrine, 0·5 mg, is usually administered intravenously as soon as the placenta is removed, and if bleeding is free 0·5 mg is given intramuscularly at the same time; otherwise it may be administered half an hour later.

Haemorrhage is usually present, and the treatment is therefore that of atonic postpartum haemorrhage: the placenta, in the majority of cases, being partially adherent.

# RETAINED PLACENTA

The placenta has left the upper uterine segment but is not expelled from the vagina.

With the use of controlled cord traction retained placenta occurs less frequently.

**Faulty technique.** An inexperienced midwife may try to expel the placenta, by using fundal pressure, e.g. downwards but not backwards or she may be trying to expel the placenta before it has separated completely. This may induce spasm of the lower uterine segment.

**A full bladder** will interfere with the midwife's efforts to expel the placenta.

**Constriction ring (hour-glass contraction)** usually arises during the treatment of third stage haemorrhage. Too vigorous massaging and squeezing of the uterus may cause spasm of the muscle fibres at the level of the physiological retraction ring or at the internal os, and prevent the expulsion of the placenta. A constriction ring is diagnosed vaginally, usually when an attempt is being made to remove the placenta manually.

If it is imperative to remove the placenta because of haemorrhage, a drug to relax the spasm will be administered, e.g. the inhalation of one ampoule of amyl nitrite. A general anaesthetic is usually administered to relax the spasm.

### *Treatment of Retained Placenta*

If after 30 minutes, with no bleeding, the placenta is still retained in spite of using controlled cord traction, medical aid should be obtained.

The placenta will be removed manually under aseptic precautions. *Pushing on the fundus is not recommended.*

The midwife on district should, before summoning the 'Flying Squad', determine by vaginal examination whether the placenta is partly trapped in the cervix or lower uterine segment. In such circumstances she could grasp the placenta and remove it.

# COLLAPSE DUE TO HAEMORRHAGE

## *Hypovolaemic Shock*

This condition is also known as low cardiac output state. Shock in obstetrics occurs most frequently during the third stage of labour and is usually associated with haemorrhage. When blood loss is rapid and severe the situation becomes extremely grave, and if not remedied promptly an irreversible stage of shock is reached from which the woman may not recover even after the transfusion of several litres of blood.

## SIGNS

**The pulse is rapid** (over 120), thready and soft; it may be imperceptible.

### The blood pressure falls

In a moderate degree of shock the systolic pressure will be below 100 mm Hg.
In a severe degree of shock the systolic pressure will be below 90 mm Hg.
In a very severe degree of shock the systolic pressure will be below 80 mm Hg.
When the systolic pressure is below 60 mm Hg the condition is critical.
In desperate cases it cannot be estimated.

**Marked pallor** or an ashen grey hue of the face is noticed; the mucous membranes become blanched; the skin feels cold and clammy.

**Respirations are at first shallow** and later deep and irregular (air hunger).

**The woman is apathetic** with occasional bouts of restlessness.

## PROPHYLAXIS

### Good physical condition

During pregnancy the woman should be brought into good physical condition to enable her to withstand the unavoidable blood loss that will occur postpartum; the prognosis in cases of haemorrhage always being more grave when the woman's health is poor.

### Rectification of anaemia

Whether nutritional or due to blood loss, anaemia should always be rectified. It is prudent to repeat the haemoglobin test at the 36th week to ensure that it is at a safe level for delivery, i.e. 12·6 g/dl.

**Avoidance of prolonged, exhausting labour** with its concomitant dehydration and metabolic acidosis. Modern methods of acceleration by i.v. oxytocin infusion are recommended.

#### TREATMENT OF COLLAPSE BY THE COMMUNITY MIDWIFE

Haemorrhage must first be brought under control (p. 425). (*The doctor will have been summoned on account of postpartum bleeding.*)

Reassure the patient by keeping calm, handling her gently, working quietly and expeditiously, so that the woman is not aware that an urgent situation has arisen. Remove the blood-stained linen. Excessive heat should not be applied in these circumstances: sufficient warmth for comfort is all that is required.

**Elevate the foot of the bed** 30 cm to treat shock; this does not control haemorrhage. Raising the legs is more effective than lowering the head, and will raise the blood pressure 10 mm Hg and, by gravity, blood will flow to the vital centres in the brain. (The hand should always be kept on the fundus while the patient is in this position because, if bleeding recommences, the uterus may fill up with blood clot and the inexperienced midwife may not be aware of this.)

**Administer fluid.** If facilities for giving an intravenous drip are not available tap water (600 ml) may be given rectally. If run in slowly with a catheter, the dehydrated patient will readily absorb that amount, and as the foot of the bed is elevated, she ought to be able to retain it. To give fluid by mouth is not advisable, even if the patient is thirsty; sips of water are useless and, if sufficient is given to be of any avail, vomiting will be induced.

*(In remote areas, in desperate cases as a first aid measure, the lower limbs may be bandaged from the feet to the thighs, and the legs elevated to direct more blood to the brain, heart and lungs.)*

## ACTIVE TREATMENT

SPEED

**This is vital in:** the first-aid measures instituted by the midwife: obtaining medical assistance: arranging for blood replacement.

RESTORATION OF BLOOD VOLUME

The 'Flying Squad' will give the patient blood group O, Rh negative or positive as required. Rh positive blood is only given if the patients Rh factor has been confirmed as positive. Fresh blood is administered if a blood clotting disorder is suspected. Synthetic blood substitutes such as Macrodex, Intradex or Dextraven are used to restore blood volume until whole blood is available. Glucose, 5 per cent, or Ringer's lactate solution may be used.

The first 1,200 ml of blood are given rapidly, i.e. in 30 minutes, using the Baxter disposable blood administration set with pressure pump, or the Martin transfusion pump. The central venous pressure is monitored. The doctor remains with the patient during this time.

TRANSFER TO HOSPITAL

Blood is always given prior to, and in some cases during, her removal by ambulance. The woman will not be transferred to hospital while in a state of collapse.

DRUGS

Hydrocortisone, 100 mg, is given in a slow intravenous drip, of glucose, 5 per cent, if suprarenal failure is present or suspected. This occurs most commonly in cases of prolonged labour when dehydration, ketoacidosis and electrolyte imbalance have not been corrected. A sedative may be necessary to calm a restless or apprehensive patient. Morphine has no beneficial action in the treatment of shock; some think it is harmful.

Oxygen is administered in severe cases. For duties re transfusion, see page 435.

OBSERVATION

The pulse should be recorded in graph form every five minutes.
The blood pressure is recorded every 15 to 20 minutes.

Only on rare occasions are instruments for cutting down required, but they should always be in readiness because for the collapsed patient they may be urgently needed.

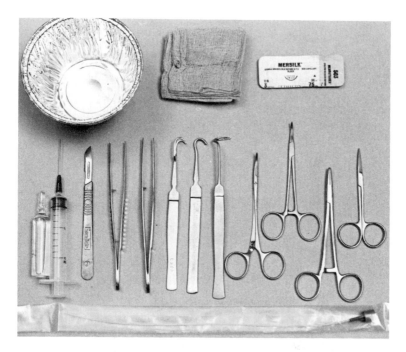

Fig. 25-4   Intravenous set for cutting down.
*Aberdeen Maternity Hospital.*

**Instruments**

2 Towel clips
1 Bard Parker handle No. 3
1 Bard Parker blade No. 10
1 pr. fine toothed dissecting
  forceps
1 pr. non-toothed dissecting
  forceps
1 Aneurysm needle
2 prs. Mosquito artery forceps
1 pr. straight iris scissors

**Needles: sutures**

No. 2 Mersilk suture size 2
Cutting needle
Ethicon 503
2 needles 259, 219
1 Syringe 10 ml
1 amp. 1 per cent lignocaine 10 ml
1 Intravenous cannula
Chlorhexidine 0·5 per cent in
  70 per cent spirit and foil
  gallipot

**Linen: dressings**

1 Aperture towel. 1 Impermeable sheet. 10 gauze swabs, 2 dressing towels. Gown, cap, mask, gloves, hand towel.

## THE 'FLYING SQUAD'

### *Obstetrical Emergency Service*

The team consists of an obstetrician, resident obstetric officer, an experienced midwife and student midwife. An anaesthetist should be one of the team. Speed in answering calls and dealing with the situation is imperative, and an ambulance equipped for the purpose is ideal (Fig. 25-5).

### NON-STERILE TABLE

Two giving-sets with pressure pump for blood. Plastic packs of glucose, blood or blood substitute as required. Tourniquet, sphygmomanometer and stethoscope, C.V.P. manometer. Stand for packs of blood, equipment for examining blood. Hibitane, 0·5 per cent, in spirit. Lignocaine (Duncaine), 1 per cent. Bag for soiled swabs. 5 cm bandage. Adhesive tape, 2·5 cm.

### THE MIDWIFE'S DUTIES

The midwife should have some knowledge of the care of blood to avoid wastage of this very precious fluid. Blood can only be used for three weeks after withdrawal from the donor and should not be removed from the refrigerator or insulated box for longer than 30 minutes. When large amounts of blood are administered it is sometimes necessary to warm the blood prior to transfusion in circumstances in which shivering would be induced in a shocked patient; room temperature is usually adequate; overheated blood may cause death.

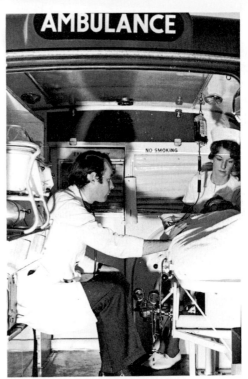

Fig. 25-5  Ambulance equipped exclusively for obstetric emergencies. Note blood transfusion being given. Midwife holding baby. By two-way radio control, contact with labour ward is maintained.

*Bellshill Maternity Hospital, Lanarkshire.*

The community midwife should, while awaiting arrival of the team, prepare adequate supplies of hot and, more especially, cold sterile water. She should keep a five-minute pulse chart and record the blood pressure every 15 minutes. A concise history of the case should be written. Placenta, blood and blood-stained linen are kept for inspection.

Resident doctor takes blood to the ambulance in insulated carrier: **2 packs blood, patient's group;** *or* **2 packs group O Rh negative; 2 packs group O Rh positive.**

Portable incubator, anaesthetic case.

Scrub up and 'prep.' pack; 2 polythene sheets; 6 paper towels; 6 paper masks; 6 paper caps; 2 plastic aprons; sphygmomanometer; stethoscope; thermometer; gastric suction equipment; Pinard's stethoscope.

Transfusion equipment; i.v. puncture set; 'cut down' set; box of syringes, needles; dressing pack.

Drugs; lotions, locked drug box; bowl pack; linen pack; delivery pack.

Instruments; sutures; 6 pairs gloves; pudendal needles; perineal repair set; catheter pack.

Spare gowns, drapes, dressings; catheter pack. Eclampsia requirements.

Baby resuscitation equipment; neonatal laryngoscope; disposable mucus extractors; endotracheal tubes; fine suction catheters; syringes; drugs; swabs.

Powerful light. Anaesthetic machine and equipment.

Bed clothes (in polythene wrap). Oxygen cylinders. Infusion fluids.

Centrifuge; suction apparatus; drip stand. 2 plasma protein solution, 1 sterile water; 1 glucose × 5 per cent. Ringer's lactate solution.

*A complete detailed list of equipment is not given.* Some do not carry Rh positive blood.

### Management by Midwife during Blood Transfusion

Strict asepsis to be maintained.

Flow of blood as directed, usually 1·2 to 2·4 ml per minute.

To facilitate the flow of blood the limb should be kept warm by a well-wrapped hot-water bottle.

Displacement of needle to be avoided.

Pulse to be recorded every 5, 15 or 30 minutes
Temperature every 1 or 2 hours ⎫ recording depends on con-
Blood pressure every 15 or 30 minutes ⎬ dition of patient.
Colour of woman to be noted. ⎭

Fluid balance to be recorded during and for 24 hours after transfusion.

Urine analysis. Observe for haematuria and test each specimen for protein and specific gravity during, and for 24 hours after, transfusion.

Watch for signs of reaction to blood transfusion.

#### TRANSFUSION REACTION

This may be due to giving incompatible blood or using outdated blood or blood haemolysed by overheating, freezing or infection. The reaction usually occurs during the transfusion, but may be delayed for some hours.

### In a severe case of incompatibility the following may occur:

Shock; acute lumbar pain; rigor; a feeling of constriction of the chest; dyspnoea; pyrexia. Haematuria follows soon after the preceding signs. Anuria may occur. Jaundice occurs a few hours or days later.

Rapid improvement may take place, but acute renal failure can ensue, sometimes resulting in death. Recovery from this phase is heralded by diuresis.

### Treatment

The midwife must stop the transfusion immediately, send for the doctor, and prepare for treatment of shock if present. Alternative fluid will be given using a fresh giving-set.

A fluid balance chart is kept; each specimen of urine is saved for analysis.
Piriton, 10 to 20 mg, may be administered for a mild reaction.
For treatment of acute renal failure see page 219.

### SHOCK IN OBSTETRICS

Although there is no such entity as 'obstetric shock' many conditions associated
with obstetrics cause shock and more than one factor may be involved.

**Hypovolaemia (low blood volume) is the most common cause,** due to postpartum
haemorrhage.

### *Causes other than Haemorrhage*

**Tissue trauma** due to accidents such as rupture or inversion of the uterus, difficult
instrumental delivery.

**Oxygen deprivation** may be due to serious obstruction of the pulmonary artery by
an embolus, e.g. blood clot or amniotic fluid.

**Endotoxic** (bacteraemic) shock occurs most commonly in association with septic
abortion (see p. 170).

**Anaesthesia** when induced by non-experts may cause hypoxia and hypotension
which are contributory factors.

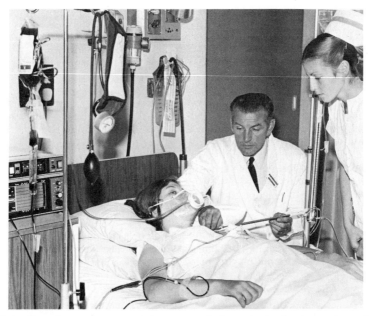

Fig. 25-6   Central venous pressure being measured. Anaesthetist showing student midwife,
pointer directed to the sternal angle (manubrio-sternal joint). Patient is receiving blood,
warmed and pressure aided as necessary using the Fenwal apparatus. Oxygen is being
administered.

*Royal Maternity Hospital, Rottenrow, Glasgow.*

## CENTRAL VENOUS PRESSURE

This is the pressure within the right cardiac atrium. Measurement of the C.V.P.
gives an indication of the amount of blood circulating within the body so

intravenous fluid replacement in cases of hypovolaemia is based on C.V.P. Without such an index patients may be given insufficient blood: conversely if given too much blood the heart would be overloaded and pulmonary oedema could occur. Blood is transfused until the C.V.P. reaches the upper limit of normal—6 to 12 cm of water. The range of C.V.P. readings varies depending on whether (a) the mid-axillary line or (b) the sternal angle is the anatomical level used as zero reference points to locate the right cardiac atrium.

**To locate the level of the right cardiac atrium** the hypovolaemic patient is positioned (usually supine) and the pointer leading from zero on the manometer scale is placed on a level with the right atrium. The doctor may direct the pointer to one of two zero reference levels. When the mid-axillary line (see Fig. 25-7) is used the C.V.P. registers 6 to 12 cm of water (saline solution) and blood is administered to reach 12 cm of water. When the sternal angle (manubrio-sternal joint; see Fig. 25-6) is used the C.V.P. would register 1 to 7 cm of water and the patient is given blood to reach 7 cm of water.

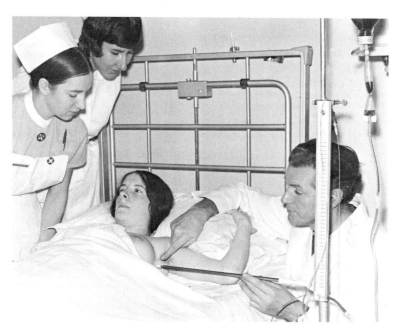

Fig. 25-7   Measurement of central venous pressure. Anaesthetist showing student midwives the pointer directed to the mid-axillary line.

*Royal Maternity Hospital, Rottenrow, Glasgow.*

**Measurement of central venous pressure**

The venous pressure manometer is set up; a radio-opaque catheter is inserted via the antecubital vein and passed into the superior vena cava until its tip overlies the right atrium. The pointer of the manometer is positioned level with either the sternal angle or the mid-axillary line. The catheter is connected to the intravenous saline infusion set at a 3 way stop-cock; the indicator of which is set at the 12 o'clock position and by changing the stop-cock indicator to the 3 o'clock position the saline will enter the manometer tubing. The fluid in the manometer falls with the fluctuations corresponding to the patient's respirations. The C.V.P. is read when the fluid ceases to fall.

Strict aseptic technique is mandatory. Kinks in the tubing must be avoided.

The patient lies on her back when readings are taken.

The stop-cock must not be left at the 3 o'clock position for longer than is absolutely necessary or the blood may clot in the cannula. The doctor is notified if the fluid level in the manometer does not fluctuate with the respirations.

---

## QUESTIONS FOR REVISION
### COMPLICATIONS OF THE THIRD STAGE
### *Oral Questions*

**Postpartum haemorrhage**

Which women are more likely to have postpartum haemorrhage?

How by good management of the second stage could you try to prevent postpartum haemorrhage? How may blood coagulation disorders complicate the third stage? Why is undue kneading and squeezing of the uterus harmful? State the average blood loss during the third stage. What constitutes postpartum haemorrhage?

How would you know that a succenturiate lobe had been retained? What are the dangers? What would you do?

*Differentiate between:* atonic and traumatic postpartum haemorrhage; adherent and retained placenta; hypovolaemic and endotoxic shock.

*Describe:*

Mismanagement of the third stage as a cause of haemorrhage.

The midwife's duties as a member of the 'Flying Squad' team.

The use of oxytocic drugs in the prevention and treatment of postpartum haemorrhage.

*Explain how you would:*

Do manual removal of placenta. Do internal bi-manual compression.

Cope with traumatic postpartum haemorrhage in a remote area. Recognise a blood transfusion reaction.

**Explain** (*a*) How good management of the second stage of labour prevents haemorrhage. (*b*) How the use of Syntometrine and controlled cord traction has reduced P.P.H. from 7 to 3 per cent. (*c*) How you would carry out manual removal of placenta.

**N. Ire. 30-min. question.** How would you distinguish between atonic and traumatic postpartum haemorrhage? Give the treatment of the atonic variety.

**N. Ire. 30-min. question.** What are the possible causes of severe haemorrhage from the uterus half an hour after the placenta has been delivered? What is the management of such a case?

**C.M.B.(Scot.) 30-min. question.** What natural processes prevent haemorrhage after delivery? Give the management of third stage haemorrhage.

**N. Ire. 30-min. question.** How does the placenta separate during the third stage of labour? What complications may occur and how would you deal with them?

**C.M.B.(Eng.) 30-min. question.** What are the causes of postpartum haemorrhage? How would you deal with a postpartum haemorrhage occurring before the delivery of the placenta?

**C.M.B.(Scot.).** Describe the management of the third stage of labour. What complications may occur during the third stage and immediately afterwards.

**C.M.B.(Scot.).** Describe the management of a patient with third stage haemorrhage.

**C.M.B.(Eng.).** Define postpartum haemorrhage and list the predisposing causes of this condition. What emergency measures should a midwife take if a woman bleeds profusely during the third stage of labour?

**C.M.B.(Scot.).** What measures should be taken during pregnancy, during labour and in the first 24 hours following delivery to prevent the occurrence of postpartum haemorrhage?

### *C.M.B. Short Questions*

**Eng.:** Atonic postpartum haemorrhage. **Scot.:** Traumatic postpartum haemorrhage. **Eng.:** The importance of the obstetric 'Flying Squad'. **Eng.:** Vulval haematoma. **Eng.:** Causes of postpartum haemorrhage. **Eng.:** Factors predisposing to postpartum haemorrhage. **Scot.:** Third stage haemorrhage.

# 26
# The Normal Puerperium

*Involution. Psychology. Management. Rooming-in. Third-degree tear. Planned 48-hour transfer from hospital. Good posture. Minor disorders. Postnatal examination. Family planning. Tubal ligation. Vasectomy.*

---

The puerperium is the period following labour, characterised by the following three features:

**The generative organs return to their pregravid state.**

**Lactation is initiated.**

**Recuperation** from the physical hormonal and emotional experience of parturition takes place.

The puerperium begins as soon as the placenta is expelled, and lasts for six to eight weeks. The process by which the generative organs return to their pregravid state is known as 'involution.' The main changes occur in the uterine muscle and decidua, but the ligaments also return to the condition they were in prior to pregnancy. The stretched vagina, pelvic floor and perineum regain their tone, but in some instances a degree of laxity persists.

## INVOLUTION OF THE UTERUS

On the completion of labour, the uterus measures $15 \times 12 \times 7 \cdot 5$ cm and weighs 900 g. At the end of the puerperium it has almost returned to its pregravid size of $7 \cdot 5 \times 5 \times 2 \cdot 5$ cm and weight of 60 g. The marked reduction in size is most rapid during the first week, the uterus losing half of its bulk during that time; this being brought about by autolysis of the muscle fibres and ischaemia of the uterus. The muscle fibres, which during pregnancy increase 10 times in length and 5 times in thickness, are reduced to normal dimensions. Whether the factor producing autolysis is a uterine hormone or enzyme is not known, but some of the protoplasm in the fibres is broken down, absorbed into the blood-stream and excreted by the kidneys. The contraction and retraction of the uterine muscle fibres compress the blood-vessels and reduce the uterine blood supply.

## Reduction in the size of the uterus

At the completion of labour the fundus is about 5 cm below the umbilicus or 12 cm above the symphysis pubis. Twenty-four hours later it has risen to the level of the umbilicus. One week after labour the fundus is approximately 7·5 cm above the symphysis pubis. Twelve days after labour the fundus is not usually palpable.

*The following list gives comparative findings:*

|  | Weight of uterus | Diameter of placental site | Cervix |
|---|---|---|---|
| End of labour | 900 g | 12·5 cm | Soft, flabby |
| End of 1 week | 450 g | 7·5 cm | 2 cm |
| End of 2 weeks | 200 g | 5·0 cm | 1 cm |
| End of 6 weeks | 60 g | 2·5 cm | A slit |

The remains of the spongy layer of decidua, to which the placenta and membranes were attached, are shed; the basal or unaltered layer regenerates a new endometrium and at the end of eight weeks the placental site is healed. A further four weeks or longer may elapse before menstruation recommences.

## THE LOCHIA

Lochia is the term given to the discharge from the uterus during the puerperium. They have an alkaline reaction in which organisms flourish more readily than in the acid vaginal secretion. The amount of lochia varies in different women and is rather more in quantity than what is lost during the menstrual flow; the odour is heavy and unpleasant, but not offensive.

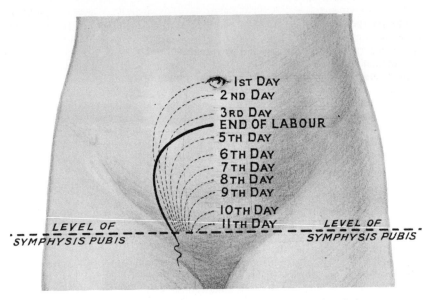

Fig. 26-1   Showing fundal height during the postnatal period.

**Lochia rubra** (red), 1 to 4 days. For the first three days the lochia consist mainly of blood. They also contain shreds of decidua and fragments of chorion, amniotic fluid, lanugo; vernix caseosa and meconium may also be present.

**Lochia serosa** (pink), 5 to 9 days. The discharge is paler and brownish in colour, containing less blood and more serum as well as leucocytes and organisms.

**Lochia alba** (white), 10 to 15 days. The discharge is creamy-greenish in colour and contains leucocytes, organisms, cervical mucus and debris from the healing process in the uterus and vagina. Slight blood discoloration may be seen for as long as three weeks. Persistent red lochia (fresh blood) is a warning sign that products of conception have been retained *in utero*, and of the likelihood of severe puerperal haemorrhage occurring. It is important that midwives realise the danger of retained products and that persistent red lochia be reported to the doctor (see p. 447).

## THE PSYCHOLOGY OF THE POSTNATAL WOMAN

The midwife should have some appreciation of the sensitivity of the woman's nervous system and the emotional turmoil to which she is subjected during the adjustment to motherhood in the puerperium. Her nervous, as well as her physical energy may have been depleted by the stress of labour, and while in this weakened condition she is faced with the care of what appears to her to be a very fragile human being.

## THE MATERNAL INSTINCT

The young mother is overwhelmed with joy in having her precious infant safely in her arms: rather awed at being entrusted with such responsibility and acutely aware of the inadequacy of her knowledge and experience of babies. It is to the midwife she looks for guidance and advice, and, if neither is forthcoming, she becomes apprehensive and dismayed.

The maternal instinct at this time may be very strong, and the mother should be given ample opportunities to express this by caressing and cuddling her baby. But this natural urge, which should be loving and protective, may very readily develop into a state of acute anxiety, particularly if the infant does not appear to her to be thriving. In a minority of women the maternal instinct is delayed and they should be assured that this is a temporary phase. Any bad news should be withheld, if possible, and especially regarding the baby: the father being told when serious illness occurs and consulted regarding informing the mother.

## THE ATTITUDE OF THE MIDWIFE

The psychological and educational aspects of puerperal care must be woven into the very fabric of the student midwife's education and become an integral part of her practical training.

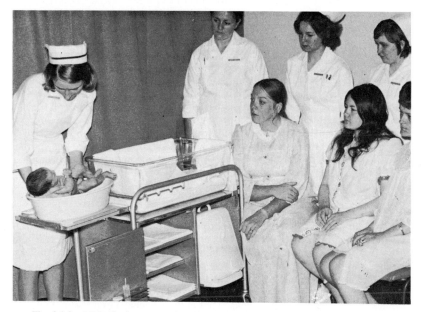

Fig. 26-2   Midwife demonstrating bathing baby to mothers and student nurses.
*Simpson Memorial Maternity Pavilion, Edinburgh.*

The midwife should try to foster a good relationship between mother and baby. Mothers vary in age, maturity, experience, intelligence, temperament, socio-economic status and marital stability. Patience, kindliness and compassion are needed.

It is essential that, by attitude, word and action, the midwife shows her deep understanding and her willingness to be helpful. A kindly approach is appreciated by all women on occasions such as these, and any advice or counsel regarding the baby's or her own welfare is usually received with gratitude and appreciation. Assurance and assistance should be given when necessary, with all procedures concerning the baby, and a certain flexibility of mind should be exhibited. The midwife must refrain from dictating or dominating. Mothers should be encouraged to change napkins, bath and dress their babies; this builds up morale and gives them confidence in their ability to cope with their infants at home.

### A Tranquil Atmosphere

Student midwives who are trained nurses, when assigned to care for postnatal women require to alter their conception of what they may consider to be good ward administration. The ward should have a home-like quality in which mothers with a feeling of contentment can relax and enjoy their babies. The ward should be a pleasant, even casual place where mothers move at their own pace while tending their infants. Rigid routine, rush and bustle are detrimental to the calm atmosphere which should prevail. Where rooming-in is practised, it is not possible to have an immaculately tidy ward, but the contentment of the mothers and the quietness of the babies more than compensate for this.

## THE MOTHER'S EMOTIONAL REACTIONS

Women react during the postpartum period in different ways. The majority are happy and contented unless for some niggling fear or anxiety regarding their babies. The temperament of the woman has an important bearing on her reactions. The happy-go-lucky woman of average intelligence is usually a successful mother. The ultra-intelligent, the imaginative or the highly-strung types are more likely to encounter or create difficulties. Certain mothers may desire to carry out ideas that they have used on previous occasions, or which have been recommended to them. A minority feel very deeply regarding having to conform to hospital ideas and methods which concern the baby, e.g. whether he should be beside her all the time; on self-regulated, three-hourly or four-hourly feeding. If 'reasons why' are given and advantages explained, such mothers would be less resentful than when they are dominated without being consulted. The midwife should try to see the mother's point of view, guiding rather than directing her. Some women are slower and more awkward in handling their babies than others. Allowance must be made for this. If made to feel incompetent they become perturbed, even depressed.

#### A PROCESS OF ADJUSTMENT

The woman with her first baby goes through a process of adjustment that for the well-balanced woman presents no problem. The pampered type may resent the transfer of attention from herself to the baby, and such feelings may be manifest as tantrums or in the making of unjustifiable complaints to redirect attention towards herself. The immature may tend to reject the responsibilities involved in parenthood and object to the curtailment of their social activities. Some may wish to return to their careers in a few weeks. That is their decision and the midwife must not criticise it.

## POSTPARTUM TEARS *(FOURTH DAY BLUES)*

This condition may be due to a temporary endocrine imbalance following childbirth: a few may have short periods of mild depression and mood swings. The women can be assured that this is a transitory state; the 'blues' occurring in about 50 per cent of postnatal mothers.

Women are psychologically vulnerable after childbirth and the susceptibility to tears is undoubtedly present. It is the duty of the midwife to do all in her power to prevent the occurrence of this. Her confidence should be built up regarding the care of her baby by knowledge given at parentcraft classes during pregnancy and continued in the postnatal ward. During the first week of the puerperium the woman should not be subjected to worry or excitement. The baby may be the main cause of worry: the visitors the cause of excitement.

### The following causes should be avoided

**Too many visitors.** Relatives, friends and sometimes acquaintances are eager to offer personal congratulations to the mother and to see the new baby. When, as happens in some countries, there are practically no restrictions on visiting hours, the patient is deprived of the recuperative power of rest and quietness and subjected to a protracted social experience that her nervous system is not in a state to cope with.

**Too little sound sleep.** In hospital this is a common complaint. The baby requires food early in the morning and late in the evening. The depletion of the nursing staff on duty at those periods delays settling down for the night and necessitates an early start which shortens the period available for sleep. The remedy is obvious. Inevitable and unavoidable maternity hospital noises bombard the nervous system. Most midwives remove crying babies from postnatal wards at night to allow the short period of sleep available to be sound.

**Anxiety about the baby** occurs if there is difficulty with breast feeding: the good midwife will spend extra time with mother and baby at feeding times. If the baby is in the intensive care unit the mother needs assurance and should visit her baby 3 or more times daily.

### Advice to Husbands

**Husbands need counsel** on how to deal with the situation, i.e. giving encouragement regarding care of the baby; refraining from expressing resentment that the baby is upsetting the household; assisting with domestic duties if needed; ensuring that sufficient rest, sleep and good food are available; above all he should give tender loving care.

## MODERN IDEAS REGARDING POSTNATAL CARE

The postnatal woman is no longer regarded as an invalid but a normal woman recovering from a natural physiological process. Supervision of the recuperative processes that follow childbirth is necessary in order to detect and correct the abnormal, but actual nursing care is not required after the first 48 hours unless complications arise. The mother's needs are physical, psychological, social and educational, and in many respects they dovetail into each other. Her physical requirements are well catered for, but her psychological needs are neither fully recognised nor met on all occasions. Her educational needs, as the inexperienced mother of a young baby, are sometimes ignored. Good human relationships are most important and must be maintained. Early ambulation has transferred many of the midwife's nursing duties to the patients themselves. This will entail lucid instruction and unremitting supervision. Intelligent and assiduous observation must still proceed, daily routine examination of breasts, bladder, lochia and the perineal suture line is most necessary.

#### INSTRUCTION OF INEXPERIENCED MOTHERS

The need for the education of postnatal mothers is a challenge and student midwives should be orientated during their midwifery training to the role of teacher, supervisor and counsellor.

It would seem reasonable to instruct new mothers regarding the care of their babies. During pregnancy, labour and the puerperium doctors foster and supervise the health and wellbeing of the baby, yet he is permitted to go home under the complete jurisdiction and care of a mother with neither knowledge of baby behaviour nor experience of baby care.

With the discharge of women from hospital during the first week of the puerperium, many at 48 hours, it is even more urgent that prenatal and postnatal teaching programmes be inaugurated to enable them to cope successfully with their babies at home.

### Education geared to meet Social Needs

**The social aspect of postnatal care should deeply concern the midwife;** the adjustment from wife to mother and the establishment of the family unit should be kept in mind and the mother advised as to coping with her new responsibilties. (1) By trying to establish a satisfactory feeding-sleeping routine. The baby who is fed satisfactorily during the day usually sleeps at night. It is most distressing for the parents to have to cope with a crying baby at night when they do not understand the cause or know the remedy. (2) By making an endeavour to instruct the mother regarding breast or bottle feeding prior to discharge. The hospital staff should prescribe the strength and amount of milk and demonstrate the correct procedure in the preparation of feeds, also stressing that babies can be thirsty when they cry, they are not always hungry. (3) By using equipment similar to what will be found in the homes when demonstrating baby-care procedures in hospital and advocating techniques applicable in the home, e.g. bathing baby on the knee rather than on a table.

Much of the teaching on baby care given during pregnancy can be revised and consolidated during the puerperium, and when applied to the mother's own baby it becomes real, worthwhile and infinitely more effective.

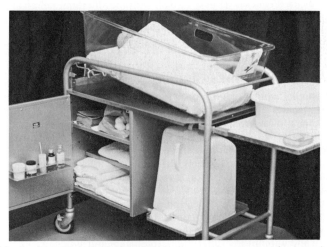

Fig. 26-3  Locker with individual bath, baby linen and equipment for 'rooming-in'.
*Simpson Memorial Maternity Pavilion, Edinburgh.*

## THE ROOMING-IN PLAN

Under this system the baby in his cot remains at the mother's bedside for the greater part of the 24 hours; mother and baby being treated as a unit. At its best rooming-in is an excellent educational project with psychological and physical advantages to both mother and baby. On demand feeding can be practised successfully.

### Educational advantages

The inexperienced mother can study her baby, and so gain knowledge, experience and assurance that will be invaluable when she goes home. Confidence is engendered by handling her infant and in carrying out procedures such as changing napkins, bathing and dressing. By observing his behaviour she notes and can enquire about incidents, e.g. the pallor of the sleeping baby, irregular or shallow breathing, hiccough, green stools, that would worry her at home. She sees her baby handled, napkins changed, bathed, and does all those things herself prior to going home. Her questions can be answered as the need arises; problems would otherwise remain unsolved at home with no adviser available.

Rooming-in is a real-life situation which provides the best possible environment for the learning process.

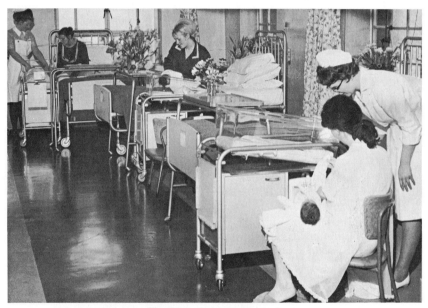

Fig. 26-4   Rooming-in ward.
*Simpson Memorial Maternity Pavilion, Edinburgh.*

### Psychological advantages of rooming-in

The infant gets more mothering than he would get in a nursery: cuddling, warmth and physical contact are necessary as an expression of love and to give emotional security to the baby. Reduction in the length of hunger-crying and frustration, by the proximity of the mother and the prompt provision of food, may have a beneficial influence on the temperament of the child. A more satisfactory and satisfying mother-child relationship can be established. The mother is happy and contented to have her baby near her, to see him when she wishes and to be given the opportunity to express her maternal instinct. During visits of the father both parents are more conscious of the family unit.

**Physical advantages**

Breast feeding is more successfully initiated. The dangers of neonatal cross-infection are lessened if adequate individual equipment is provided. The contact of baby and nursing staff is reduced to a minimum and this also reduces cross-infection.

## THE MIDWIFE, A TEACHER

The midwife is well endowed with obstetric knowledge, skill and experience, and the tuition in parenthood now required, during training, by the Central Midwives Boards will enable her to instruct mothers in a practical manner. Zeal and an abiding interest in mothers and babies make the effort worth while; the satisfaction in preparing mothers to care for and enjoy their babies is immense.

Teaching requires patience to allow for lack of comprehension, and because of the inevitability of much repetition. Fortunately more teaching time is now available since midwives are relieved of many of the nursing duties incumbent on those who care for patients confined to bed.

A curriculum should be drawn up giving daily talk-demonstrations of at least thirty minutes' duration to groups of mothers. Incidental teaching should proceed throughout the day, mainly in a supervisory capacity. Rounds should also be made to discuss non-urgent individual difficulties and to give advice where indicated.

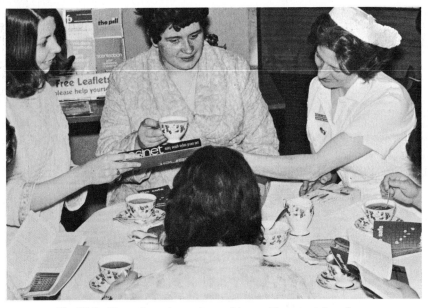

Fig. 26-5   Sister discussing various subjects with postnatal mothers.
*Maternity Hospital, Stirling.*

### SUBJECTS FOR TALKS OR DISCUSSION

**Advice when mother goes home.** Food, sleep, rest, tranquillity, recreation. (*By Nursery Sister.*)

**Baby care.** Feeding, fresh air, sleep, exercise, stools, sore buttocks, crying.

**Bathing baby as in the home.** (*Talk demonstration.*)

**Attending the child health clinic.** Immunisation, safety in the home. (*By Health Visitor.*)

**Family planning.** (*By Doctor.*)
**The new father.** **Enjoy your baby.** (*By Midwife.*)
**Planning baby's day.** (*Now we are three—or four.*)
**Morning or evening bath times.**
**Self-demand feeding;** three- or four-hourly feeding.
**How to deal with the toddler.**

# MANAGEMENT OF THE PUERPERIUM

The management of the puerperium consists in providing the means whereby the woman can recuperate physically and emotionally, and gain supervised experience in the feeding and care of her infant; this embraces the following principles:

**The advancement of physical wellbeing.** Good nutrition: correction of anaemia: comfort: cleanliness: sufficient physical activity to ensure good muscle tone.

**The establishment of emotional wellbeing.** Quietness: freedom from excitement and worry: the proper psychological approach.

**The prevention of infection** and other avoidable complications.

**The promotion of breast-feeding** (p. 497).

**The provision of baby-care teaching.**

### IMMEDIATE CARE

Although the puerperium begins immediately the placenta is born, the first hour is usually included under the management of labour. The woman is made comfortable, a light meal served and a sedative given to ensure rest and sleep.

The uterus should be of cricket-ball consistency, the blood loss normal in amount, the pulse below 90. Should bleeding occur, or if the uterus is believed to contain blood clots, it should be massaged until it contracts, the clots expressed and an oxytocic preparation, such as ergometrine, 0·5 mg or Syntometrine, 1 ml given intramuscularly. If the bleeding is not brought under control, medical aid must be summoned.

### ASEPSIS AND ANTISEPSIS

Asepsis must be maintained, especially during the first week of the puerperium because the woman is particularly vulnerable to infection at this time.

The uterus provides an ideal environment for the multiplication of organisms. The lacerated or bruised tissues of the vulva and vagina, being devitalised, are unable to resist the invasion of organisms. The vaginal orifice is gaping and organisms can readily enter. The woman's resistance is lowered because of depletion of energy, lack of sleep and food. Blood loss may have been excessive.

#### Domestic cleanliness

The adequate use of soap and water is the first requirement. In hospital modern appliances are used to minimise the spread of infected dust. The room and bed-linen, the woman's skin and clothing should be clean.

### TEMPERATURE AND PULSE

Temperature and pulse are two excellent guides as to the woman's condition, and both should be normal throughout the puerperium. Any rise in temperature during the first week should be attributed to puerperal sepsis until proved otherwise. The temperature is unstable during the puerperium and tends to rise because of minor disorders, such as engorgement of the breasts, or due to excitement, but such an elevation is transient and should not be above 37·7°C.

The pulse rate should be slow, ranging between 60 and 80, but, if over 90, it is advisable to record it on the chart in red to draw attention to the fact. Excitement and fatigue may accelerate the pulse temporarily, but when pulse and temperature are both increased, puerperal sepsis or other infection is the most likely cause.

Temperature and pulse are taken every morning and evening, and if the temperature is 38°C once, or 37·4°C on two occasions, or if the pulse is over 90 on more than two instances, temperature and pulse should be taken four-hourly and medical advice sought. An endocervical or high vaginal swab, midstream specimen of urine and throat swab are sent to the laboratory. (*In some hospitals the temperature is taken twice daily for three days and then once daily, in the evening.*)

### PALPATING THE UTERUS

In a training school, student midwives should be taught to recognise the normal decrease in size of the involuting uterus. The fundal height need not be measured other than to instruct the novice. The decrease in size is approximately 1 cm daily and not until the 11th or 12th day is the fundus no longer palpable. Any tenderness is noted and reported. Palpating the fundus also draws attention to an overdistended bladder. With early ambulation this is less likely to occur but can very readily be overlooked unless there is a specified daily examination.

The author is aware of a postnatal patient being admitted to hospital on the fourth day with acute abdominal pain: 3 litres 360 ml of urine were withdrawn by catheter. Another hospital patient had 1 litre 860 ml of urine withdrawn on the fifth day postpartum. (Cases of ruptured bladder have been reported.)

The bladder should be emptied prior to uterine palpation, because a full bladder may displace the uterus upwards, as will a loaded rectum. If the fundal height remains stationary, or is higher than on the previous day, the bladder should be percussed to ascertain whether it contains residual urine. A plastic 15 cm ruler should be used, being more accurate than a tape measure which may curve down behind the fundus.

### *Dealing with the Lochia*

Vulval pads should be removed by the midwife with her hand inserted into a 15 cm plastic bag.

### ABNORMALITIES OF THE LOCHIA

| Note and record | Report to Doctor | Significance |
| --- | --- | --- |
| **The amount** ..... | Excessive ..................... | Retained products. |
| | Scanty (*with pyrexia*) ........... | Puerperal sepsis (*septicaemia*). |
| **The colour** ...... | Persistently bright red .......... | Danger of haemorrhage |
| | Brown and profuse (*with bulky uterus*) ..................... | Subinvolution. |
| **The consistence** .. | Pieces of membrane or placenta . | Retained products. |
| **The odour** ...... | Offensive .................... | Retained products. |
| | Offensive (*with pyrexia*) ........ | Puerperal sepsis (*local uterine infection*). |

## RETENTION OF URINE

Retention of urine is less common since early ambulation was inaugurated, but occasionally occurs following a difficult delivery.

An overdistended bladder may have been bruised by the fetal head, and the tissue at the base of the bladder is sometimes oedematous. Bruising of the urethra and bladder neck may take place if the second stage has been prolonged, and the subsequent oedema of the vulva, as well as the suturing of the perineum, interfere with the act of micturition. The pain and discomfort in the vulva prevent relaxation of the urethral sphincter, which may go into spasm. To avoid urinary tract infection, retention of urine should be treated actively: the doctor being consulted before passing a catheter.

The woman should be encouraged to void within 12 hours of confinement, but must never be forced to wait for that period before catheterisation is carried out. The experienced midwife is never eager to pass a catheter unnecessarily, and will do all in her power to avoid this. Nevertheless, the woman must not suffer, and if the simple remedies do not succeed and she is obviously in pain a catheter should be passed. It is the overdistended bladder as much as the procedure of catheterisation which predisposes to urinary tract infection.

The inexperienced midwife may overlook the possibility of residual urine, because the woman is apparently passing adequate amounts. The bladder should be percussed every day. If there is any doubt about residual urine the doctor will ask for a catheter to be passed after micturition and an accurate measurement of the retained urine made: over 60 ml being significant.

## THE BOWELS

The bowels tend to be sluggish during the puerperium. When the diet contains sufficient roughage and fluid, the bowels need less artificial stimulation, but a mild aperient, a small prepacked enema, a glycerine, or bisacodyl (Dulcolax) suppository, is usually given if the bowels do not move before the third morning after delivery and on every subsequent third day. The modern tendency is to pay less attention to the bowels if the woman is well and comfortable.

### DIET

The nursing mother needs a liberal nourishing diet to build up her strength and to enable her to produce sufficient breast milk. Good wholesome food is essential, containing sufficient proteins (80 g) daily, minerals and vitamins, as the production of an adequate supply of breast milk is believed to be influenced by the intake of protein and vitamin B. Many women are anaemic at this time so the midwife must ensure that foods rich in iron are included in her diet.

Additional fluid is required, but excessive quantities of fluid will not increase the milk supply. Milk is high in proteins and calcium, and as the woman is losing calcium from her body when she produces milk, 1,200 ml should be taken in her diet every day. Fruit or vegetables should be served at every meal. The traditional idea that fruit and vegetables upset the baby is no longer recognised.

### HAEMOGLOBIN ESTIMATION

Twenty-four hours after delivery the haemoglobin level is estimated. If 11·5 g/dl or less, ferrous sulphate tablets are given. If low, Jectofer would be considered: if 7·5 g/dl or less a transfusion of packed cells may be prescribed. The haemoglobin level is checked again prior to discharge. Iron is usually continued at home for one month and as required.

### REST AND SLEEP

A sedative, such as nitrazepam (Mogadon), 5 or 10 mg is usually necessary to ensure sleep for the first few nights; rarely should it be necessary after then, except in cases of high blood pressure. If kept awake by some discomfort, such as after-pains, haemorrhoids, or engorged breasts, the midwife should treat the cause: the doctor will prescribe an analgesic.

Persistent insomnia in the absence of pain should be viewed with concern as a warning sign of oncoming mental illness. The woman needs adequate rest, quietness and sleep, because of the hypersensitive state of her nervous system, but without organisation this is not easily achieved in a postnatal ward. The day begins early and ends late, with an almost incessant round of routine visits and treatment. The ward should be closed morning and afternoon for one hour; the patients requested to relax and keep silent if they cannot sleep.

### What to Report to the Doctor

The midwife should be prepared to report on the following points.

Temperature and pulse.    Condition of sutured perineum.
Appetite: sleep.    Pain, e.g. in the breast; abdomen; leg; head.
Bowels: bladder.    Any peculiarity in behaviour.
Character of lochia.

## EARLY AMBULATION

Free movement of the legs is essential to avoid venous thrombosis: the woman being encouraged to walk rather than sitting in a chair. Six hours after normal delivery women may have a shower bath with a mobile hand spray or a tub bath in the kneeling position. Patients having had epidural analgesia are assessed before being allowed out of bed. Some keep patients, delivered by mid-forceps and after Caesarean section in bed for 12 hours.

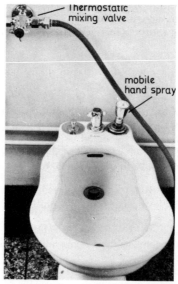

Fig. 26-6  Bidet with mobile hand spray.
*Queen Mother's Hospital, Glasgow.*

## VULVAL TOILET

Swabbing is only carried out on patients confined to bed, i.e. Caesarean section, difficult instrumental delivery for hygiene and comfort.

Details in technique vary from hospital to hospital. Groins, thighs and buttocks should be thoroughly washed with soap and water prior to swabbing. The haemolytic streptococcus, although dormant at present, is a potential threat which should not be ignored: it is harboured in the nose and throat as is the staphylococcus pyogenes. Intelligent mask-wearing is a precautionary measure. If masks are not worn the midwife should not speak while swabbing the vulva.

It is important that observation of the perineal suture line be carried out daily until healed; pads must be inspected daily.

### TREATMENT OF THIRD-DEGREE TEAR

The sutured perineum must be kept clean, antiseptic and dry. The vulva is swabbed in the usual way and dried carefully. A piece of gauze is placed between the labia. The vulva may be exposed to the air or to the light of an ordinary electric lamp, the anglepoise type being very convenient. With the woman's legs in the position for swabbing, the light is placed 30 cm from the vulva; the gentle heat is soothing to inflamed tissues, and dries the area. The exposure is given for 15 minutes and repeated every eight hours.

Avoidance of strain on the sutures. The woman should not sit bolt upright; she may roll over on to her side to feed her baby.

Nestosyl ointment is useful to allay discomfort and reduce inflammation. Codis or pentazocine (Fortral) tablets (2) may be necessary. Marked inflammation or oedema should be reported; (*the application of magnesium sulphate or sodium chloride soaks will lessen such inflammation and swelling*). Bromelain (Ananase), 20 mg every 6 hours for 48 hours is useful to relieve inflammation, bruising and oedema. Some apply cubed ice to the perineum in a plastic bag occluded with a knot. A sterile gauze swab is applied to the wound to prevent an 'ice burn'. An incontinence pad under the buttocks will absorb accidental leakage. If there are signs of sloughing, if the wound is infected, or when the tissues are being cut by the sutures they should be removed. Faeces passed vaginally indicate lack of healing by first intention and the formation of a recto-vaginal fistula (see Glossary).

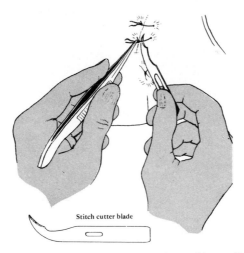

Stitch cutter blade

Fig. 26-7   Removal of perineal sutures, using Swann Morton Stitch Cutter.

The bowels need not be confined; giving milk of magnesia, 8 ml twice daily, beginning on the second day and increasing the dose to 15 ml on the third day. A glycerine suppository or a small water enema given with a catheter, will result in an easy evacuation of the bowels. A high residue diet is given. A soft bulky stool being less traumatic and painful than a dry hard one.

### REMOVAL OF SUTURES

Non-absorbable sutures are removed on the sixth day or sooner, depending on the wishes of the obstetrician: the woman first having had a shower or bath.

A mask is worn, gloves are not absolutely necessary. The perineum is first swabbed with Hibitane 1-2,000, the knot held with dissecting forceps, and the stitch snipped with a stitch cutter and gently removed. The number of sutures should be checked with the record of the number inserted.

### The Break-down of a Sutured Perineum

**If clean.** Hibitane sitz baths are given twice daily for not longer than five minutes. Exposure to an ordinary electric light four-hourly.

**If septic.** In addition to Hibitane sitz baths cleanse with hydrogen peroxide: a small piece of gauze soaked in Eusol is inserted into the broken-down area.

While resuturing the perineum most obstetricians prefer a general anaesthetic.

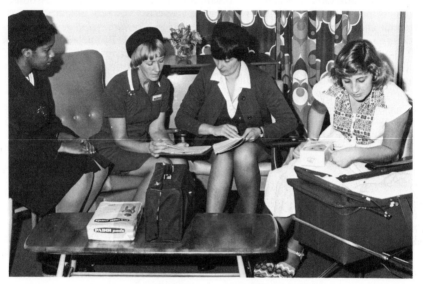

Fig. 26-8 Community midwife transferring care of mother and baby to the Health Visitor. Student midwife observing.

*Community Midwifery Service, Bellshill Maternity Hospital, Lanarkshire.*

## PLANNED EARLY TRANSFER FROM HOSPITAL TO HOME

Healthy mothers and babies are allowed home after 24 to 48 hours if certain conditions are met. Arrangements must be made when the woman comes to book in early pregnancy: her family doctor having signified his willingness to undertake or arrange for postnatal care. Her reproductive history and current wellbeing must be satisfactory.

A prenatal visit is paid by the midwife to assess the home conditions and discuss domestic arrangements. Overcrowding is not acceptable. The question of heating is important during cold weather; the mother-to-be being advised regarding the need for a warm room for baby day and night: a wall thermometer is loaned if necessary and the national pamphlet on cold injury supplied. The question of a home help is discussed and arrangements made if desired. The husband may plan to be on holiday but in some cases the help of a reliable woman is acceptable for washing, cooking and caring for any small children.

About the 36th week an evening visit is paid to confirm that arrangements have been completed and to gain the husband's co-operation. The house must be warm when mother and baby arrive home, food and other requirements on hand. The midwife explains that she will visit on the evening of the day of transfer and daily until the 10th day, when the Health Visitor takes over. Should the 10th day fall on a Friday the midwife visits until Monday.

On the 8th day the Guthrie test is done: perineal scar inspected and any non-absorbable perineal sutures removed.

Prior to transfer home the hospital midwifery service notifies the community midwifery service. The health visitor is notified by the Area Medical Officer (via the notification of birth form). Community midwives and health visitors have a close relationship with the hospital.

Careful screening of babies is carried out prior to and on the morning of 48-hour discharge, more babies than mothers having to be readmitted. The hospital-based community midwife is more conversant with new ideas in baby care and in recognising signficant signs that indicate an abnormality such as hypernatraemia or hypocalcaemia. She has easy access to expert paediatric advice and for readmission to hospital without delay. Arrangements are made for a postnatal examination.

## GOOD POSTURE FOR AMBULANT MOTHERS

### Notes to Midwives

Since most mothers are ambulant from the first postpartum day, bed exercises are unnecessary: group teaching is now more readily accomplished so a programme of health education combined with good posture and rehabilitating exercises should be inaugurated. For patients confined to bed, deep breathing exercises are beneficial. To prevent venous thrombosis, raising and lowering the knees, flexing and rotating the ankles, flexing and stretching the toes can be done repeatedly during the day. The approach with greatest appeal to young mothers is via health and beauty, special emphasis being laid on restoration of the figure and the creation of a feeling of wellbeing. To arouse and maintain interest the exercises should be linked with some domestic or baby care activity rather than being presented as bald physical exercises.

#### POSTNATAL EXERCISES FOR NON-AMBULANT PATIENTS

All movements should be made gently, smoothly and rhythmically.

The midwife should grade the exercises carefully, beginning with 'deep breathing' the day after delivery; then 'strengthening of the abdominal muscles': then 'exercises for the pelvic floor muscles'. To tone up the pelvic floor muscles the woman is told to stop the flow of urine midstream: also to tighten the pelvic floor frequently. On the third postpartum day ambulant exercises may be started. Deep breathing facilitates the circulation of blood and may diminish the risk of venous thrombosis: this should be practised prior to each lesson.

#### HEALTH EDUCATION

Good nutrition plays a very important part in the maintenance of good health so a diet high in proteins, minerals (including iron) and vitamins should be advocated and, when possible, displayed. Mental and emotional health contribute to physical wellbeing as well as the enjoyment of life and good human relationships. This aspect of health education should not be neglected.

Specific instructions regarding the lifting of heavy weights should be given and the method of avoiding back strain while so doing demonstrated. The nursing chair should be without arms and low enough to make a comfortable lap for baby without the need for a foot stool. Baby's bath could be placed on a stool to bring the edge to knee level.

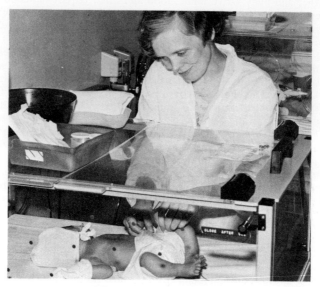

Fig. 26-9 Mothers visit their babies in the neonatal intensive care unit at least three times daily and are encouraged to caress the baby, give a bottle feed or change the napkin.
*Queen Mother's Hospital, Glasgow.*

### Advice on Personal Matters

Many women are reluctant to mention certain subjects although they are eager for advice concerning them:

**When may sexual intercourse be resumed?** Four weeks should elapse after childbirth but opinions differ on this.

**Family planning?** Clinics are held in maternity and other hospitals. Attendance not later than three weeks after delivery is necessary for advice re contraception.

**How long will vaginal discharge continue?** Slight blood-stained discharge may continue for three or more weeks after childbirth.

**When does menstruation restart?** Usually menstruation returns in two or three months after childbirth: pregnancy may occur prior to this.

## MINOR DISORDERS

### After-pains

These are due to spasmodic uterine contractions, and have been likened to dysmenorrhoea. They occur during the first 48 hours of the puerperium and are more commonly experienced by multiparae. In some cases they are due to the presence of blood clots in the uterus; if the uterus is bulky, clots are usually present and should be expressed. When a piece of membrane is known to have been left *in utero* one of the ergot preparations should be given. To relieve the pain an analgesic drug such as Distalgesic will be necessary. Panasorb or pentazocine (Fortral) 2 tablets are good. Pethidine, 50 mg by mouth, repeated in two hours, if necessary, is also effective.

### Haemorrhoids

With the pressure of the baby's head on the anus during the perineal phase of labour, haemorrhoids sometimes prolapse and give rise to pain and intense discomfort. To relieve the engorgement, magnesium sulphate or hypertonic sodium chloride soaks may be applied for 48 hours. The application of some soothing ointment such as Nupercainal or Anusol cream is very comforting. An analgesic drug such as pentazocine (Fortral) 50 mg will relieve pain: elevation of the foot of the bed is helpful in acute cases.

#### SUBINVOLUTION

In this condition there is delay in the return of the uterus to normal; the fundal height remains stationary for a few days (check for full bladder); the uterus is soft and boggy, the lochia are reddish brown and profuse. Subinvolution may be caused by any condition which interferes with good uterine contractions, such as retained products, fibroids, or which interferes with the ischaemic state of the uterus, e.g. local uterine infection. The midwife should ensure that the uterus is empty at the end of labour and facilitate good uterine drainage by early ambulation and avoiding a distended bladder or loaded bowel.

**Retroversion,** which is usually associated with subinvolution, does not occur until after the seventh day of the puerperium as the uterus is too big to enter the pelvic brim until then. It is more commonly found at the postnatal clinic. The woman complains of a bearing-down or dragging sensation in the pelvis. Pelvic floor exercises are recommended.

## POSTNATAL EXAMINATION (*on discharge*)

The first postnatal examination is carried out by the doctor on the day prior to discharge. A vaginal examination is not now usually made: the breasts are examined, uterus palpated, perineum inspected and the calves of the legs palpated. If a family planning clinic at the hospital is available she is invited to attend, otherwise the doctor advises her to see her family doctor for contraceptive advice within two or three weeks.

A liberal nourishing diet should be advocated and the need for 'body building' foods stressed. Iron tablets are usually prescribed for four weeks. The need for adequate rest should be impressed on her as well as the avoidance of lifting heavy weights.

An appointment for a second examination, six weeks postpartum, is made.

*At many hospitals each patient is interviewed by a Health Visitor prior to her discharge.*

## POSTNATAL EXAMINATION (*sixth week or later*)

This examination may be delegated to the patient's family doctor under the general practitioner co-operation scheme.

Prior to examination the bladder is emptied and the urine tested for protein: if a urinary infection occurred during pregnancy a mid-stream specimen is obtained for bacteriological examination; the woman is weighed, blood pressure taken. A haemoglobin estimation is made and iron therapy prescribed if necessary. The patient's records should be at hand. It is a psychological error not to ask how the baby is progressing (having first made sure he survived).

A vaginal examination is made; the tone of the pelvic floor muscles being noted; a speculum examination is made to detect cervical lacerations or erosion.

**Requirements**

| | |
|---|---|
| Sterile gloves.   Swabs. | Pessaries: Hodge, ring. |
| Swabbing lotion: obstetric cream. | Bivalve and Sims' specula. |
| Paper bag, for used dressings. | Uterine dressing forceps. |

Special follow-up clinics are conducted for women who have had pre-eclampsia or who have such conditions as tuberculosis, cardiac disease, anaemia or urinary tract infection.

### POSTNATAL COMPLAINTS AND CLINICAL FINDINGS

Slight red lochia may still be present for three or four weeks. Bleeding may be due to the resumption of menstruation, but this is not usual until two or three months after childbirth or even later.

Erosion of cervix is considered by some to be hormonal in origin. It may regress spontaneously within two months of confinement. If persistent, with an offensive discharge, thorough cauterisation under general anaesthesia is carried out. Vaginal discharge may be due to infection or erosion of the cervix.

Prolapse and retroversion of the uterus are often associated with cystocele and rectocele. The woman complains of pelvic discomfort with a dragging or bearing-down feeling. The knee elbow position for 10 minutes twice daily and the adoption of the prone position for sleep may prove beneficial. If not a pessary is inserted at the 12th week and worn for two months. Additional rest is essential, and constipation should be corrected if present.

Urinary tract conditions such as frequency, urgency, dysuria, if due to infection, respond well to antibiotics; in some centres women with such symptoms are referred to the Urological Department. Stress incontinence is usually associated with a lax pelvic floor and cystocele.

### BACKACHE

This is a common complaint among poorly nourished, overworked multiparous women whose muscles are lax and easily fatigued. The remedy (*not easily provided*) is good food, rest and fresh air; a well-fitting corset gives much relief.

Sacro-iliac strain, due to laxity of the sacro-iliac ligaments, causes severe backache, which is often relieved by physiotherapy, e.g. radiant heat, massage, remedial exercises and the rectification of faulty posture. A suitable supporting belt is sometimes advocated but orthopaedic advice may be necessary. Pelvic conditions are no longer considered to be the cause of lumbo-sacral backache.

# ORIENTATION TO FAMILY PLANNING

It would seem to be a fundamental human right that parents should control their fertility and limit the size and spacing of their family, for involuntary parenthood creates many problems, social and financial as well as physical and emotional. To establish a family is still the earnest desire of most married couples although the modern idea is to limit the number of children. Three is suggested as a satisfactory number and they are usually spaced at intervals of about two years. This concentrated period of childbearing enables the mother to resume her career at an earlier date than was previously possible.

## Family planning services

The National Health Service makes statutory provision for family planning services through Area Health Authorities. (Health Boards, Scotland). These services are provided free, and include medical examination, family planning advice, supplies and appliances. They are available to the married and unmarried on medical or social grounds, and are provided through NHS hospitals, clinics, general practitioners and a community service.

During the examination prior to discharge after confinement the obstetrician discusses the question of contraception and advises the woman to see her family doctor within three weeks or to attend a family planning clinic. Midwives trained in family planning techniques visit postnatal women in some hospitals to motivate them regarding contraception, mentioning reliable methods, answering questions and referring them to doctor or F.P. clinic.

## METHODS OF CONTRACEPTION
### COITUS INTERRUPTUS

This is a primitive, old method which is widely practised. Although better than taking no precautions at all it should not be recommended because it is so unreliable. The method consists in withdrawal before ejaculation takes place but a small quantity of semen may escape before this and impregnate the woman: the self-discipline required is not always attained. When taking the sexual history, midwives should be aware that coitus interruptus is meant when the woman uses such terms as 'being careful', 'taking care'.

### THE OCCLUSIVE RUBBER CAP
*(Failure rate is said to be 12 per cent)*

No contraceptive appliance is absolutely reliable so it is essential that the woman fully understands the instructions she is given and carries them out faithfully.

There are various types of cap that are inserted into the vagina prior to coitus and removed not less than eight hours afterwards; the diaphragm or Dutch cap being most frequently prescribed. It consists of a thin rubber dome encircled by a coiled wire spring 50 to 100 mm in diameter and by covering the cervix and fitting snugly against the walls of the vagina it prevents the spermatozoa from entering the cervical os. At the clinic a vaginal examination is made to assess the required 'cap' size, and the woman is shown how to insert and remove it. She is told to avoid constipation. Before insertion 4 ml of spermicidal jelly or cream is smeared on the inside and outside of the cap for additional protection. Too much cream makes it slippery and difficult to insert. Aerosol foams cause less irritation than some creams and jellies.

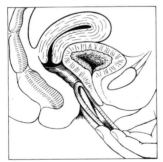 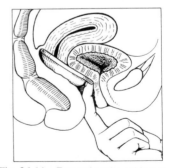

Fig. 26-10   Inserting the rubber cap.     Fig. 26-11   Removing the rubber cap.
*Ortho Pharmaceutical Ltd.*

### To insert the cap

The cap is inserted not more than three hours before intercourse.

The woman usually stands with the left foot on a chair, thigh at right angles to the body. Spermicidal jelly is smeared on the diaphragm as an additional safeguard.

The rim is squeezed and the cap directed along the posterior vaginal wall, into the posterior fornix; then the anterior rim is pushed up behind the symphysis pubis.

### To remove the cap

The cap should not be removed for at least eight hours after intercourse.

The finger is hooked into the rim behind the symphysis pubis and the cap is pulled downwards. In some cases the vaginal walls and pelvic floor muscles are lax, not having recovered from the effects of parturition, and the cap will not remain in position. A vault cap (Dumas) or an alternative method of contraception will be recommended.

### THE CONDOM OR RUBBER SHEATH

This thin latex rubber appliance (like a finger stall) is worn by the husband. For maximal safety spermicidal jelly is introduced into the vagina as well as being smeared on the outside of the condom. The failure rate when used with spermicidal jelly is 5 per cent.

### *Condoms are often recommended*

Until the woman can insert the diaphragm satisfactorily.

Until the vaginal walls are involuted after childbirth.

Neither cap nor condom is absolutely reliable, but detailed advice on their use is given at the F.P. clinic.

### THE RHYTHM METHOD

### *(erroneously known as the safe period)*

This method limits coitus to the periods when no ovum is available for fertilisation (see Fig. 26-14). The nine days surrounding the day of ovulation are unsafe, so coitus must not take place on the five days before, on the day of, and on the three days after ovulation, a total of nine days. Ovulation usually occurs 14 days prior to the first day of the menstrual period but may occur earlier or later.

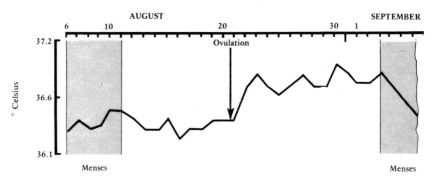

Fig. 26-12   Chart showing that by taking the temperature daily the date of ovulation can be determined by the rise of about 0·3°C manifest at that time.

### *Determining the day of ovulation*

A slight rise in basal body temperature 0·3°C, occurs on the day following ovulation and if sustained for a few days denotes that ovulation has occurred, so by taking the temperature in the mouth every morning before getting up for a few months the day of ovulation can be established; the temperature is recorded in graph form. A detailed menstrual record is kept for at least six months; the days of abstinence from coitus are then adjusted to allow for irregularities in the time of ovulation. Limiting coitus to the safe period is utilised where other methods are condemned on religious grounds but the failure rate is high.

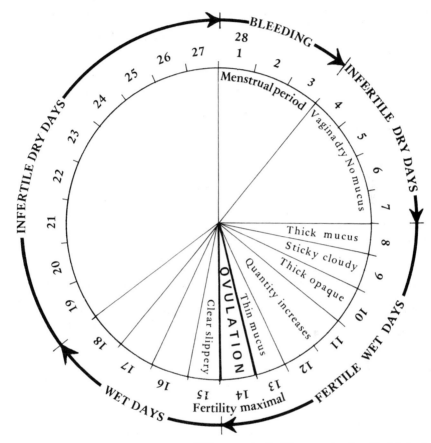

Fig. 26-13 Cervical Mucus Pattern (Billings method). Diagram showing 'dry' infertile days and 'wet' fertile days.

### Cervical mucus pattern (Billings method)

Cervical mucus, under the influence of the ovarian oestrogenic hormones, can on certain days be favourable or hostile to spermatozoa.

The woman notes before retiring whether the vaginal entrance is dry or wet using toilet paper. Following menstruation there are 4 dry days and 9 dry days during which the woman is infertile. See diagram (Fig. 26-13).

### Injectable contraceptives

Depo Provera (medroxyprogesterone acetate) is used in over 70 countries but in Britain is only prescribed as a single injection in selected cases, e.g. for the wives of men having recently undergone vasectomy or in the postpartum woman being immunised against rubella. The injection is given intramuscularly and is effective for 12 weeks.

## ORAL CONTRACEPTIVE PILLS

The pills inhibit ovulation in the menstrual cycle during which they are administered. For the purpose of taking the pill the first day is calculated from the first day of the menstrual period. One pill is prescribed daily for 21 days from the 1st day. They are dispensed in packs of 21 or 22. Withdrawal bleeding occurs when the monthly course of pills is stopped, usually described to patients as 'a period'. Contraceptive pills are prescribed only under strict medical supervision and are on the Prescription Only Medicine List. Unless the woman agrees that her general practitioner be informed, the F.P. clinic do not prescribe oral contraceptive pills.

**Side effects** are nausea, headaches, breast discomfort, and weight gain.

In order to detect precancerous cells in the cervix a Papanicolaou smear is taken prior to starting the course.

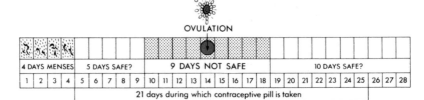

Fig. 26-14  Diagrammatic representation of the 15 safe days and of the 21 days during which the contraceptive pill is taken. The pills are started on the first day of the menstrual period.

### Lower risk pills are available

Because of the incidence of venous thrombosis, oral contraceptives containing not more than 50 micrograms of oestrogen are now prescribed.

Orthonovin 1/50; Gynovlar 21; Minilyn Minovlar; Norinyl-1; Anovlar 21; Norlestrin 21; Ovulen 50; Demulen 50.

Low dose pills with oestrogen 30 micrograms are: Microgynon, Eugynon and Minovular. Loestrin contains 20 micrograms.

Tablets containing *no oestrogen* are now available, i.e. Progestogen only pills. They are taken continuously, one tablet every day. Micronor (Ortho) and Noriday (Syntex) both contain 350 micrograms norethisterone.

#### ABSOLUTE CONTRAINDICATIONS

Oral contraceptive pills are not prescribed in the following circumstances:

History of deep venous thrombosis or of severe liver disease especially when jaundice is manifest during pregnancy. Malignant disease of the breast.

Episodes of motor or sensory loss should be reported at once.

#### SECONDARY AMENORRHOEA (*post pill*)

A number of women have had amenorrhoea for 6 to 12 months after ceasing to take the pill. (In persistent cases Clomiphene has been prescribed to stimulate ovarian function.) When pregnancy does occur it is difficult to estimate the expected date of delivery so the woman should be told to look for the early signs of pregnancy and to record the date of quickening.

### INTRA-UTERINE DEVICE (I.U.D.)

This method has its greatest advantage in developing countries to control population explosions, minimal co-operation being required from those using it. The mode of action is not completely understood; fertilisation occurs but embedding is inhibited.

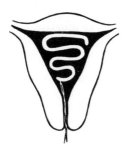

Fig. 26-15   Lippes loop.

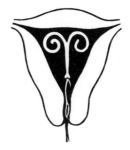

Fig. 26-16   Saf. T. Coil.

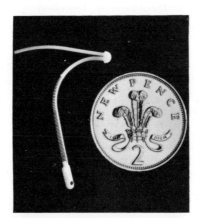

Fig. 26-17   The Gravigard copper-device.
Figs. 26-15–26-17   Intra-uterine contraceptive devices.

A pliable plastic loop is introduced into the uterine cavity by straightening and passing it through a 3 mm plastic cannula. The device remains *in utero*: Lippes loop and the Saf. T. Coil are both effective. A newer appliance is the Gravigard copper-7 device which is small and can be used for the nullipara. That the device is still *in utero* is indicated by the strand of thread hanging from the cervix and this should be checked regularly by the user. Pregnancy has occurred while the device was *in situ*: in rare cases it has perforated the uterine wall and entered the pelvic cavity. Insertion of the device is recommended at the end of a menstrual period when some cervical dilatation exists or after confinement or abortion. The Lippes loop can be inserted immediately after the placenta is delivered. The perforation rate is high for six weeks postpartum (after immediate insertion). In Britain the doctor is responsible for the insertion of these devices.

### Insertion of an Intra-uterine Device

The device is not inserted if the uterus is abnormal, if pelvic infection is present or if pregnancy is suspected. The vulva is swabbed, cervix cleansed with antiseptic lotion. The anterior lip of cervix is grasped with a single-toothed teneculum and a sound introduced to determine the size of the uterine cavity and diagnose retroversion if present. The I.U.D. is inserted slowly and carefully and the woman should remain recumbent for a few minutes. Low abdominal pain is usually relieved by an analgesic and a cup of tea. Slight bleeding is usual after insertion: very rarely pallor and thready pulse are manifest if introdution of the device has been hurried or the woman gets up too soon. Treatment of this vaso-vagal collapse is to place the woman in the supine position with her head low and to maintain a clear airway.

Uterine cramp may be troublesome for a few days; later there may be heavy menstrual periods with spotting between them. The woman returns for a 'check up' after three periods. Expulsion of the I.U.D. sometimes occurs and follow-up is needed to encourage women to continue. Simple remedies and reassurance should be tried before resorting to removal of the device but this may have to be done for severe pain or free bleeding. The woman is told to report a purulent discharge, an unpleasant odour, or absence of the thread through the cervix.

## STERILISATION

### Tubal Ligation, Vasectomy

Sterilisation is a final method of contraception and this fact should be clearly explained to the parents concerned. Very rarely can the operation be reversed.

There is no statutory requirement under English or Scottish law that the consent of the spouse must be obtained to sterilisation of the partner but the British Medical Association solicitor advises that the signature of both spouses be obtained whenever possible.

### Tubal Ligation

Ligation of the Fallopian tubes, unless done at Caesarean section, is carried out one to three days after delivery, the tubes being readily accessible then. Through a small abdominal incision the tubes are ligated and a segment excised under general

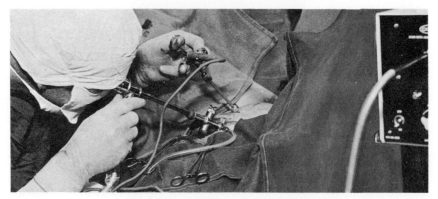

Fig. 26-18   Sterilisation by laparoscopy.
*Simpson Memorial Maternity Pavilion, Edinburgh.*

anaesthesia. The woman is discharged on the 7th day or sooner. Some postpone ligation until 3 months postpartum to avoid the risk of thrombosis and to ensure that the baby survives.

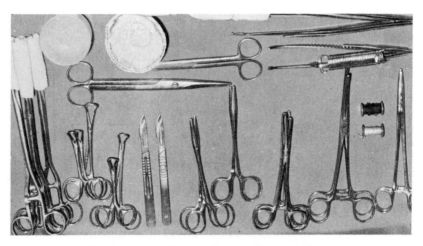

Fig. 26-19   Requirements for postpartum tubal ligation.
*Simpson Memorial Maternity Pavilion, Edinburgh.*

**Instruments**

   3 or 4 Rampleys swab holders.
   4 towel clips. 6 Spencer Wells forceps.
   2 B.P. handles No. 4; blades No. 23.
   3 Allis's tissue forceps.
   1 dissecting forceps toothed.
   2 Mayo curved forceps. 2 Mayo scissors.
   2 Mayo needle holders.
   1 Michel clip gallery and applicator.

**Gown Pack**

   4 gowns, hand towels, caps, masks.

**Sutures**

   Chromic catgut No. 2/0; No. 1.
   Linen thread No. 60. Mersilk No. 0.
   No. 1 Mersilk on Colt's needle
   *or* half-circle round-bodied needle No. 1 Chromic.

**Linen and Dressing Pack**

   1 laparotomy sheet.
   6 dressing towels 90 × 90 cm.
   2 packs (5) Raytec swabs 20 cm.
   2 packs (5) Raytec swabs 10 cm.
   1 gauze dressing for Mastisol *or*
   aerosol plastic dressing spray.
   2 gallipots, foil dish.

*Peritoneum*   Eyeless needled suture
   (No. 1 chromic catgut on round bodied needle Mayo's No. 2).

*Muscle sheath*   Eyeless needled suture
   (No. 1 chronic catgut on $\frac{1}{2}$ circle tapercut needle).

*Skin*   Eyeless needled suture
   (No. 1 Mersilk on 90mm curved cutting needle).

### *Laparoscopic Sterilisation*

The bladder is emptied. Three to five litres of carbon dioxide gas is injected abdominally into the peritoneal cavity by means of a special trocar and cannula: the incision is enlarged to one cm and the laparoscope inserted. A second stab incision is made in the abdomen; the Palmer biopsy drill forceps introduced and a coagulation current passed. The centre of the area of the Fallopian tube that has been coagulated is severed by means of the forceps drill. Through the same incision the other Fallopian tube is dealt with. This operation is performed 6 weeks after confinement. The women are discharged home in 9 hours if no condition exists warranting further hospital care.

<h2 style="text-align:center">VASECTOMY</h2>

Vasectomy is a safe, simple and reliable form of male contraception, and there has been an increasing demand for this operation in recent years. Vasectomy can, since 1972, be done free of charge on the National Health Service on social as well as on medical grounds. Those considered eligible are married men with a stable marital relationship and having at least two children. The object is to limit the family to the number of children they want and to eliminate constant apprehension over an unwanted pregnancy: the physical, emotional and social welfare of the family group being enhanced.

Sexual desire and activity are not affected. Vasectomy produces a mechanical barrier to the passage of sperms but there is no endocrine deprivation. Husband and wife should have the purpose and effect of the operation explained to them and it is advisable for both to sign a consent form.

The vas, the tube that carries the spermatozoa from the testes, unites with the duct of the seminal vesicle from which the seminal fluid is derived. If the vas on both sides is ligated and a length of 6 cm is excised, the sperms produced cannot mingle with the semen and enter the ejaculatory duct; they eventually become absorbed by phagocytosis.

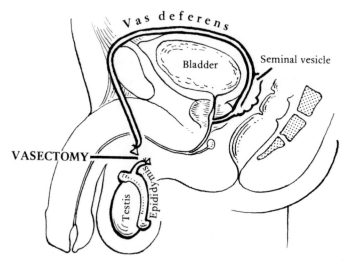

Fig. 26-20   Male generative organs: showing vasectomy.

The operation can be done under local or general anaesthesia; a small incision being made on each side of the scrotum.

The man rests for three or four hours after the operation. Discomfort may be present for 24 to 72 hours. Full contraceptive measures must be carried out until 2 semen analyses at intervals of one month show no sperms. A minimum of 12 ejaculations should be made prior to examination of the first semen specimen.

The promotion of family planning is an essential component of health education and an integral part of preventive medicine. Because of the midwife's specialised knowledge of all aspects of the reproductive process and her intimate contact with the childbearing woman she is the logical person to participate as a member of the family planning team. Having received an orientation course in family planning during her training as a midwife she should have sufficient knowledge to counsel her patients regarding fertility control, spacing and limiting the size of their families. She should be able to discuss the available facilities and the various methods of contraception, their effects and side effects. Religious objections must be respected. Midwives who intend to specialise in the promotion of family planning must undergo a much more comprehensive course of instruction combined with adequate clinical experience of contraceptive techniques (e.g. Course 900. The Joint Board of Clinical Nursing Studies). Those who elect to work in developing countries need additional knowledge and experience to enable them to undertake the insertion of contraceptive devices and the prescription of 'the pill': and to understand cultural and religious customs and taboos, building on and improving existing beliefs and practices rather than substituting more sophisticated methods.

## MOTIVATION

The family planning midwife must first and foremost be highly motivated so that she can persuade and convince. This entails awareness of the wider aspects of the subject to fortify her conviction and her endeavours. Parents who already have more children than they can provide for, are usually eager for reliable contraceptive advice. The midwife will find the less responsible parents need more persuasion and 'follow-up'. Their vocabulary is limited, so to communicate successfully she must learn the local colloquial terms used to describe the various contraceptive practices. Population control is unlikely to appeal to the less intelligent as a motive for regulating conception, whereas the more responsible parents are cognisant of this. A high birth rate is no longer necessary for man's survival and any scheme that lowers the stillbirth, neonatal and infant death rates must be accompanied by a programme of birth control to keep population growth in balance. Seventy years ago families of 12 were common: the infant death rate was 150 per thousand live births; now it is less than 15 per thousand.

### PROMOTION BY MIDWIVES

The degree of participation in contraceptive practice depends on Government policy and local medical opinion. Where doctors are in short supply and a population explosion exists, midwives may be given a course of instruction to enable them to participate actively. In Britain it is doubtful whether the midwife would be permitted legally to insert the contraceptive device or to prescribe the pill. She may undertake cervical smears, fit the cervical cap, take sexual histories and assist the doctor as required: answer questions, explain procedures. She may participate in research projects, undertake community field work, e.g. case finding and 'follow-up'.

## Educating and Counselling Parents

Special qualities of personality are needed in motivating women to attend the clinic and encouraging them to carry out the prescribed procedure.

In future more time will be spent in case finding and follow-up as well as in communicating and teaching. It is essential that midwives who undertake this function have more than a rudimentary knowledge of the principles of education, for they cannot communicate successfully unless they understand how to teach and how people learn. Women of lower grade mentality need much explanation and repetition: conversely the intelligent woman will be knowledgeable and expect well informed answers to her questions, biological, psychological and pharmacological.

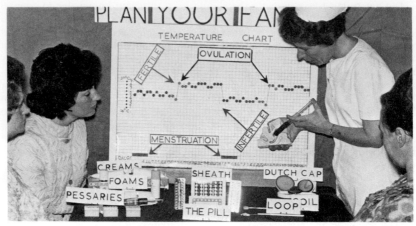

Fig. 26-21  Family planning counselling.
*Bellshill Maternity Hospital, Lanarkshire.*

### THE SOCIAL ASPECT OF CONTRACEPTION

In a country with multiracial immigrants, information should be obtained regarding the cultural and religious beliefs that influence the contraceptive practices of the various ethnic groups in order to enhance understanding of their customs. Their methods may seem primitive and unreliable but a simple method that is used, will be more effective than a safer method that is too complicated or is unacceptable. Tact and patience are needed when introducing procedures that are foreign to the immigrant. The question of abortion being used as a method of family planning is causing concern: religious and moral objections exist.

Family planning by reducing the number of children gives those born an opportunity of better care, housing, nutrition and education, so the quality of life is improved. The dangers of childbearing increase with age and after the fourth child irrespective of age. Two or three children is now considered an adequate family: when spread at two-year intervals the woman can recuperate sufficiently, is not subjected to overwork and can complete her childbearing role within six years and return to her former employment as and when she wishes.

### QUESTIONS BY PATIENTS AND ANSWERS BY MIDWIVES

What are the chances of becoming pregnant if no contraceptive is used?
*Sixty per cent of women having regular intercourse will become pregnant within four months.*

Is the Dutch cap more reliable than the condom?
*If the condom is in good condition it is better.*

Is there any danger that the diaphragm will be lost inside the body?
*No! None whatsoever.*

How long does a diaphragm last?
*It should be examined weekly by the user and at the clinic every year.*

Are sea sponges and pieces of foam an effective barrier to the sperm?
*They are not reliable and should not be used.*

After having a baby can I become pregnant before my periods start?
*Yes! Because ovulation (when your egg is liberated) occurs before menstruation.*

Does a condom prevent venereal disease?
*It helps to protect the man who has sexual relations with an infected woman.*

Can I have the intra uterine device inserted before I go home after my baby is born?
*Some devices are inserted then.*

How many children must you have before being sterilised?
*Opinions differ. Some say four, other doctors do so for two or three.*

At what time of day do I take the pill?
*At night.*

If I forget to take it at night?
*Take it next morning and again that night.*

If I miss night and morning?
*Use another method of contraception for the rest of the period, e.g. the condom.*

Does vasectomy diminish sexual pleasure?
*Not at all. By removing anxiety about unwanted pregnancy it is beneficial.*

What happens to the sperms after vasectomy?
*They are absorbed but your husband will still pass semen during intercourse.*

Must the pill be stopped for a while every two years?
*No!*

Which is the least irritating: foam, jelly, cream?
*Aerosol foams are the least irritating.*

Will douching after intercourse prevent pregnancy?
*It is not reliable and seldom used today.*

Is there danger of cancer with the pill?
*No evidence of this. The dose of the drug is too small to be harmful.*

When on the pill, for what reason should I stop it and see the doctor?
*Sudden severe headache, severe pain in chest or leg.*

Will an excessive dose of contraceptive pills cause abortion?
*No! But they might damage the fetus.*

Which method is most commonly used?
*This varies. Probably the condom, withdrawal and the pill in that order.*

Do many women in Britain use the intra-uterine device?
*About 3 per cent of women using contraception have one inserted.*

If I breast feed my baby will this prevent my becoming pregnant?
*You are less likely to, but it is not reliable.*

---

## QUESTIONS FOR REVISION

### THE PUERPERIUM

What do you understand by rooming-in? State the advantages.
What would you report to the doctor regarding the postnatal woman?
Why are temperature and pulse important during the puerperium?
What abnormalities of lochia may occur and what is their significance?
What can you learn from palpating the lower abdomen of the postnatal woman?
How soon can a woman, delivered normally, have a shower bath?
What advice or help could you give for the following: (a) after pains; (b) oedema and bruising of the perineum; (c) backache; (d) restoration of the figure?
What would you do in the following circumstances: If the pulse was 90 one hour after delivery? If the

uterus was larger than you thought it ought to be on the 3rd postpartum day? If the lochia were bright red on the 8th day? If the woman is upset and crying? If the perineal sutures are cutting out?

**N. Ire. Council. 30-min. question.** What observations would you make in the early postnatal period? Why are they important?

**C.M.B.(Eng.) 30-min. question.** What disorders of micturition may occur in the puerperium? Describe the management of each.

**C.M.B.(Eng.) 30-min. question.** Describe the physiological changes which occur during the puerperium.

**N. Ire. Council 30-min. question.** What is a complete tear of the perineum? Give in detail the nursing 'after-care' in such a case.

**C.M.B.(Eng.) 30-min. question.** Outline the basic needs and nursing care of the mother during the first ten days after delivery. What fears does the mother commonly experience during this time?

**C.M.B.(Eng.) 30-min. question.** Discuss the emotional stresses of the puerperium.

**N. Ire. M. Council.** Describe the care given by the midwife visiting a mother and baby at home on the 10th day of puerperium. For what reasons might it be necessary for the midwife to continue visiting after the 10th day.

**C.M.B.(Scot.).** What is the puerperium? Which complications may occur in the mother during this period? Describe the management of a patient who develops a temperature of 40°C on the second postnatal day.

**N. Ire. M. Council.** (a) Enumerate the main causes of pyrexia in the mother during the early postnatal period. (b) Describe the diagnosis and treatment of *one* condition you mention in part (a).

**C.M.B.(Eng.).** Discuss the care given by the community midwife to the mother and baby transferred home early following delivery in hospital.

**N. Ire. M. Council.** (a) What observations should be made of the mother during the 'lying in' period. (b) Describe the nursing care during the 'lying in' period. (c) Enumerate the complications which may arise.

**N. Ire. M. Council.** (a) Describe the urinary bladder. (b) Discuss the disorders of micturition which may occur during (i) pregnancy; (ii) the puerperium.

**C.M.B.(Scot.).** Define the postnatal period. How may the daily observations and examination of a postnatal patient be used to detect abnormalities?

**C.M.B.(Scot.).** What are the factors which should alert the midwife to the onset of postnatal depression? Describe the management of a patient with this condition with particular reference to the role of the midwife.

**C.M.B.(Eng.).** Postnatal examination six weeks after delivery.

**C.M.B.(Scot.).** What are the daily observations made by the midwife on a patient during the first ten days following delivery? What findings may indicate deviation from normal?

**C.M.B.(Eng.).** How would you assess the suitability of a patient's home for the early transfer from hospital of a mother and baby?

In which cases would this not be advisable? What previous arrangements must be made? For which reasons might the baby not be permitted to go home on the morning of intended discharge? When does the midwife visit?

## C.M.B. Short Questions

**Eng.:** Whom do you inform when a mother and baby leave hospital? **Eng.:** Arrangements for early transfer home of mother and baby. **Eng.:** The records kept by a midwife following early transfer home of a mother and baby. **Eng.:** Assessment of the mother prior to early transfer home after hospital delivery. **Eng.:** Disturbances of micturition in the puerperium. **Eng.:** Postnatal clinic. **N. Ire.:** Minor psychological disorders of pregnancy and the puerperium. **Eng.:** Retention of urine in the puerperium. **Eng.:** Postnatal depression. **Eng.:** 6th week postnatal visit. **Eng.:** Puerperal anaemia. **Eng.:** Superficial thrombophlebitis. **Eng.:** Observation of the mother during the first six hours after labour. **Scot.:** The lochia. **Eng.:** Urinary tract infection in the puerperium. **Eng.:** Observation of the mother in the first 24 hours after delivery. **Eng.:** Failure of mother to pass urine after delivery.

## Terminology

| Description | Term |
|---|---|
| Cervical cytology to detect early cancer | |
| Raw area of cervix | |
| Bladder prolapsed into vagina | |
| Localised anaemia of the uterus | |
| Faeces being passed vaginally | |
| Delay in return of the uterus to normal size | |
| Breaking down of uterine fibres by hormone or enzyme | |

State what you know regarding: (a) the psychology of the puerperal woman; (b) the social aspects of puerperal care; (c) the education of the young mother; (d) treatment of a third degree tear.

**FAMILY PLANNING**

(1) Who is responsible for providing family planning clinics? (2) What are the risks associated with (a)

using the rhythm method? (b) intra-uterine devices? (c) the oral pill? (3) How is the day of ovulation determined? (4) When should the woman attend the F. P. clinic after confinement?

**C.M.B.(Scot.) 30-min. question.** Describe the methods currently available for family planning.

**C.M.B.(Eng.) 30-min. paper.** How are the family planning services provided? Describe briefly the methods available.

**C.M.B.(Scot.).** Describe the purposes and benefits of counselling on family planning.

**C.M.B.(Scot.).** What would you tell a postnatal patient about: (a) oral contraception, (b) intra-uterine contraceptive device, (c) rhythm method of contraception.

**C.M.B.(Eng.).** Explain the various factors which may influence a patient's decision concerning her choice of contraception.

**C.M.B.(Eng.).** What family planning services are provided? Describe briefly the methods available.

**C.M.B.(Eng.).** What information and advice would you give to a recently delivered mother who asks you about family planning?

**N.Ire. M. Council.** Discuss family planning under the following headings: (a) Methods. (b) Family Planning services. (c) The midwife's role in family planning.

## C.M.B. Short Questions

**Eng.:** Vasectomy. **Scot.:** What is the presently prescribed maximal amount of oestrogen in the contraceptive pill? **Eng.:** Male and female sterilisation. **Eng.:** Outline talk on family planning. **Eng.:** Family planning.

**Eng.:** Ideal arrangements for early transfer of mother and baby to home from hospital. **Eng.:** Planned early transfer of mother and baby from hospital. **Eng.:** Home assessment for 48-hour early transfer of patients. **Eng.:** What preparations would you make to ensure continuity of care? **Eng.:** Postnatal exercises. **Eng.:** Haemorrhoids in the puerperium. **Eng.:** Perineal wound care. **Eng.:** The contraceptive pill. **Eng.:** Barrier methods of contraception. **Eng.:** Intra-uterine contraceptive device. **Scot.:** Laparoscopic sterilisation.

# 27
# Complications of the Puerperium

*Puerperal sepsis. Urinary tract infection. Breast infection. Venous thrombosis. Pulmonary thromboembolism. Puerperal haemorrhage. Incontinence of urine. Psychiatric disorders. Fourth day 'blues'*

## PUERPERAL SEPSIS (PUERPERAL FEVER IN SCOTLAND)

Puerperal sepsis is an infection of the genital tract by organisms, occurring within 14 days (Eng. and Wales) and 21 days (Scot.) after abortion or childbirth. In England the condition is not notifiable. In Scotland the doctor notifies the Chief Administrative Medical Officer of the Health Board (or the appropriate Community Medical Specialist acting on his behalf) when the temperature 38°C is sustained during a period of 24 hrs or has recurred during that period. The maternal mortality rate from puerperal sepsis has been lowered since the introduction of sulphonamides and antibiotics. But during 1970–1972 in Britain 15 women died of puerperal sepsis.

The *haemolytic streptococcus group A* is still potentially the most dangerous organism for the postpartum woman because of its ability to invade the blood stream. Fortunately it is sensitive to certain antibiotics, and if treated promptly the infection can usually be brought under control. The habitat of the haemolytic streptococcus group A is in the nose and throat.

*Staphylococcal infection* tends to be localised, and abscess formation is common, but fatal septicaemia may occur.

The *Clostridium welchii* is occasionally found in the vagina and in the presence of bruised or necrosed tissue may become aggressive and cause septicaemia. Haemolysis of red cells occurs, resulting in profound anaemia, anuria is sometimes present, and the infection may become rapidly fatal.

The *Escherichia coli*. Genital tract infection by this organism is usually confined to the uterus and gives rise to foul-smelling lochia. Septicaemia sometimes occurs.

### Control of the spread of infection

Efficient mask wearing. The use of paper handkerchiefs followed by hand-washing.

Scrupulous domestic cleanliness. Fresh air. Modern methods of dust control.

Impeccable obstetric aseptic and antiseptic technique.

#### LOCAL UTERINE INFECTION

The temperature steps up gradually and rarely goes beyond 38·8°C.

The pulse is over 90 and rarely over 120.

The lochia are profuse, brownish, offensive and frequently contain pieces of chorion.

The uterus is large (subinvoluted), soft in consistence and tender to touch.

The woman may complain of headache and general malaise.

In this condition the leucocytes in the wall of the inflamed uterus destroy many of the invading organisms and limit the spread of infection. With prompt antibiotic treatment the condition usually resolves within three or four days.

470

### GENERAL OR BLOOD-STREAM INFECTION

## *Septicaemia*

The temperature rises sharply to 39·4°C or over and may be continuous or remittent. Rigors are common, especially with anaerobic organisms.

The pulse in severe cases may be 140 to 160 and is the best guide to the patient's condition. (A fall in temperature with a rapid pulse is not a sign of improvement.)

The lochia are sometimes pale and scanty; they may have a fetid odour.

The uterus involutes normally and may not be tender to touch.

Pallor, due to anaemia, becomes marked, and the skin sometimes has an icteric tinge; skin rashes may be evident.

Vomiting may be persistent, and, on occasions, diarrhoea is troublesome.

Loss of appetite and sleeplessness are usual, delirium is not uncommon.

Endotoxic (bacteraemic) shock may occur (see p. 170).

## *Management of Puerperal Sepsis*

Barrier nursing should be employed by the midwife in cases of puerperal pyrexia, prior to the patient being seen by the doctor, who will then order isolation of the patient.

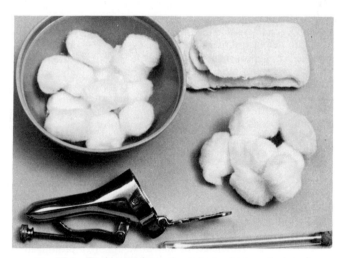

Fig. 27-1   Equipment for endocervical or high vaginal swab.
Swabbing lotion without antiseptic. Vaginal speculum. Test-tube for swab.
*Aberdeen Maternity Hospital.*

### INVESTIGATION OF PUERPERAL SEPSIS

The type of labour and delivery, including any vaginal interference, is noted. The temperature and pulse chart is studied. The breasts, chest, throat and legs are examined for signs of infection. The abdomen, lochia, and vulva are inspected.

An endocervical swab for culture, mid-stream specimen of urine, nose and throat swabs and, in some cases, blood cultures are taken. The sensitivity of the infecting organism to the antibiotics is also tested. When taking an endocervical swab the woman is placed in the lithotomy or cross-bed position and the vulva swabbed with sterile water to which no antiseptic has been added. The use of a speculum is essential to avoid contamination from the lower vagina.

Blood investigation is made because anaemia is common in puerperal sepsis, due to blood loss and to the haemolysis of red cells by certain organisms and toxins.

## MEDICAL TREATMENT

The administration of ampicillin (Penbritin) is started as soon as endocervical swab, throat swab and mid-stream specimen of urine have been obtained. Cephradine (Velosef) 250 mg may be prescribed prior to the diagnosis being confirmed. The appropriate antibiotic is prescribed when the bacteriological report is received.

Metronidazole (Flagyl) has been used in cases of non-clostridial anaerobic infections prophylactically. Therapeutically it is given in conjunction with antibiotics.

The need for iron is great. A transfusion of packed cells is given if the haemoglobin is under 7·4 g/dl.

Electrolyte control is carried out daily. A good diuresis is attained by giving an i.v. infusion of glucose 5 per cent with added vitamins and potassium chloride, depending on the degree of imbalance.

### NURSING CARE

Good nursing is absolutely essential and may be a life-saving measure. Sleep is imperative and sedatives are usually necessary.

It is advisable to give a mild laxative such as Senokot 2 tablets at night followed by a bisacodyl (Dulcolax) suppository or small prepacked enema, next morning.

A fluid balance chart should be kept, and the bladder gently palpated and percussed daily to detect residual urine.

The patient is propped upright with pillows to encourage uterine drainage; the adoption of the prone position for half an hour twice daily will also facilitate drainage from the uterus.

The diet should have a high calorie, high vitamin content and be easily digested: the woman is coaxed to eat. Adequate protein is essential. Vitamins are very necessary: vitamin C aids healing and blood formation.

## EXTRA-GENITAL INFECTIONS

URINARY TRACT INFECTION

Pyelonephritis occurs in a number of cases during the puerperium, but the efficient treatment of pyelonephritis during pregnancy helps to prevent recrudescence of the condition. It may sometimes follow prolonged difficult labour. Rigors may occur; pain and tenderness in the kidney region are present.

**Treatment** is similar to that given during pregnancy (p. 216) prophylactic measures are:—(1) the avoidance of (a) anaemia, (b) prolonged labour, (c) catheterisation, (2) the active treatment of retention of urine, (3) Cephalexin (Keflex) (Ceporex) 250–500 mg 6 hourly.

RESPIRATORY INFECTIONS

Respiratory infections and tonsillitis may cause puerperal pyrexia, but the possibility of puerperal sepsis must not be disregarded even when signs of other infections are apparent, for both might be present.

## BREAST INFECTIONS

Mastitis is inflammation of the breast, which if not treated may proceed to abscess formation. In mild cases which are superficial and localised the term 'flushed breast' is commonly applied. The condition rarely occurs prior to the eighth day of the puerperium and most frequently arises during the second or third week.

The most common infecting organism is the *Staphylococcus aureus*: the infant's eyes and nose may be the source of infection or the multiplication of organisms which are always present in the breast. This is commonly due to stasis of milk brought about by engorgement; imperfect emptying of the breast; bruising of breast tissue by rough or prolonged expression of milk. A cracked nipple permits the introduction of organisms.

### SIGNS AND SYMPTOMS

A sharp rise in temperature, 38·3° to 40°C.
Rapid pulse. Throbbing pain and tenderness in the breast.
A diffuse or wedge-shaped, indurated, reddened area.
General malaise with headache and shivering.

### *Treatment*

A sample of milk is sent for bacteriological examination.

Prompt recognition of the early signs and immediate administration of antibiotics offer the greatest hope in the prevention of abscess formation. Antibiotics such as cloxacillin are most effective when given early. In hospital the *Staphylococcus aureus*, the common infecting organism, is penicillin resistant, so methicillin (Celbenin) is usually prescribed. To relieve pain and induce sleep analgesics are given, e.g. Codis 2 tablets; or Panasorb 2 tablets; or pentazocine (Fortral) 2 tablets.

Lactation is suppressed. A supporting binder should be applied (*while the woman is lying flat on her back*), the breasts being supported by large pads of cotton wool. It is definitely harmful to apply a firm binder over unsupported inflamed breasts; stasis in the dependent area results, and this favours abscess formation which is treated in the Surgical Department.

## VENOUS THROMBOSIS

In this condition clot formation occurs in the veins usually of the lower limbs.

### *Susceptibility of Puerperal Women to Thrombosis*

#### Increased viscosity of the blood after the 28th week

This is often intensified because of dehydration and haemorrhage during labour.

#### Stasis of blood in the veins

Varicose veins predispose to stasis. The recumbent position and disinclination to move, e.g. following Caesarean section, haemorrhage, shock.

#### Changes in the walls of the veins

These may be due to varicosities, inflammation or trauma.

#### Age over 35 and high parity

##### PROPHYLAXIS

#### During pregnancy

In women with thrombo-embolic disorders oestrogen preparations are contra-indicated. All women, should during their pregnancy, be encouraged to take plenty of exercise and in the latter stages to avoid sitting with legs dependant. Those with marked varicose veins or symptoms of venous insufficiency should wear anti-embolism stockings or crepe or blue line bandages. Surgical treatment of varicose veins is not carried out during pregnancy.

Low dose subcutaneous heparin (5,000 units 8 hourly) can be used for those who are at considerable risk of developing venous thrombosis or pulmonary embolism. There is no contra-indication to the use of heparin throughout pregnancy. Warfarin sodium can also be used, but because of potential teratogenic effects its use during the first trimester is avoided.

**During labour**

The avoidance of exhaustion, dehydration and haemorrhage.

The avoidance of trauma to limbs, due to pressure by stirrup rods when in the lithotomy position. Bruising of limbs in moving an unconscious patient on to the trolley.

Avoidance of overdistension of the bladder which along with the large uterus can cause pressure on or angulation of iliofemoral venous segments.

Dextran 70 (Macrodex or Lomodex 70) can be used during any operative procedure such as a Caesarean section: the most popular Dextran regime being 500 ml during the operative procedure and then further doses of 500 ml on the next one to three days. Dextran decreases both the blood viscosity and platelet adhesiveness.

**During the puerperium**

To avoid venous stasis all women should be encouraged to move their legs as much as possible whilst in bed. Early ambulation has reduced but not eliminated thrombosis. Patients who need assistance must be helped and encouraged to walk along the ward. Merely sitting, immobile, in a low chair with the legs dependant has less therapeutic value than ankle exercises, leg elevation and freedom of leg movement in bed.

For those who are at a special risk of developing a deep venous thrombosis, prophylaxis with low dose subcutaneous heparin (5,000 units 8 hourly) may be started 6 hours after delivery. This should be continued until the patient is fully ambulant.

## Observation

Successful treatment depends on early diagnosis. The midwife must be 'leg conscious' in susceptible cases. The legs should be examined, while bathing or bed-making, without producing a phobia. Localised pain or tenderness in the calf or groin should be reported to the doctor.

## SUPERFICIAL VEIN THROMBOSIS

Mild cases in which the superficial leg veins are affected may be associated with varicose veins. The involved veins can be palpated and are tender to touch: redness of the overlying skin may be evident. Temperature and pulse are both slightly increased. The condition may be manifest as early as the fourth day postpartum, but usually around the 10th day. The risk of pulmonary thromboembolism is slight unless extension occurs along the long saphenous vein in the thigh. Tenderness in the thigh should be reported.

## Treatment

Anticoagulants are not necessary. If there is extensive superficial thrombophlebitis then the leg should be elevated. Either phenylbutazone or oxyphenbutazone can be given to try to reduce the inflammation and discomfort. It is usually unnecessary to limit the patient's movements: some find that a crepe or blue line bandage and subsequently support tights are beneficial.

DIAGNOSIS

The clinical signs of a deep vein thrombosis are pain and discomfort in the calf or thigh. Swelling of these areas will be evident if the thrombus is occlusive. If the thrombus is non-occlusive there will be no swelling. Homan's sign (pain felt in the calf muscles when the foot is dorsiflexed with the leg extended at the knee), and a slight rise in temperature to 37·2°C may also occur.

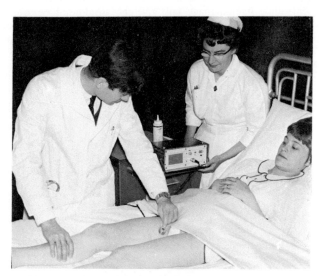

Fig. 27-2   Ultrasonic screening for deep vein thrombosis.
*Simpson Memorial Maternity Pavilion, Edinburgh.*

Deep vein thrombosis is usually manifest during the second week of the puerperium, but may arise during the first week. The danger of a portion of the blood clot becoming detached and giving rise to pulmonary thromboembolism exists.

The diagnosis of deep vein thrombosis can be extremely difficult. Some patients may have no peripheral signs of a deep vein thrombosis and yet have a pulmonary embolism. Conversely a patient who complains of discomfort in the calves may not in fact have a deep vein thrombosis.

The most accurate diagnostic method is ascending venography. This procedure can, however, be uncomfortable and may not be available. Ultrasonic scanning (Fig. 27-2) is useful when there are occlusive clots in the ilio-femoral segments; below that level it is of no use.

## *Treatment*

ANTICOAGULANT DRUGS

The anticoagulant drugs heparin and warfarin sodium (Marevan) are used. Heparin which will prevent further thrombus formation is given intravenously by a pump or in boluses of roughly 7,500 to 12,000 units six hourly. The thrombin clotting time can be measured to estimate the amount of heparin required. The heparin can be continued for a period of ten days and then stopped. In some cases the doctor will start the oral administration of warfarin sodium after two to three days. The dosage of this drug can be controlled by measuring the prothrombin time.

If the patient does not have a pulmonary thrombo-embolism, then the warfarin can be stopped after three to four weeks.

### Side effects

Heparin may, if given for a period with inadequate control during the first week of the puerperium, cause haemorrhage from the placental site or the formation of a haematoma in an abdominal incision. The doctor is notified and he will, if other means of controlling haemorrhage fail, give the antidote, 1 per cent protamine sulphate solution, 5 to 10 ml, intravenously, to counteract the effect of heparin.

The antidote to warfarin is Vitamin $K_1$ (phytomenadione). It is given in the dose of 10 to 20 mg slowly intravenously. As this drug may take a few hours to have any effect, fresh blood can be used if speed is essential.

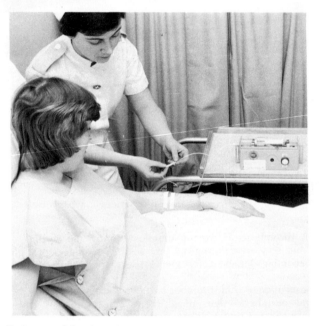

Fig. 27-3   Patient receiving heparin by Handley clockwork slow infusion pump. Note patient's gown with buttons on both sides for i.v. infusions.

LEG ELEVATION AND MOVEMENTS

For deep vein thrombosis confined to the calf no restriction of movements is necessary. The patient can move about the ward as much as she wishes and movements of her legs in bed should be encouraged. If an ilio-femoral thrombosis is present the patient should be confined to bed until most of the swelling has subsided. The legs in the latter case should be elevated to facilitate the return of blood to the heart. This is done in such a manner that the leg is not immobilised and free movement is possible. A cradle to support the bedclothes is necessary (Fig. 27-4). Both groups of patients should wear anti-embolism stockings or other forms of support when they are up and about. Depending on the degree of swelling at the time of discharge the patient should continue to wear some form of support.

A piece of blood clot becomes detached from a thrombus in the veins of the pelvis or lower limbs and travels by the inferior vena cava to the right side of the heart and via the pulmonary artery to the lung.

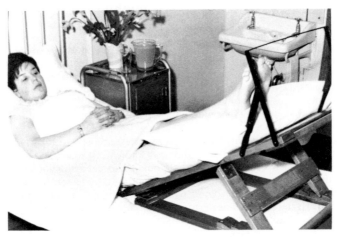

Fig. 27-4   Leg elevator. Used in cases predisposed to or having developed venous thrombosis

*Note.*—(1) Elevation of feet to above heart level. (2) Provision by metal cradle for freedom of movement. (3) Affords maximal comfort.

*Aberdeen Maternity Hospital.*

### Signs and Symptoms

Pain in the chest which catches the breath is an important early symptom of pulmonary embolism: breathlessness is common and haemoptysis is present in 40 per cent of cases. Depending on the size of the embolus the patient will be pale, dyspnoeic, sweating, hypotensive and distressed. Collapse, respiratory failure and cardiac arrest may occur. The outcome will depend on the size of the embolus; in rare cases death occurs within a few moments.

The diagnosis of pulmonary thrombo-embolism will be made on clinical grounds with the help of an ECG.

### Treatment

**Medical aid should be summoned urgently;** the patient given extra pillows, oxygen; the bed is screened: the patient's relatives are notified of serious illness. A drip should be set up—heparin in a dose of 10 to 15 thousand units should be given. If the patient is very distressed, small doses of morphine or diamorphine may be given i.v. The patient's condition will usually improve over the next few hours. The blood pressure usually returns to the normal range and the arterial blood gases will also tend towards normal. If the condition does not improve then the decision regarding pulmonary angiography followed by either a pulmonary embolectomy or streptokinase infusion will be made.

If the embolus is small, apart from some chest discomfort and pleuritic pain, the patient may have no physical signs of an embolus. The diagnosis is made by isotope lung scanning. Once the diagnosis has been made anti-coagulation with heparin and then warfarin is initiated and continued for three to six months. If there is no pulmonary embolism anti-coagulants would be given for only three to four weeks. Some doctors give an antibiotic to diminish the risk of pulmonary infection.

## PUERPERAL HAEMORRHAGE

### (Secondary Postpartum Haemorrhage)

Bleeding may take place from the 24th hour up to the sixth week of the puerperium, but commonly occurs between the 10th and 14th days. This is due to retention of a piece of placenta, which when it sloughs off opens up the large uterine sinuses. (Ultrasonography is used to detect retained products of conception.) In some cases no products of conception have been retained. The haemorrhage may or may not be associated with sepsis. Persistent red lochia is a warning sign.

Severe haemorrhage is usually due to the presence of a succenturiate lobe or large cotyledon of placenta. The author has known of three fatal cases from this cause, two of which occurred after the women had been discharged. In another case, 12 litres of blood were given over a period of days to replace the blood lost. One patient lost 1,200 ml of blood while in the 'toilet' on the ninth day of the puerperium. Hysterectomy was performed in a case in which the bleeding could not be controlled.

### TREATMENT OF SEVERE HAEMORRHAGE BY THE MIDWIFE

She should massage the uterus, express the clots, send urgently for medical assistance ('Flying Squad'), give ergometrine, 0·5 mg, or Syntometrine, 1 ml, intramuscularly, and repeat if necessary. If the situation is critical bimanual compression of the uterus must be carried out to control the bleeding and ergometrine given i.v. The 'Flying Squad' will, if necessary, give blood and when the woman has rallied she will be transferred to hospital for digital exploration of the uterus.

## INCONTINENCE OF URINE

Paradoxical incontinence due to retention of urine with overflow may not be diagnosed by the inexperienced midwife.

Stress incontinence occurs in multiparous women with laxity of the pelvic floor and urethral sphincter which has occurred due to parturition; cystocele may also be present. Incontinence in such cases is not complete, and consists in the dribbling of urine during coughing, sneezing or sudden exertion. The condition sometimes clears up as the woman's health improves. Nourishing food, iron, and pelvic floor exercises will help to increase muscle tone. If incontinence persists, operation may be necessary.

### VESICO-VAGINAL FISTULA

This is an artificial opening between the bladder or urethra and vagina. The condition is rare in countries where good obstetric care is available.

When incontinence occurs immediately after the birth of the baby, it is usually due to laceration of the bladder during a difficult instrumental delivery. When incontinence begins five or six days after labour, it is due to sloughing of a damaged area of bladder, caused by prolonged pressure by the fetal head during labour. To avoid such an occurrence the bladder should be emptied every two hours throughout labour and prolonged labour should be avoided; more especially the second stage.

### Treatment

An indwelling catheter is inserted and left *in situ* for ten days or longer with sealed drainage. Fluids are given up to 3 litres daily; antibiotics are prescribed. The fistula usually heals without operation, but if it persists the woman is referred to the gynaecological department for operation, usually about 8 to 10 weeks later when her health has been built up.

# PSYCHIATRIC DISORDERS

These occur in about one per 1,000 births, more commonly in primigravidae and may be manifest during pregnancy, the puerperium and the ensuing year: rarely during labour. There is no special type of mental disorder peculiar to the childbearing woman.

Normal pregnancy and labour may impose a degree of emotional strain on the woman of nervous temperament, and severe stress may precipitate psychiatric disorders, especially if she has a family history of mental instability. But many such women go through the experience of childbearing without a mental breakdown if other contributory factors are not superimposed. If the woman is happy in her home life and is not subjected to severe conflict or anxiety she is less likely to develop psychiatric symptoms. The maladjusted personality when subjected to gross disharmony is liable to break down.

#### THE ROLE OF THE MIDWIFE

(1) **During pregnancy,** the midwife should try to inculcate in all her patients a confident, serene outlook regarding childbearing and childrearing. She should help the woman to clarify her misapprehension and try to dispel her fears as far as is possible.

(2) **The midwife is mainly concerned with** (*a*) the preventive aspect; (*b*) recognising early signs and (*c*) giving supportive care in mild cases of depression.

(3) **Certain 'high risk' factors** may be manifest during pregnancy which indicate the possibility that the woman may become depressed during the puerperium. The midwife should be alert to such signals and report them to the doctor.

(i) A family history of mental illness.

(ii) Previous depression in the puerperium.

(iii) Death of, or a disturbed relationship with, the patient's mother.

(iv) Excessive anxiety exhibited during the first trimester of pregnancy.

(4) **Giving advice and support for the fourth day blues.** The emotional state experienced by some women during the early days of the puerperium, characterised by tearfulness and mild depression, is commonly known as 'the blues'; and should not be regarded as a psychiatric disorder. The cause is not fully understood and may be due to endocrine imbalance, metabolic adjustment, physiological and psychological adaptation at a time when the woman has suffered the emotional trauma of labour and may be apprehensive regarding her ability to cope with the responsibilities of baby care. Breast and perineal discomfort add to her feelings of misery. In about one per cent cases of 'the blues' the depression becomes more severe and persistent, with anxiety and irritability; such cases are usually treated successfully by the general practitioner. When the depression is associated with abnormal thought processes, i.e. delusions, there is a risk of suicide and infanticide; treatment by a psychiatrist is essential.

Postnatal women may be dismayed when 'the blues' occur and some consider they should have been made aware of this possibility. Midwives should therefore advise expectant mothers that the condition is common, benign and transient, usually clearing up within a few days. Husbands should also be told that their wives may be sad and weepy, with feelings of inadequacy, and should be advised to be encouraging, patient and attentive.

The midwife has a most important influence during the postnatal period and should endeavour to give 'tender loving care' blended with helpful assurance. Adequate quietness to ensure rest and sleep should be achieved: sedatives may be necessary.

## DEPRESSION

This is the most frequent neurosis occurring during the puerperium and is more severe and persistent than 'the blues'.

SIGNS AND SYMPTOMS

(a) **Insomnia** with no apparent cause such as noise or pain.
(b) **Unusual sadness,** anxiety or irritability.
(c) **Excessive self-doubt** about her ability to care for her baby.
(d) **Ideas of guilt** or self blame.
(e) **Thoughts of harming herself or her baby.**

Suicidal or infanticidal threats must always be taken seriously and the mother should be closely observed until medical help is obtained.

### *Treatment*

This is usually carried out by the general practitioner. The mother is encouraged to talk about any negative feelings she may have towards her baby. The husband should be assured that the majority of women respond to treatment within three to six weeks.

#### PSYCHOSES OCCURRING DURING THE PUERPERIUM

These are serious disorders in which the mother may lose contact with reality. She may have delusions (i.e. false beliefs firmly held against all evidence to the contrary) and also experience false perceptions such as hearing voices or seeing imaginary persecutors. Confusion, disorientation and lability of mood are also particularly characteristic of the psychoses occurring at this time. There are three major disorders. (1) Schizophrenia, (2) manic-depressive psychosis and (3) organic psychosis.

The treatment of these disorders is undertaken by psychiatrists. The midwife should however record her observations regarding the mother's mood or behaviour. When the following symptoms are present the possible onset of a psychosis is likely.

(i) **Insomnia** with no adequate cause.
(ii) **Unusual lability of mood,** e.g. sudden depression or unexpected laughter.
(iii) **Unwarranted suspiciousness** and persecutory ideas.
(iv) **Delusions or hallucinations.**
(v) **Sullen withdrawal or excessive restlessness and elation.**
(vi) **An altered or 'odd' way** in which the mother relates to or handles her baby.

#### MANAGEMENT

The mother is admitted to a psychiatric unit accompanied by her baby if this is considered advisable. Any physical puerperal complications are investigated and adequately treated.

Major tranquillisers such as chlorpromazine (Largactil) may be given by injection or orally and if the mother is seriously depressed anti-depressant drugs and/or electro-convulsive therapy may be required.

Early treatment in suitable surroundings by experts gives the greatest opportunity for rapid and complete recovery. The necessary nursing care is highly specialised and ought to be given by nurses qualified in psychiatric nursing.

Until skilled nursing care is available, the midwife should arrange for the patient to be nursed on the ground floor in a quiet single room and never left alone. The woman is fed with a spoon; knives and forks are not used. The danger of gas, matches and antiseptics must be kept in mind but such precautions should not be obvious to the patient. Attractive, digestible food should be served and the woman coaxed to eat and drink. The bladder should be emptied regularly. Persuasion and patient reassurance are required; it is futile to attempt to convince the woman by argument. Midwives should be aware that certain anti-depressant drugs such as phenelzine (Nardil) may potentiate the action of pethidine and might produce coma. The anti-depressant drug amitriptyline (Tryptizol) is commonly used for depression in the postnatal period but not during early pregnancy because of possible teratogenic effects on the developing embryo: side effects are blurred vision, dry mouth.

The majority of women with puerperal psychoses are discharged from a psychiatric unit within six weeks but all will require careful follow up as an out patient. In women with an organic psychosis or a manic depressive psychosis, the prognosis is usually good. For those with schizophrenia the prognosis may be less favourable.

**The midwife has a significant role to play in the prevention,** detection and early management of psychiatric disorders that occur during pregnancy and the early postnatal period. Her relationship to the mother is an important factor in psychiatric treatment.

---

## QUESTIONS FOR REVISION

### COMPLICATIONS OF THE PUERPERIUM

For what reasons are the following drugs prescribed? Heparin; amitriptyline, phenelzine. What are the causes of vesico-vaginal fistula? What is the treatment? What are the signs of pulmonary thrombo-embolism? What could the midwife do pending the arrival of the doctor? What precautions would you take when nursing a puerperal patient with depression? How would you apply a supporting breast binder? How would you take an endocervical swab?

**Define** stasis; flushed breast; anaerobic organism; puerperal haemorrhage.

**C.M.B.(Scot.) 30-min. question.** On the ninth day of the puerperium the patient has a sudden vaginal haemorrhage. What is the cause of this? Give the emergency and subsequent treatment.

**C.M.B.(Eng.) 30-min. question.** What urinary tract complications may occur in the puerperium? Indicate briefly how these might be avoided and treated.

**C.M.B.(Scot.) 30-min. question.** A woman is found to have a temperature of 38·5°C on the third day after a forceps delivery. Discuss the possible causes and the investigation of this pyrexia.

### PUERPERAL SEPSIS

**Differentiate between:** local uterine infection and septicaemia; thrombus and embolus; paradoxical and stress incontinence.

**Describe:** investigation of puerperal sepsis; nursing care in puerperal sepsis; incontinence of urine; the cause of mastitis.

**C.M.B.(Eng.) 30-min. question.** Enumerate the main causes of pyrexia during the puerperium. Describe the diagnosis and treatment of one condition you mention.

**N. Ire. Council.** Discuss the causes of pyrexia in the postnatal period. Describe the investigations that would be made.

### C.M.B. Short Questions

**Eng.:** Investigations made when a patient has a temperature of 38°C puerperal thrombo-phlebitis on the fifth day of the puerperium. **Eng.:** The common causes of pyrexia during the puerperium. **N. Ireland:** Discuss the management of a patient who develops a pyrexia on the fifth day of the puerperium. **Eng.:** The diagnosis and treatment of deep vein thrombosis in the puerperium. **Scot.:** Thrombo-embolism. **N. Ire.:** Superficial thrombophlebitis. **Eng.:** Puerperal thrombophlebitis. **Eng.:** Anticoagulant drugs. **Eng.:** Superficial venous thrombosis. **Eng.:** Secondary postpartum haemorrhage. **Eng.:** The predisposing factors in secondary postpartum haemorrhage. **Eng.:** Deep vein thrombosis. **Eng.:** Recognition of puerperal psychosis. **Eng.:** Pulmonary embolism in the puerperium.

Discuss the role of the midwife in the prevention of psychotic episodes in the puerperium.

How should the midwife deal with 'fourth day blues'?

# 28
# Physiology, Management and Minor Disorders of the Newborn

*Initiation of respiration. Digestion. Temperature regulation. Reaction to organisms, Examination. Neurological responses. Screening. Physical needs. Daily observation. Stools. Daily care. Psychology. Vomiting.*

In order to appreciate the need for gentleness and patience in handling the newborn baby student midwives should consider:

**The sheltered life he has led in utero.**
**The ordeal to which he has been subjected.**
**The physical adjustments he must make to extra-uterine life.**

For nine months the fetus has lived in a warm environment, protected by fluid, obtaining nourishment without using the intestinal tract and receiving oxygen without pulmonary respiration. Fetal breathing movements have been seen on the real-time ultrasonic scanner. The fetus has not been called on to produce heat, and has encountered only a very few organisms.

The process of labour causes injury and death to many babies, so because of the strenuous ordeal to which the infant has been subjected, involving pressure on the brain and some degree of hypoxia, he should be handled with infinite gentleness, wrapped up warmly and left quietly in a heated cot to recover from the trauma of birth.

The main physiological adjustments to be made are (1) the initiation of pulmonary respiration, (2) the establishment of changes in the circulation, (3) the inauguration of digestion, (4) the regulation of heat and (5) the reaction to organisms.

## (1) THE INITIATION OF RESPIRATION

Breathing is the first function to be established. The lungs *in utero* are solid, because they have not been inflated and aerated, the alveolar cells secrete a substance, surfactant, that prevents the walls of the alveoli from adhering. Breathing is initiated in response to lack of oxygen and the high level of carbon dioxide in the blood stream, which stimulates the respiratory centre in the medulla. But if the $CO_2$ level is too high it depresses instead of stimulates. Respiration is aided by compression of the chest wall during actual birth, the impact of cool air on the face and the handling of the limbs and body. The healthy baby cries almost as soon as he is born, but he must breathe in order to cry: with the first breath the blood vessels in the lungs expand.

The initial respiratory movements are shallow and almost imperceptible, then comes a gasp, followed by crying. The respirations are rapid (around 40 per minute) and may be irregular for some hours. To facilitate lung expansion *healthy babies are encouraged to cry* lustily at birth; otherwise complete aeration of the lungs may be delayed for hours or days, as occurs in preterm and asphyxiated babies. Breathing in the newborn is almost entirely abdominal.

### (2) DIGESTION

The baby has to suck, swallow, digest and absorb food as well as defaecate.
**Colostrum.** Nature has provided this food which is easily digested, the protein

consisting of lactalbumin, but not caseinogen as in milk. It is nutritive, quenches thirst, is laxative in effect, and contains immune bodies and vitamins.

**Meconium.** The baby's first stool is meconium which is present in the intestine from about the 16th week of intra-uterine life. It is dark green/greenish-black in colour, being composed of bile-pigment, fatty acids, mucus and epithelial cells.

### (3) TEMPERATURE REGULATION

Heat regulation in the newborn is unstable and because of the low metabolic rate heat production is poor. The baby leaves an environment of 37·7°C and enters one of about 21·1°C; being wet, he will lose heat by evaporation. The baby should therefore be received into a warm Turkish towel, dried, wrapped in a cotton cellular blanket which covers the head and laid into a warmed cot. Even with such treatment his temperature may fall to around 35·5°C within an hour and it may be some hours before it rises to the normal level.

The first bath should be delayed for at least 12 hours and carried out in a room at a temperature of 21° to 26·6°C, with water at 37·7°C. Towels and clothing should also be warmed. If the baby's hands, feet and lips are blue after the first bath, it has been carried out too soon or the baby has been chilled.

**Neonatal hypothermia** in which the baby's temperature may fall as low as 30°C, is the result of exposure to cold (see p. 543). Low-reading rectal thermometers, ranging from 25°C to 40°C should always be used for newborn babies in order to detect temperatures below 35°C.

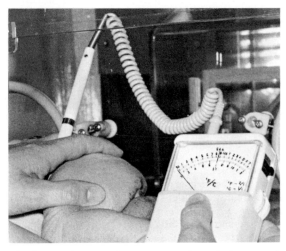

Fig. 28-1   Electronic thermometer registers in five seconds.
*Maternity Hospital, Stirling.*

### (4) REACTION TO ORGANISMS

Passive immunity to many specific infectious diseases is inherited from the mother, but some weeks elapse before the baby produces an active immunity to various organisms. During passage through the birth canal skin abrasions may occur and the baby's face is exposed to organisms. The eyes, umbilicus and skin are all vulnerable to infection. Gram-positive and gram-negative organisms are important causes of neonatal infection.

The *Staphylococcus aureus* is the organism to which babies have least resistance.

Thorough domestic cleanliness when handling babies is the finest safeguard against infection.

### Heart beat

The heart rate is 120–140 beats per minute usually ascertained by auscultating the apex beat. The heart is higher in the newborn than in the adult so the diaphragm of the stethoscope is placed at the left sternal edge in the midclavicular line but the point of maximal intensity is variable, sometimes over and above the left nipple. There is little difference between the sounds at apex or base in the newborn. If a separate stethoscope is not available for each baby the diaphragm should be wiped with a medi-swab.

### Blood

The number of red cells necessary during intra-uterine life is in excess of what is required after birth, so the extra cells are broken down and the haemoglobin stored by the liver. The number of red cells at birth is approximately 6,000,000 per cu mm and haemoglobin 18 g/dl.

The clotting power is low because newborn infants are nearly always deficient in vitamin K, a substance needed by the liver in the production of prothrombin, one of the elements necessary for the clotting of blood.

### Urinary function

The bladder of the baby at term contains urine which is usually expelled during birth. No concern need be felt if the baby does not pass urine for 24 hours. The kidneys of the newborn do not excrete fluids nor chlorides efficiently, and if insufficient fluid is given, the urine may be dark yellow in colour and may leave a brick-dust-like deposit on the napkins which at first glance appears to be blood, but is due to uric acid crystals.

### (5) EXAMINATION OF THE NEWBORN BABY

It is now considered essential that the baby is examined by a paediatrician or doctor during the first 24 hours. (Babies who need special care are admitted to the neonatal special or intensive care unit.) The need for warmth at this time must be observed; i.e. room, cot, clothing, towels. Transferring the baby from the labour ward to the nursery or postnatal ward in a portable incubator or a warm covered plastic cot is commendable.

**On admission from the delivery ward note:** Appearance, activity, regular breathing. Any abnormality in colour such as cyanosis, pallor or jaundice should be reported to the doctor.

**Check.** Name and identification bracelet, sex, Apgar score, and other relevant facts from the delivery chart (see p. 343).

**Check** for cord bleeding and religature if necessary. Record the baby's temperature. A detailed examination is carried out, usually prior to the first bath, beginning at the head and working downwards. Unless deliberately and systematically done some abnormality may be overlooked.

### Weight

The average weight at birth is 3 kg, but babies at term may weigh from 2·2 to 5·4 kg. Boys are slightly heavier than girls, and in the third and subsequent babies the weight tends to increase.

During the first three days a physiological loss of 100 to 200 g occurs. The bigger the baby the more he will lose, and when feeding is not satisfactory the loss may be as much as 400 g. The decrease in weight is due to the loss of tissue fluid, a deficient food and fluid intake as well as the loss of meconium. When the milk supply becomes adequate, a slow steady increase in weight occurs, but infants do not all regain their birth weights by the 10th day: 160 g weekly is the usual amount gained during the first months.

## Measurements

The average length of the baby at term is 50 to 52 cm and may be as much as 58 cm in babies over 4·5 kg. Length is considered to be a more reliable criterion of gestational age than weight. A plastic ruler should be used and the baby measured from the vertex to the heels or crown to rump as required. For accuracy a measuring box is available. Crown–rump 34 cm, head circumference 35 cm, and biparietal diameter 9·5 cm being useful for basic growth measurements.

### THE HEAD

The average circumference is 34 cm.

Excessive moulding and a large caput arise during difficult labour and suggest the possibility of intracranial injury. Depressed skull fractures are very rare. The mongoloid appearance of a baby with Down's syndrome is characteristic.

**The eyes.** Nystagmus is not uncommon in normal babies. Small subconjunctival haemorrhages, bright red in colour, are frequently seen; they disappear spontaneously within a week.

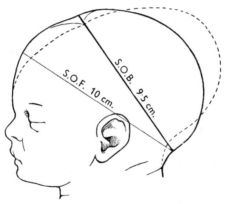

Fig. 28-2   The type of moulding in a vertex presentation, head well flexed, is shown by the dotted line.

The mouth should be inspected in a good light for cleft palate, which may only involve the soft palate. Cleft lip is readily seen. The mouth may be drawn to one side, due to facial paralysis. Excessive frothy mucus suggests an oesophageal atresia.

**Tongue-tie.** In this condition the frenulum of the tongue is attached almost to the tip. Paediatricians do not advocate snipping it and the mother should be told that it will be all right, as older relatives are apt to advise having it cut.

**Teeth.** Very occasionally babies are born with the two lower incisors erupted. They are sometimes soft and loose, and are always easily extracted.

### THE ARMS AND HANDS

The infant should be moving both arms freely, and, if not, the question of fracture, dislocation or paralysis must be considered.

Fingers should be counted, the hand being opened out, as an extra little finger attached by skin may be lying in the palm: the application of a tight ligature (by the doctor) will remove it by necrosis. Webbed fingers are rare but may be missed: they are operated on some months later.

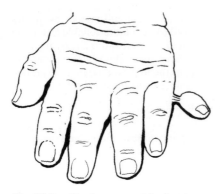

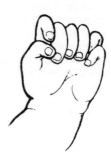

Fig. 28-3b   Polydactyly requires surgical operation.

Fig. 28-3a   Can be removed by ligation.

Fig. 28-3   Extra digit.

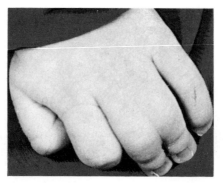

Fig. 28-4   Webbed fingers. Hand of new-born baby.

### THE BODY

**The cord** should be examined for oozing, and another clamp or ligature applied if necessary.

**The external genitalia.** More than a cursory glance is needed to establish the sex; pseudohermaphroditism may be present and conditions such as hypospadias. A degree of narrowing of the foreskin (phimosis) is natural and the prepuce is non-retractable during the first year. Forcibly pulling back the foreskin is apt to cause minor lacerations, and is not advocated: the orifice grows satisfactorily during the first year. Paediatricians do not now recommend circumcision.

**The anus** may be imperforate, and to prevent this being overlooked the first temperature should be taken rectally—gentleness is essential to avoid injury.

**The back** is inspected for spina bifida, the hips for dislocation. (*Some centres do not permit midwives to carry out the Ortolani test.*)

### THE LEGS

Fractures are rare: paralysis, if present, usually accompanies spina bifida. Talipes and congenital dislocation of the hips should be recognised early so that corrective treatment is given as soon as possible. The legs may appear to be bent, but this is normal. The toes should be counted: webbed toes are not uncommon and are usually ignored. The pad of fat on the instep is normal and gives an erroneous impression of flat foot.

## The special senses

Parents often ask when the baby will see, hear, etc., and for that reason the following facts are given:

**Taste.** The lips and tongue are very sensitive; the sense of taste is not very well developed, but babies seem to prefer sweeter foods.

**Hearing.** Loud noises cause the baby to cry, but the ability to discriminate between sounds is not developed for two or three months.

**Sight.** True vision is not present at birth, but some psychologists consider that babies have perceptive sight within one hour of birth. At one month the baby looks towards a bright light. The eyes do not focus properly for some weeks, and squint may persist for as long as six months. The eyes are of a bluish-grey colour and may change to brown during the first year. Tears are not present unless the eyes are inflamed; smiles and tears appear at from four to six weeks.

## The umbilical cord

The stump of umbilical cord shrivels by a process of necrosis or dry gangrene, and separates from the skin at a line of demarcation. The umbilical vein inside the abdomen becomes thrombosed. To aid separation of the cord, it is kept clean and dry.

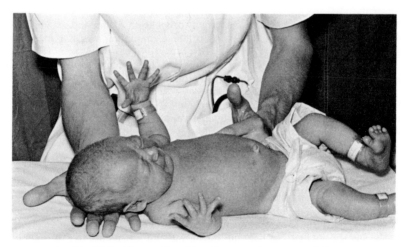

Fig. 28-5 Moro reflex. Note fingers and toes extended.
*Neonatal Intensive Care Unit, Royal Maternity Hospital, Rottenrow, Glasgow.*

## The skin

The skin is very delicate, easily irritated, abraded and infected. It is covered at birth with a substance—vernix caseosa, secreted by the sebaceous glands—which acts as a lubricant during birth, protects the skin and retains heat. To remove the vernix the finger tips smeared with mild soap should gently massage the area and the substance will rapidly dissolve.

Lanugo, a downy fluff, is seen mostly on the skin of the preterm baby.

### (6) NEUROLOGICAL RESPONSES IN THE NEWBORN

To elicit reflex behaviour, all babies have a neurological estimation made 24 hours after birth: in some centres only preterm, light for date and those suspected of intracranial damage or defect are assessed. An aggregate of criteria is more reliable in estimating gestational age than any one individual response.

**Moro reflex.** This may be incomplete in the preterm baby: complete absence suggests intra-cranial damage. The baby's body and head are supported in the supine position. When the head is allowed to drop back one or two cm the baby throws out his arms briskly with extension of elbows and fingers followed by an arm embracing movement (see Fig. 28-5).

**Rooting response.** When a flat surface, e.g. palm of the hand, is brought in contact with the baby's cheek he turns his head to that side searching for the mother's nipple—no such movement is made by the preterm infant.

**Grasp response.** The baby grasps firmly a finger placed in the palm of his hand.

**Traction response.** When the baby is raised to the sitting position, by traction on the wrists, the preterm baby does not resist: the full term infant offers strong resistance.

**Stepping response.** The baby when grasped by the body in a standing position with his feet on a flat surface makes stepping movements.

### NEONATAL SCREENING

**Routine examination by the midwife,** of the baby at birth, is a familiar screening process. The Apgar score evaluates the immediate condition of the baby. Recognition of the absence of one artery in the umbilical cord suggests other congenital abnormalities. Cleft soft palate, congenital dislocation of hip and an imperforate anus could be overlooked if the appropriate examination was not made on all babies.

**Neurological tests** are made by the paediatrician 24 hours after birth, e.g. the Moro reflex to assess gestational age, intracranial defect or damage. Tests to detect errors of metabolism, e.g. the Guthrie test is made on all babies for excess phenylalanine in the blood; further biochemical tests being made to confirm the diagnosis. The Dextrostix test for hypoglycaemia is made on infants of diabetic mothers, light for date babies and in those with certain abnormal conditions, e.g. intracranial injuries, convulsions. Screening tests are also available for a number of rare disorders, i.e. maple syrup urine disease, cystic fibrosis.

## (7) THE BABY'S PHYSICAL NEEDS

**Warmth** is very necessary until the infant has recovered from the ordeal of birth and food is being taken. Loss of heat by evaporation and particularly from the baby's head at birth should be avoided. The room should be between $21 \cdot 1°$ and $23 \cdot 8°C$ and the cot clothing light but warm. There is a tendency to over-heat babies in summer; on the other hand, they are not always kept warm enough during the winter nights, especially at home. **Chilling must be avoided to prevent neonatal hypothermia.**

**Nourishment.** See Breast and Bottle Feeding, page 497.

**The need for fluid** is imperative during the first two days: 150 ml fluid per kg body weight being required daily after the third day.

**Babies sleep** for 20 out of the 24 hours during the first two months. Mothers should be advised to avoid noises such as a blaring radio, to which the infant will become accustomed, but which by bombarding the nervous system may produce irritability.

**Fresh air** is necessary but draughts must be excluded. In warm weather healthy babies can be taken out of doors after the first few days.

**Exercise is essential** for newborn babies: arms and legs should have freedom to move, and babies should not be tightly bound up. They must be allowed to squirm, wriggle and kick, to stimulate the circulation of blood and strengthen their muscles for sitting, standing and walking later on.

**Mothering,** i.e. love and affection. Rooming-in provides greater opportunities for mothering and bonding. Mothers with no respiratory infection are encouraged to handle 'long stay' babies, feed and caress them: clean hands are essential. Nursery midwives are expected to 'mother' the babies in their care.

### (8) PROTECTION

Babies need protection from infection, suffocation, bright lights and strong wind.

To avoid suffocation by inhalation of vomitus, babies should be laid on their sides or in the prone position after feeds, as vomitus may be inhaled if lying on their backs. At home the young baby should sleep in the same room as the mother during the first year of life.

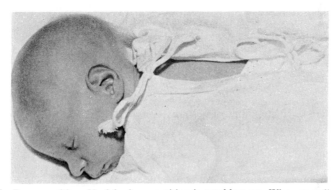

Fig. 28-6   Prone position. Useful when vomiting is troublesome. When complications are present necessitating close observation of respiratory activity the prone position is not advisable.

*Simpson Memorial Maternity Pavilion, Edinburgh.*

**Choking** may occur when milk flows too quickly through a rubber teat, therefore propping of bottles during feeding is strongly condemned.

**Smothering on a soft pillow.** Babies who are tightly wrapped up may roll over onto their faces, which they burrow into the pillow. A young baby does not require a pillow and, because of the risk of suffocation, it should not be used. Plastic bibs are also potentially dangerous.

**Overlaying.** This will only occur in the home, and the mother should have been instructed to provide a separate cot. She must be warned of the danger should she inadvertently lay her arm or the blankets over the baby's face. The midwife must always improvise a cot when one is not provided. The danger of cats must be kept in mind; they have been known to lie on the baby's face, with fatal results due to suffocation.

**Babies' eyes** should be shaded from brilliant sunshine; glaring ceiling lights should be dimmed when possible.

**Strong wind** blowing on a baby's face will 'take its breath away'. Mothers should be advised to protect the baby's face when exposed outside on a windy day.

# DAILY OBSERVATION OF THE NEWBORN BABY

The thriving baby has a clear, pink skin, firm muscles, a vigorous kick and a lusty cry. He takes his food eagerly, has a clean tongue, normal stools, bright eyes, gains in weight and sleeps well. (*Signs of illness are described under their respective headings.*)

During the first 24 hours close supervision is necessary as the majority of complications are manifest during this time. The doctor depends on the vigilant observation of the midwife to detect abnormalities and early signs of illness, and on the careful recording of her findings.

**Respirations.** The rate and type of respirations are most important during the first 48 hours of life; the normal rate being around 40 per minute; usually respirations are regular, smooth and quiet. Periods of apnoea, grunting respirations, flaring of the nasal alae or indrawing of the chest wall should be reported to the doctor at once.

**Temperature** taken once daily. **Weight** every third day.

**Feeding.** Time, whether three-hourly or four-hourly or self-regulated.

Time, whether three-hourly or four-hourly or self-regulated.

Breast-fed, whether wholly or partly; amount of milk in any test feeds.

Bottle-fed, type of milk and the amount taken.

Cyanosis or exhaustion during or after feeding should be reported; regurgitation noted.

**Medicines,** oxygen and treatment.

Other facts such as the passage of urine; the number and character of the stools; day on which the cord comes off; excessive crying, anorexia, any signs of illness.

## THE STOOLS

**Meconium** (see p. 483). When the baby is given milk the meconium stool becomes greenish-brown, then yellowish-brown.

After the fourth day the typical soft, yellow semi-fluid stool of the breast-fed baby is usual, the bowels moving three, four or more times daily. The acid stool of the breast fed baby inhibits the growth of *E. coli*. Cow's milk produces a firmer, paler stool of putty-like consistency, with a slightly offensive odour.

Green stools occur occasionally in healthy babies, and if the infant is hungry and not feverish they may be ignored. Persistent green stools with mucus should be reported. Greenish-yellow, frothy, loose stools, with a sour odour, are due to too much sugar and tend to cause sore buttocks.

Greenish-yellow, loose, frequent stools with curds, causing sore buttocks, are due to overfeeding.

Pasty, greenish stools with small firm curds, often causing colic, are due to too much protein.

**Yellow or green frequent watery stools** may be due to epidemic gastro-enteritis (p. 563).

**Small dark** brownish yellow stools, often accompanied by mucus, are due to gross under-feeding.

**Pale, greasy,** offensive, bulky stools with large soft curds often accompanied by vomiting, may be due to cow's milk too rich in fat.

**Mucus.** A trace of mucus is normal and may be due to underfeeding and, if excessive, usually denotes enteritis.

**Melaena** (see p. 574).

# DAILY CARE

**The eyes.** Because of the risk of ophthalmia neonatorum the eyes must be inspected several times daily: inflammation and any discharge noted.

*A midwife must call in medical aid if there is any discharge from the eyes of an infant.* To avoid infecting the eyes it is advisable to wash and dry the face with cotton wool, using a small bowl of sterile water.

**The mouth** does not require cleansing, but should be examined daily for thrush after the fourth day: the small glistening spots sometimes seen on the posterior area of the palate are not due to thrush. The nose needs no attention, unless to wipe away any visible smudges with a piece of cotton wool.

### The umbilical cord

Daily inspection is essential: a thick cord may be very moist and this predisposes to infection. The umbilical area is cleansed with Hibitane, 0·5 per cent, in spirit 70 per cent, and dusted with antiseptic cord powder.

The cord usually comes off between the sixth and tenth day, delay commonly being due to a low-grade infection. Inflammation, discharge, or an offensive odour should be reported.

**The temperature** is taken every day and each infant in hospital should have his own low reading thermometer. The axilla or groin may be used instead of the rectum. To detect neonatal hypothermia taking the temperature is particularly important during the winter months.

*Bathing, handling and dressing the baby are described in the teaching of parenthood section. Care of the buttocks* (p. 492).

### Crying

Crying is the baby's only language, and the newborn baby cries vigorously, looking as though he is suffering extreme pain. But babies cry because of the slightest discomfort, and the midwife can merely surmise the cause, for different cries are not easily recognised in the first two weeks of life, except for the high-pitched cry of the baby who has sustained intra-cranial injury. A feeble whimper is abnormal.

## PSYCHOLOGY OF THE NEWBORN BABY

Midwives and mothers are apt to consider the baby's welfare entirely from the physical angle; but the health and happiness of each individual is dependent on psychological and mental as well as physical factors. Psychological defects account for more of life's failures than do physical defects. The newborn baby is an individual, having certain inherited tendencies which will to some extent influence his behaviour, but he is also influenced by the environment into which he is born. He has no knowledge of the world, and he will build up his impression of it and form habits of reacting to it, according to whether he finds it pleasant or otherwise. Certain primal needs must be met in order to survive. The baby's reaction to hunger and thirst is vociferous crying, and when these needs are not met the response is one of uncontrolled frustration; crying is his only language. The persistent thwarting of a natural urge which the infant is unable to satisfy may sow the seed of a disgruntled personality.

### NEWBORN BABIES NEED LOVE

Nature has provided the mother with a maternal instinct which she expresses by cuddling and caressing her infant. Much of a baby's experience is centred round feeding, and when nestled in the mother's arms he feels warm, comfortable and infinitely secure.

The average baby is more likely to develop into a well-balanced personality under the care of a mother who gives expression to her maternal instinct rather than one who subordinates her instinct to scientific principles (see Self-regulated Feeding, p. 502). Babies will not thrive without mothering (*mother love*); although there are mothers who give too much love, they can be guided and it is safer to give too much than too little.

Midwives should try to foster a happy relationship between mother and baby by helping with the difficulties of feeding and creating a serene atmosphere, for it seems reasonable to expect the baby who finds the world a pleasant place, to respond to it positively. Mothers should be given scope for the expression of their love. Some condemn any attempt to comfort a crying baby as 'spoiling', but much harm can accrue from leaving a baby alone crying for long periods.

## MINOR DISORDERS OF THE NEWBORN

### SORE BUTTOCKS

Reddening of the napkin area is caused by the napkins not being changed frequently enough; material too rough e.g. (Turkish towelling, dried too quickly); using strong soaps in washing napkins and not properly rinsing them. Localised excoriation and ulceration of the area between the buttocks is usually caused by frequent loose irritating stools. A candidial buttock rash may be seen in babies who have had antibiotics; the macerated appearance and raised edges of the lesions are typical. A swab should be taken from any resistant napkin rash and sent for culture. If positive the administration of nystatin orally combined with the application of nystatin cream is curative; gentian violet is cheaper but stains the linen.

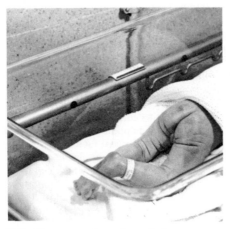

Fig. 28-7   Treatment of sore buttocks by exposure to air.

### *Prophylactic Care of the Buttocks*

Meconium should not be permitted to dry on the buttocks as it becomes firmly adherent to the skin. Even if the napkin feels dry, it should be inspected for meconium. The napkins should be changed before and after feeds if soiled or wet: the buttocks washed with soap and water, mopped dry and a little emollient substance massaged into the buttocks.

*Curative Treatment*

The cause, if known, should be remedied. To avoid urine and stool irritating the lesions, napkins should be changed as soon as possible if the baby is awake. The buttocks are gently washed with soap and water, the excoriated area may be wiped with olive oil if preferred. If the skin is red, Thovaline cream, Massé or benzalkonium (Drapolene) cream, Eucerin anhydrous or titanium (Metanium) ointment and Vasogen a silicone cream or centrimide (Cetavlex) cream are soothing. The old-fashioned zinc and castor oil is still popular.

**Exposure of the buttocks to the air.** The infant is laid prone or on his side upon a napkin, for an hour or two, three times daily. Exposure to sunshine for 10 minutes daily is also helpful. Some use an electric hair dryer (Coolair) with good results.

## Marking ink poisoning

Deaths have occurred by absorption of marking ink through the skin from napkins that have been issued without having been boiled to fix the aniline dye. Cyanosis is manifest.

## Skin rashes

Because of the risk of staphylococcal infections, babies should be examined daily and segregated, if necessary, to avoid epidemics. The commonest skin rash in the newborn is erythema toxicum or urticaria neonatorum: areas red and blotchy with small white centres. A wool rash consists of blotchy red patches which make the infant cross. The affected area should be dabbed with baby talcum powder. A heat or sweat rash is evident as pin-point spots, sometimes having a hard transparent centre also reddened areas between skin folds. It is more common in summer when babies are sometimes swaddled in layers of wool. After bathing, a bland antiseptic dusting powder is applied.

## Nail-fold injuries, scratches

Babies' fingers should be dried gently, as the nail-folds are easily torn. To prevent babies from scratching their faces the use of mittens is favoured by some nursery midwives. Mitts should be made of fine cambric. Wool, gauze, lint and nylon have loose threads that have been known to wind around the baby's finger, causing gangrene and loss of a finger.

## Dehydration fever

When given insufficient fluid and kept too warm the temperature rises to 38°C; the mouth and skin are dry, the baby is flushed, thirsty and cross. The urine, being concentrated, leaves a stain on the napkin, which feels gritty. Blood electrolytes should always be determined. Where no laboratory facilities are available, the prepacked electrolyte solution for oral administration may be available.

## Physiological jaundice

About 20 to 30 per cent of newborn babies develop jaundice during the third or fourth day, due to inefficient hepatic function; bilirubin in the blood rises and this is evident as jaundice. Extra fluid should be given because the unconjugated bilirubin which crosses the blood-brain barrier makes the infant drowsy and disinclined to suck. The use of phototherapy which lowers the serum bilirubin in the jaundiced newborn has reduced the need for replacement transfusion in cases where the serum bilirubin has been over 255 micromol/l in the preterm or compromised baby and 340 micromol/l in the well baby at term.

## Engorged breasts

The breasts of male, as well as female, babies may become swollen, hard and hot, mostly commonly on the third day. The condition is due to breast stimulation by the withdrawal of maternal oestrogens from the baby's blood and is rarely seen in preterm babies. The breasts should not be squeezed or compressed. The condition will subside spontaneously.

## Pseudo–menstruation

A blood-stained vaginal discharge is occasionally seen in girl babies, and is thought to be due to the withdrawal of oestrogens which have passed into the fetal blood stream from the placenta.

## Constipation

This is rare in breast-fed babies. The term should only be applied when the stools are infrequent and hard, causing the infant to strain in passing them. No concern need be felt if the bowels only move once in two or three days, so long as the motion is soft and easily passed. It is better to avoid using laxatives; extra water is usually effective; milk of magnesia, 4 ml, is suitable if this fails. Midwives should not resort to the drastic stimulus of inserting catheters or soap suppositories into the rectum.

## VOMITING

Vomiting is common in young babies for no apparent reason, and during the first 24 hours the vomitus may consist of mucus, sometimes streaked with blood, which the infant has swallowed during labour: giving isotonic saline (0·9 per cent) orally acts as a stomach lavage. Vomiting, occurring at intervals of a few days, in a thriving infant may be ignored. Possetting, which is the regurgitation of a few ml of milk after feeds should not be described as vomiting.

Faulty technique in feeding is one cause. The infant gulps the milk too quickly, is not given an opportunity to bring up wind, or is handled roughly after feeding. If bottle fed, the amount or the strength of the food may be excessive.

Vomiting may be mechanical, in that the cardiac sphincter of the stomach is too relaxed, a condition which usually improves in a week or two.

**Vomiting may be a serious sign** and is found not only in systemic infection, but in alimentary and urinary tract infection as well as in mechanical intestinal obstruction. Bile staining almost always indicates intestinal obstruction. If persistent, electrolyte imbalance must be corrected. Grass-green vomitus is usually serious.

### The following should be noted:

The day of onset? Are other signs of illness present? Check the temperature and respiratory rate. The colour of the vomitus (*particularly bile*). Is the vomiting forcible? Is the whole feed returned? Length of time after feed. Is the baby constipated? Is the appetite poor? Is diarrhoea present? Loss of weight.

---

## QUESTIONS FOR REVISION

### PHYSIOLOGY AND MANAGEMENT OF THE NEWBORN BABY

State a normal baby's temperature, respirations, heart rate, length, weight.

**Describe** the following: The psychology of the newborn baby; the establishment of respiration; the thriving baby; the baby's needs; examination of the newborn baby; daily observation of the newborn.

What would make you surmise that a baby crying in the night during the second week of life is: too hot; thirsty; too cold; in pain; hungry? Give other reasons for discomfort.

**C.M.B.(Scot.) 30-min. question.** What congenital malformations may be found during the sytematic examination of the newborn?

**Define the following terms:** surfactant; hypothermia; passive immunity; phimosis; nystagmus; vernix caseosa; overlaying; frenulum; lanugo; webbed fingers; meconium; tongue-tied.

The cord comes off about the ......... day; keeping the stump dry aids ......... ; the cord separates by a process of ......... ; plastic clamp is removed on the ......... day; inflammation of the umbilicus is known as ......... ; delay in separation may be due to .........

## C.M.B. Short Questions

**Eng.:** Examination of the head of the newborn. **Eng.:** The characteristics of a normal, healthy fulltime infant. **Scot.:** What is the duration of the neonatal period? **Eng.:** What daily observations of the baby does a midwife make? **Scot.:** Describe the routine examination of a newborn baby. **Eng.:** Meconium. **Scot.:** Colostrum. **N. Ireland:** Vernix caseosa. **Eng.:** The significance of the cry of a baby. **Eng.:** Care of the stump of the umbilical cord.

**Eng.:** Failure of the newborn child to gain weight. **Eng.:** Causes of failure to thrive in a six-day-old infant. **Scot.:** Describe the causes of vomiting. **Scot.:** Describe the management of vomiting in the newborn. **N. Ireland:** Napkin dermatitis. **Eng.:** Stools of the newborn. **N. Ireland:** Melaena in the newborn. **Eng.:** Sore buttocks. **Eng.:** How may sore buttocks be prevented and treated?

**Eng.:** Abnormal temperature of the neonate. **Eng.:** Normal stools during the first week of life. **Scot.:** Routine care of the umbilical cord. **Eng.:** Care of the stump of the umbilical cord. **Scot.:** Excoriated buttocks. **Eng.:** Weight loss in the mature infant during the first few days of life. **Scot.:** Identification of a baby. **Eng.:** The skin of the neonate. **Eng.:** Neonatal vaginal bleeding. **Eng.:** Neonatal screening tests. **Eng.:** Physiological jaundice. **Eng.:** The infant's stools in the first week of life.

### BABIES' STOOLS

*Place Correct Number of Cause Against Sign*

| | Cause | Signs | Number |
|---|---|---|---|
| 1 | gross underfeeding | pasty, greenish, tough curds, mucus (colic) | |
| 2 | meconium | black | |
| 3 | too much sugar | bulky, pale, greasy (offensive odour) | |
| 4 | breast fed | pale yellow, firm (slightly offensive odour) | |
| 5 | overfeeding | yellowish-green, watery | |
| 6 | too much fat | greenish-yellow, loose, small curds (sore buttocks) | |
| 7 | gastro-enteritis | greenish, frothy, loose (sour odour) | |
| 8 | melaena | greenish-black | |
| 9 | fed on cow's milk | yellow, semi-fluid | |
| 10 | too much protein | small-brownish-yellow, mucus | |

### MINOR DISORDERS OF THE NEWBORN

How would you (a) prevent (b) treat sore buttocks? Describe the various skin rashes which may occur and state how they may be prevented. How would you recognise and treat the following: engorged breasts; constipation in a bottle-fed baby? What are the common (*not serious*) causes of vomiting? What observations would you make and report to the doctor regarding this sign?

**N. Ire. Council 30-min. question.** Discuss the care of the skin in the neonatal period, mentioning the commoner abnormalities which may be met.

**C.M.B.(Scot.) 30-min. question.** State the causes of vomiting in the newborn. What observations should be made and how may these conditions be treated?

**C.M.B.(Eng.) 30-min. question.** What abnormal conditions may develop in an apparently normal baby in the first forty-eight hours following its birth? Briefly discuss their management.

**N. Ire. Council 30-min. question.** A week old infant fails to gain weight. What steps would you take to determine the cause and to correct this?

**C.M.B.(Eng.) 30-min. question.** Describe how you would examine a newborn baby. What congenital abnormalities might you find?

**C.M.B.(Scot.).** Describe in detail the examination of the baby's head and neck following the birth of the baby. What abnormalities may be detected in these areas within the first seven days of life?

## Miscellaneous Questions

**N. Ire. Council.** (*a*) Enumerate the minor disorders which may occur in the new born infant. (*b*) Describe the management of any three you mention in (*a*).

**N. Ire. Council.** How may mother/child relationships be established? (*a*) When the infant is normal. (*b*) When the infant is pre-term and requires special care.

**C.M.B.(Scot.).** A baby fails to gain weight during the first 14 days of life. Describe the possible causes and what investigations should be made.

**N. Ire. M. Council.** (*a*) What problems may parents with a first baby encounter when the mother is discharged from hospital? (*b*) How may they be helped to overcome these problems?

**C.M.B.(Scot.).** Give a detailed description of the routine examination of a newborn baby.

**C.M.B.(Scot.).** What observations of the baby should be made by a midwife during the first ten days of life? Indicate the purpose of each observation.

**C.M.B.(Scot.).** What are the causes of vomiting in the first week of life? Describe the investigation and management.

# 29
# Breast Feeding–Bottle Feeding

*Preparation for, benefits, and management of breast feeding. Self-regulating feeding programmes for breast and bottle-fed babies. Cracked nipples. Suppression of lactation. Comparison of human and cow's milk. Forms of modified cow's milk. Vitamin supplements*

It is universally agreed that breast milk cannot be excelled as a food for babies.

Breast milk is suited to the baby's needs and digestion; it is almost germ-free when produced; goes directly to the consumer without being handled; is always fresh: and has a lower renal solute content than cows' milk.

Breast milk contains protective antibodies, anti-viral properties and vitamins. Lactoferrin in breast milk has a bacteriostatic effect on *E. coli*.

Breast-fed babies get more mothering and when cuddled at the breast they feel loved and secure. They have fewer illnesses during the first year of life.

Breast feeding reduces the risks of hypocalcaemia and milk allergy.

Breast feeding is beneficial for mother-baby bonding.

Breast feeding causes less work: no modification of milk, no cleaning of pans and bottles, no heating of feeds. Breast milk is cheap to produce, but expensive to buy.

The danger of the mother giving the baby grossly concentrated dried milk feeds and causing hypernatraemia is eliminated. Cot deaths do not occur so frequently in breast-fed babies. Breast feeding delays the return of ovulation and may give a longer period of infertility.

### ANATOMY AND PHYSIOLOGY OF THE BREAST

The breasts are compound secreting glands, composed mainly of glandular tissue which is arranged in lobes, approximately 20 in number. Each lobe is divided into lobules that consist of alveoli with secreting cells which produce milk. The breasts are richly supplied with blood. Small lactiferous ducts, carrying milk from the alveoli of each lobe, unite to form about 20 larger ducts: these, before opening on the surface of the nipple, widen to form ampullae which act as temporary reservoirs for milk.

The nipple, composed of erectile tissue, is covered with epithelium and contains plain muscle fibres which have a sphincter-like action in controlling the flow of milk. Surrounding the nipple is an area of loose skin known as the areola.

Oestrogens and progesterone induce alveolar and duct growth as well as stimulating localised milk secretion. The production of milk is held in abeyance during pregnancy by the high level of oestrogens, which keeps the hormone prolactin in check. Oestrogens are produced by the placenta as well as the ovary, and when the placenta is expelled, the level falls. Prolactin concentration in maternal plasma reaches maximal levels during the puerperium.

By some neuromuscular mechanism involving oxytocin, the act of sucking a lactating breast stimulates the flow of milk. The 'let down' (draught reflex) whereby milk flows freely may be impaired if the mother is anxious or worried: the atmosphere should therefore be one of calm assurance. The expulsion of milk is controlled by the ejection reflex.

## PREPARATION FOR LACTATION

The maternal instinct is not always dominant until after the birth of the baby, and the woman during pregnancy may have no inclination towards breast feeding. If the mother-to-be states that she has no intention of attempting breast feeding, she may be persuaded to try, but she should not be forced to do so against her will.

During pregnancy the expectant mother should be told about the advantages of breast feeding and encouraged to breast feed. Husbands ought to be persuaded to give the necessary approval and emotional support. Fortunately breast feeding is on the increase and midwives should foster this tendency.

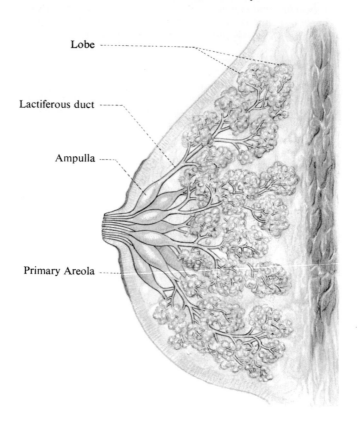

Lobe

Lactiferous duct

Ampulla

Primary Areola

Fig. 29-1   Diagram of the lactating breast.

To give the woman confidence the midwife should advise her regarding preparation for and the general management of breast feeding. The minor details of management are best taught when actually feeding the baby. The breasts should be supported with a firm brassière which does not depress the nipples.

**Inverted nipples.** The nipples may be below the level of the skin surface and great difficulty experienced in everting them. Sometimes they are 'flat' (on a level with the skin surface) and in both cases they may be improved by the use of plastic Woolwich shells.

### Prevention of nipple cracks

During pregnancy an effort should be made to toughen the nipples and get them accustomed to friction, in readiness for the vigorous sucking to which they will be subjected: the nipples being massaged by rolling them between the finger and thumb and drawing them out every day during the last two months, using a good face-soap and water.

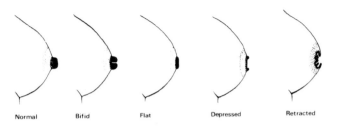

Fig. 29-2  Types of nipples.

# MANAGEMENT OF BREAST FEEDING

The midwife should be willing to give advice, help, encouragement and emotional support during the early postnatal days; this may require time, patience and a strong desire to achieve success.

Cleanliness is the first essential, the midwife explaining to each mother that her nails should be short and clean and that she must not touch her nipples with unwashed hands nor wipe them with her handkerchief. The woman's hands are washed before each feed, and the midwife must always wash her hands before touching the breasts. The modern tendency is to reduce nipple cleansing to a minimum and to wash the breasts once daily. Spirit and antiseptics should not be used: they dry and irritate the epithelium of the nipple and predispose to excoriation. The routine application of nipple cream is not advised unless the nipples are painful. Clean supporting brassières should be worn.

Before the infant is taken to the breast, any discharge from the eyes or nose ought to be removed; the napkin must be changed, and the gown should not be stained with stool. Attention to such details will reduce the number of breast infections.

## THE TECHNIQUE OF BREAST FEEDING

The woman should be given a few moments to admire her baby before putting him to the breast, unless he is crying. The breast feeding experience ought to be one of pleasure as well as business for mother and baby, the midwife giving help and advice, if necessary, but not dominating the situation. The mother ought to be serene and calm, and there should be no bustle, hurry or tension; she should give her undivided attention to her infant. Serenity facilitates the 'let down' reflex.

Mother and baby should be in a comfortable position. If the baby is held almost upright, head extended rather than flexed, the swallowing of air is minimal and eructation facilitated; his cheek in contact with the breast stimulates the 'search' reflex. The mother, sitting up and leaning slightly forwards, supports the breast in the palm of her hand, allowing the nipple to pass between her first two fingers. In this way she directs the nipple into the baby's mouth and keeps the breast away from the baby's nose.

### Fixing and sucking

The baby draws the nipple back to the posterior region of the tongue; the loose tissue around the nipple (the areola) is in the baby's mouth, therefore the ampullae are also in the mouth. The lips are wide apart, not pursed. The gums compress the ampullae and the milk flows along the tongue. The baby's neck should not be hampered by blankets, in order that free movement of the lower jaw is possible. The head should be at such a level that too much pull is not exerted on the nipple. There is no necessity to bind the baby's arms firmly except when he is struggling and refusing to fix, but once having got hold of the nipple the infant should be given freedom to squirm and kick.

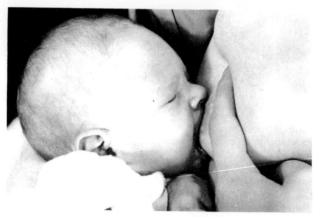

Fig. 29-3   Note that the areola is in the baby's mouth and that his lips are wide apart.

**FIXING AND SUCKING**

The mother may, because of perineal sutures, be unable to sit up to handle her baby properly. The baby can feed equally well when the mother is lying on her side (see Fig. 29-5). She might be highly strung and nervous, especially if the baby is proving difficult. Calmness and reassurance are necessary as well as patience.

The nipples may be flat. If so, the areola should be gently stroked and stretched away from the nipple which is then pulled out with the fingers or a breast pump used to draw it out. To encourage the baby to persevere, some colostrum should be expressed into his mouth. Nipple shields, whether made of rubber, or glass and rubber, are of little value; the baby can rarely suck sufficient milk through them. (Flattened nipples, due to acute engorgement, are discussed on page 505.)

### Prevention of cracked nipples during the puerperium

Ensure that the baby has 'fixed' properly, to avoid bruising the nipple with his gums. The nostrils must be clear, or the baby will let go of the nipple in order to breathe, and repeated catching hold of the nipple will bruise it.

Do not pull the baby off the breast when he has finished sucking; press the cheeks and depress the lower jaw to avoid trauma to the nipple or lift the outer border of the upper lip to break the suction; holding the nostrils is unkind. The nipples should be dried thoroughly after each feed and if tender a soothing ointment such as Massé cream is applied, especially in the case of the blonde or red-haired primipara.

The baby should not sleep at the breast in any case, but, if the nipple is in his mouth breathing on it will cause it to become excoriated in the same way that improperly dried hands become chapped.

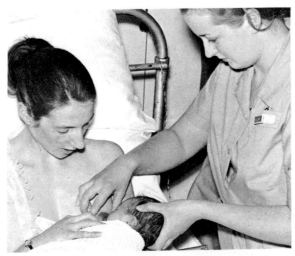

Fig. 29-4   Midwife helping mother to fix baby.
*Maternity Section, Ayrshire Central Hospital, Irvine.*

### SELF REGULATION BREAST FEEDING

## On Demand

In feeding newborn infants the modern trend is to adopt a more flexible routine with fewer restrictions on the number of feeds and in the length of sucking time.

**Babies are now given some preference** as to how often they will be fed and how much milk they will take. This concept appears to be more in line with what nature intended and is commonly practised in unsophisticated lands.

### THE LENGTH OF SUCKING TIME

**Sucking time is no longer limited.** The act of sucking stimulates the flow of milk, so ample sucking is essential during the first days of life when lactation is being initiated and established.

Observation of newborn animals indicates that they are permitted to suck, during the first few days, as often and for as long as they want.

### FEEDING ON DEMAND

Under the Self Regulation regime the programme of feeding is no longer under complete maternal jurisdiction: the baby participates regarding the times of feeding and the amount of milk he wants.

**The rooming-in plan** (p. 444) is recommended in order that mother and baby can be in close proximity to each other. This facilitates bonding and enables the baby's urge to suck and his hunger to be gratified without delay. Having to scream for long periods before being fed teaches him nothing and only arouses frustration and annoyance. The baby should not be fed every time he cries as crying may be due to some slight discomfort. He may be thirsty and need water 15 to 20 ml.

### THE FEEDING PATTERN

**Babies have individual characteristics** regarding their feeding patterns. Some object to being regimented by the clock and want to be fed more frequently than every three or four hours: this tendency being most apparent during the first weeks of life. Under the relaxed regime a more loving relationship between mother and baby is created and a successful feeding programme established.

**The first feed is given as soon as possible** and within a few hours of birth. During the period of colostrum secretion the infant may suck the breast for only four or five minutes. He may, during the early days, take seven or eight short feeds: the sucking time being extended daily. When he takes enough milk to satisfy him for three or four hours he adopts a regular feeding pattern.

**When lactation is established** most babies take what they want in approximately 15 minutes, i.e. 8 to 10 minutes at the first breast and 4 to 5 minutes at the second breast; the next feed being started with the second breast. Babies are no longer curtailed or cajoled to conform to a prescribed feeding schedule.

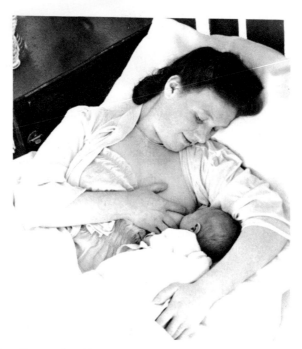

Fig. 29-5  A mother comfortably feeding her baby while lying on her side. (Note how the breast is being held away from the baby's nose.)

*Simpson Memorial Maternity Pavilion, Edinburgh.*

### THE INTERVAL BETWEEN FEEDS

**This should not be permitted to exceed 5 hours.** Some small or jaundiced infants may sleep for long periods if allowed to do so. Babies at home who are bathed during the forenoon may sleep afterwards for a prolonged period. Mothers should be advised that when the infant does not wake to take his feeds, during the day disturbed nights will ensue.

### NIGHT FEEDS

The mother needs counsel regarding how to deal with her baby at night and particularly when he is crying. A night feed is now advocated to avoid an interval between feeds of over 5 hours which is the limit recommended.

It has been found that the night feed also eliminates excessive filling and hardening of the breasts as well as ensuring sound sleep for the baby.

Babies have no cognisance of day and night and it may be some weeks before they settle into a rhythmic 3 or 4 hourly feeding pattern. The infant who is fed adequately during the day is more likely to sleep well at night and the night feed is an additional assurance. Eventually when lactation is properly established he will sleep throughout the night.

Babies cry for the slightest reasons. If he has recently been given a feed and is otherwise comfortable merely turning him over on to his other side, and giving him a friendly pat, will usually pacify him.

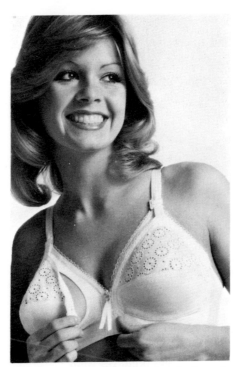

Fig. 29-6   Balance nursing bra of cool crisp cotton.

### AMOUNT OF FOOD REQUIRED

The amount of milk given to the baby is gradually increased according to the amount he takes. It has been calculated that average requirements would be about 100 ml/kg/24 hours on the third day and 150 ml/kg/24 hours on the 10th day, but these are only guidelines: the baby takes as much as he wants. In hot weather and if the stools are loose the infant will require more fluid.

### *Diversity of Opinion*

There is much diversity of opinion concerning feeding of the newborn at the present time. More liberal attitudes to first week breast feeding are being promulgated and this involves rooming-in. Bottle fed babies are given similar gratification. Enforced three and four hourly feeding times during the first weeks of life are now discouraged. Such changes will necessitate giving up some cherished ideas and procedures, but if by research traditional methods have been outmoded the proposed system could be tested and adopted if successful, beneficial to babies and acceptable to mothers.

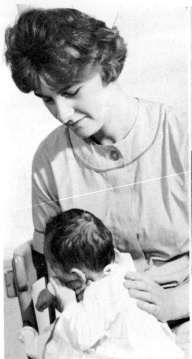

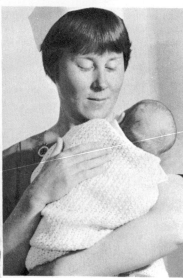

Fig. 29-8

Fig. 29-7

Breaking the wind.

*Aberdeen Maternity Hospital.*

#### BREAKING THE WIND

All babies swallow air while sucking, and the baby who is not fixed properly or who sucks an empty breast swallows more than usual. To bring up wind the baby is held upright against the left chest, and when the back is gently patted the slight jogging movement releases the air in the stomach; as the air escapes the baby belches. The advantage of the upright position is that no milk is expelled. Some sit the baby on the mother's lap making him bend forwards and to the left to bring the air bubble under the cardiac orifice of the stomach. If the infant is laid in his cot without first bringing up wind, he will bring it up later and milk as well, or it will pass down and give rise to 'colicky pain'.

Wind should be broken half-way through the feed, because if the stomach is distended with air the infant will not take a sufficient amount of milk. The procedure is repeated at the end of the feed.

**Possetting** is the regurgitating of a mouthful of milk by the baby and should not be described as vomiting. It may occur when wind is broken, with hiccoughs, or because of clumsy or rough handling after a feed. Possetting is also a safety valve when the infant has taken too much.

## DIFFICULTIES IN BREAST FEEDING

### (*Maternal*)

Many of the difficulties are preventable and surmountable.

**Unwillingness.** A mother who is unwilling to breast feed her baby rarely succeeds, but if handled with tact and understanding she may be persuaded to do so.

**Over-anxiety.** In cases where breast feeding has previously failed, or in the older primipara, the woman's anxiety to succeed may inhibit successful lactation. The midwife can impart knowledge and try to instil a placid and hopeful outlook.

**General health.** The woman may be in poor health. (See Contra-indications to Breast Feeding, p. 506).

**The breasts.** The difficulty may be functional when the breasts are incapable of secreting an adequate amount of milk. The supply is sometimes scanty from the beginning, or it fails after two or three weeks. This may be due to mismanagement.

## ENGORGED BREASTS

This is a conditon varying in degree from slight to severe, commonly occurring between the third and fifth day of the puerperium. The breasts are full, heavy and hard, due to venous and lymphatic engorgement and oedema and not to an abundant supply of milk. The muscular mechanism by which milk is expelled is inhibited and when breast tension rises excessively the cells cease to produce milk.

### *Treatment*

SLIGHT ENGORGEMENT

Bathe the breasts in hot water before feeds and gently stroke them with soapy hands towards the nipple.

Put baby to the breasts for a few minutes and then express the remaining milk. Apply ointment (Massé cream) to the nipples and use a firm supporting brassière.

SEVERE ENGORGEMENT

Do not put the baby to the breast or use manual expression if the breasts are so tense, hard and swollen that the nipple is flattened and the baby cannot grasp the areola. Stilboestrol is not prescribed by as many obstetricians as formerly. It may be necessary to give an analgesic such as Panasorb or pentazocine (Fortral) or Distalgesic 2 tablets to relieve pain. The baby is put to the breast as soon as the nipple can be grasped, and an effort made to keep the milk flowing and the breasts soft.

## CRACKED NIPPLES

The mother should be told to report if her nipples are tender, and, if so, they should be examined under a magnifying glass for fissures. Early recognition and prompt treatment will result in more rapid healing. The baby should be taken off the breast for 24 hours if the nipples are cracked. In the interval the milk is expressed manually. Exposure to an electric lamp 30 cm distant or to the air for 20 minutes every six hours will promote healing.

*Various Remedies are Advocated and Many are Successful*

Ointments are soothing, but must be applied sparingly or the nipple will become soggy, e.g. Massé cream, lanoline.

The midwife should be aware that cracked nipples often bleed during sucking and cause melaena; the infant may vomit the blood.

#### DIFFICULTIES DUE TO THE BABY

Serious defects, such as cleft lip or cleft palate, prevent the infant from sucking, but breast milk should be expressed and fed by bottle or spoon. A sore tongue, due to thrush, makes the child disinclined to feed. Snuffles, usually due to a nasal infection, interferes with breathing during sucking. Mentally subnormal babies do not use their tongues effectively.

Asphyxia and intracranial injury may necessitate the administration of oxygen and the infant may be too ill to be moved from the cot. Jaundice causes lethargy and disinclination to suck.

#### CONTRA-INDICATIONS TO BREAST FEEDING

**Psychiatric disorders.** Because of the danger of the mother doing harm to her child and because her own nutritional wellbeing is particularly important the infant may be weaned. Severe epilepsy may also result in injury to the child.

**Tuberculosis.** In cases of active tuberculosis the baby should be isolated from the mother because of the risk of infection by handling. In developing countries mother and baby are both given anti-tuberculosis agents: the baby being fed at the breast (see p. 210).

If a woman who is nursing her baby becomes pregnant the baby should be weaned.

## THE SUPPRESSION OF LACTATION

This is more easily accomplished when treatment is started on the first day of the puerperium, as when stillbirth occurs. It is much more difficult to suppress lactation when the baby has been sucking the breast for five or six days.

Many authorities do not approve of giving oestrogens to inhibit lactation. Women of high parity, over 35 years of age and particularly when having had a major operative delivery are predisposed to thrombo-embolism: oestrogens may intensify this risk. Bromocriptine (Parlodel) is effective and non-oestrogenic. It takes effect within 48 hours.

The baby is taken completely off the breast and under no circumstances must he be allowed to suck the breast again. Neither manual expression nor extraction of milk by breast pump should be performed even although the breasts are hard, heavy and painful. (*The temptation to do so is great but it must be resisted.*) The removal of milk by either sucking, expression or extraction will stimulate the flow of milk.

To prevent stasis in the dependent areas of the breasts they are elevated by pads of cotton wool and supported by a firm brassière or binder. This must be applied while the woman lies flat on her back holding her breasts inwards and upwards.

Applying a firm binder to breasts, without first elevating them, produces stasis in the lower area and this may predispose to mastitis due to multiplication of the organisms that are inevitably present in the breasts.

Analgesics are given for pain, e.g. pentazocine (Fortral) or Distalgesic or Panasorb tablets (2).

### OVER-FEEDING

This is occasionally seen towards the end of the first week. Vomiting may occur and the stools are usually loose and greenish, with undigested curds, the buttocks become excoriated. The baby behaves as though hungry, crying and sucking his fist, possibly he is thirsty; he may lose weight because of indigestion and frequent loose stools.

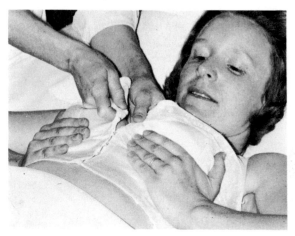

Fig. 29-9    Applying brassière when suppressing lactation. Breasts elevated; brassière fastened from below upwards.

*Maternity Section, Ayrshire Central Hospital, Irvine.*

### UNDER-FEEDING

**A breast-fed baby may be under-fed if:**
The supply of milk is inadequate. He vomits the milk.
He does not take the required amount.

#### Signs of under-feeding

The baby usually, but not always, cries a great deal and fails to gain weight.
The stools may be brownish green and small, occasionally they contain mucus: the urine may be insufficient in quantity.

#### Investigation

Is the tongue clean and the baby eager for food? Does he vomit? Are the stools normal? The midwife should supervise a feed, watching if the baby is sucking and swallowing properly. Manual expression of both breasts is carried out to see if the baby has emptied the breasts.

**Test-feeding** will reveal whether the baby is taking too much or too little food; the infant being weighed after sucking for, 5, 10 and 15 minutes. If he gets sufficient milk in five minutes, subsequent feeds will be limited to that time. The interval between feeds should be lengthened.

**Test-feeds** should be carried out over a period of at least 24 hours. Accurate scales are necessary. The infant is weighed with his clothes on before being fed at the breast and again in the same clothes at the conclusion of the feed, without changing the napkin if it is soiled. The difference between the two weights indicates the amount of milk obtained from the breast.

### Treatment of under-feeding

The mother should be reassured and complementary feeds given temporarily.

If the milk supply is inadequate, an endeavour is made to stimulate the breasts to produce more milk. See that the woman is having three substantial meals daily with sufficient proteins and vitamin B with an adequate but not excessive fluid intake.

### Manual expression of milk

The midwife washes her hands and stands behind the woman, who is sitting up; lifts up the breast by placing the fingers of the right hand under it and the thumb above, grasping the outer border of the primary areola. With a deep, inward compressing movement she squeezes the reservoirs about thirty times per minute, moving the areola but not the fingers and avoiding touching the nipple. The milk flows from a lactating breast in a steady stream.

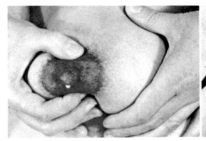 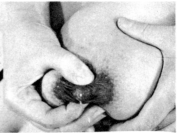

Fig. 29-10   Fingers directed inwards and          Fig. 29-11   Fingers brought slightly forwards
                     backwards.                                    without moving them on the skin.

Figs. 29-10 and 29-11   Manual expression of milk.

### Complementary feeding

This method consists in giving the baby additional milk immediately after a deficient breast feed to complete it. The milk should not be too sweet, or the baby may prefer it to breast milk. He should be offered 60 ml (*or more*) of prepacked formula feed or modified dried milk, and permitted to take as much as he wants.

### Supplementary feeding

This method consists in giving milk in place of a breast feed, and should not be used in cases of under-feeding as it tends to inhibit the production of breast milk. Occasionally it may be used if breast feeding is well established and the mother wishes to be absent at feeding time.

## BOTTLE FEEDING

There is no perfect substitute for breast milk. Cow's milk can be modified so that the percentage of its constituents approximates to those of human milk, and although it does not completely meet the nutritional requirements of the infant it provides a satisfactory food. Dried modified cows milk is used during the first year of life, because it is fortified with vitamins and iron. Modification should produce low protein, low solute feeds.

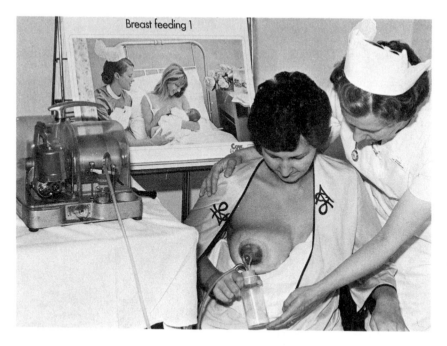

Breast feeding 1

Fig. 29-12   Electric breast pump.
*Queen Mother's Maternity Hospital, Glasgow.*

### Basic Principles

The milk must be clean and free from organisms.

The milk should be modified to meet the infant's requirements for growth, energy and heat. It ought to be capable of digestion by the infant.

The amount given should be in a concentration to satisfy the infant's needs without giving an excessive amount of water.

**COMPARISON OF HUMAN AND COW'S MILK**

*grams per 100 ml*

| Grams | Sugar | Fat | Protein | Minerals | Water | Kilocalories |
|-------|-------|-----|---------|----------|-------|--------------|
| Human milk | 7 | 4 | 1·2 | 0·4 | 89·7 | 67 |
| Cow's milk | 4·7 | 3·8 | 3·3 | 0·75 | 88 | 67 |

**Sugar.** The amount of sugar in cow's milk is less than in human milk, therefore sugar must be added.

**Fat.** The fat globule in cow's milk is coarse and more difficult to digest than human milk.

**Protein.** There is more than twice as much protein in cow's as in human milk, and the ratio of caseinogen to lactalbumin is six times greater. The tough caseinogen curd of cow's milk is made more digestible for babies by drying or boiling.

**Sodium.** There is three times as much sodium in cow's milk as in human milk. When mothers pack or heap the scoop of powdered milk the baby may get 4 times the required amount of sodium. The baby cries with thirst, the mother thinks he is hungry and gives more milk. Excess sodium in the blood (hypernatraemia) can damage the brain cells. Midwives must warn mothers about this.

**Caloric requirements** are 110 calories per kg of body weight per day, but calories alone are not a physiological method of calculating the amount of infant food needed. 100 ml of human or cow's milk has a calorie content of 67. Sugar provides 4 calories per gram.

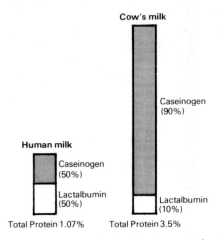

Fig. 29-13   Diagrammatic representation of ratio of caseinogen to lactalbumin in human and cow's milk.

## FORMS OF COW'S MILK

Fresh cow's milk is not now recommended as a food for infants under one year old. Modification and sterilisation have to be carried out in the home and these may be neither adequate nor accurate. The casein curd is tough, the fat globule large and coarse, so digestive upsets are more common. The essential vitamins and iron are deficient.

### DRIED MILK

Dried or powdered milk is produced from fresh cow's milk which is subjected to heat; the fluid being removed by evaporation. The process renders the casein curd more digestible. The milk powder is free from bacteria; it should be protected from flies by placing the opened carton in a glass jar or tin with a lid.

## LOW SOLUTE MILK

**Modified dried milks** are those in which the protein, sodium and phosphate content have been reduced to levels approaching those of human milk. The butterfat is replaced by vegetable fats that are more digestible. Dried milk is fortified to an International Standard with vitamins A, C, D, E and B complex. Iron is added and some contain additional zinc and copper.

**The following modified dried milks having a low solute content are available**

Cow and Gate Premium baby food, SMA Gold Cap, Osterfeed. These resemble human milk closely; the fat is a mixture of vegetable oil and butterfat.

Cow and Gate V Formula and SMA Regular have had all the butterfat removed and replaced by vegetable oil.

Cow and Gate Babymilk plus, Ostermilk Complete Formula and Ostermilk Improved Number 2 have had less modification.

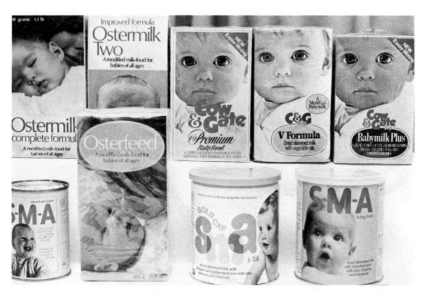

Fig. 29-14   A selection of dried milks modified to approximate standards of human milk.

### To reconstitute Dried Milk

The scoop provided in the carton must be used to measure the powder. It is essential that the less intelligent mothers are shown how, and understand the importance of accurately measuring the dried milk and the water. (For demonstration see p. 786). One level measure of power is added to each 30 ml water.

## SELF REGULATING REGIME

### On Demand Bottle Feeding

Bottle fed babies are now given the same Self Regulating Regime as is used for breast fed babies (p. 501). This allows them to participate regarding how frequently they will be fed and how much milk they will receive.

### The first feed

As soon as possible and within four hours of birth the baby is offered 30 ml of modified prepacked food or reconstituted modified dried milk. The amounts taken is recorded on the baby's chart.

**Rooming-in is practised** and the mother calls the midwife when the baby appears to want food. She is told that the interval between feeds should not be longer than $4\frac{1}{2}$ to 5 hours and that babies who receive adequate food during the day are more likely to have peaceful nights.

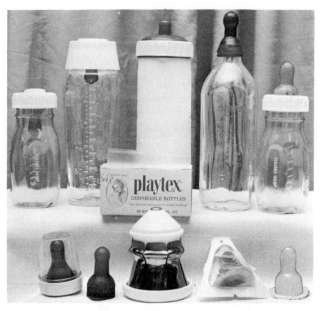

Fig. 29-15   Bottles and teats in current use.

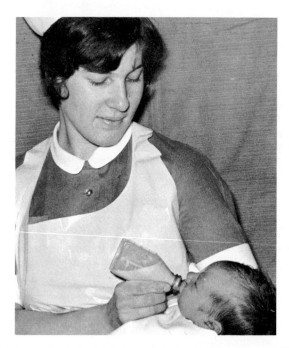

Fig. 29-16   Student midwife feeding baby as instructed. Giving her undivided attention to baby. Holding bottle 'as a pencil'. Bottle neck full of milk. Baby's head well supported. Bib in position. Student wearing disposable apron.

*Simpson Memorial Maternity Pavilion, Edinburgh.*

## MODIFIED PREPACKED FEEDS

These feeds, in disposable bottles have been modified to conform to the constituents of human milk. The protein and mineral content has been adjusted to give a low renal solute load, e.g.

**Cow and Gate** Premium, sterilised, modified, prepacked feed 120 ml.

**SMA Gold Cap** Ready to feed system provides 100 ml sterile modified milk feeds are now given at living room temperature in many hospitals.

**Modified Dried Milk** having a formula similar to prepacked feeds is preferred in some hospitals and is recommended on discharge home.

## VITAMIN SUPPLEMENTS

*Note. The Government issue of Children's Vitamin Drops are stated to contain approximately 35 drops per ml.*

Vitamin A, 5,000 i.u.; vitamin C, 150 mg; vitamin D, 2,000 i.u. per 35 drops.

Babies who are breast fed should be given 3 drops of children's vitamin drops daily from 4 weeks; increasing to 7 drops at 4 months.

Mothers should be warned that a high intake of vitamin D will cause excess absorption of calcium (hypercalcaemia) with deposition of calcium in the kidneys and walls of blood vessels.

Additional vitamins are not necessary for babies on dried milk that has been modified to resemble human milk; the vitamins having been added to the modified milk. Mothers should be told not to boil orange juice.

---

# QUESTIONS FOR REVISION

### BREAST FEEDING

How would you persuade a woman to breast feed her baby? What are the benefits to the baby? How do you 'fix' a baby at the breast? How often does the baby go to the breast during the first 3 days?

**Describe or discuss** prevention and treatment of cracked nipples; treatment of engorged breasts; the modern attitude to breast feeding; advantages of breast feeding.

**Define the following terms:** colostrum; lactiferous ducts; search reflex: Hypernatraemia.

**How would you differentiate between:** over-feeding and under-feeding; vomiting and possetting; weighing and test-weighing?

**C.M.B.(Eng.) 30-min. question.** Describe your routine management of breast feeding in the first ten days of life. What do you understand by the term 'engorgement of the breasts'?

**N. Ire. Council 30-min. question.** What would you think that a breast fed baby was underfed? How would you deal with this problem?

**C.M.B.(Eng.) 30-min. question.** What are the advantages of breast feeding? Discuss the attitudes of modern mothers to breast feeding.

**Scot.** What advice would you give regarding breast feeding: (*a*) in pregnancy, (*b*) in the postnatal period?

**N. Ire. M. Council.** (*a*) Describe the anatomy of the breast, including the changes which occur during pregnancy. (*b*) What anatomical defects of the breast may make natural feeding difficult, and how would you deal with these difficulties?

**N. Ire. M. Council.** (*a*) Discuss the factors which may influence a woman to breast feed her baby. (*b*) What psychological problems may arise during breast feeding?

**N. Ire. M. Council.** Describe the physiology of lactation. What problems may arise in the establishment of successful breast feeding? How would you help a mother to overcome these problems?

## *C.M.B. Short Questions*

**Eng.:** Engorgement of the breasts. **Eng.:** Factors necessary for successful breast feeding. **Eng.:** Demand feeding. **N. Ire.:** Suppression of lactation. **Eng.:** Prevention of sore nipples. **N. Ire.:** Breast engorgement. **Eng.:** Establishment of breast feeding. **Eng.:** Anatomy of the breast. **Eng.:** How is lactation initiated? **Eng.:** What can be done to encourage successful lactation?

**Eng.:** The onset of lactation. **Eng.:** Painful breasts in the puerperium.

**Scot.:** Describe the risks associated with bottle feeding of the baby.

**Scot.:** Describe in detail the advice given to a mother regarding bottle feeding.

**Scot.:** Complementary and supplementary feeds.

## BOTTLE FEEDING

**Discuss the advantages and disadvantages of:** Three-hourly, four-hourly, self demand feeding. Fresh cow's milk; dried milk.

How could a mother give her baby too much sodium? What is the danger of this?

**Differentiate between:** complementary and supplementary feeding; caseinogen in cow's and human milk; vitamins A, C and D.

What advice would you give to a mother: (*a*) whose baby cried for long periods during the night? (*b*) whose baby was bottle fed, appeared to be healthy but was not gaining weight? How would you apply a supporting breast brassière while inhibiting lactation?

### *C.M.B. Short Questions*

**Eng.:** How to instruct mothers to make up a feed. **Eng.:** Care of baby's feeding equipment in the home. **Eng.:** What are the dangers associated with artificial feeding of the newborn? **Eng.:** Artificial feeding requirements of a normal mature infant in the first week of life. **N. Ire.:** What guidance would you give to a young primipara on infant feeding? **Eng.:** Enumerate the points you would emphasise in your instructions to mothers who elect to feed their babies artifically.

**C.M.B. Scot.:** Describe (*a*) the anatomy of the breast, (*b*) the hormonal stimuli which prepare the breasts for lactation and promote milk production.

**C.M.B. Scot.:** What are the advantages of breast feeding and how could this be successfully achieved?

**C.M.B. (Eng.).** Give the anatomy of the mammary glands and discuss the advantages of breast feeding.

# 30
# Low Birth Weight Babies

*Definition of low birth weight, preterm and light for date. The preterm baby—signs, treatment, maintenance of temperature. Feeding: oro-gastric, naso-gastric, jejunal, intravenous. Expert nursing. Observation. Oxygen therapy. Disorders. Light for date babies: clinical features, complications*

---

The management of preterm babies, being highly specialised is directed by a paediatrician. Nevertheless a grave responsibility rests on the midwife, for the survival of these infants, whose hold on life is slender, depends greatly on expert nursing: they need special care in regard to environment and feeding. This can be given with greater efficiency in a neonatal intensive care unit where incubators and mechanical monitoring devices are available and paediatricians and skilled midwives are on constant duty. The first 48 hours are the most dangerous.

In a national survey 8 per cent of babies were found to weigh 2500 g or less.

### DEFINITION

**The low birth weight baby** weighs 2500 g or less at birth regardless of the estimated period of gestation. But not all babies of low birth weight are preterm: some are light for date. Differentiating between the two is important because the treatment and the complications are not similar.

**The preterm baby** is one born before 37 completed weeks of gestation calculated from the onset of the last menstrual period. This baby is not well equipped to adapt to life outside the uterus. Two-thirds of low birth weight babies are preterm.

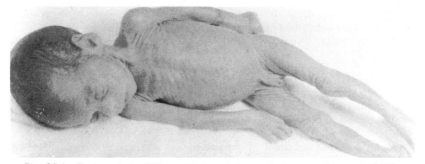

Fig. 30-1   Preterm baby 700 g at birth, weight on discharge at 16 weeks 2400 g.
*Simpson Memorial Maternity Pavilion, Edinburgh.*

**The light for date baby** is one whose birth weight is below the 10th centile for its estimated gestational age. This condition reflects intra-uterine malnutrition and growth retardation of the fetus. One-third of low birth weight babies are light for date and it is possible for the baby to be both preterm and light for date.

Certain neurological tests which elicit reflex behaviour are utilised to differentiate between preterm and light for date babies. Many responses are absent in the preterm infant, e.g. **the traction reflex:** when the baby is raised, by traction on the arms, the preterm baby does not attempt to raise his head, the light for date baby does. The Moro reflex may be incomplete or absent in the preterm baby. See Fig. 28-5.

### CONDITIONS ASSOCIATED WITH PRETERM BABIES

Severe cardiac diseases; pre-eclampsia; antepartum haemorrhage; twins; fetal malformations; low social class.

In 50 per cent of cases no cause is apparent. (Socio-economic factors are important, e.g. insufficient rest during the last 8 weeks of pregnancy).

### SIGNS OF PRETERM BABY

**Length,** 45 cm or less.
**Weight,** 2500 g or less.
**Sutures** and fontanelles wide.
**Pinnae** of ears soft and flat.
**Nails** are soft but not always short.

**Skin,** red, within a few hours it is tight and shiny. Skull bones soft.
**Lanugo** plentiful, absent in very small babies. Vernix scanty. Eyes closed.
**Plantar creases** are not visible under 34 weeks.

### AVERAGE WEIGHTS AND LENGTHS

| Weeks | Grams | Centimetres |
|-------|-------|-------------|
| 28 | 1100 | 40 |
| 32 | 1900 | 44 |
| 36 | 2800 | 48 |

### PRINCIPLES OF TREATMENT

**Prevention. Good management during labour. Efficient care at birth. Maintenance of body temperature. Observation. Suitable feeding. Expert nursing. Oxygen therapy. Avoidance of infection.**

### PREVENTION

Because of the serious loss of life in preterm babies, an effort is being made to recognise and treat early the medical and obstetrical conditions which induce preterm labour. Expectant mothers should be advised regarding good nutrition and to cease employment outside the home at 28 weeks.

## Arrest of Threatened Preterm Labour

Labour can be suppressed by giving the uterine relaxant ritodrine (Yutopar) i.v.

The infusion is continued until 24 hours after the arrest of threatened labour. A maintenance dose of 10 mg (one tablet) may then be given orally every 4 to 6 hours for 14 or more days.

Yutopar is contra-indicated in pre-eclampsia, antepartum haemorrhage and diabetes.

Cases of very premature labour in which the cervix is dilating have been arrested for 48 hours to allow betamethasone to be administered. This drug stimulates the production of surfactant in the immature fetal lungs.

### GOOD MANAGEMENT DURING PRETERM LABOUR

To avoid depression of the fetal respiratory centre, sedatives of the opium group should not be used. Cyanosis must be avoided. Continuous fetal heart rate monitoring is carried out.

An episiotomy is made under local analgesia when the fetus is expected to weigh under 2500 g, to shorten the perineal phase and so prevent the intracranial congestion or injury which may occur because of the soft skull bones and wide sutures.

### Transfer to hospital

If the woman in preterm labour cannot be transferred to hospital, the baby should be admitted to a special or intensive neonatal care unit if he weighs less than 2500 g. It is recommended that a resuscitation team (neonatal 'Flying Squad'), consisting of a paediatrician and nursery midwife, be available to treat and transport to hospital for further supervision low birth weight babies and other neonatal emergencies.

Wrapping the infant in a Silver Swaddler (aluminium coated plastic) (the baby first being wrapped in a warmed cotton blanket) prevents loss of heat if the incubator must be opened en route to suck out mucus from the pharynx. A portable incubator should have the temperature constantly maintained at 32°C in readiness to transport a baby from labour ward to the special care nursery or from home to the hospital neonatal intensive care unit.

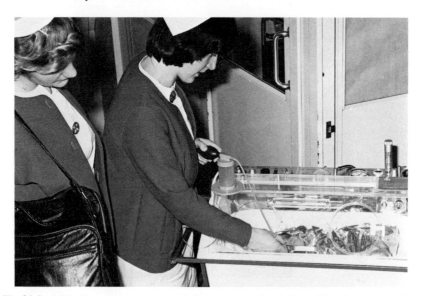

Fig. 30-2    Midwife sucking out mucus during transportation in heated incubator to hospital. Preterm baby wrapped in Silver Swaddler.

*Royal Maternity Hospital, Rottenrow, Glasgow.*

## EFFICIENT CARE OF THE BABY AT BIRTH

### Warmth

The delivery room should be at a temperature of 24°C. Two warm towels should be in readiness, one into which the baby is received and the other with which to dry him: the head being large must not be exposed while wet. The infant should be wrapped and warm while any necessary treatment is being carried out. A paediatrician is present when the baby is expected to weigh less than 2500 g or if not immediately available, a midwife from the neonatal intensive care unit.

### Establishment of respiration

Preparations should be made to assist in the establishment of respiration, for the respiratory centre in the medulla is immature. The lungs tend to be atelectatic and are not well developed; the diaphragm and chest muscles are weak, therefore the baby is often asphyxiated. Mucus catheters are used to clear the air passages. The cord is clamped and cut. The gastric contents are aspirated if polyhydramnios was present. Babies of 28 weeks gestation who do not breathe within 30 seconds should be intubated.

The infant is transferred to the special nursery in the portable incubator then placed in an incubator, given oxygen, in the lowest concentration needed to relieve any cyanosis.

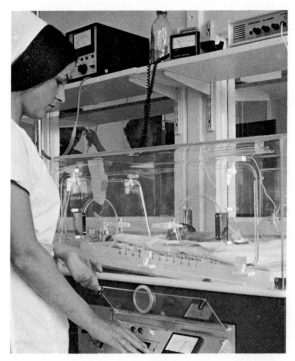

Fig. 30-3   Model 79 servo incubator provides continuous monitoring of the temperature of preterm or sick babies: automatically alters the environmental temperature to compensate for changes in the temperature of the infant: audible and visual alarms for overheating, power supply or air circulation failure.

*Courtesy of Vickers Ltd., Basingstoke, Hampshire.*

Bathing is contra-indicated.

An aqueous solution of vitamin $K_1$, preferably Konakion, 1 mg, may be injected intramuscularly to minimise the risk of haemorrhage.

### The maintenance of body temperature

Preterm babies are unable to maintain body temperature because of their immature heat regulating centre in the medulla. Heat production is poor because of the limited food intake and low metabolic rate; heat loss is excessive because of the large surface area, lack of subcutaneous fat and sluggish muscular activity.

The smaller the baby the greater is the risk of hypothermia. The body temperature should not be permitted to fall below 36·5°C. A rectal temperature of 37·2° is desirable.

The skin temperature is important during critical periods and an electronic thermistor probe attached to the baby's skin records this: 36·6°C being aimed at. The difference between skin and central temperature indicates the degree of metabolic activity.

### INCUBATOR TEMPERATURE

This depends on the size and postnatal age of the infant. Charts are available giving a range of neutral thermal environment. The smaller babies are usually naked so the temperature should be 32° to 34°C, with relative humidity maintained at 60 per cent. Perspex heat shields may be necessary to conserve body heat.

The incubator room temperature should be maintained at 24°C to 30°C.

When incubators are not available the room temperature should be 26·6°C to 29·4°C for the smaller babies and 23·8°C for the larger ones.

Electric blankets should be used with great caution if at all, because of the risk of burns and electric shock.

Cooling rooms 18·3°C are necessary to acclimatise the baby to ordinary room temperature.


# FEEDING

### Choice of Milk

Breast milk is ideal, because of its digestibility, but in some cases of preterm labour the mother is unable to produce a satisfactory supply of milk, and if pooled breast milk is not available, suitably modified milk, e.g. prepacked low protein, low solute formulae such as SMA Gold Cap, Cow and Gate Premium, can be used.

The practice of withholding oral fluid or food for 24 or more hours is no longer approved of: the dehydration and hypoglycaemia that ensues are believed to produce impairment of the cerebral circulation which may adversely affect intellectual function.

## METHOD OF FEEDING

The feeding of small preterm infants should be undertaken only by skilled experienced nursery midwives.

The method used depends on the size and vitality of the infant and his ability to suck and swallow.

The sucking and swallowing reflexes are sometimes poorly developed and inco-ordinated; fluid placed in the mouth may run down the trachea. The vomiting and coughing reflexes are also inadequate and regurgitated food is inhaled into the lungs; vomiting must therefore be avoided.

## NASOGASTRIC FEEDING

Many preterm babies suffer from some degree of respiratory difficulty or intracranial injury and the effort of sucking may increase any cyanosis and induce exhaustion.

Babies of 34 weeks gestation or less, and those with heart disease, cyanosis, dyspnoea, exhaustion or any serious illness should be 'tube fed'.

**Approximate volume of food.** (*Baby 2000 g: 34 weeks gestation*)

The baby would be given within 3 hours of birth, 10 ml of undiluted breast milk (if available) or suitably modified prepacked milk formula, e.g. SMA Gold Cap, by tube.

| Day of life | 1 | – | 3 | – | 5 | – | 7 | – | 10 |
|---|---|---|---|---|---|---|---|---|---|
| Ml/kg/24hrs. | 60 | – | 100 | – | 150 | – | 175 | – | 200 |
| Ml per feed | | | | | | | | | |
|   12 feeds | 10 | – | 15 | – | 25 | – | 30 | – | 33 |
|   10 Feeds | 12 | – | 20 | – | 30 | – | 35 | – | 40 |

If this volume of food causes vomiting the amount is reduced. Slightly more can be given with a maximum of 200 ml/kg/24 hrs on the 14th day. Three-hourly feeds may be started after 36 weeks gestation.

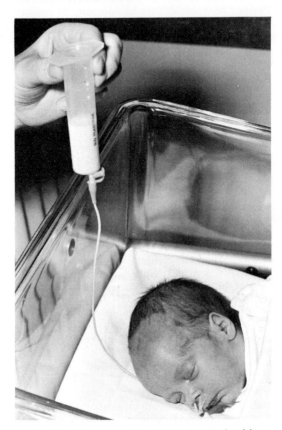

Fig. 30-4   Nasogastric feed given by gravity drip.
*Aberdeen Maternity Hospital.*

### A Suitable Regime Would Be:-

**First feed** given two to four hours after birth.
**Hourly feeds** at 32 weeks gestation and under.
**Two-hourly feeds** at 32–36 weeks gestation.
**Three-hourly feeds** can be attempted after 36 weeks gestation.

Midwives should not 'tube feed' babies until they have had a practical demonstration and carried out the procedure under supervision. The dangers are inhalation pneumonia, overfeeding and vomiting: all of which are preventable. Some are apprehensive in case they pass the catheter into the trachea but if due care is taken this is unlikely, as the opening of the larynx is very small. The baby would cough and become cyanosed so a careful watch is maintained on the colour of the infant during the procedure.

### Requirements for Nasogastric Feeding

1 polyvinyl indwelling feeding tube, 3½ FG for babies weighing less than 2000 g: a 6 FG tube being used for larger babies. Milk container 5 or 10 ml. a gallipot with sterile water. 2 gauze swabs; bottle of modified milk; micropore tape; blue litmus paper.

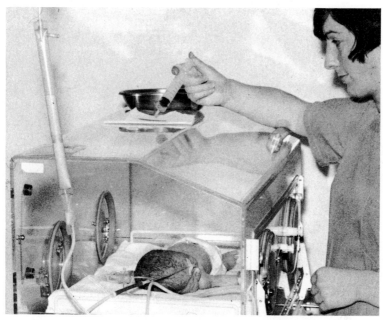

Fig. 30-5   Testing gastric aspirate with litmus paper. If acid to litmus, this confirms that the tube is in the stomach.

*Simpson Memorial Maternity Pavilion, Edinburgh.*

## *Method*

The tube is measured from the bridge of the nose to the xiphisternum. The baby's neck should be extended but not hyperextended: the tube is introduced via the nostril into the stomach: micropore tape being used to attach the tube to the forehead. Milk does not flow readily through a feeding tube of 3½ FG so very slight pressure may be necessary at the start of the feed, using a 5 or 10 ml syringe. For larger babies the 6 FG catheter requires no pressure: the milk flows by gravity. When removing the tube it should be withdrawn slowly, not whisked out: pinching the catheter near the baby's lips to avoid milk being inhaled. The head end of the incubator is raised and the baby propped over on his right side for 15 minutes after feeds.

#### JEJUNAL FEEDING

By this means more fluid and nutrients can be given. A radio opaque duodenal tube 5 FG and 125 cm long with a metal tip is introduced as for naso-gastric feeding. To check that it is in the stomach a specimen of gastric juice is withdrawn and tested for acidity. The tube is then inserted a further 12 cm: the outer end being attached to the forehead with micropore tape.

To facilitate entry into the duodenum the baby is propped over on to his right side. The tube is introduced a further 1 cm every 20 minutes until the aspirate is yellowish green and alkaline.

Breast milk (preferably) is given continuously by slow pump or intermittently by funnel.

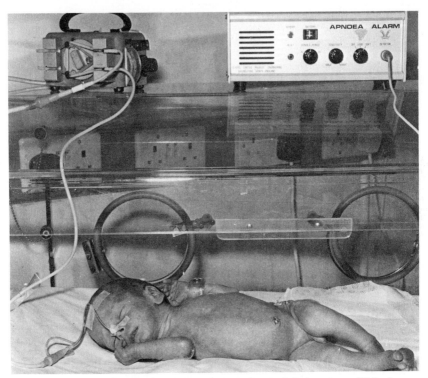

Fig. 30-6   Naso jejunal feed given by slow continuous infusion pump. (Holter)

### PARENTERAL NUTRITION

In some centres in Britain very low birth weight infants unable to tolerate tube feeding are given plasma concentrations of nutrient materials: carbohydrates, lipids (Intralipid), amino acids (Vamin) and electrolytes. The majority of babies weighing less than 1500 g at birth have arterial catheters introduced into an umbilical artery to monitor arterial oxygen tensions. This route is utilised for giving nutrients. After 4 or 5 days, scalp and other peripheral veins are used. Daily estimations of plasma pH, bicarbonate, sodium, potassium, chloride, osmolality, glucose and urea are necessary: adjustments being made in the light of biochemical findings. Plasma calcium, phosphorus, magnesium, ammonia and amino acid are estimated twice weekly. A clinical assessment is made twice daily including oedema, weight, tachycardia and tachypnoea. Abnormalities are assessed: arterial and venous pressures measured. Culture of the alimentary fluid on a daily basis is less exsanguinating than blood culture. The baby is nursed naked in an incubator and an ECG monitor utilised. A broad spectrum antibiotic such as cephalothin (Keflin) or cephalexin is given im or iv. Various complications may arise, i.e. metabolic acidosis, septicaemia, circulatory overload, phlebitis.

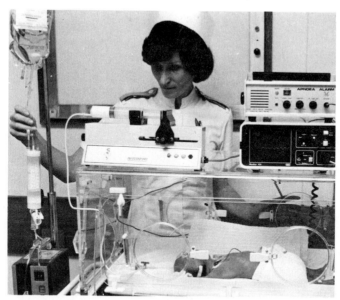

Fig. 30-7   Intravenous alimentation using slow syringe pump. Apnoea and cardiac monitors in use.

*Aberdeen Maternity Hospital.*

## BOTTLE FEEDING

An admirable method of holding the bottle, with the forefinger under the tip of the chin assisting the 'up and down' movement of the lower jaw is shown in Figure 30-8. Sucking lip movement may occur before the baby is vigorous enough to be given bottle feeds. If allowed to suck too soon the infant may become limp or cyanosed. The attempt should be abandoned at once. Progression from tube to bottle should take about one week.

### Pipette feeding

This method now condemned is sometimes used by midwives not experienced in tube feeding. Only about 0·6 ml is given at a time and this must be swallowed before the next 0·6 ml is given. It is a slow process so the milk should be kept warm. The pipette should have a bulbous tip. Syringes with a teat and rubber bulb to inject the milk into the mouth are dangerous: inexperienced midwives may squirt the milk into the pharynx and cause choking.

#### GENERAL POINTS ON FEEDING THE PRETERM BABY

Scrupulous cleanliness should be observed.

Wind is brought up by raising baby to the sitting position or by gently rolling him over on to the left hand and rubbing his back with the right hand. Tube-fed babies do not require to have wind brought up.

After feeds the baby should be laid on his right side, with the head of the cot raised, for 15 minutes to facilitate emptying of the stomach and to allow any vomited milk to run out of his mouth. An aspirator ought to be readily available to remove regurgitated milk from the nasopharynx.

The amount of food actually taken should be recorded as well as the amount offered.

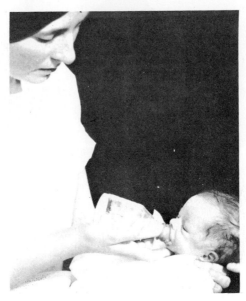

Fig. 30-8  Note forefinger under chin to assist the up and down movement of the lower jaw when a baby is reluctant to feed.

*Aberdeen Maternity Hospital.*

### VITAMIN REQUIREMENTS

The preterm baby requires vitamin A 2500 i.u. daily: vitamin D 600–800 i.u. daily after the second week. (*This amount must not be exceeded because of the risk of hypercalcaemia*). Vitamin C, 25 mg: vitamin $B_1$, 0·5 mg: vitamin $B_2$, 0·2 mg.

To avoid the risk of aspirating oily vitamin preparations, water miscible or concentrated forms should be used.

A useful preparation containing vitamins A, B, C and D is Abidec, 0·6 ml being given daily from the 7th day if baby is feeding well.

Folic acid, 1 mg daily, is given to infants 1500 g or less, starting at 7 days and finishing at 12 weeks.

## EXPERT NURSING

**Infinite patience and devoted care are essential;** meticulous attention to detail imperative. The midwife must understand the basic principles of treatment, if she is to carry them out intelligently and be able in the doctor's absence to change or withhold treatment when necessary.

**All changes should be made tentatively** and gradually whether in feeding or the environmental temperature.

**The infant should be handled as little as possible** and with great gentleness; dexterity comes with practice.

**The baby should lie on alternate sides following feeds:** a folded towel behind the back helps to maintain position which should be changed at hourly intervals.

**It is advisable to allow a period of rest between undressing and feeding,** as the necessary handling, followed by the effort of sucking and swallowing, may produce cyanosis and exhaustion.

**The cord is swabbed four-hourly** with Hibitane in spirit or Thiomersil 1 per cent
**The face and buttocks are washed daily.**

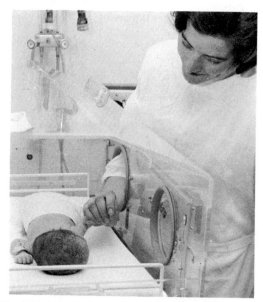

Fig. 30-9    Mothers are encouraged to caress their babies.
*Simpson Memorial Maternity Pavilion, Edinburgh.*

### Mothering

Even tiny babies thrive better when cuddled and the mother should be permitted to do this. In some centres the mothers in hospital visit their babies 3 or more times daily to stroke and caress them: they are encouraged to bottle feed, change napkins and do other simple tasks. But if the mother is not available mothering should be given by the midwife as soon as the baby is well established. Nursery midwives must avoid being too possessive as some mothers resent this.

### OBSERVATION

During the critical first 48 hours the small baby needs constant supervision. Accurate observation, prompt recognition and timely reporting of abnormal signs will enable the doctor to interpret their significance and prescribe the appropriate and often life-saving treatment.

### Colour

Cyanosis, greyness, pallor, jaundice should be reported.

### Respirations

The respirations may be 50 to 60 per minute recorded when quiet, sometimes shallow, frequently irregular and occasionally Cheyne-Stokes.

### Attacks of apnoea should be reported at once

Such episodes lasting over 15 seconds or recurring at frequent intervals are of serious importance. Apnoea occurring during the first 48 hours of life is usually treated as due to infection until proved otherwise: biochemical and intracranial causes together with severe respiratory failure are also considered. The baby who is overheated in an incubator may develop apnoea.

Flicking the sole of the foot or directing a stream of oxygen on the face will usually stimulate respiration: the airway is cleared. The apnoea monitor (Electrodyne Contactless) is placed under the mattress. Inflatable apnoea monitors are in common use.

Apnoea associated with bradycardia or colour change must be investigated and treated vigorously.

### Temperature

The temperature is taken morning and evening, with a low-reading thermometer, per rectum, axilla, or groin; the usual range is 36·5° to 37·5°C. The temperature of an ill baby is taken 4-hourly or continuously by using a skin probe.

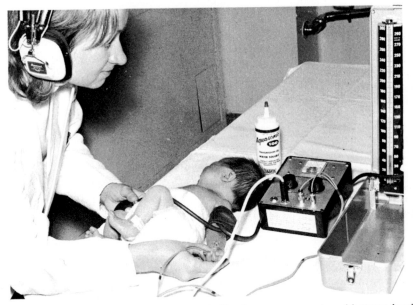

Fig. 30-10  Transcutaneous Doppler electronic blood-pressure apparatus with stereo headphones. Used for babies with cardiac disease, respiratory distress syndrome and when having intravenous nutrition (aquasonic 100 for skin contact).

*Simpson Memorial Maternity Pavilion, Edinburgh.*

### Stools

The stools are inspected, their frequency and consistency noted: meconium tends to persist for three or four days.

### Oedema

Oedema of the face, abdomen and legs is common; if severe, this should be reported.

**Weight-gain**

Preterm babies gain weight slowly. Daily weighing indicates whether the baby is over or under-hydrated. Excessive gain alerts one to the possibility of a renal or cardiac problem.

### FAVOURABLE SIGNS

**Pink colour** with absence of cyanosis.
**Good muscle tone,** increasing vigour in movements.
**Hearing the cry in very small babies,** lusty crying in larger ones.
**Eagerness for food;** gain in weight. Lessening of oedema.

### LESS FAVOURABLE SIGNS

**Cyanosis** may be due to some serious condition such as congenital heart disease, respiratory distress syndrome, intracranial injury, or both. Increasing cyanosis should be reported at once.

Greyness is due to a combination of cyanosis and pallor, and indicates collapse, extreme exhaustion, severe infection or intracranial haemorrhage. Babies who are ill should not be required to suck and swallow; aspiration of milk may occur.

## OXYGEN THERAPY

Oxygen should only be administered when needed and not as a routine procedure.

Midwives should be aware of the potential dangers in administering oxygen and particularly in concentrations of over 30 per cent. Blindness in preterm babies due to retrolental fibroplasia appears to be related to the administration of oxygen; nevertheless the baby must get sufficient oxygen to relieve cyanosis. The concentration should be reduced to the lowest level that will maintain a pink colour.

### REGULATION OF OXYGEN CONCENTRATION

This should be carried out at hourly intervals as a routine measure: the use of the IMI oxygen analyser gives satisfactory results.

**The most accurate method of controlling oxygen therapy** is to measure the partial pressure of oxygen in arterial blood and to adjust the inspired oxygen concentrations accordingly. An arterial catheter, $3\frac{1}{2}$ FG, is introduced through an umbilical artery into the aorta with strict aseptic precautions; then sutured in position. Samples of blood, 0·3 ml, are withdrawn into a heparinised syringe and analysed. For convenience a 3-way tap is attached to the catheter which is flushed after the sample has been obtained and kept filled with a heparinised saline solution.

## AVOIDANCE OF INFECTION

Infection is one of the greatest dangers to preterm babies, and is preventable. In addition to the precautions taken to avoid infection of all newborn babies (p. 556), the following are recommended.

Hand washing is vitally important between handling each baby and always after changing napkins and before feeding. Paper or other individual towels should be used.

Feeds should be prepacked or prepared and given under conditions similar to surgical asepsis. Disposable napkins are placed in destructible containers and removed from the nursery as soon as possible.

### PSEUDOMONAS AERUGINOSA (PYOCYANEA)

**The pyocyanea group** of organisms is causing serious infections in preterm babies: urinary, gastro-intestinal and other lesions. Pseudomonas aeruginosa have been found in incubators, aspirators and resuscitating machines (disposable tubing is recommended); humidity and moisture favour growth. Sudol (phenol, 50 per cent) is bactericidal to pyocyanea.

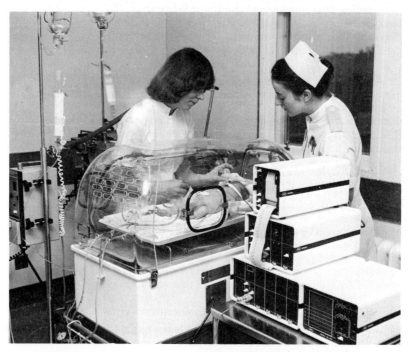

Fig. 30-11 Baby with enlarged heart and bilateral pleural effusion. Top cabinet: blood pressure recording strip. Middle cabinet: oscilloscope for visual recording of blood pressure. Bottom cabinet: ECG tracing. Glucose drip 5 per cent by Tekmar.

*Aberdeen Maternity Hospital.*

## Disinfection of Incubators

The inside of the incubator should be cleaned and the water changed daily; they should be replaced every week and on discharge of the baby, in order to cleanse and disinfect them thoroughly after which they are aired for 48 hours. Cleansing should always precede disinfection because the gases used will not penetrate 'dirt'. An incubator provides an ideal environment for organisms as well as for preterm babies.

### INSTRUCTION TO MOTHERS OF PRETERM BABIES

Before the infant is discharged the mother should be given adequate instruction and practice in feeding, bathing and the general care of her infant. She should be shown how to give iron and vitamin supplements, and advised on how to avoid respiratory and gastro-intestinal infections. Some hospitals have furnished a room in which the mother can reside with her baby for a few days while gaining supervised experience under home-like conditions: an admirable educational project.

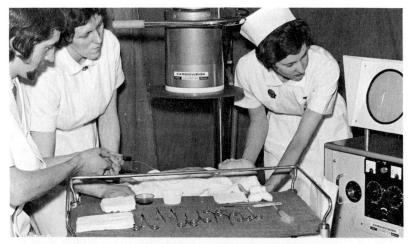

Fig. 30-12   Cardiovision. Introducing intravenous umbilical catheter proximal to the right atrial chamber by radiological control for intravenous alimenation. Also used in respiratory distress syndrome when obtaining blood samples for biochemistry findings. Sister is looking at the image intensifier.

*Neonatal Intensive Care Unit, Royal Maternity Hospital Rottenrow, Glasgow.*

## DISORDERS OF PRETERM BABIES

### *Idiopathic Respiratory Distress Syndrome*

This condition is one of the major causes of death in preterm infants of less than 34 weeks' gestation, 2000 g; those who had asphyxia; babies of diabetic mothers and babies delivered by Caesarean section. Avoidance of intrauterine anoxia and birth asphyxia would reduce the incidence of IRDS.

**These babies have a deficiency of surfactant,** a substance necessary to facilitate lung expansion, prevent pulmonary collapse and control capillary permeability and pulmonary blood flow.

Lecithin is a component of surfactant and the lecithin/sphingomyelin ratio in the amniotic fluid has a predictive value regarding fetal lung maturity and the likelihood of idiopathic respiratory distress syndrome developing in the newborn. Lecithin levels below 3·5 mg per 100 ml amniotic fluid, obtained by amniocentesis, indicate that the fetus would be at risk of IRDS if delivered then.

**Steroids such as betamethasone** may stimulate the secretion of surfactant in the fetal lungs if given to the woman when preterm delivery is advisable or inevitable, e.g. for severe pre-eclampsia, diabetes or intrauterine growth retardation.

#### SIGNS OF IDIOPATHIC RESPIRATORY DISTRESS SYNDROME

**Difficulty in respiration is apparent from birth** and is very definite at 4–6 hours with inspiratory retraction and moist expiratory grunting, recession of sternum and indrawing of lateral chest wall. Tachypnoea (over 60 per minute), irregular respiratory rhythm; apnoea occurring early is an ominous sign indicating the need for pulmonary ventilation. The blood pressure is low: normal being 65/40.

Cyanosis of face and body or grey colour with cyanosis of lips, hands and feet are usually present.

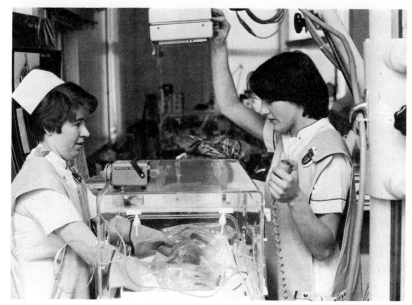

Fig. 30-13    Fetus having chest X-ray for RDS. Midwife wearing lead gloves in plastic bags.
*Aberdeen Maternity Hospital.*

## Diagnosis

**A chest radiograph** is taken and the ground-glass mottling of the lungs and clear outline of the bronchial tree are characteristic.

**Blood gas studies** will demonstrate hypoxaemia. Low $pO_2$.

**Biochemical abnormalities**: respiratory and metabolic acidosis, and rise in serum potassium and low blood oxygen concentration.

### Silverman retraction scoring

This method is concerned with the degree of chest retraction; in cases of idiopathic respiratory distress syndrome, a score of 10 at a single observation indicates maximal retraction: a serious state of affairs.

| | |
|---|---|
| **See-saw sinking of upper chest** with rising abdomen | 2 |
| **Marked sinking of intercostal spaces** on inspiration | 2 |
| **Marked xiphoid retraction** | 2 |
| **Chin descends,** lips apart | 2 |
| **Expiratory grunt audible** | 2 |
| | 10 = serious |

The criteria are scored $0-1-2$ depending on the severity.

Absence of all these signs would give a score of 0 = favourable.

Sternal recession may persist for days after respiratory distress syndrome.

### TREATMENT OF IDIOPATHIC RESPIRATORY DISTRESS SYNDROME

**The infant is nursed in a warm incubator** with high humidity and sufficient oxygen to abolish cyanosis. Suction to clear the airway is essential

**Umbilical arterial catheterisation is carried** out as soon as the clinical diagnosis of IRDS is made, i.e. one or two hours after birth. Into one of the umbilical arteries an arterial catheter 3½ FG, with 3-way tap, is inserted. The catheter is utilised for infusion of fluids, nutrients and electrolytes: sampling and monitoring of the infant's blood. By syringe, blood samples are obtained for the estimation of pH, $pO_2$, $pCO_2$, base excess (see Glossary) and electrolytes daily or as required. From the findings respiratory and metabolic acidosis are diagnosed and rectified; oxygen therapy accurately controlled.

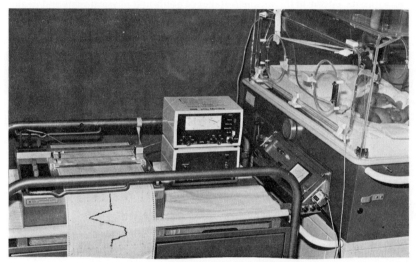

Fig. 30-14  Baby receiving partial pressure of oxygen recorded via an indwelling umbilical arterial catheter.

*Queen Mother's Hospital, Glasgow.*

**Blood gas analysis** permits calculation of the pH of the blood and other biochemical factors in 5 minutes and this procedure is now used in preference to the Astrup apparatus. Acidosis and other disturbances can be combated promptly by the administration of glucose 10 per cent and sodium bicarbonate 8·4 per cent. The intra-arterial drip is regulated by means of a peristaltic pump the amount usually being 72 ml/kg body-weight/24 hours.

**Antibiotics** may be administered 6-hourly for 5 to 7 days, when umbilical catheters are in use.

**CPAP** (continuous positive airway pressure) is sometimes used to supply constant oxygen-enriched air by nasal prongs, endotracheal tube or head box. (See p. 553.) This pressure, up to 12 cm of water, counteracts the tendency of the lung to collapse due to surfactant deficiency. Severe IRDS may require ventilation with PEEP (positive end expiratory pressure). (See Fig. 32-12.)

### NURSING CARE

**Maintenance of a clear airway.** Blocked catheters are dealt with. Endotracheal tubes cleared hourly by suction catheter.

**Apnoeic episodes are detected and treated.** Contactless apnoea alarm in use.

**Giving ventilator care** for CPAP and PEEP as indicated on p. 554.

**Ensuring that body and incubator temperatures are maintained** at the required level: warmth is essential but clothing must not impede respiration.

**Checking that warmed humidified oxygen is administered** at the prescribed concentration.

**Carrying out feeding via umbilical arterial catheter** as directed: umbilicus cleansed with Hibitane in spirit or Thiomersil one per cent.

**Baby positioned and supported** to provide greatest respiratory ease; top of incubator elevated: baby's head slightly extended: infant turned every hour.

**Recognising the significance of electronic monitor panel readings** re heart beat, respirations, blood pressure.

**Notifying the doctor** in the incipient stages of abnormal physical signs and dealing with emergencies such as apnoea until his arrival.

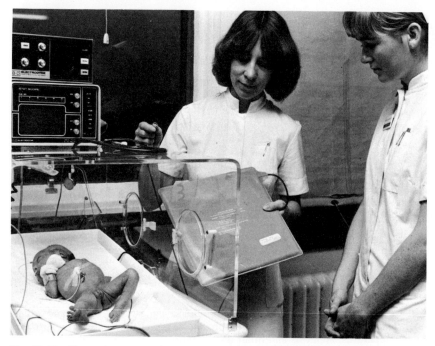

Fig. 30-15  Electrodyne contactless apnoea monitor. IMI model 5500. Clinical instructor showing student midwife a contactless monitor similar to the one under the cot mattress. The indicator panel and control cabinet is placed on top of the ECG cardiorater.

*Aberdeen Maternity Hospital.*

### OBSERVATION

**Hourly checks** of respiration, oxygen concentration, fluid in umbilical arterial giving set.

**Four-hourly checks** of temperature and heart rate.

**Weighing twice daily** for fluid balance.
**Silverman retraction score** noted repeatedly.
**Colour and general condition** under vigilant surveillance.

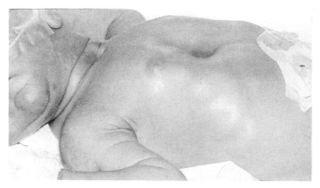

Fig. 30-16   Baby with xiphoid recession.
*Queen Mother's Hospital, Glasgow.*

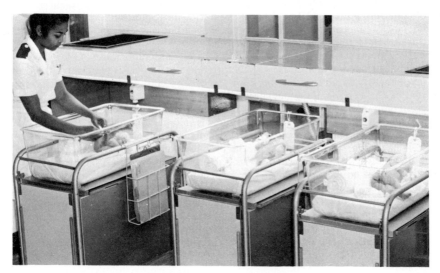

Fig. 30-17   Phototherapy unit.
*Aberdeen Maternity Hospital.*

### PHOTOTHERAPY FOR JAUNDICE

**Jaundice is more severe and prolonged in preterm babies** and many paediatricians advocate phototherapy as a prophylactic measure for all babies less than 34 weeks' gestation. If persistent over 36 hours the serum bilirubin test is made. When the concentration reaches 175 micromol/l in the preterm baby and 205 micromol/l in the baby at term, phototherapy is given and discontinued when the serum bilirubin is below 175 micromol/l. Earlier feeding of preterm babies and phototherapy have reduced the need for replacement transfusion.

**To reduce hyperbilirubinaemia** the baby with jaundice is exposed (naked) to high density fluorescent light: fluorescent tubes above the incubator emit 'blue light' and a fall of about 20 micromol/l serum bilirubin can be expected after 12 hours' exposure.

**Phototherapy** is also given to infants with physiological and ABO incompatibility jaundice. Phototherapy should be commenced as soon as possible and the hours of exposure recorded; the baby being turned at feed times. The eyes must be protected: a Netelast tubular elastic netting worn as a cap is effective in maintaining a light-proof eye shield in place. To avoid hypothermia adequate warmth and monitoring of body and cot temperatures are necessary: overheating must also be guarded against. The napkin is placed under the baby to allow maximal skin exposure. Loose stools may occur.

**Oedema** in which the tissues are hard is sometimes present in small preterm babies. This is probably due to electrolyte imbalance, and immaturity of kidney function.

**Infections** of the respiratory tract and pneumonia due to inhalation of food are serious. Gastroenteritis is particularly lethal. Systemic candidiasis can be fatal to preterm infants.

### Anaemia

The small preterm baby is deprived of the store of iron that the infant at term obtains during the last 12 weeks of intra-uterine life. Some authorities estimate the haemoglobin at birth, then every two weeks and, if it is less than 7·4 g/dl, a blood transfusion is given.

The administration of iron is of no value until the second month of life as it is not utilised for haemoglobin formation before that time, but it is imperative that iron supplements are given after the fourth week and continued throughout the first year of life. Ferric ammonium citrate, 60 mg, or ferrous sulphate, 30 to 60 mg, are given daily, starting with smaller doses to avoid digestive upsets. Fersamal syrup, 2 to 4 ml, is well tolerated. Sytron, 2 ml daily, is suitable for small babies. Iron should always be given after feeds to avoid gastric irritation. Folic acid is given to babies weighing under 1500 g because of the possibility of megaloblastic anaemia.

**Rickets** is liable to occur in preterm babies so vitamin D must be given after the second week to aid the absorption of calcium and maintain the concentration of phosphorus.

**Retrolental fibroplasia,** in which an opaque membrane forms behind the lens resulting in blindness, occurs in preterm babies under 2000 g in weight. The cause is related to the administration of concentrations of oxygen above 40 per cent over an extended period. The skilful administration and accurate analysis of the concentration of oxygen has decreased the incidence of this catastrophe in recent years. Cyanosis must be relieved.

## LIGHT FOR DATE BABIES

The term 'light for date' refers to babies whose birth weight is below the tenth centile for their estimated gestational age; this being obtained from a graph (see Fig. 7-14). The condition reflects intra-uterine malnutrition and growth retardation of the fetus, which may be due to placental dysfunction, as might occur in pre-eclampsia, and essential hypertension.

### CLINICAL FEATURES DURING PREGNANCY

**Small baby syndrome.** After the 30th week, on abdominal palpation, the fetus appears to be small for date and does not increase in size at the normal rate. The amount of amniotic fluid is below average and maternal weight and abdominal girth are stationary.

**Plasma or urinary oestriol assays** are made after the 30th week to assess fetoplacental vitality. A slow rise in oestriol excretion suggests intra-uterine growth retardation.

**Ultrasonic cephalometry** is employed to measure fetal growth rate when the fetus is suspected of being at risk from placental insufficiency. If the bi-parietal diameter does not show a normal increase, intra-uterine growth retardation is suspected.

**During labour** fetal blood sampling and electrocardiograph monitoring of the fetal heart are usually carried out. Caesarean section may be necessary.

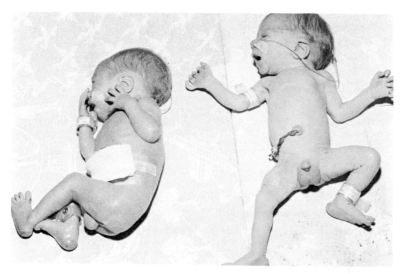

Fig. 30-18
Preterm Baby.
30 weeks' gestation, 1480 g.

Light for date baby.
39 weeks' gestation, 1480 g.

*Simpson Memorial Maternity Pavilion, Edinburgh.*

### DIAGNOSIS OF LIGHT FOR DATE BABY AT BIRTH

It is imperative that the midwife recognises the light for date baby at birth so that treatment can be given without delay.

**A history of pre-eclampsia** during pregnancy would arouse suspicion.

**If the small baby syndrome had been manifest during pregnancy.**

**The clinical appearance of the baby.**

The skin is dry and wrinkled giving a wizened 'old man' look in severe cases. No oedema is present. The baby is long and thin. The nodule of breast tissue is not considered to be an accurate sign of a light for date baby. The plantar creases are well defined on stroking the sole of the foot from toes to heel. The Moro and the traction reflexes are present. In the preterm baby they are not. Pinna of ear has cartilaginous ridges.

Gross discrepancy between the weights of twin babies, one 10 per cent less than the other is strongly suggestive that the smaller baby is light for date.

### *Treatment*

**The Dextrostix test** is carried out and if the blood glucose is below 1·1 mmol/l, glucose solution 10 per cent is given into a scalp vein.

### Early feeding

The baby should be given a feed of milk modified to human standards within 2 hours after birth and fed two hourly for 48 hours.

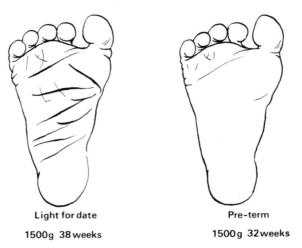

|  |  |
|:---:|:---:|
| Light for date | Pre-term |
| 1500g 38 weeks | 1500g 32 weeks |
| Deep indentations present at birth | Faint marks present at birth |

Fig. 30-19  Plantar creases are only one manifestation of gestational age. (No one sign is definitive.)

### COMPLICATIONS OF LIGHT FOR DATE BABIES

**Asphyxia.** There is a high incidence of asphyxia but respiratory distress syndrome rarely occurs as in the preterm baby.

**Hypoglycaemia.** This is a very hazardous state that must be diagnosed and dealt with at once because if low blood glucose persists for more than 36 hours it may cause permanent brain damage. Delayed or low glucose feeds favour hypoglycaemia.

**Hypothermia** is more common in light for date babies especially if environmental warmth is inadequate and feeding delayed.

**The mortality rate is lower** in light for date babies than in babies of similar weight but earlier gestational age.

---

## QUESTIONS FOR REVISION
### PRETERM AND LIGHT FOR DATE BABIES

What percentage of babies are of low birth weight? How could a midwife try to prevent preterm labour? Why is delayed feeding no longer practised? How would you transfer a preterm baby 20 miles to hospital? What incubator temperature is advisable for a baby 1,360 g?

Discuss advice to a mother on taking her baby home weighing 2,500 g; incubator nursing; prevention of infection; feeding a baby weighing 1,360 g.

*For what reason may the following drugs be given* to preterm babies: Konakion; Sytron; Abidec?

*For what reason might the following appliances be used* and what are the midwives' responsibilities: apnoea monitor; silver swaddler; constant i.v. infusion pump; phototherapy unit; arterial catheter?

*Why are the following carried out:* Silverman retraction scoring; positive pressure respiration; continuous naso-gastric feeding?

*What do you suspect from the following observations* and what would you do: baby twitching; cyanosed; (*a*) with frothy mucus (*b*) after a feed; apnoeic episode lasting 15 seconds; respirations 80 per minute; inspiratory recession?

*Discuss as a means of preventing infection:* mask wearing; use of disposable napkins; the method you prefer in cleaning incubators.

*Why do preterm babies develop the following?* What can be done to prevent them? Anaemia; rickets; retrolental fibroplasia; hypothermia.

*What precautions* would you take during preterm labour to preserve the life of the fetus?

*Why should* an inexperienced midwife not take charge of the feeding of a preterm baby? How would you pass the naso-gastric tube? **What would you note** and record regarding a preterm baby? What are your responsibilities when administering oxygen?

In what conditions would you: (*a*) anticipate; (*b*) recognise a light for date baby? What complications may arise? Describe the feeding of such a baby. What is the normal newborn blood glucose level?

**C.M.B(Eng.) 30-min question.** Enumerate the factors which may cause low birth weight. What may a midwife discover in the course of antenatal care that would suggest that the fetus may be 'at risk' in this respect?

**C.M.B.(Scot.) 30-min question.** What are the risks associated with preterm birth? Describe the management of a preterm baby weighing 1680 grams at birth.

**C.M.B.(Eng.) 30-min question.** Describe the care of a baby weighing 1580 grams at birth, for the first 10 days of its life.

**(N. Ire.) Council 30-min question.** What are the special risks to which a preterm baby is exposed? Describe the nursing care of such an infant.

**C.M.B.(Scot.) 30-min question.** What are the differences between a preterm and a light for date baby? Give the basic principles in the management of each.

**N. Ire. Council** (*a*) Define what is meant by the pre-term infant? (*b*) What are the clinical features of such an infant? (*c*) Discuss the management during the first two weeks of life.

**C.M.B.(Eng.)** Following a period of unsatisfactory intra-uterine growth a baby is born at 36 weeks gestation. Describe the care that may be necessary during the first week of life.

**Scot.:** Discuss the problems associated with heat regulation in the newborn.

**N. Ire. Council** (*a*) Define the 'light for date' baby: (*b*) describe the clinical features of such a baby: (*c*) discuss the management of this baby during the first seven days of life.

**N. Ire. Council** What is idiopathic respiratory distress syndrome? In what circumstances may this occur? Describe the management of a baby with this condition.

**Scot.:** Give an account of the care in the first week of life of a baby born at 34 weeks gestation who weighs 1·5 kg at birth.

**N. Ire. Council** Describe the nursing care of the preterm baby.

## C.M.B. Short Questions

**Eng.:** Describe a baby suffering from respiratory distress syndrome. **N. Ireland:** Tube feeding in the preterm infant. **Scot.:** Give the management of respiratory distress syndrome.

**Eng.:** How may the 'small for date' baby be recognised after birth? **Eng.:** 'Small for date' babies.

**Scot.:** Detail the advantages of a 'special care' nursery.

**Scot.:** Discharge of a baby from hospital: **Scot.:** Moro Reflex. **Eng.:** Demand feeding.

**C.M.B.(Eng.)** Respiratory distress syndrome. **Scot.:** Self demand feeding.

**C.M.B.(Scot.)** What is:–

(*a*) a prematurely born (pre-term) baby; (*b*) a light for date baby

Describe the complications which may occur in each.

# 31

# Neonatal Metabolic Disorders

*Baby of diabetic mother. Hypoglycaemia. Hypocalcaemia. Hypomagnesaemia. Hypernatraemia. Convulsions. Phenylketonuria. Hypothermia*

## THE BABY OF THE DIABETIC MOTHER

Some of these babies are unduly large (over 4 kg), fat with bulky cheeks. This may be due to inadequate maternal diabetic control during pregnancy. The overweight babies tend to develop idiopathic respiratory distress syndrome, their condition deteriorating within three or four hours with laboured, rapid breathing, poor lung expansion, pallor, cyanosis and limpness. In spite of their size and weight these babies need special care and should be nursed in an incubator.

### MANAGEMENT

Initially this is concerned with the prevention of respiratory complications: the lecithin sphingomyelin ratio test being a useful precautionary measure against idiopathic respiratory distress syndrome. Admission to a special care nursery is essential. A paediatrician and an experienced nursery midwife take charge of the infant who is placed in a humidified environmental temperature of 32°C with oxygen of sufficient concentration to relieve any existing cyanosis. Vitamin $K_1$ (Konakion), 1 mg, is given i.m.

A marked and rapid fall in blood glucose, from over 5·5 mmols/l to 0·8 mmols/l occurs within two hours of birth. Routine monitoring of plasma glucose levels is carried out by Dextrostix every half hour for 3 hours and then before each feed for 48 hours or more: when below 2·5 mmols/l a true plasma glucose test is made: if below a critical level 10 per cent glucose solution is given i.v. into a scalp vein. If the infant's condition does not improve the blood serum is examined for low calcium and low magnesium concentrations.

**By early feeding** an attempt is made to avert hypoglycaemia. Starting within three hours after birth the baby is given orally 72 ml/kg body weight, modified milk (SMA Gold Cap) 2 hourly for 12 hours then 3 or 4 hourly. If unable to suck, the nasogastric route is utilised. All feeds should be given by a midwife experienced in the handling of such infants.

### Observation

A midwife sits constantly beside the incubator, observing colour and general condition, recording respirations and the apex beat.

**Intubation may be needed** so equipment should be readily available. Every precaution is taken to prevent infection.

## NEONATAL HYPOGLYCAEMIA

The condition of low blood glucose (less than 1·6 mmols/l in a mature baby and 1·1 mmols/l in a low birth weight infant) commonly occurring during the first 48 hours of life, is a hazardous state that must be anticipated, recognised and dealt with at once. Should hypoglycaemia persist for over 36 hours, permanent brain damage may be done.

**Prevention is the important factor.** Early feeding of babies 'at risk' has reduced the incidence of hypoglycaemia. The midwife must be aware of the conditions predisposing babies to this low blood glucose state and utilise the Dextrostix blood glucose screening test. Early feeding is mandatory by naso-gastric tube if necessary: SMA or other modified milk being given.

### Dextrostix glucose screening test

The midwife carries out this test in suspected babies within 2 hours of birth and before each feed for 72 hours. The risk of hypoglycaemia is even greater on the

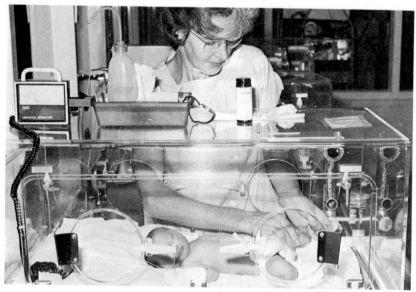

Fig. 31.1   Midwife doing Dextrostix test.
*Queen Mother's Hospital, Glasgow.*

second day. Blood is obtained by heel prick. The foot should be warm; the heel cleansed with Hibitane, 0·5 per cent, in spirit, 70 per cent, and dried. With a sterile disposable lancet a puncture 3 mm deep is made parallel to the sole, avoiding bone. One large drop of blood is allowed to drip on to the reagent area and after exactly 60 seconds it is washed off using a 'squeezy' bottle not the water tap. The strip area is compared with the colour chart according to instructions on the bottle. If the result is under 2·5 mmols/l, the doctor does a blood glucose estimation.

Babies liable to develop hypoglycaemia are those with diabetic mothers: small preterm and light for date babies: those with intracranial injury, severe asphyxia, and idiopathic respiratory distress syndrome.

The diagnosis is made by blood glucose estimation: there are no diagnostic clinical signs. The baby may be jittery with twitching, eyerolling, apnoeic or cyanotic episodes, reluctance to feed and convulsions.

### Treatment

When the blood glucose level is below 2 mmols/l, glucose, 10 per cent, is administered via a scalp vein 10 ml per hour by constant infusion-pump or micro-drip set to achieve an accurate glucose and fluid intake. The response is usually rapid and oral feeds with breast milk or modified pre-packed milk are commenced before the i.v. infusion is discontinued.

# HYPOCALCAEMIA

In this condition the serum calcium level falls below 1·9 mmol/l (a safe level is 2·2 mmols/l). It usually occurs in preterm, light for date, asphyxiated infants and the baby of the diabetic mother. (The condition is not seen in breast fed babies). The high phosphate content of cow's milk leads to a lowering of serum calcium levels: full-cream milks, allowing calcium to be excreted in the stools along with the high fat, may play some part. Hypocalcaemia may follow replacement transfusion.

**Signs.** Irritability, fine rapid tremor of fingers, jerky limb movements. If convulsions occur the baby between seizures is normal and alert.

### Treatment

The response to calcium is rapid. 10 ml of 10 per cent calcium gluconate or calcium syrup is administered. Rarely is calcium given intravenously because it is irritant to tissues so great care must be exercised to avoid spilling or leakage.

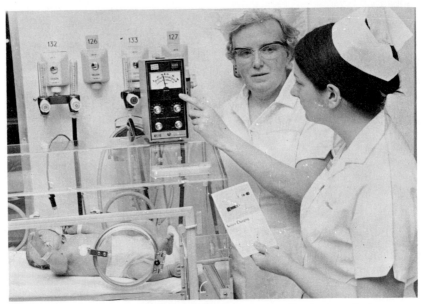

Fig. 31-2   Student midwife being shown how to use the oxygen analyser.
*Maternity Hospital, Stirling.*

## HYPOMAGNESAEMIA

Magnesium depletion may occur in newborn babies with vomiting or diarrhoea and in those who are grossly underfed: twitching and convulsions being exhibited. The condition may be suspected when the infant with hypocalcaemia does not respond adequately to calcium therapy. The baby is pale, limp, reluctant to feed, passing loose stools. Treatment consists in the administration of magnesium sulphate i.m. or i.v.

### HYPERNATRAEMIA (*High Blood Sodium*)

This condition is commonly due to carelessness or ignorance in making up dried milk feeds and in giving cereals during the first or second month of life. When the baby is given too much sodium, this dehydrates the brain cells and may cause mental retardation. Cow's milk contains four times as much sodium as breast milk and if the mother heaps or packs the scoop of powder the infant gets six times the amount of sodium he requires. The infant cries with thirst; 'mouthing' and fist sucking; the mother thinking he is hungry increases the volume or the strength of the feed. Death has occurred due to renal damage. An episode of vomiting or diarrhoea by increasing dehydration could precipitate hypernatraemia in babies fed on cow's milk. The condition is rare in breast fed babies.

Midwives have a responsibility to teach mothers how to make up feeds accurately and to warn them of the dangers of giving too much milk powder, and better still to breast feed their babies.

## NEONATAL CONVULSIONS

The three commonest causes during the first weeks of life are asphyxia, intracranial injury and biochemical imbalance.

**First Day.** Severe asphyxia; the convulsion usually occuring at the termination of an apnoeic episode due to hypoxia of the brain cells; metabolic acidosis as well as respiratory acidosis may be present (see p. 552). Intracranial injury causes cerebral depression: which may be followed by tonic convulsions during the subsequent period of cerebral irritation.

**During the first 72 hours.** Hypoglycaemia (see p. 538).

**5th to 8th day.** Hypocalcaemia (see p. 540). The infant being alert between convulsions.

**During the second week.** *Meningitis.* The baby looks ill, some have an elevated temperature: head retraction: bulging fontanelle: vomiting. Lumbar puncture is made to determine the causative organism.

### Signs of a convulsion

Premonitory signs such as twitching of the muscles of the face, hands and feet may be manifest. Rigidity of the limbs and spine with head retraction usually occurs: the eyes roll or stare: cyanosis deepens rapidly due to spasm of the diaphragm interrupting respiration. Generalised convulsive movements follow; head, arms and legs jerking spasmodically; strabismus may be present: froth appears on the lips. Following the seizure the infant is unconscious for a few minutes, limp and pale or ashen grey in colour. Convulsions vary in length, severity and type and the stages are not clearly defined.

### Observation

The midwife should note (a) which areas of the body are involved, (b) duration of the convulsion and (c) behaviour after or between convulsions.

| Convulsion Chart (Simpson Memorial Maternity Pavilion, Edinburgh) | | | | | | |
|---|---|---|---|---|---|---|
| Date | Time | Type (tonic, clonic) | Region(s) involved | Apnoea | Cyanosis | Duration |
| | | | | | | |

## TREATMENT OF A CONVULSION

**The doctor is notified.** If milk is being regurgitated the baby is turned face downwards. Mucus is removed from mouth and nose: the baby being propped over on one side to prevent the tongue from blocking the larynx. Oxygen is administered to relieve cyanosis. Warm blankets are applied. The midwife obtains blood and does the Dextrostix test for glucose after a convulsion occurs during the first 48 hours of life. **Sedatives are prescribed,** e.g. phenobarbitone, 2 to 3 mg 8 hourly or paraldehyde: or an anticonvulsant such as phenytoin (Epanutin): biochemical imbalance and metabolic acidosis are diagnosed and corrected: urine analysis and urine culture, blood culture and lumbar puncture are done as is deemed necessary. The baby is nursed in a quiet room and protected from external stimuli; being handled as little as possible. Close observation is essential.

### The Jittery Baby

**Various conditions give rise to tremor,** twitching and jerky limb movements; the diagnosis being facilitated by the midwife's meticulous observation and reporting.

**Intracranial injury:** twitching of facial muscles and fingers, eye rolling, nystagmus, clenched fists, periods of twitching of limbs. Rigidity of the trunk, rapid darting movements of the tongue are preceded by irritability and a piercing shriek.

**Hypoglycaemia:** twitching, hyper-alertness, irritability, apnoeic episodes, convulsions, limpness.

**Hypocalcaemia:** irritability, twitching, hyper-alertness, fine rapid tremor of fingers, waving limb movements occurring between 5 and 8 days of life. The infant is alert between convulsions

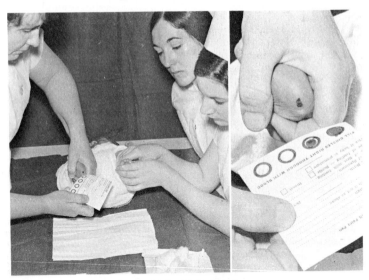

Fig. 31-3   Guthrie test.
*Maternity Section, Central Hospital, Irvine, Ayrshire.*

### PHENYLKETONURIA

This condition is an inborn error of the metabolism of amino acids occurring in about 1–7500 births. Deficiency of an enzyme causes disordered amino-acid metabolism and an increase of phenylalanine in the blood which gives rise to severe mental retardation.

The Guthrie inhibition assay for phenylalanine in the blood is the most efficient diagnostic method available. The test is made not before the 8th day (the baby having had milk feeds for 48 hours), and prior to 14 days. Further biochemical tests are made to confirm a positive diagnosis before low phenylalanine dietary therapy is begun. Early provision of a low phenylalanine diet will diminish mental retardation.

### Collection of blood samples for the Guthrie test

The baby's foot should be warm; massaging the heel improves the circulation. Cleanse the heel with Hibitane in spirit or a mediswab and wipe it dry. With a sterile disposable lancet a puncture not more than 2·4 mm deep is made parallel to the sole, avoiding bone. Touch the reverse side of the filter paper lightly on to the drops of blood without making contact with the skin. Fill the other circles with blood if possible. Allow the blood to dry before placing the card in the envelope. Dry heel and apply pressure for a few seconds.

### Maple syrup urine disease

The urine has the odour of maple syrup. This condition is a severe inborn error of amino acid metabolism. During the first week of life the infant may be lethargic and have persistent vomiting: Convulsions may occur. A special diet is prescribed. The condition is detected when the Guthrie or Scriver blood tests are done in a neonatal screening programme.

# NEONATAL HYPOTHERMIA

### (This Condition Gives Rise to a Metabolic Disturbance)

The normal baby's temperature may fall to 35°C or less within one hour of birth unless precautions are taken to avoid chilling. The term 'neonatal cold injury' is applied when hypothermia is severe and a dangerously low level is reached, 30° to 33°C. Babies at risk are preterm: hypoxic brain damage is a common cause. Hypoglycaemia may complicate the situation.

## SIGNS

Baby feels cold to the touch: rectal temperature is below 35°C.

Respirations may be slow: cry feeble, lethargy, reluctance to feed.

Excessive redness of face and extremities. Solid oedema (sclerema) is an ominous sign.

#### PREVENTION

The labour ward temperature should be maintained at 21° to 24°C: the cot to receive the baby kept constantly warm. Immediately the baby is born he should be received into a warm towel and dried. This is particularly important during resuscitation. A warmed Turkish towelling wrap, that envelopes the whole infant, is recommended (see Fig. 19-12). During transfer to ward or nursery the baby should be in a heated plastic cot with lid, otherwise, properly wrapped. Some transport preterm babies within the hospital in a portable incubator. During transport from home to hospital the baby is wrapped in warm towels inside a silver swaddler and placed in a heated portable incubator or substitute warm conveyor.

Bathing should be postponed until the baby's temperature is 36·3°C at least. The room, towels and clothing should be warm.

**Low reading thermometers** 25° to 40°C should be used (C.M.B. rule), the baby's temperature taken once daily at least. The mother must be instructed re the need for warmth and given the national leaflet. The room temperature should be 18° to 21°C particularly at night. A wall thermometer should be loaned if necessary.

### Treatment of Hypothermia

Rewarm the baby slowly 1°C per hour in an incubator at 32°C until the rectal temperature reaches 36·6°C. If warmed too quickly, convulsions may occur. The Dextrostix test is made every 6 hours. Low blood glucose or signs of hypoglycaemia, i.e. twitching or convulsions, indicate the immediate need for milk feeds.

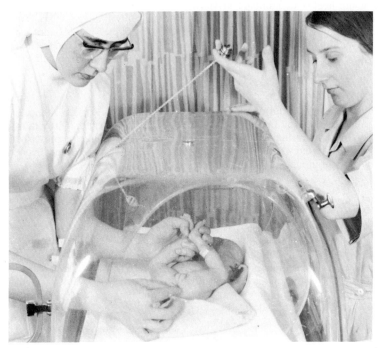

Fig. 31-4   Use of radiant heat shield to conserve heat round the infant. Temperature being recorded per rectum.

*Royal Maternity Hospital, Rottenrow, Glasgow.*

### CYSTIC FIBROSIS (Mucoviscidosis)

This is a genetic disorder in which the mucous glands throughout the body produce thick tenacious mucus. The effect on the pancreas, intestine and lungs causes serious complications. Failure to pass meconium indicates meconium ileus which causes intestinal obstruction. When there is a family history of the disorder, and in a screening programme, the midwife is required to test the first meconium passed for high protein; an Albustix reagent strip being used, a further sweat test is made to detect the high sodium and chloride secreted by the sweat glands.

---

### QUESTIONS FOR REVISION

Write notes on: the Dextrostix test; signs and treatment of hypoglycaemia: nursing care of a light for date baby.

**Define:** intra-uterine growth retardation; hypoglycaemia; hypothermia.

Differentiate between low birth weight and light for date: Silverman and Apgar scoring: Moro and traction reflex: hypocalcaemia and hypoglycaemia. What causes hypernatraemia and how can the midwife help to prevent this?

## METABOLIC DISORDERS

Describe the appearance of the baby of a diabetic mother. Why are they nursed in an incubator? What are the dangers during the first 48 hours?

Describe the treatment of the baby of the diabetic mother in detail. What are the causes of hypernatraemia? How do you collect a blood sample for the Guthrie test?

Write not more than 10 lines on each of the following: observation, feeding, nursing care of the baby of the diabetic mother.

**(N. Ireland) 30-min question.** What are the special risks to which the infant of a diabetic mother is exposed? Outline the management of the respiratory distress which often affects these infants.

How would you deal with a convulsion? What observations would you report to the doctor? Name the diagnostic tests that will be made.

What are the signs of hypothermia? How would you prevent and treat the condition? What is the range of a low reading thermometer?

## C.M.B. Short Questions

**Eng.:** The baby of a diabetic mother. **Eng.:** Hypoglycaemia in the newborn. **Scot.:** Diagnosis and treatment of hypoglycaemia. **N. Ireland:** Neonatal hypoglycaemia.

**Scot.:** Diagnosis and treatment of hypothermia. **Eng.:** Hypothermia (neonatal cold injury). **Eng.:** The neonatal cold syndrome.

**Eng.:** What is the Guthrie test? Why and when is it carried out? **Eng.:** The test for detecting phenylalanine? **Eng.:** Phenylketonuria. **Scot.:** The Guthrie test.

### Neonatal hypothermia

A hypothermic baby feels............to the touch, has a............cry: respirations are............he is............to feed, his temperature is below............

# 32
# Serious Neonatal Disorders

*Asphyxia: mild, severe: resuscitation, intubation, apnoea. Acid base status. Mechanical aids to respiration. Infections, prevention, ophthalmia neonatorum, urinary tract, thrush, epidemic gastro-enteritis. Rh haemolytic disease: prevention, management, intra-uterine and replacement transfusions. Haemorrhagic states*

## INTRA-UTERINE HYPOXIA

During intra-uterine life the mechanism of pulmonary respiration is held in abeyance by the fore-brain (slight respiratory movements do take place). If, during labour, the oxygen supply to the fetus is diminished, the respiratory centre is stimulated and the fetus breathes and inhales amniotic fluid which may be meconium stained: should oxygen lack continue, the fetus will die of anoxia. Slight intra-uterine hypoxia may have persisted over a long period or it may present as a sudden more severe episode as in prolapse of cord.

The main signs of intra-uterine hypoxia are slowing of the fetal heart rate and the passage of meconium (*causes and signs are discussed under fetal distress, p. 300*). Monitoring the fetal state during labour is essential in order that delivery takes place before oxygen lack causes brain damage or death. Fetal scalp blood sampling gives evidence of metabolic acidosis and the need for immediate intervention.

Pulmonary respiration is initiated when the respiratory centre in the medulla is stimulated by oxygen lack. This occurs when the uterine contraction that expels the baby's body causes the placenta to become partly detached from the uterine wall. The mechanism of respiration is also aided by compression of the thorax during the expulsion of the body, and the impact of the relatively cool air on the baby's skin.

## ASPHYXIA NEONATORUM

In this condition the baby at birth does not breathe. Asphyxia is usually classified under two main types, mild and severe, which are in actual fact clinical stages of the same condition.

### CAUSES

DYSFUNCTION OF THE RESPIRATORY CENTRE

**Immaturity**—as occurs in the smaller preterm baby.
**Depression**—due to narcotic drugs and general anaesthetics.
**Damage**—intracranial injury, haemorrhage or oedema.

OXYGEN LACK

**Blockage of airway** by thick mucus, meconium-stained amniotic fluid or blood.
**Maternal cyanosis**—as in eclampsia.
**Placental insufficiency** as in pre-eclampsia and postmaturity—premature separation as in antepartum haemorrhage.
**Cord**—Prolapse or true knot.

# MILD ASPHYXIA

This condition may be due to any of the causes mentioned, which have been of short duration or mild. It is frequently due to blockage of the airway with mucus. Response to treatment is usually prompt.

### SIGNS

The cord is pulsating strongly and feels firm. Apgar score 5 to 7.

The period of apnoea is usually short (less than 30 seconds); the infant makes an attempt to breathe.

Colour is a dusky, bluish red. Muscle tone is good.

## *Treatment*

**Clear the airway immediately** with a mucus extractor using short sharp sucks to prevent the inhalation of mucus during the first gasp and to allow the infant to obtain air. Mechanical suction should be gently used.

**Stimulate crying** by flicking the sole of the foot.

**Administer oxygen** by baby funnel or mask, not closely applied to the face, at 2 litres per minute. A stream of oxygen directed on the baby's face will stimulate respiration and provide high $O_2$ for the baby's first breaths.

**Clamp and cut the cord.** Wrap the infant in a warm towel and remove to the Resuscitaire.

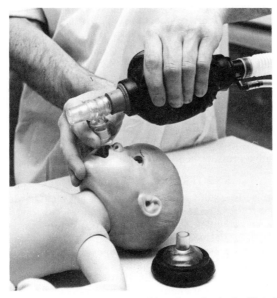

Fig. 32-1   Demonstration of use of Ambu bag with endotracheal tube. Note finger supporting lower jaw by pressure on bone (not on the soft tissue under the chin).

**For apnoea** when pethidine or morphine has been administered to the mother within three hours of birth neonatal naloxone (Narcan) 0·01 mg/kg may be administered i.v. or i.m.

**Summon medical aid** if the baby does not respond in one minute to the treatment given; prolonged oxygen lack will give rise to severe asphyxia.

# SEVERE ASPHYXIA

When shock is present at birth it is possible that intra-uterine hypoxia has existed or intracranial injury occurred. Hypoxia produces venous engorgement and capillary haemorrhage in the brain, lungs, heart, liver and other tissues: biochemical changes in the blood occur, i.e. respiratory and metabolic acidosis. Prolonged hypoxia will damage the brain cells and may give rise to mental retardation.

### SIGNS OF SEVERE ASPHYXIA

**The baby is not breathing.** (Later shallow breaths with occasional gasps may occur.)

**Colour is bluish white or grey. Apex beat** weak and slow.

**Cord feels flabby;** pulsations are feeble.

**Muscle tone is poor,** the infant cold and limp. **Apgar score 0 to 2.**

## *Resuscitation Equipment.*

**Baby laryngoscope.** Pharyngeal and endotracheal disposable mucus aspirators.

**Warne's endotracheal tubes** 10, 12, 14 FG. Suction catheters 5 FG aspiration tube 12 FG, stomach tube 12 FG, oesophageal tube 14 FG.

**Guedel neonatal airways** sizes 0, 00, 000.

**Syringes:** four 5 ml; six 2 ml with assorted needles; No. 19 **Venflon 25 FG, scalp vein needles.** Three way taps, micropore tape, scissors.

**Drugs:** naloxone neonatal (Narcan); vitamin $K_1$ (Konakion.)

**Fluids**—sterile water 100 ml for injections; Glucose 10 per cent for i.v. infusion, Isotonic saline in 100 ml bottles, sodium bicarbonate 8·4 and 5 per cent.

### TREATMENT OF SEVERE ASPHYXIA

**Send for medical aid.**

**Aspirate the pharynx,** then the nostrils using a mucus extractor.

Clamp and cut the cord. Keep baby warm. Handle gently.

When respiratory depression is due to opiates given to the mother during labour, neonatal naloxone (Narcan) 0·01 mg/kg is injected into the umbilical vein.

**Acid base status** is ascertained and dealt with. (For details see p. 550). IPPV intermittent positive pressure ventilation may be necessary (see p. 553).

## ENDOTRACHEAL INTUBATION

This procedure is carried out when the baby does not breathe within one minute of birth or sooner if the condition of the baby is causing anxiety. The stimulus of inserting the tube may stimulate the baby to make respiratory efforts. If necessary it should be done without delay.

**The Central Midwives Boards permit the midwife to carry out intubation** in appropriate cases if she has been properly trained in the procedure and has obtained permission from the health authority under whom she is working. Midwives should be aware that endotracheal intubation should not be undertaken without due need as well as adequate instruction and practise under supervision. Inexpert intubation may cause soft tissue damage and induce laryngeal spasm.

## *Procedure*

**The baby is placed on a Resuscitaire** or high table with an overhead radiant heat source. He is laid on his back on a downward inclined plane, head slightly extended.

**An infant laryngoscope** held in the left hand is passed gently over the dorsum of the tongue which is depressed until the epiglottis is seen.

**Mucus in the glottis is carefully aspirated.** An endotracheal tube 10 or 12 FG is inserted into the glottis and a fine mechanical suction catheter 5 FG is used to clear the trachea; the laryngoscope is removed.

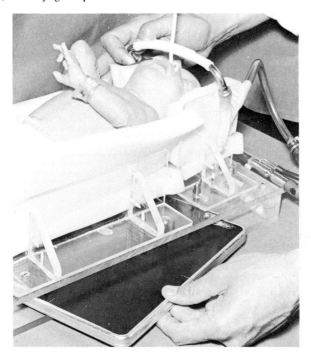

Fig. 32-2   X-raying a baby on artificial ventilation. The infant, attached to a Jackson-Rees endotracheal tube, lies in a perspex foam-lined cradle which stabilises his head and, being radiolucent, allows X-rays to be taken without disturbance.

*Neonatal Intensive Care Unit, Simpson Memorial Maternity Pavilion, Edinburgh.*

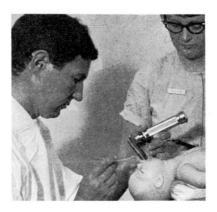

Fig. 32-3   Paediatrician demonstrating position for holding the laryngoscope prior to insertion of endotracheal tube. Note pillow under shoulders to hyperextend the head.

*Neonatal Paediatric Unit, Royal Maternity Hospital, Rottenrow, Glasgow.*

**The endotracheal tube is connected to the oxygen and IPPV** (intermittent positive pressure ventilation) **apparatus** to expand the lungs, deliver oxygen-enriched air and initiate respiration. (See page 553.) 1 mg Vitamin $K_1$ (Konakion) is given i.m. in cases of asphyxia.

## ADMISSION TO THE INTENSIVE CARE UNIT

**Following resuscitation, intensive incubator care is essential.** Electronic cardiac monitoring is carried out. Arterial blood pressure is assessed and hypotension combated. In some centres, blood gas tensions and pH are estimated and biochemical status controlled by sodium bicarbonate 8·4 per cent and glucose 10 per cent. An Electrodyne contactless apnoea monitor is recommended.

### *Observation*

**The rate and type of respiration,** apnoeic episodes, indrawing of sternal region and chest wall.

**Colour changes.**

**The apex beat,** particularly bradycardia.

**The rectal temperature** is recorded 4-hourly, and maintained within the neutral thermal range 36·5° to 37·5°C to reduce oxygen consumption and acidosis.

### *Nursing Care*

**Skilled, devoted nursing** is mandatory with intelligent observation and sufficient knowledge to cope with emergencies.

**Warmth and quietness** are essential. Minimal handling with great gentleness is of cardinal importance.

**Oxygen,** which is warmed and humidified, is administered in sufficient concentration to relieve cyanosis as required.

**Head and shoulders are raised:** the baby being propped over on his side and turned every two hours.

**The Dextrostix test is made** before feeds for 24–72 hours if hypoglycaemia is anticipated and early feeding by nasogastric tube carried out.

When inhalation of meconium stained amniotic fluid has occurred, a broad spectrum antibiotic is given as a prophylactic measure.

#### APNOEA

Apnoea is more common in the preterm infant and may be due to various causes: respiratory, intracranial, biochemical, infection and overheating. When apnoeic episodes occur a contactless Electrodyne apnoea monitor is used: a red light will flash and stay on to show that an apnoeic episode is occurring or has occurred: an audible alarm also sounds.

In mild cases flicking the foot, arching the chest by placing a hand under the back at about shoulder level, will often stimulate respiratory effort. The airway should, of course, be cleared of mucus or vomitus as necessary.

When cyanosis is present immediate resuscitation using oxygen, bag and mask is performed followed by the use of CPAP (continuous positive airway pressure) or by aminophylline as a respiratory stimulant: some combine the two. If apnoea recurs or if the pH is less than 7.2, mechanical ventilation is recommended.

#### ACID BASE STATUS

This should be ascertained by blood sampling and analysis by a gas analyser or more rarely the Astrup machine.

**Respiratory acidosis** occurs when the infant is unable to excrete carbon dioxide:

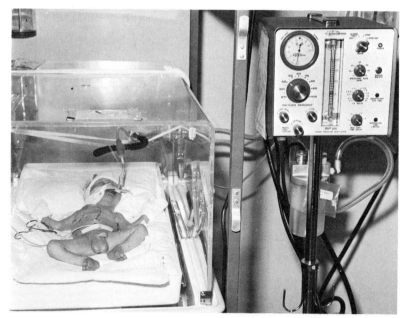

Fig. 32-4  Baby having assisted ventilation with Bourne's ventilator. Umbilical catheter inserted for blood gas analysis.

*Queen Mother's Hospital, Glasgow.*

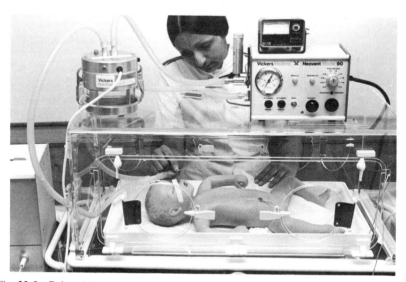

Fig. 32-5  Baby with asphyxia and low Apgar score having assisted ventilation in Vicker's incubator 79 model. Neovent, humidifier and oxygen analyser on top of model. Midwife adjusting nasotracheal tube.

*Aberdeen Maternity Hospital.*

carbonic acid is produced in the blood, the infant becomes acidotic, the pH falls. The condition is dealt with by pulmonary ventilation.

**Metabolic acidosis,** is caused by acute oxygen lack and inhibits respiratory centre function. The situation must be dealt with urgently. Biochemical monitoring of the blood is carried out and to correct the acid base balance glucose 10 per cent and sodium bicarbonate 8·4 per cent, depending on the pH of the blood, is given via an umbilical artery. Oxygen is administered in sufficient concentration to relieve cyanosis.

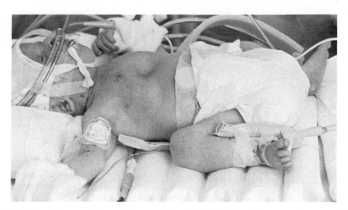

Fig. 32-6   Baby with sternal recession receiving CPAP using rubber nasal prongs. Orogastric tube in situ to keep stomach deflated. Electrode on right arm attached to cardiac monitor. Indwelling venous catheter in right foot for Cockburn cocktail. Baby lying on apnoea alarm mattress.

*Royal Maternity Hospital, Rottenrow, Glasgow.*

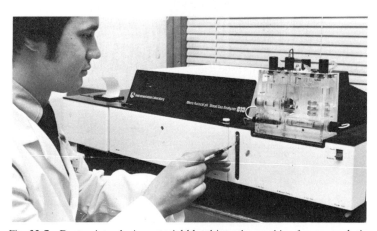

Fig. 32-7   Doctor introducing arterial blood into the machine for gas analysis.

*Aberdeen Maternity Hospital.*

**Hypoglycaemia** occurs during severe asphyxia and may cause brain damage: glucose 10 per cent is administered intra-arterially.

## IPPV

**Intermittent positive pressure ventilation is** utilised when the baby fails to breathe or when the Apgar score is 0–1 at birth or below 6 at five minutes. IPPV may also be employed if breathing is not sustained following intubation. To expand the lungs and initiate respiration, oxygen or oxygen-enriched air is delivered at 30 cm water pressure, which is reduced in a few minutes to 15–10 cm and maintained until spontaneous respiration is established. The oxygen flow lasts one second and is repeated at two second intervals. A simple water manometer that blows off at 30 cm is used when sophisticated equipment is not available. Pressure above 30 cm might rupture the alveoli of the lungs. An inflation bag or T-piece may be connected directly to the endotracheal tube. Subsequently the airway is sucked out and kept clear of mucus: the baby is turned every hour, pressure areas on the ears and other vulnerable areas are dealt with.

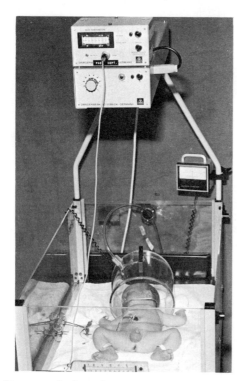

Fig. 32-8  Baby in Draegar unit. Servo heat control; oxygen head box; oxygen analyser; umbilical catheters in situ.

*Royal Maternity Hospital, Rottenrow, Glasgow.*

## CPAP

**Continuous positive airway pressure** is applied to assist respiration and prevent the alveoli of the lungs from collapsing on expiration in a baby who is breathing spontaneously. The oxygen pressure is maintained during the inspiratory and expiratory phases of respiration to improve oxygenation. CPAP may be applied via rubber nasal prongs, endotracheal tube, face mask, or less frequently a perspex head box (which has a disposable collar seal that fits snugly around the neck but should not constrict the neck veins). The positive pressure and flow-rate of the warmed humidified oxygen is controlled. Oxygen-enriched air, warmed and humidified, flows into the head box which contains a thermometer, hygrometer and oxygen analyser. The head is stabilised by sand bags and rests on a foam rubber pad to prevent occipital pressure sores.

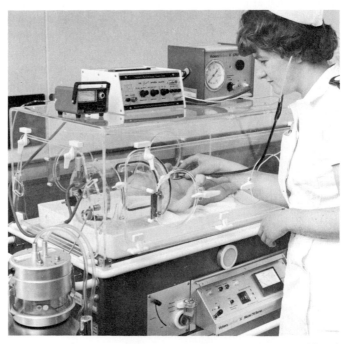

Fig. 32-9   Baby with respiratory difficulty having CPAP (continuous positive airway pressure). On top of incubator is the oxygen analyser, apnoea alarm. CPAP cabinet. Humidifier at foot of incubator.

*Aberdeen Maternity Hospital.*

An Electrodyne contactless apnoea monitor is placed under the mattress.

**Nasal rubber prongs,** may be used as a means of applying CPAP. To prevent nasal sores Naseptin cream is introduced into the nostrils every two hours. Babies receiving CPAP are not fed orally because of the danger of inhaling vomitus in the supine position; the i.v. route is preferred. A cardiac monitor is utilised.

Hourly checks are made of respiration, oxygen concentration, humidity, i.v. fluid in the giving set. Four-hourly: body and incubator temperature. Twice daily weighing is carried out to assess fluid balance.

## CNP

**Continuous negative pressure** is an alternative to CPAP and provides continuous distending pressure within the lungs; the baby's body being placed in a negative pressure chamber. The intrathoracic pressure is then higher than the pressure surrounding the baby's chest: a blow off valve is provided. The infant's head is readily available for intubation and other treatment. See Fig. 32-15.

**PEEP. Positive end expiratory pressure** may be employed when in cases of respiratory distress syndrome CPAP does not attain the desired results. PEEP prevents the end phase of expiration from reaching zero pressure and prevents collapse of the alveoli.

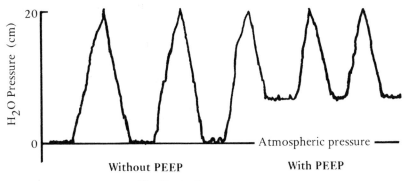

Fig. 32-10   Drawing—PEEP.

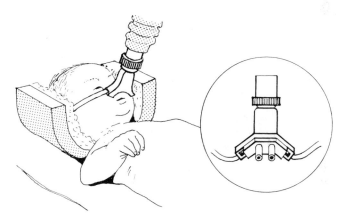

Fig. 32-11   Nasal rubber prongs used to give oxygen by CPAP.

**Artificial respiration.** The Bourne and the Draeger are well-known respirators used when other methods are inadequate for the baby who does not breathe spontaneously.

### Face mask and bag

The pharynx and then the nostrils must first be cleared of mucus. A neonatal face mask and inflating bag can be used to deliver oxygen or oxygen-enriched air under pressure (a) to expand the lungs when the baby has not breathed and (b) to sustain ventilation for short periods when the infant fails to breathe properly. The range of pressure depends on the rate and vigour with which the bag is squeezed: 40 times per minute being average. An inbuilt pressure-limiting valve present in some models, prevents over-inflation (and rupture) of the alveoli. Masks should only be closely applied to the face when a blow off valve is provided or the inflation bag is soft.

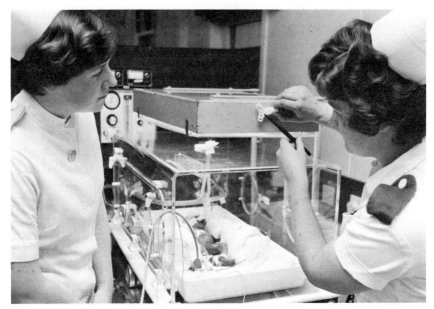

Fig. 32-12   Nursing officer showing nasal prongs to student midwife. Baby in incubator receiving oxygen by CPAP.

*Aberdeen Maternity Hospital.*

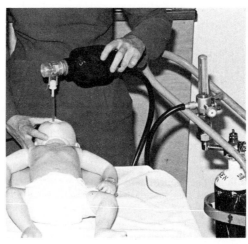

Fig. 32-13   Demonstration of Ambu bag and endotracheal tube to administer oxygen under IPPV (intermittent positive pressure ventilation).

If a Guedel or other oropharyngeal airway is not available, the lower jaw must be firmly supported; pressure being applied to the jaw bone not to the soft tissue. In some models a small aperture is blocked and unblocked by the finger every two seconds to provide IPPV (intermittent positive pressure ventilation). When a positive pressure apparatus is operated by a finger occluding an open T-piece, a blow off manometer is essential.

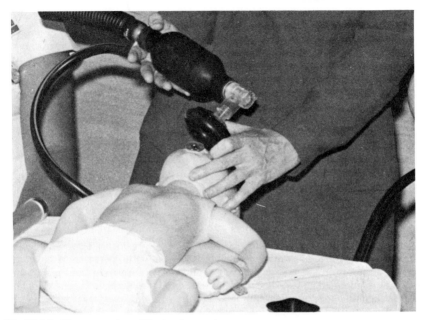

Fig. 32-14   Demonstration of Penlon bag and mask with oral airway to deliver 100 per cent oxygen.

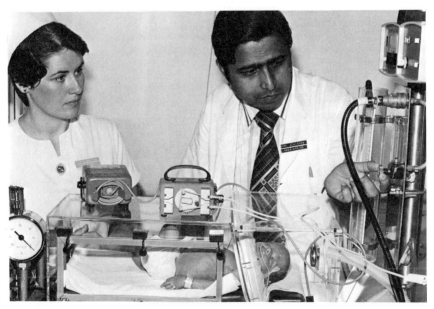

Fig. 32-15   Draeger continuous negative pressure chamber, (baby's body is exposed to negative pressure) the head is exposed for giving duodenal naso gastric feeds and is resting on a foam pillow. An oxygen analyser, and Holter pump to regulate milk of i.v. fluids, are on top of the chamber: a negative pressure 'blow off' is at the foot of the chamber.

*Royal Maternity Hospital, Rottenrow, Glasgow.*

**Mouth to mouth breathing**

This procedure, which requires no equipment, can be used when a better method is not available. The airway must first be cleared by mucus extractor. Gauze may be placed over the baby's mouth and nose. The midwife fills her mouth with air, holds her breath and expels air into the baby's mouth using as much force as it would take to blow out a small candle: undue force would rupture the alveoli of the lungs. If oxygen is at hand a catheter placed in the midwife's mouth will increase the oxygen content of the air delivered to the baby.

# INFECTIONS OF THE NEWBORN BABY

**The prevention and control of neonatal infection is a major problem** in maternity hospitals in which the common infecting organism, the staphylococcus aureus, is penicillin resistant. Non-haemolytic streptococci are now causing infection in the neonate. Infection is spread from baby to baby via the hands and clothing of the staff and also by air and dust.

The pseudomonas aeruginosa (pyocyanea) group of organisms, a contaminant of humidifying systems is causing neonatal infection with increasing frequency: urinary, respiratory and umbilical. Suction and oxygen apparatus and respirators should be dismantled and washed with hot water and a suitable detergent. Sudol or Tego is recommended for cleansing incubators, sinks and other surfaces.

The provision of a cubicle for mother and baby with individual equipment including toilet and hand basin is ideal: rooming in is recommended. Nurseries should be small with not more than four cots and at least 60 cm of space between them. Admission of patients beyond the optimal number should be avoided: invariably this results in the nursing staff being overworked and unable to carry out good barrier-nursing technique.

**No person who is suffering from a respiratory infection,** diarrhoea, or who has any septic focus, should be in contact with babies.

### THE NEED FOR CLEANLINESS

Domestic and personal cleanliness with the liberal use of soap and water is the first essential. Vacuum cleaners are employed to avoid the dissemination of dust; daily scrubbing of floors and damp dusting of furniture are essential, sinks and their plug holes scrubbed. Incubators and individual equipment must be cleansed daily and replaced by clean ones at least weekly and on discharge of each infant. Adequate supplies of clean baby and cot clothing as well as bed linen for the mother should be provided.

Facilities for handwashing in sluice rooms are essential.

**Vigilant observation**

Babies should be inspected thoroughly every day while naked, and isolated for a septic lesion. Prompt reporting to the doctor is necessary in order that the appropriate investigations and treatment can be carried out.

### NURSING TECHNIQUE

**Hand washing is most important**

Between the handling of babies the hands are washed for 30 seconds and dried with disposable towels; wrist watches prevent thorough hand washing and should not be worn. Hand washing should follow immediately after the use of paper handkerchiefs, which are used once only and discarded.

### Making up feeds

Cleanliness and surgical aseptic technique are essential.

Terminal sterilisation of feeds is recommended.

Teats on bottles should have individual covers.

The staff who make up or issue feeds should not change napkins or attend to puerperal women.

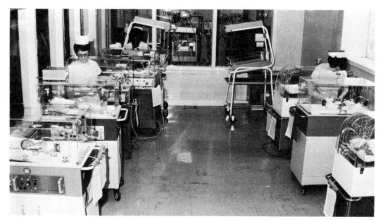

Fig. 32-16   Neonatal intensive care unit.

*Queen Mother's Hospital, Glasgow.*

### Modified barrier nursing

The rooming-in plan provides a means whereby handling of the baby by the nursing staff and consequent risk of infection is reduced. Perspex cots on metal trolleys are available with adequate storage space for equipment and ample linen for the individual baby. The wearing by nurses of a separate gown for each baby ought to, but has not proved to, be an effective means of limiting the spread of infection, probably because of staff shortage and insufficient time to observe the proper technique of gown-wearing. The wearing of simple short-sleeved dresses issued daily, is commendable.

Napkins can be changed and babies sponge-bathed in their cots. When a midwife must change the napkins of a series of infants in their cots, she ought to wear a gown which is subsequently discarded: disposable aprons are available: they should be worn for feeding only or bathing and changing napkins only. Hands must be washed between handling each baby.

### Mask wearing

Mask wearing has not proved an efficient means of reducing neonatal infections. When worn for long periods the mouth becomes an incubator for organisms.

Talking should be reduced to the absolute minimum if masks are not worn when handling babies in order to avoid droplet infection; the midwife should turn her head away from the baby if talking is necessary.

### Handling napkins

Soiled napkins should be placed immediately in a covered receptacle, removed after a 'changing round' and sent directly to the laundry where they are boiled as well as washed: disposable ones are destroyed. Feeding-bibs used in incubators should be disposable and must not come in contact with the napkin area. Baby clothes should be boilable and laundry methods subjected to critical appraisal. Cotton cellular blankets can be autoclaved.

### Isolation

A self-contained unit should be available for babies suffering from an infectious condition, with adequate individual equipment, disposable napkins and other means for limiting the spread of infection. Units for mother and baby are essential for some cases: some recommend removing the baby from the midwifery department.

## OPHTHALMIA NEONATORUM

Ophthalmia neonatorum is a notifiable disease, and the doctor notifies the Chief Administrative Medical Officer of the Area Health Authority (Health Board, Scot.).

#### DEFINITION

**(England).**—'A purulent discharge from the eyes of an infant commencing within 21 days of its birth.'

**(Scotland).**—'Any inflammation that occurs in the eyes of an infant within 21 days of birth and is accompanied by a discharge.'

#### CAUSE

The baby's eyes may be infected during his passage through the birth canal, or later by the mother's hands. The midwife may infect the eyes by failing to observe prophylactic measures.

A number of cases of neonatal conjunctivitis are due to the *B. proteus* and *Staphylococcus aureus,* which produce a profuse yellow discharge. Pneumococci and streptococci are sometimes found, but the gonococcus is most dreaded because of its destructive action. The *Ps. aeruginosa* causes severe ophthalmia; blindness having been reported.

**The TRIC agent conjunctivitis** now known as **chlamdial** ophthalmia neonatorum occurs at about the 6th to 10th day with a watery discharge. It is treated with tetracycline drops or ointment. If resistant Vibramycin is prescribed. A cervical smear is taken from the mother.

### MANAGEMENT OF OPHTHALMIA NEONATORUM

#### Prophylaxis

The treatment of vaginal discharge during pregnancy.

The midwife, with clean hands, should wipe the eyes at birth with large pledgets of dry sterile cotton wool. (Some bacteriologists consider that this procedure is ineffective.)

The midwife should always wash her hands before touching the baby's face, which ought to be washed before the head and body, and cleanse the buttocks last. The mother ought to be told not to use her handkerchief to wipe the baby's eyes.

Midwives must carry out the methods of prevention and treatment as laid down by their employing authority.

**Active treatment**

Medical aid is sought, the infant isolated.

The midwife notifies the local supervising authority of ophthalmia neonatorum.

A smear and culture of the discharge is sent to the bacteriological laboratory, where the causal organism is identified and tested for sensitivity to the antibiotics. *Some use Stuart's transport medium. (When the baby of an unbooked mother develops a 'sticky eye' a smear and culture is taken immediately and examined for gonococci.)*

An antibiotic preparation such as neosporin or chloramphenicol eye drops 0·5 per cent are instilled into the conjunctival sac hourly for 8 hours and 4 hourly thereafter for 5 days. Framycetin ointment is used in some centres.

For *Pseudomonas aeruginosa*, Polymyxin (Neosporin) eye drops are specific.

## GONOCOCCAL OPHTHALMIA

### SIGNS

**Ophthalmia neonatorum** may be manifest by the 4th day as a sticky, watery discharge, with slight reddening of the conjunctiva. The inflammation quickly spreads, the conjunctiva covering the eyeball and lining the lids being congested and often oedematous; the discharge becomes copious in amount and purulent. The eyelids also may be inflamed and swollen and are kept tightly shut.

The immediate transfer of cases, infected by the gonococcus, from the neonatal department to an isolation unit is imperative. Strict precautions and prompt treatment are essential because of the danger of blindness.

**When swabs have been taken, penicillin eye drops 2500 units/ml** (2 drops) are instilled into both conjunctival sacs every 5 minutes during the first hour, then hourly for 24 hours and 2-hourly until the purulent discharge ceases. Benzyl penicillin 50,000 units/kg/day intramuscularly is given for 7 days.

Neomycin, gramicidin or Terramycin ointment by preventing the eyelids from becoming adherent ensures good drainage from the conjunctival sac. Bathing the eyes is not necessary unless the discharge is profuse, and should consist in gentle wiping of the lids with large pledgets of wool. The baby should be laid on the side of the infected eye, so that the pus will drain on to a dressing laid under the head.

### *Blindness*

In serious neglected cases of gonococcal ophthalmia milkiness of the cornea ensues, followed by ulceration and subsequent impairment of vision: occasionally perforation of the cornea takes place, giving rise to blindness.

## UMBILICAL INFECTIONS (Omphalitis)

**The common infecting organism is the E. coli.** Cases of tetanus have occurred following the use of unsterile cord powder. Some authorities spray all cords at birth with polymyxin (Polybactrin) and daily until the cord separates. Inflammation, discharge or an offensive odour should be reported to the doctor.

### *Spread of and Treatment of the Infection*

The infection spreads into the cellular tissue, and an area, the size of a coffee cup, may be red and indurated (in some cases there is no visible inflammation). Neomycin bacitracin (Cicatrin) powder or Thiomersil 1–1000 is useful for a sticky umbilicus. The antibiotic to which the organism is sensitive is administered systemically, e.g. penicillin and gentamicin. Hexachlorophane powder may be applied.

The infection may spread via the umbilical vein to the liver causing hepatitis. Jaundice arising in the second week, even when no local signs of infection are manifest, is suggestive of this condition. Septicaemia usually follows. The association with abdominal distension is particularly ominous; blood culture is carried out without delay.

### Umbilical polypus

A reddish brown tag, about 1·25 cm long and 0·3 cm in diameter, occasionally develops when there has been a low grade umbilical infection, and is seen three or four weeks after birth. The doctor will apply copper sulphate or a silver nitrate stick or ligate it.

## PEMPHIGUS NEONATORUM (BULLOUS IMPETIGO)

Pemphigus, a highly contagious skin disease of the newborn, characterised by watery blisters, is rarely seen in the severe form today. The organism is usually the *Staphylococcus aureus* and the initial lesions are pink macules, which rapidly form vesicles and then pustules surrounded with a red ring.

### *Treatment*

Notify the doctor promptly. A swab is taken from one of the blebs to test the organisms for sensitivity to the antibiotics: the baby is isolated.

Administration of an antibiotic, both local and systemic, as indicated by the sensitivity tests. Cloxacillin or erythromycin may be used in severe cases pending the result of sensitivity tests.

Wipe the blebs with Thiomersil 1–1000, remove epidermis from the blebs.

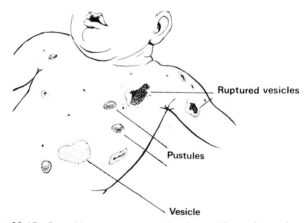

Fig. 32-17   Pemphigus neonatorum, showing vesicles and pustules.

#### URINARY TRACT INFECTION

This gives rise to attacks that look like fainting in which the infant becomes limp and grey. The temperature may not be raised; vomiting may be present. (*To obtain a specimen of urine the Sterilon paediatric urine collector is useful for boy or girl babies.*) This is sent to the laboratory within one hour. When a baby is 'off colour' a bag specimen of urine is obtained and if positive suprapubic aspiration of bladder is carried out using a size 21 needle. When the sensitivity test is received the appropriate antibiotic is given e.g. gentamicin. A urinary anti-infective such as cephalexin (Ceporex) is beneficial.

*Ps. aeruginosa* (pyocyanea) is resistant to many antibiotics. Colistin (Colomycin) i.m., 50,000 iu. per kg, in 24 hours is effective or carbenicillin (Pyopen). The condition may take six weeks or longer to clear up and may be associated with congenital renal tract abnormality. Radiological investigation is carried out when the acute pyelonephritis has subsided: intravenous pyelography will usually be carried out.

## KIDNEY AND URINARY TRACT ABNORMALITIES (non-infectious)

These may be suspected in cases where the ears are low-set or there is only one umbilical artery. Failure of urinary secretion is associated with oligohydramnios.

**Bladder extrophy** (ectopia vesicae). The bladder is exposed on the lower abdomen with urine oozing from it. Treatment may be transplant of ureters into the rectum.

**Renal agenesis** (imperfect development) is associated with other malformations.

**Epispadias.** Urethra opens on the upper surface of the penis. Treatment: surgical repair later.

**Hypospadias.** Urethra opens on the under surface of the penis near the tip. Treatment: surgical repair later.

## THRUSH *(Candidiasis)*

Oral thrush is characterised by white patches in the mouth, that are composed of epithelial cells; the causal organism is the *Candida albicans*. Thush does not occur prior to the fourth day. The mother's vagina, the baby's mouth and hands, and the midwife's hands are sources or means of spreading infection.

The greyish-white raised patches, often surrounded by a zone of inflammation, are seen inside the cheeks, on the gums, palate and tongue. A milky tongue looks like grey paint and has an even distribution, but spots on the edges of the tongue are diagnostic, as sucking would remove milk curd from that region. A raw area is left on removing one of these lesions which are more adherent than milk curds. In mild cases the infant is not upset, but in severe cases he goes off his feeds, vomits, becomes irritable, looks greyish and may have loose stools and sore buttocks. The condition may be fatal to preterm babies, the lungs and intestinal tract being involved.

### Treatment

Treat vaginal candidiasis in the pregnant woman. Good nursery technique, daily inspection of mouths.

Notify the doctor: use barrier nursing.

If the mouth is very dirty it must first be swabbed with sodium bicarbonate solution. Apply dequalinium (Dequadin) paint, three-hourly, or nystatin (Nystan), 100,000 units per ml, (which must be shaken vigorously prior to each application), four times daily 4 to 7 days. In resistant cases gentian violet, 0·5 per cent aqueous solution, is applied twice daily for three days and once daily until the lesions disappear; cotton wool on Spencer Wells' forceps is used. Gentian violet, 0·06 ml (one minim), is dropped with a pipette on the back of the tongue. Staining of tissues and linen is a disadvantage. Gentian violet is very drying, and if applied too frequently will cause sloughing of the mucous membrane. Nystaform cream is suitable for sore buttocks due to candidiasis.

## EPIDEMIC GASTRO–ENTERITIS *(Neonatal)*

This is a treacherous scourge because of its insidious onset and rapid course. Unless the midwife recognises the early signs, other babies will be infected before the disease is diagnosed; successful treatment depends greatly on its being started early. Epidemics still occur: various strains of *E. coli* being involved.

The condition rarely develops before the end of the first week. The stools are not always green, neither are they invariably offensive. The temperature is seldom elevated.

**First day.** The earliest sign is sudden loss of appetite; the infant is listless and pale; the stools may or may not be loose at this stage: an abrupt loss of weight occurs.

**Second day.** The stools are watery and yellow, like urine, as many as 10 daily, or they may be uncountable.

Signs of dehydration occur, such as dry mouth, sunken fontanelle and overlapping of the skull bones; the face is pinched, eyes dull and sunken with dark rings.

Metabolic acidosis is common: clinically this being manifest by rapid, deep, respirations.

Vomiting may be present; abdominal distension develops in severe cases. The infant becomes collapsed, greyish-blue in colour, and if untreated death may ensue.

### *Treatment*

**Prophylaxis.** Breast-feeding; impeccable nursery technique; scrupulous cleanliness in preparing bottle feeds.

**Strict isolation** and the use of destructible napkins. Preferably the baby is transferred to the isolation unit of a children's hospital.

**Rectal swabs** are taken for stool culture and sensitivity tests. (Swabs also taken from contacts.)

Milk is withheld for 24 hours at least. The fluid intake must be maintained.

Correction of dehydration is accomplished in mild cases by the oral administration of fluid: giving 120 ml per 450 g body-weight for the first 24 hours.

Replacement of electrolytes is essential in severe cases and is effected by the administration of isotonic saline or plasma with glucose 5 per cent then give 0·18 per cent saline with 5 per cent glucose by slow intravenous drip or as indicated by biochemical investigation. Intravenous fluid is given until vomiting ceases.

Kaomycin (which contains neomycin and kaolin) is excellent in most cases of intestinal infection, dose 4 ml every six hours.

When improvement is noted in about three days, by the diarrhoea lessening and the appetite returning, skimmed breast milk, or modified dried milk, 1 in 3 is given.

## RESPIRATORY INFECTIONS

Babies are readily infected from the mother or a member of the nursery staff who has a 'cold,' if precautions are not taken. Nasopharyngitis is recognised by snuffles, and if the infection spreads downwards the cry becomes hoarse. The baby should be isolated, given extra fluid and kept comfortably warm. Bronchopneumonia may develop and is sometimes fatal.

Nose and throat swabs are taken, the usual infecting organism being the staphylococcus aureus. If there is any question of the baby having inhaled meconium-stained amniotic fluid broad spectrum antibiotics are given prophylactically, e.g. four neonatal vials per day for five days; the baby may require oxygen and high humidity.

### PNEUMONIA

This condition is more common in preterm babies (probably due to inhalation of vomitus), in hypoxic babies who have inhaled much amniotic fluid, and on the rare occasions in which the membranes have been ruptured for 36 hours prior to birth. Group B streptococci the common infecting agent is sensitive to penicillin.

Respirations are rapid, over 60 per minute, and may be grunting or laboured. Cyanosis is manifest in severe cases.

The temperature may not be high. Listlessness. Diarrhoea or vomiting may be present. Refusal to feed is common.

In severe cases the infant is in a shock like state with apnoeic attacks.

A radiograph of the chest is obtained to confirm the diagnosis.

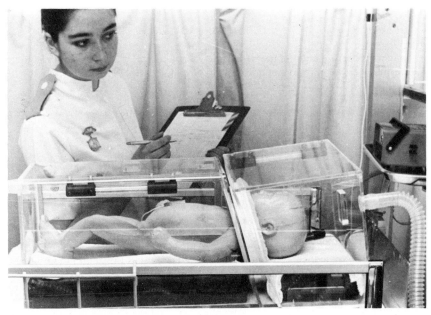

Fig. 32-18  Baby with respiratory infection. Head box to provide oxygen. Negative pressure applied to body and chest to expand the lungs.

*Aberdeen Maternity Hospital.*

### Treatment

The baby should be isolated in a warm room, 21°C, with a humid atmosphere or, if cyanosed, nursed in an incubator (oxygen concentration sufficient to abolish cyanosis). Pulmonary ventilation may be necessary.

**Antibiotics** are administered e.g. ampicillin 200 mg/kg/day and gentamicin 5 mg/kg body weight, per day.

The baby is turned from side to side (propped with a small pillow) every hour or two.

**Mucus should be removed** by suction from mouth and nostrils to keep a clear airway. For apnoeic episodes mechanical ventilation may be employed.

**Feeding** must be carried out by an experienced nursery midwife to avoid choking or exhaustion: feeds should be small; naso-gastric feeding is advisable. If sucking causes respiratory distress or exhaustion, intravenous fluids are given.

**Clothing** must be warm but light to prevent excessive perspiration. The infant should not be tightly wrapped to avoid hampering the movement of the thoracic and abdominal muscles used in respiration.

### Meningitis

This infection is three times more common in babies of low birth weight and is frequently caused by enteric organisms.

**Signs are non-specific,** e.g. vomiting, diarrhoea, lethargy. Only a few have a bulging fontanelle and neck stiffness: diagnosis is confirmed by lumbar puncture. Antibiotic therapy is given according to the organism isolated and its sensitivity. The intrathecal route may be utilised.

## SUPERFICIAL INFECTIONS

These must be controlled as they may be the source of more severe infections.

### Rhinitis

To relieve engorgement of the nasal mucosa ephedrine, 0·25 per cent, in isotonic saline, may be applied by dropper for 2 or 3 days. Oily drops should never be used.

### Septic spots

The baby must be isolated to prevent cross infection. The spots should be wiped with Thiomersil 1–1000, and framycetin (Soframycin) cream applied.

### Nailfold infection (paronychia)

Injury to nailfolds by rough drying and sucking the fingers predispose to infection.

The fingers should be wiped with Thiomersil 1–1000 or gentian violet 1 per cent aqueous solution and the hand enclosed in a cotton mitten.

### Neonatal mastitis

Abscess formation may result from squeezing engorged breasts. The area is red, hard, shiny. *Treatment:* Incision and drainage. (The author saw 4 ml pus evacuated from the breast of a baby two weeks old.)

# HAEMOLYTIC DISEASE OF THE NEWBORN

## *Due to Rhesus Incompatibility*

Rhesus haemolytic disease of the newborn is an important immunological disorder. The rhesus factor is an antigen present on the red blood cells of 83 per cent of the population: those having this antigen are classified as Rh positive; the 17 per cent who do not have the antigen are known as Rh negative. Rhesus incompatibility occurs mainly in the pregnant woman who is Rh negative.

### INHERITANCE OF THE Rh FACTOR

**The Rh factor is transmitted in the genes of the chromosomes of both ovum and spermatozoon.** If both parents are Rh− the fetus would be Rh−; if both parents are Rh+ the fetus would be Rh+ and in both instances there would be no incompatibility.

Rh incompatibility only arises when the mother is Rh− and the father is Rh+. The fetus always inherits the positive gene rather than the negative one. A further problem arises because the father may have inherited an Rh− gene from one of his parents and an Rh+ gene from his other parent: his genotype would be heterozygous. In such a case half of his genes will be Rh− and compatible with an Rh− mother; the other half being Rh+ will be incompatible. The father's genotype may be homozygous when he inherits from both his parents an Rh+ gene: all his genes will be Rh+. The father's genotype may be tested during his Rh− wife's pregnancy to find out whether he is homozygous or heterozygous to predict whether all subsequent babies are likely to be incompatible.

There are three pairs of Rh antigens: Cc, Dd, Ee; the D antigen being the cause of immunisation in 95 per cent of cases. The capital letter = Rh positive: the small letter = Rh negative.

## IMMUNISATION OF THE Rh− PREGNANT WOMAN

**If the Rh− woman has an Rh+ fetus in utero** it is possible that fetal red cells, which contain the Rh antigen, will enter her circulation. Normally fetal and maternal blood does not mix during pregnancy, but on occasions partial placental separation occurs and a 'feto-maternal bleed' ensues. This could happen during abortion, amniocentesis, version or antepartum haemorrhage, but is much more likely to take place during the third stage of labour. In many cases 2 ml of fetal blood enters the maternal circulation during the third stage of labour but no difficulty arises unless the woman is Rh− and her fetus is Rh+.

The Rh antigens on the fetal red cells stimulate the maternal reticulo-endothelial system to produce antibodies which will destroy the fetal red cells containing the Rh antigen. The woman immunises herself against the Rh antigen and will continue to produce antibodies during any subsequent pregnancy. That the feto-maternal bleed most commonly occurs during the third stage of labour explains why there is no incompatibility with the first Rh+ baby unless the Rh− woman had been immunised previously by inadvertently receiving a transfusion of Rh+ blood.

Transfusing an Rh− woman with Rh+ blood does not take place today: laboratory techniques are designed to ensure that no Rh− female from babyhood to the menopause will receive a transfusion of Rh+ blood. The formation of antibodies is the natural response of the Rh− woman to the invasion of Rh+ blood into her circulation. These antibodies are liable to pass from the maternal to the fetal circulation via a leak in the placenta and will haemolyse the red cells of the fetus that carry the Rh antigen.

**Haemolysis** is the excessive destruction of red cells and this causes severe anaemia in the fetus. One of the end results of haemolysis is manifest as jaundice: anaemia and jaundice being characteristic of Rh haemolytic disease of the newborn.

## *Prevention of Maternal Immunisation*

(1) **Preventing Rh− women from producing antibodies** will reduce if not abolish Rh haemolytic disease of the newborn: the most effective means of prevention being an immunological one. When the Rh− woman has been subjected to conditions in which a feto-maternal bleed would be expected to occur, e.g. abortion, placental abruption or most likely the third stage of labour, it is usual to do the Kleihauer test which reveals the presence of fetal red cells in maternal blood.

Within 72 hours of the feto-maternal bleed, the Rh− woman is given an i.m. injection of Rh anti-D immunoglobulin (IgG) which coats the offending fetal Rh+ red cells in the maternal circulation before her reticulo-endothelial system is stimulated to produce antibodies.

The current arrangements in the United Kingdom are: The Rh− woman without antibodies is given within 72 hours after delivery of an Rh+ fetus, 100 micrograms of Rh anti (D) immunoglobulin i.m. If the Kleihauer test for detecting fetal cells in maternal blood shows that a large 'bleed' has occurred, a larger dose of 1 gG would be administered.

Following an abortion up to 12 weeks' gestation, 50 micrograms of anti-D IgG would be given. Following an abortion after 12 weeks she would receive 100 micrograms. Should anti (D) IgG not be given, the woman will form antibodies.

(2) **Avoidance of giving Rh+ blood to an Rh− female** from her birth to the menopause.

(3) **Reducing the incidence of 'feto maternal bleeds'** (a) doing a sonar scan prior to amniocentesis to locate and avoid penetrating the placenta; (b) using gentle manipulation when performing version or manual removal of placenta; (c) refraining as far as possible from abdominal palpation in cases of placental abruption.

CLINICAL MANIFESTATIONS OF Rh HAEMOLYTIC DISEASES

## (1) Hydrops fetalis

This is the most serious form of Rh haemolytic disease. Fetal anaemia is so severe that cardiac failure may ensue: the baby at birth is grossly oedematous with an enlarged abdomen due to ascites, usually stillborn and macerated. If born alive, the baby occasionally survives. The mother will have had polyhydramnios which in an Rh− woman with antibodies should give rise to suspicion of hydrops fetalis. An X-ray film may (rarely) show a Buddha-like fetus with a halo round its head due to the oedematous scalp. The placenta is large and pale with fluid oozing from it: the author having seen one weighing 2,500 g, the baby weighing 3,200 g.

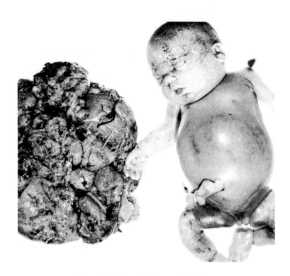

Fig. 32-19    Hydrops fetalis.

## (2) Congenital haemolytic anaemia.

This is the mildest form of Rh haemolytic disease. Anaemia which produces a wax-like pallor and jaundice giving a pale, lemon tint to the skin, may be manifest as early as the fourth day but sometimes may not not be apparent until the third or fourth week. The liver and spleen are enlarged. The haemoglobin may be as low as 6 g/dl. 'Top up' transfusions of packed cells are usually necessary.

## (3) Icterus gravis neonatorum.

This severe form of jaundice is usually manifest within 12 to 24 hours of birth. Mild cases may be missed unless examined in strong daylight. Golden amniotic fluid and yellow staining of the umbilical cord may be manifest and could be confused with the greenish discoloration of amniotic fluid and umbilical cord due to meconium staining.

Jaundice is not present at birth because during intrauterine life the breakdown product bilirubin from the haemolysed fetal red cells, is excreted via the placenta into the maternal circulation. After birth, the baby must cope with the elimination of unconjugated bilirubin which is detoxicated (conjugated) by a liver enzyme and excreted in the baby's urine and faeces. If untreated, icterus gravis leads to the serious condition kernicterus (see p. 573).

**To detect patients 'at risk'** the blood of every pregnant woman is examined, for ABO Group and Rhesus type, at her first visit to the prenatal clinic. If Rh negative, her blood is examined for antibodies. When no antibodies are present, the test for antibodies is repeated at 26–28 and 34–36 weeks.

When Rh antibodies are found on doing Coomb's test, an indirect antiglobulin test (IAGT), the titre (quantity of antibodies) is estimated:–

every 4 weeks to the 24th week
every 2 weeks to the 32nd week
every week to the 40th week and at delivery.

If the antibody titre reaches a critical level, amniocentesis is performed and the amniotic fluid examined to assess the level of bilirubin.

## Spectrophotometric Scanning of Amniotic Fluid

**Amniocentesis is performed usually about 28 weeks,** to assess the severity of the condition by estimating the amount of bilirubin excreted by the fetus into the amniotic fluid. The placenta is localised by sonar prior to the tap. The bladder is emptied. Five ml of amniotic fluid is withdrawn using a 5 to 9 cm, 22G spinal needle. Light must be excluded from the fluid en route to the laboratory. By spectrophotometric analysis of the amniotic fluid, bilirubin level is assessed, the severity of the condition estimated and subsequent management planned. At intervals as indicated the test is repeated.

### Supervision

The Rh– woman with antibodies is supervised throughout pregnancy by an obstetrician who has expert knowledge and experience in the management of such cases. She is booked for delivery in a centre where replacement transfusion can be undertaken if necessary

The Rh– woman with no antibodies will be given Rh anti-D immunoglobulin if she gives birth to an Rh positive baby.

### Intra Uterine Blood Transfusion

This highly specialised treatment is seldom necessary today. When amniocentesis indicates a severely affected fetus, whose immaturity precludes delivery, intrauterine transfusion may be the only hope of achieving a live baby. Twenty-four hours prior to the transfusion a radio-opaque substance is injected into the amniotic sac: the fetus swallows some of the dye which provides a target area for inserting the needle into the fetal peritoneal cavity: 40 to 120 ml Rh– packed red cells are then slowly injected.

#### PRETERM INDUCTION OF LABOUR

The Rh negative woman with antibodies, or the history of a previously affected child, is an absolute indication for delivery in a hospital equipped for replacement transfusion. Labour may be induced at the 35th to 38th week depending on the findings on amniocentesis. Paediatricians, blood transfusion service and laboratory staff are alerted.

At birth the cord is clamped at once to avoid giving the infant more blood containing the offending antibodies. Five ml of cord blood should be allowed to drip from the placental end of the cord via a small funnel into a dry sterile blood bottle and an anticoagulant tube. The cord must not be squeezed because Wharton's jelly upsets some of the laboratory tests: metal or cord clips should not be used. No cord powder should be applied to the umbilicus: wet dressings favour sepsis.

(Blood may be withdrawn with a dry sterile syringe and needle from the umbilical cord vein. To avoid haemolysis the needle should be removed before injecting blood into the test tubes.)

### The Following Tests are Carried out on Cord Blood

**Haemoglobin estimation.** If below 14·8 g/dl this suggests red cell destruction. If the level of cord haemoglobin is below 10 g/dl, immediate replacement transfusion is likely to be necessary.

**Coombs' direct antiglobulin test** (DAGT) demonstrates the presence of maternal antibodies on the fetal red cells; a positive result signifies haemolytic disease in the baby and the need for serial estimations of serum bilirubin levels.

**Rh typing. ABO grouping.**

**Serum bilirubin.** If the cord blood level is over 60 micromol/l, serial estimations are made at 4 to 6 hourly intervals. Should the level reach 170 micromol/l within 24 hours and particularly if the infant is preterm, replacement transfusion would be considered. Subsequently, should the level of 340 micromol/l or more be approached the danger of kernicterus exists, and replacement blood transfusion is carried out to prevent serious brain damage.

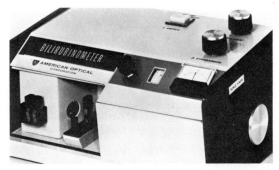

Fig. 32-20   Bilirubinometer. Developed for measurement of the level of serum bilirubin in the newborn.

*Courtesy of Optical Co. Ltd., 39 Hatton Garden, London, E.C. 1.*

### Clinical Examination of the Baby with Icterus Gravis

Respiration may be slow in being established and frothy mucus troublesome.

Jaundice usually develops within 12 hours and becomes rapidly deeper until the fifth or sixth day. (*Pressure on the skin by the diaphragm of a stethoscope produces a blanched ring which makes the yellow staining obvious.*)

The baby is lethargic and pallor of the mucous membranes is sometimes noted.

Enlargement of the liver and spleen will be detected by the doctor.

#### Phototherapy

If babies in whom icterus gravis is anticipated are given phototherapy immediately after birth, fewer replacement transfusions are required.

Replacement transfusions are now less necessary since Rh− women have received injections of Rh anti-D immunoglobulin when conditions are present that would give rise to a 'feto-maternal bleed.

Written permission is obtained from the parents prior to giving the transfusion:they are informed and assured.

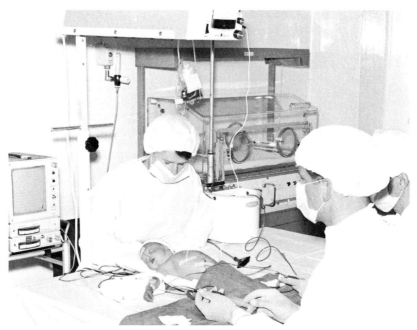

Fig. 32-21  Two paediatricians giving replacement transfusion. Skin temperature probe attached to heating device above.

**Cardiac rate meter** (Cardiorater): heated incubator. Drip stand.
**Cruciform padded splint** (*sloped*): Kling bandage 10 cm.
Overhead heating panel servo controlled.
**Preset tray** (contents in Fig 32-22), blood warmer: waste blood container 500ml.
**Disposable equipment:** adult blood administration set with pump: blood transfusion tubing: extension tubing Luer fitting: umbilical cannulae, arterial 3·5 and 5, venous 6 and 9: two 3-way taps: 5 syringes 20 ml: oesophageal tubes FG 6: mucus extractors: Warne endotracheal tubes 12 and 14: eyeless needled sutures with 3/0 silk.
**Drugs:** ampoules Lanoxin, frusemide (Lasix), Konakion, Calcium gluconate, 10 per cent, Heparin, glucose 10 per cent, Hibitane, 0·5 per cent, in spirit, Vacolitre isotonic saline, sodium bicarbonate 8·4 per cent.
**Sphygmomanometer,** 2 baby cuffs, stethoscope, strapping 2·5 cm, electronic thermometer.
**Blood investigation tubes,** Sequestrene, lithium heparin, fluoride oxalate, dry.
**Record chart.**

*Simpson Memorial Maternity Pavilion, Edinburgh.*

To replace the baby's blood, which contains a reduced number of normal red cells, many haemolysed red cells, low haemoglobin, high serum bilirubin and maternal antibodies, a replacement transfusion is carried out. This should be done within six hours of birth or as soon as possible. Ten ml of blood is withdrawn and discarded. The blood is given by plastic catheter via the umbilical vein. Each subsequent syringeful of blood taken off is immediately replaced by a similar volume of fresh donor blood. If venous pressure is high 15 ml are taken off first and replaced by 10 ml. The remainder is taken off and replaced in 10 ml amounts. A specimen of blood is taken at the beginning and the end of the transfusion for haemoglobin, haematocrit and serum bilirubin tests.

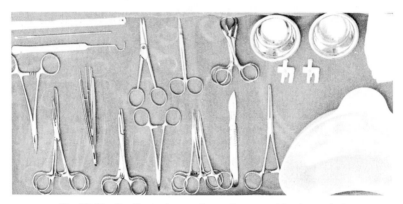

Fig. 32-22   Sterile equipment for replacement blood transfusion.

**Linen**
  2 gowns: sheet with operating aperture.
  gauze swabs 4 packs of 5.

**Equipment**
  receiver; 2 gallipots.
  metal ruler 15cm.

**Disposable**
  Umbilical cannulae FG6 and 9: 3½ and 5. 5 syringes 20 ml: eyeless needled suture with 3/0 silk: Two 3-way stopcocks. Luer fitting extension tubing, blood transfusion tubing.

**Instruments**
  2 small towel clips.
  straight Mayo forceps 15 cm.
  Bard Parker handle 4, blade 23.
  small aneurysm needle: probe.
  fine dissecint forceps plain.
  fine dissecting forceps toothed.
  3 straight mosquito forceps.
  1 curved mosquito forceps.
  2 find Allis's forceps.
  2 Spencer Wells forceps.
  1 pair iris scissors: 1 needle holder.
  1 pair stitch forceps.

*Simpson Memorial Maternity Pavilion, Edinburgh.*

**The blood must be fresh** (not stored) and have an ABO group compatible with the baby's. Partially packed cells are given because donor blood may only contain 85 per cent haemoglobin. Rh negative blood is given because the maternal antibodies in the baby's circulation would destroy Rh positive blood. (It does no harm to give an Rh positive individual Rh negative blood.)

It should be noted that the baby is not only getting blood: the offending antibodies, haemolysed red cells and bilirubin are also being withdrawn and anaemia corrected. This tides the infant over the first two weeks, until he can produce sufficient of his own Rh positive blood and get rid of the maternal antibodies. Giving the baby Rh negative blood does not alter his Rh factor, the baby will continue to produce Rh positive blood.

Blood is warmed by placing in water not above 37°C or haemolysis may occur; the Bristol blood warmer is sometimes used.

**Hypothermia must be avoided** so the procedure is carried out in a room with a temperature of 28°–32°C: an overhead radiant heater being useful. The baby is immobilised on a crucifix splint; rarely is a sedative necessary.

The stomach is aspirated if a feed has been given within three hours, mechanical suction or mucus extractors should be at hand.

### OBSERVATION

A midwife sits at the baby's head concentrating on observation and recording of the condition of the baby. It is essential that an accurate record is made of each syringeful of blood withdrawn or replaced, so that the infant's blood volume is maintained.

**A MIDWIFE RECORDS INTAKE AND OUTPUT AS FOLLOWS:**

| Name | | Date | | Blood used | Baby No. |
|------|------|------|------|------|------|
| **Time** | **Vol. out (ml)** | **Vol. in (ml)** | **Heart rate** | **Drugs** | **Clinical Comment** |
| | | | | | |

**To monitor the heart beat** a cardiorater is invaluable but if not available apex beat recordings are made every 5 minutes: the diaphragm of the stethoscope being strapped to the baby's chest.

**An electric thermometer** records the body temperature.

*The doctor is notified of:*

Progressive increase, decrease, sudden drop or irregularity in heart beat rate; cardiac arrest is usually heralded by bradycardia.

**Cyanosis,** greyness, pallor. If very anaemic, heart failure may occur; sudden quietening of the baby may indicate impending collapse.

Respiratory difficulty: particularly tachypnoea.

Tremors or twitchings which might indicate hypoglycaemia or hypocalcaemia;

### POST TRANSFUSION CARE

**The baby is placed in a warm cot or incubator** and 'specialled' for 6–8 hours. The parents are told about the baby's progress.

**The umbilicus is inspected** for bleeding every 30 minutes for 3 hours, then 3–hourly for 24 hours.

**Serum bilirubin** is estimated 6 hours after transfusion and subsequently as indicated by the rate of rise in the unconjugated bilirubin: usually 6-hourly.

**Hypoglycaemia** is detected by 4-hourly Dextrostix estimations.

For subsequent transfusions one ml calcium gluconate 10 per cent is administered after each 100 ml of blood.

## Follow-up

All babies who have suffered from haemolytic disease are prescribed iron, folic acid and Abidec on discharge and attend a special 'follow up' clinic for 2 months at weekly intervals for the detection of such conditions as anaemia, deafness, cerebral palsy and mental retardation.

## KERNICTERUS

This serious condition, now rarely seen since Rh incompatibility can be prevented, is manifest by signs of cerebral irritation and deepening jaundice due to the effect of high levels of unconjugated bilirubin on the brain cells. When the serum bilirubin, which is normally under 34 micromol/l in the newborn, rises above 68 micromol/l, jaundice becomes visible. Should unconjugated bilirubin reach the critical level of over 340 micromol/l, kernicterus is liable to occur with yellow staining and necrosis of brain cells.

### Signs

Jaundice deepens. The baby is lethargic and disinclined for feeds.
Cerebral irritation is manifest, with head retraction. Convulsions may occur.

### Treatment

Serum bilirubin estimations are made twice daily in cases where a high bilirubin level exists; if rising, every 6 hours.

Replacement blood transfusion is given and repeated if necessary to lower the high serum bilirubin level.

A few of these infants recover but they may be mentally subnormal, deaf, or suffer from cerebral palsy.

### ABO Incompatibility

The clinical manifestations are mild; jaundice being present, anaemia is uncommon. The condition is seen in Group A or Group B infants of Group 0 mothers. The indirect Coombs test is positive as a general rule in the first 24 hours of life. The diagnosis is confirmed by finding anti A or anti B in Group A or Group B infants. Management is directed to the control of hyperbilirubinaemia.

#### OTHER CAUSES OF JAUNDICE IN THE NEWBORN BABY

**Jaundice (commonly known as 'physiological')** is due to immaturity of the liver which is intensified in preterm babies. Phototherapy may be employed. If jaundice persists for over 36 hours serum bilirubin is estimated and when over 340 micromol/l or rising, and clinical signs warrant it, a replacement transfusion is given.

**Sepsis.** Umbilical infection may spread to the liver, and in some instances no external signs are apparent, the jaundice usually occurring towards the end of the first week.

**Urinary infection.** If jaundice deepens when it should be fading, a causative factor such as urinary infection should be sought.

**Breast milk jaundice** is rare and may be due to an unidentified steroid in the mother's milk. It usually occurs around the 6th day. Breast feeding should be continued.

**Bruising that is severe,** as occurs when the Malmstrom extractor is applied to the scalp.

### Congenital obliteration of the bile duct

Jaundice appears after several days, deepens in colour until the skin has a greenish bronze hue, which persists for weeks. The stools are putty-coloured, the urine contains bile. Serious haemorrhage may occur, and only a few of these babies survive the necessary operative treatment.

### HAEMORRHAGIC STATES OF THE NEWBORN BABY

**Hypoprothrombinaemia** is almost invariably present during the first three days of life. Due to the low level of prothrombin in the blood: its clotting power is diminished, and when bleeding occurs, no matter what the cause, it tends to persist. Vitamin $K_1$ (Konakion 1 mg) is usually administered prophylactically to all babies at or within 4 hours of birth.

**Melaena** most commonly occurs at the meconium stage. Oozing of blood takes place from the intestinal mucous membrane and is usually slight, but a massive haemorrhage may occur. The baby is pale and collapsed in such cases, sometimes prior to the passage of blood in the stools. Save napkins for inspection, notify the doctor, treat shock. A fresh blood transfusion and vitamins $K_1$ (Konakion 1 mg) and C may be administered. It must be remembered that blood from a cracked nipple may be swallowed and give rise to melaena, but in such a case the baby is not pale and the melaena is slight. Inexperienced midwives sometimes confuse meconium with melaena; meconium is dark green, melaena is black. If there is a pink ring on the napkin surrounding the stool, or if, when the napkin is placed in water, pink staining occurs, blood is present.

**Haematemesis** is not usually severe, and may be due to the swallowing of blood during labour.

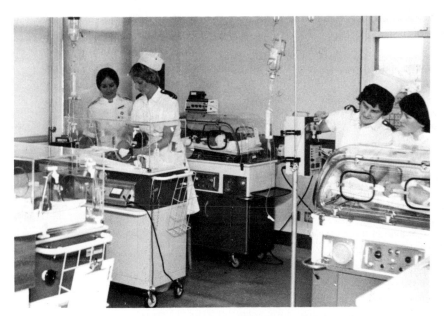

Fig. 32-23    Intensive care unit: Fluids being administered.

*Aberdeen Maternity Hospital.*

### OTHER CAUSES OF BLEEDING IN THE NEWBORN

The small blood vessels may be damaged, as occurs in intracranial injury.

In hypoxia the blood vessels throughout the body become engorged with blood and oozing may take place into the organs and tissues.

Oestrogen withdrawal causes slight uterine bleeding in female babies (see p. 494).

Omphalorrhagia (*bleeding from the umbilicus*) is usually due to shrinking of the cord or an ineffectively applied ligature, and in such cases re-ligation is indicated. Death has occurred in such cases. 30ml of a baby's blood is the equivalent of 600 ml of an adult's.

When bleeding occurs after the cord is off, it is commonly due to umbilical sepsis. The administration of vitamin $K_1$ (Konakion 1 mg) and the application of adrenaline and pressure, or, in rare cases, a pair of artery forceps, will control it.

# QUESTIONS FOR REVISION

## ASPHYXIA NEONATORUM

**C.M.B.(Scot.) 30-min question.** What are the causes of cyanosis in the new born baby? Describe the investigations necessary to establish a diagnosis.

**C.M.B.(Scot.) 30-min question.** What are the causes of intra-uterine hypoxia? Describe the principles underlying the management of severe asphyxia in the newborn.

**C.M.B.(Scot.) 30-min question.** Describe the respiratory complications which can arise in the first seven days of a baby's life.

**C.M.B.(Scot.) 30-min question.** A baby has recurrent apnoeic attacks during the first week of life. What may be the causes of these? How may such a baby be investigated and treated?

**C.M.B. (Scot.) 30-min question.** How would the midwife assess the degree of asphyxia in a baby at birth. Describe her management of an asphyxiated baby

**C.M.B.(Eng.) 30-min question.** How would you resuscitate a baby who fails to breathe at birth? Give your reasons for the treatment you would adopt.

**Council (N. Ireland) 30-min question.** A newborn infant fails to breathe. What may cause this, and what would you do?

**C.M.B.(Scot.) 30-min question.** Describe the management of a baby with an Apgar score of 4 at one minute after delivery.

Define the following (*a*) intermittent positive pressure ventilation, IPPV. (*b*) continuous positive airway pressure, CPAP. Apnoeic episodes.

Differentiate between:- metabolic and respiratory acidosis, mild and severe asphyxia. Apgar and Silverman score.

Explain how you would cope with each of the following: a mildly asphyxiated baby; administration of oxygen by: (*a*) mask, (*b*) nasal catheter, (*c*) positive pressure; endotracheal intubation; mouth to mouth breathing.

**Signs of asphyxia.** The baby's colour is..........apex beat is..........muscle tone is..........umbilical cord is..........Apgar score is..........

## NEONATAL INFECTIONS

**Define ophthalmia neonatorum** (Eng. or Scot. as applicable). Give 4 prophylactic measures. Why is the gonococcus the most dreaded organism?

**C.M.B.(Eng.)** What are the common sites of infection in the newborn: What can be done to minimise the incidence of infection?

**C.M.B.(Scot.) 30-min question.** How may infection be recognised in the first week of life? What are the common sites of infection in the newborn? What routine investigations are carried out on a baby with a suspected infection?

**C.M.B.(Eng.)** Which infections may occur during the first ten days of life? Discuss prevention of cross infection amongst babies in a maternity hospital.

**C.M.B.(Eng.)** What advice would you give a mother concerning the protection of her baby against infectious diseases and accidents?

**Council (N. Ireland).** (*a*) What daily observations should be made on a new born infant, and what is their significance? (*b*) Describe the measures which may be taken to prevent infection in the new born infant.

**For what conditions might the following drugs be used** in the treatment of neonatal infections: cloxacillin; neomycin bacitracin powder; Terramycin ointment; hibitane, 0·5 per cent, in spirit; soluble penicillin; Colomycin; dequalinium; neomycin and kaolin; framycetin cream; ephedrine.

**What early signs would suggest:** oral thrush; urinary tract infection; epidemic gastroenteritis; omphalitis; pemphigus; pneumonia?

**(N. Ireland) 30-min question.** Describe the care of the skin, the eyes and the umbilical cord of the newborn with particular reference to the prevention of infection.

**Council (N. Ireland) 30-min question.** What is ophthalmia neonatorum? Describe the prevention and treatment of this condition.

**C.M.B.(Scot.) 30-min question.** What are the signs of infection in the first two weeks of life? What are the main sources and how may the incidence of infection be minimised?

**C.M.B.(Scot.) 30-min question.** Describe the effects, local and general, of infection in the newborn. Give the investigation and management.

**Council (N. Ireland) 30-min question.** A four-day-old baby develops diarrhoea. Discuss the investigation and treatment of this condition.

**C.M.B.(Scot.) 30-min question.** What steps can be taken to minimise the occurrence of the infection in the newborn?

### C.M.B. (Short) Questions

**N. Ire.:** What is the Apgar score? **Scot.:** What is the management of asphyxia? **N. Ire.:** Briefly discuss the treatment of neonatal asphyxia. **Scot.:** Describe a baby born in a state of asphyxia. **Eng.:** Give reasons why a newborn baby may be slow to breathe.

**N. Ire.:** Discuss the significance of loose motions in the newborn. **N. Ireland:** Aspiration pneumonia in the newborn. **N. Ire.:** Oral thrush infection. **N. Ire.:** Describe the management of a baby with loose motions.

**Scot.:** Define ophthalmia neonatorum. **Eng.:** The midwife's duty when a baby in her care develops a discharge from the eye. **Scot.:** What obligations do the Rules of the Central Midwives Board for Scotland place on midwives regarding babies' eyes?

## HAEMOLYTIC DISEASE OF THE NEWBORN BABY

How would you deal with the umbilical cord if the mother has Rh antibodies? Why would sonar be used prior to amniocentesis?

What precautions are taken when transporting the amniotic fluid to the laboratory? **During replacement transfusion:** what observations does the midwife make? How is the baby kept warm? Why is the stomach sometimes aspirated?

**Define:** transplacental bleeding and state how a midwife could try to prevent this; give signs and treatment of kernicterus.

**With what techniques do you associate the following names:** Kleihauer; Coombs; Tuohy?

**Council (N. Ireland) 30-min question.** What is haemolytic disease of the newborn? Describe briefly the clinical appearance and the methods of diagnosis.

**Council (N. Ireland) 30-min question.** What are the causes of jaundice in a baby in the first week of life? Describe briefly the treatment of any of them.

**Council (N. Ireland).** A patient is expecting her third baby, and is found in early pregnancy to have a Rhesus negative blood group with antibodies. (*a*) What particular points in her history would be significant. (*b*) Describe the management of such a patient in the prenatal period.

### C.M.B. (Short) Questions

Explain why fewer replacement transfusions are now necessary. Differentiate between homozygous and heterozygous genotype.

Define the terms haemolysis: hydrops fetalis: phototherapy. State the dose of Rh anti-D immunoglobulin given following (*a*) abortion (*b*) childbirth. During replacement transfusion what observations on the baby does the midwife make?

**N. Ireland:** How may haemolytic disease of the newborn be prevented? **Eng.:** Rh Anti-D serum. **Scot.:** Rh incompatibility. **Eng.:** For what purpose may amniocentesis be performed? **N. Ireland:** Jaundice in the first 48 hours of life. **Eng.:** Kernicterus. **Eng.:** Causes and dangers of jaundice in the first week of life. **Scot.:** Hyperbilirubinaemia diagnosis and treatment. **Eng.:** Reasons for exchange transfusion of the baby. **N. Ireland:** How may haemolytic disease of the new-born be treated?

**Eng.** Cerebral irritation in the newborn. **Scot.** Phototherapy. **Eng.** Gonococcal ophthalmia. **Eng.** Prevention of Rhesus iso-immunisation. **Eng.** Cord blood testing. **Eng.** Oral thrush in the newborn. **Eng.** Anti-D immunoglobulin. **Eng.** Methods of neonatal resuscitation. **Eng.** Skin infections in the newborn. **Eng.** The postmature baby.

**C.M.B.(Scot.)** What are the conditions which cause jaundice in the newborn? A baby becomes jaundiced during the first ten days of life. What investigations will be made?

**Council N. Ireland.** (*a*) Enumerate four pathological causes of jaundice in the first ten days of life. (*b*) Discuss the treatment of any *one* condition you have mentioned in part (*a*).

**C.M.B.(Scot.)** What is a chromosome? Name two chromosomal abnormalities. Take one of these two and describe: (*a*) the cause (*b*) the appearance of the child (*c*) the effect on the subsequent development of the child.

**C.M.B.(Scot.)** What is the significance of the following in the first week of life: (*a*) a low haemoglobin level; (*b*) a low blood glucose level; (*c*) a low serum calcium level; (*d*) a low blood pH; (*e*) a raised serum bilirubin level.

# 33
# Birth Injuries—Malformations

*Intracranial injury. Caput and cephalhaematoma. Fractures. Paralysis, facial. Erb's.*
*Atresia, oesophageal, duodenal, ano-rectal. Cleft lip and palate. Genetic and*
*environmental causes of abnormalities. Hydrocephaly. Anencephaly. Spina bifida.*
*Congenital dislocation of the hip. Talipes. Down's syndrome. Dealing with parents*
*of handicapped baby. Cot deaths.*

## INTRACRANIAL INJURY AND HAEMORRHAGE

A few babies who are stillborn or who die during the first week are found at
post-mortem examination to have intracranial injuries. Physical and mental
impairment may ensue in the babies who survive, and some cases of spastic
paralysis are due to this cause: midwives should be as much concerned with
prevention as with treatment of this grave condition.

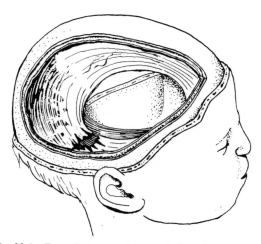

Fig. 33-1   Tear of the tentorium cerebelli and haemorrhage.

### STRUCTURES INVOLVED

The falx cerebri, a fold of meninges (dura mater), which dips down between the
two halves of the cerebrum, is liable to be torn due to excessive or rapid
compression of the fetal head during labour. The tentorium cerebelli, a fold of dura
mater, continuous with, but at right angles to, the falx cerebri and lying between the
cerebrum and cerebellum is also liable to be torn. The vein of Galen, which is in
close proximity to the tentorium, is the usual source of bleeding. The haemorrhage
is usually subdural and the presence of blood in the spinal fluid on subdural tap is
diagnostic. Ultrasound has been used for diagnosis and a mid-line shift of the falx
cerebri is manifest on the echo encephalogram.

578

### CAUSES

(1) **Preterm babies,** because of lack of protection by their soft skull bones and wide sutures as well as the delicacy of the cerebral vessels and tissues, are particularly prone to intracranial injury; the haemorrhage is usually intraventricular.

(2) **Hypoxia** causes profound venous engorgement of the cerebral vessels.

(3) **Trauma:** compression and stretching as occurs in moulding.

(a) **Excessive compression**
Contracted pelvis. Occipito-posterior position.
Large baby.

(b) **Rapid compression**
Aftercoming head in breech delivery.
Precipitate labour.

(c) **Upward compression**
Aftercoming head in breech delivery.
Face to pubes.

commonly causing subarachnoid haemorrhage.

### Prevention

Avoidance of intra-uterine hypoxia: fetal heart monitoring: use of Saling's method of blood sampling.

In the following circumstances babies should be closely observed for signs of intracranial injury for at least 48 hours, even although these are not manifest at birth.

**Prolonged labour.**  **Breech delivery.**  **Asphyxia.**
**Difficult delivery.**  **Face to pubes.**  **Preterm labour.**

### SIGNS

In severe cases at birth the infant is shocked, the eyes roll upwards or sideways with horizontal oscillation of the eyeballs (nystagmus): twitching of the facial muscles and convulsions may occur.

**Trunk and limbs may be rigid,** the fists clenched; limpness is also common. Darting, adder-like movements of the tongue are seen.

**Difficult grunting expiration,** often moist, due to excess of mucus; sometimes shallow, rapid and irregular with attacks of apnoea and cyanosis.

**Worried and anxious expression:** wrinkling of forehead; eyes wide open for long periods staring with a 'knowing look'. The infant is often pale with dark circles round the sunken eyes: feeble murmuring cry or bouts of shrill shrieking, followed by limpness, and an ashen grey colour. Head retraction, rigid neck. Tense or spongy fontanelle.

### NURSING CARE

**Incubator nursing** (with the baby naked for adequate observation) in the neonatal intensive care unit is essential. Quietness is needed: all disturbing stimuli being excluded: handling may provoke convulsions so it should be minimal. The infant is turned from one side to the other at feed times: bathing, weighing and measuring can be postponed until later. Vitamin $K_1$ phytomenadione (Konakion) one mg is given i.m. to prevent further bleeding.

**Sedatives are usually prescribed,** e.g. phenobarbitone six or eight hourly, 5–10 mg/kg/day, for the jittery baby. If the drug prescribed is not effective, the midwife must notify the doctor as it is necessary that the infant be relaxed and asleep.

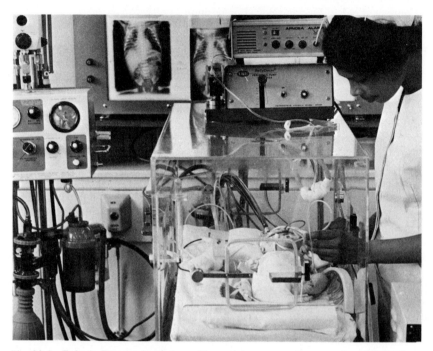

Fig. 33-2   Baby in Draegar incubator, with resolving pneumothorax and resolved pulmonary haemorrhage. Peristaltic pump and apnoea alarm on top of incubator. Bird respirator. Cardiac monitor. Midwife doing oral suctioning.

*Royal Maternity Hospital, Rottenrow, Glasgow.*

**A clear airway is imperative.** Secretions that collect in the pharynx should be removed by suction: humidifying the oxygen will help to prevent the drying of secretions.

**Feeding by the nasogastric tube is advisable;** the tube being left *in situ*. The baby is not removed from the incubator during feeding. Hypoglycaemia will cause further brain damage so must be avoided. Fluid balance should be maintained, intravenous alimentation may be utilised.

**The following equipment should be at hand:** mechanical suction or mucus extractors; oxygen; laryngoscope; endotracheal tube. In severe cases equipment for continuous positive airway pressure (CPAP).

## OBSERVATION

*Diligent Observation is Mandatory*

**Vital signs.** These are recorded 4-hourly at least; electronic monitors cause least disturbance to the infant.

**The respiratory pattern is significant** and the following are noted: increase in rate, irregularity, grunting expirations and sternal recession. Apnoeic episodes lasting over 15 seconds or recurring frequently are a serious manifestation usually associated with hypoglycaemia and hypocalcaemia as well as with intracranial injury. Apnoea mattresses giving an alarm bleep are invaluable: the Electrodyne contactless monitor being a good example. Prolonged apnoea will cause brain damage, so the midwife in charge should be competent to intubate the baby in an emergency. Serial blood gas measurements are utilised to monitor pulmonary ventilation. Cyanosis will be obvious when the oxygen uptake is defective.

**The temperature of baby and incubator** is recorded every 4 hours: Servo controlled incubators and electric thermometers being useful devices. Hypoxic brain damage is liable to cause hypothermia so chilling must be avoided.

**The apex beat** and the blood pressure are taken and recorded 2 or 4 hourly.

**Worsening of the condition** e.g. extreme lethargy, pronounced drowsiness and increasing respiratory depression are serious signs.

### Follow up

Babies who have suffered hypoxic or traumatic brain damage at birth are followed up at assessment centres where mental development and neuromuscular coordinating ability are evaluated.

### FRACTURES

Fractures in the newborn are usually complete, not greenstick, and because of rapid callus formation and bone growth permanent deformity is rare. Medical aid is necessary: attempts to elicit crepitus should not be made.

**Skull fractures are rare,** but spoon-shaped indentations may occur, due to pressure from the promontory of the sacrum in the rare cases in which a woman with pelvic deformity is allowed to go into labour. If the baby survives, the depression gradually becomes rectified as growth proceeds.

**The spine is seldom fractured,** unless by mismanagement in delivering the aftercoming head in a breech presentation, i.e. by bending the cervical vertebrae acutely backwards. Stillbirth results.

**The humerus may be fractured** in dealing with shoulder dystocia and in bringing down extended arms if the midwife does not 'splint' the humerus while so doing. Deformity is evident and the infant does not move the arm freely. Adhesive strapping is applied to the upper arm, which is then placed alongside the trunk, with a pad of wool in the axilla. The forearm is flexed, with the fingers touching the clavicle on the opposite side, and a 10 cm bandage used to bind the arm to the body, taking care not to impede respiration. Callus forms in about 10 days and the infant is then allowed free movement.

**The fractured clavicle** is treated by binding the arm to the body with the hand at the level of the clavicle on the opposite side.

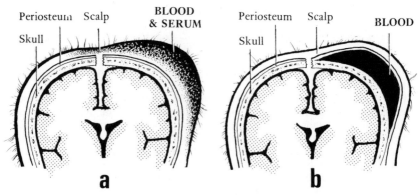

Fig. 33-3

## CAPUT SUCCEDANEUM

A caput succedaneum is an oedematous swelling on the fetal skull, a serosanguinous (serum and blood) infiltration into the scalp tissue. Due to pressure by a 'girdle of contact' which is usually the cervix; the venous blood supply is retarded, and the area lying over the os becomes congested and oedematous.

A secondary caput may form:

1. In occipito-posterior positions when the occiput rotates forwards.

2 In cases where the head is held up on the perineum.

## CEPHALHAEMATOMA

A cephalhaematoma is a swelling on the fetal skull, an effusion of blood under the periosteum covering it, due to friction between the skull and pelvis. It occurs in cases of cephalopelvic disproportion and precipitate labour, when tearing of the periosteum from the bone causes bleeding.

As the pericranium (periosteum) is adherent to the edges of the skull bones, the swelling is confined to one bone.

No treatment is necessary, the blood is absorbed and the swelling subsides. After one week a ridge of bone may be felt round the periphery of the swelling, due to the accumulation of osteoblasts.

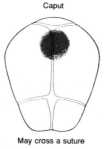

Caput

May cross a suture

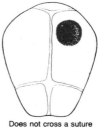

Cephalhaematoma

Does not cross a suture

Fig. 33-4

Is present at birth.
May cross a suture.
Tends to grow less.
Disappears within 36 hours.
Is diffuse, pits on pressure.
A double caput is always unilateral.

Appears after 12 hours.
Never crosses a suture.
Tends to grow larger.
Persists for weeks.
Is circumscribed, does not pit.
A double cephalhaematoma is usually bilateral (Fig. 33–5).

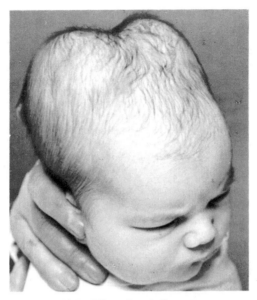

Fig. 33-5   Bilateral cephalhaematoma.

## INJURY TO MUSCLES AND NERVES

### Torticollis

The sterno-mastoid muscle in the neck may be bruised and lacerated if the head is pulled sideways in delivering the anterior shoulder, or if the neck is twisted in rotating the shoulders during breech delivery. A small haematoma forms, and a swelling the size of a pigeon's egg appears one or two weeks after birth. Gentle massage and movement, with stretching of the neck muscles carried out after feeds are sufficient to cause regression of the tumour.

#### FACIAL PARALYSIS

Facial paralysis occurs when the facial (seventh cranial) nerve is compressed unduly, as may be done with the forceps blade, or by haemorrhage and oedema round the nerve. It may occur in a spontaneous delivery if, when grasping the head, undue pressure is applied on the mastoid process or over the ramus of the lower jaw where the facial nerve is very superficial.

**The paralysed side is smooth;** the corner of the mouth droops and milk dribbles out, but sucking is not interfered with; the eye usually remains open. In crying, the mouth is drawn over to the uninjured side of the face.

**No treatment is required** other than the application of an ophthalmic ointment dressing over the eye, if open, during sleep. The condition improves in one or two weeks; should paralysis persist, the damage is probably intracranial.

#### ERB'S PARALYSIS

This condition is due to damage or stretching of the roots of the brachial plexus (a nerve junction at the side of the neck under the clavicle). Injury occurs when the neck is twisted or stretched, as might happen in delivering the aftercoming head of the breech, or in excessive lateral flexion of the neck when delivering the shoulders in a vertex presentation.

The upper arm hangs limply, close to the body, and the infant cannot lift it although he can move the hand and fingers. The arm is inwardly rotated and the half-closed hand turned outwards (the waiter's tip).

A light metal splint is procured, to maintain abduction and external rotation of the arm: the upper arm being kept at right-angles to the body, the forearm flexed, fingers pointing to the top of the cot and the palm facing the side of the head.

**The practice of pinning the sleeve to the pillow region is now condemned.** It has been known for the baby to be lifted without the safety pin having been removed: this causing pain and further nerve injury.

Massage and passive movement are usually ordered. The arm may recover in weeks, or it may be months. Severe damage may give rise to permanent 'birth palsy', the arm being short and wasted.

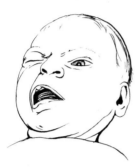

Fig. 33-6   Left-sided facial paralysis. Note that the eye is open on the paralysed side, the mouth drawn over to the non-paralysed side.

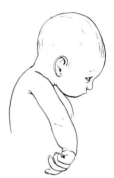

Fig. 33.7   Erb's paralysis.

### INJURY TO ADBOMINAL ORGANS

**Rupture of the liver,** which is relatively very large in the newborn, may be caused by grasping the body during a breech delivery. The baby becomes grey and shocked. More cases are now surviving with modern surgery.

## ALIMENTARY LESIONS

### OESOPHAGEAL ATRESIA

This is associated with a fistula between the oesophagus and trachea in 90 per cent of cases due to faulty development of these structures. Polyhydramnios is usually present, probably because the fetus is unable to swallow amniotic fluid.

The condition should be suspected prior to giving the first feed by the presence of fine frothy mucus in the mouth and nostrils and a history of polyhydramnios. A catheter should be passed into the oesophagus (a soft thin one may curl up); if obstructed at 5 to 7 cm oesophageal atresia is suspected. X-rays are used to confirm the diagnosis; a radio-opaque catheter being inserted into the oesophagus.

### *Treatment*

Medical aid is summoned. On no account should the baby be given water or milk to drink; he is liable to inhale it, collapse of lung may occur, pneumonia ensues, and the success of the necessary surgical operation will be impaired. If fed the baby coughs, splutters and becomes cyanosed. Suction ought to be used at once or the baby held upside down to drain off the fluid. He is then kept in a semi-raised position to prevent gastric juice from entering the trachea through a fistula; the accumulation of secretion in the nose and throat being removed by suction. The pouch should be emptied prior to transporting the infant for chest surgery; the baby is kept warm, propped up and suction used repeatedly; an oesophageal catheter being *in situ* during transport.

### Duodenal atresia

This is the commonest intestinal abnormality: volvulus, fibrous bands or adhesions may also occlude the bowel. Vomiting is persistent, first milk then bile; green vomitus, that stains what it falls on, continues. The upper abdomen may be distended, and following the passage of meconium no further stools are passed. Fluids and electrolytes must be replaced but nothing given by mouth. An immediate operation is often successful.

### Ano-rectal atresia (*Imperforate Anus*)

The anal sphincter may be closed by a membrane, in which case it can be reconstructed operatively. In certain types operation is carried out immediately; a colostomy is sometimes performed. On attempting to take the 'first' temperature rectally, no anus is found to be present. A small amount of meconium may be passed, because frequently in such cases a fistula from the intestine opens between the fourchette and the vaginal orifice in girl babies, and on the perineum in boys. The extent of the malformation may be determined by radiography.

### Exomphalos

Exomphalos is a protrusion of the abdominal organs, contained within a sac of peritoneum, through a large umbilical opening, sometimes 7 cm in diameter. A non-adherent dressing is applied and the infant transferred from the labour ward to the operating theatre; care being exercised to avoid rupturing the sac. Operative measures are usually successful, if carried out without delay, but when the sac has ruptured and the abdominal organs are exposed, heat loss is prevented by enclosing limbs and trunk in a sterile plastic bag during transport to a specialist centre.

### Umbilical hernia

Umbilical hernia consists of a small swelling which projects from the umbilicus, usually a few weeks after the cord has separated, seldom containing bowel or omentum and easily reducible. Medical advice is sought. The modern view is that no treatment (not even a pad and binder) is indicated in the majority of cases, spontaneous cure taking place within 18 months, but if not, operative repair will be necessary, preferably at the age of 18 to 24 months. If large, operation may be considered at 9 months.

### Pyloric stenosis

This condition is rare during the first week. The gastric contents are forcibly ejected: waves of gastric peristalsis, running from left to right, are usually visible abdominally after feeds. The treatment of pyloric stenosis is mainly surgical. Pyloric spasm gives rise to similar signs, but is less serious, and may start within three days of birth. The vomitus contains much mucus. The condition is amenable to medical treatment.

## CLEFT LIP: CLEFT PALATE

These can occur singly or together, and either may be unilateral or bilateral. The malformation is due to lack of union of the fronto-nasal palate, and may be slight or severe. Every newborn baby's mouth should be inspected in a good light, as the soft palate only may be cleft. In such a case choking and cyanotic attacks may occur at feeding time and milk is returned down the nose.

The cleft lip may be unilateral and very slight, or more extensive. The most severe form is manifest when bilateral (or double) cleft lip and cleft palate are both present. There is a wide gap between the nostrils, with a piece of bone projecting through it, the vomer.

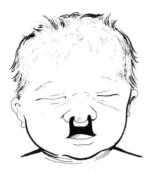 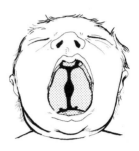

Fig. 33-8   Bilateral cleft lip and palate.          Fig. 33-9   Cleft palate.

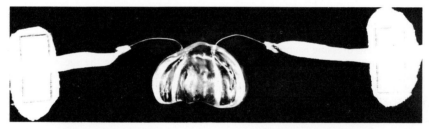

Fig. 33-10   Dental plate for newborn. The tapes fastened to the wire of the plate are held in position by a strip of adhesive which is attached to pieces of elastoplast on the cheeks. This avoids excoriating the skin during the frequent removals to cleanse the plate.

*By courtesy of Orthodontic Department, School of Dental Surgery, Edinbrugh.*

### *Treatment*

The unilateral cleft lip may be repaired during the third to sixth weeks (some are done on the 10th day) to obtain a good cosmetic result; other surgeons prefer to wait until the infant weighs 4·5 kg with haemoglobin over 11·8 g/dl and no respiratory infection. Bilateral cleft lip requires a more extensive surgical procedure and this is usually deferred until the infant is three months old. A large soft teat should be used to give the infant some of the satisfaction of sucking. Operation on the cleft palate is done when the child is about 18 months old; after then, the earlier the operation the better will the speech be. To allay their disappointment parents should be assured that the cosmetic results are now excellent and shown photographs of babies before and after successful operations. Mothers should be given ample experience while in hospital in feeding the baby (held in the upright position) and in cleansing the mouth.

**Dental plates**

For complete clefts of the lip and palate, dental plates are now being used to achieve the maximal degree of pre-surgical alignment of the segments of the maxilla prior to operation. They are applied during the first week of age, worn all the time, taken out and cleansed after feeds. Biting of the lower gum on the splint is an essential part of the treatment. The plates are remade very three or four weeks until the fourth month when the lip is repaired. This succession of progressively smaller plates pulls the cleft segment and gum margins together. The babies do not resent them. With reasonable care there is no danger of choking or of swallowing the plates. It is important to keep the areas in contact with the plate lubricated with petroleum jelly.

### Advantages of Dental Plates

**Bottle feeding is possible. There is less risk of respiratory infection.
Repositioning helps the dentist and orthodontist in their care of the teeth.**

## CONGENITAL ABNORMALITIES

Great concern is being felt regarding the congenital abnormalities that now occur in about 2 per cent of births. They may be physical or mental. The causes are not fully understood but are usually divided into two main groups:

#### GENETIC OR INHERITED CAUSES

The defect is transmitted via the genes in the ovum or spermatozoon.

**e.g. Mongolism; Anencephaly; Cleft palate; Cleft lip; Achondroplasia.** These are discussed under their respective headings.

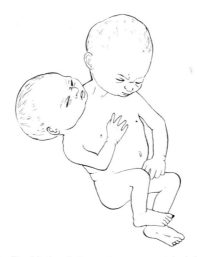

Fig. 33-11   Double-headed monster, asymmetrical disomata.

#### ENVIRONMENTAL CAUSES

**Hypoxia. Infection. Radiation. Drugs.**

In the early embryonic state, tissues are particularly vulnerable to deprivation of vital substances, i.e. oxygen, and this may impair their structure and impede function. The very small delicate organs have little resistance to infection or noxious substances and are readily damaged; the placenta, never a perfect barrier, is less effective prior to the 12th week. If the adverse factor is active during the time at which a particular tissue is being laid down or a special organ is being formed—e.g. heart, brain, limb, eye, ear—that organ is likely to be damaged. Cardiac defects, mental subnormality, absence of limbs, cataract and blindness or deafness, may result.

### Hypoxia

The embryo requires a constant supply of oxygen and lack of this may seriously affect the developing brain cells. Oxygen lack may occur if the mother's blood is deficient in oxygen due to conditions that produce cyanosis, e.g. serious cardiac or pulmonary disease, general anaesthesia inexpertly induced or if the placenta is partially separated as may occur during a threatened abortion.

### Infection

The infection rubella, occurring during the first 12 weeks of pregnancy, is the most outstanding example.

### Radiation

Exposure to radioactive substances (used in industry) is dangerous in pregnancy. Diagnostic (abdominal) radiography is avoided during the first 30 weeks of pregnancy.

### Drugs

Great caution is now being observed in prescribing drugs during the first 12 weeks of pregnancy when the developing embryo is at risk. During 1960–62 in Great Britain 244 babies were born with phocomelia and/or amelia (see Fig. 33-12).

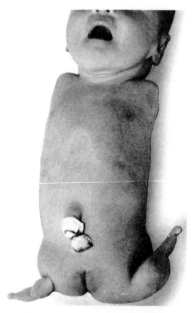

Fig. 33-12   Baby with amelia (no arms), phocomelia (long bones absent), due to Thalidomide.

*(Courtesy of Dr Spiers, Maternity Hospital, Stirling.)*

This grave tragedy was due to the action of the drug Thalidomide ingested by pregnant women during the fourth to eighth week of pregnancy as a sedative or as an anti-emetic for morning sickness. Midwives should warn expectant mothers against taking drugs other than those prescribed by the doctor.

Progestogens and adreno-corticoid hormones administered in early pregnancy have produced male type genitalia in female babies.

## ABNORMALITIES OF THE CENTRAL NERVOUS SYSTEM

### HYDROCEPHALY

The hydrocephalic head is unusually big, the sutures and fontanelles are large, the bones thinned out because of an excess of cerebro-spinal fluid in the ventricles of the brain. Hydrocephaly is mainly caused by some obstruction in the cerebro-spinal fluid pathway. The forehead is prominent.

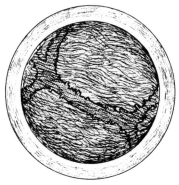

Fig. 33-13   Vaginal touch picture of hydrocephalus. Wide fontanelles and sutures.

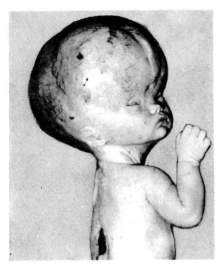

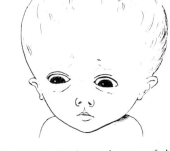

Fig. 33-15   'Setting-sun' eyes of hydro-cephalic baby.

Fig. 33-14   Hydrocephaly. Cerebro-spinal fluid, 2 litres withdrawn by Drew Smythe catheter via the spina bifida.

*Aberdeen Maternity Hospital.*

The fetus may present by the breech, and on abdominal palpation the large soft head in the fundus may be thought to be the buttocks. In cases where the vertex presents, the head is high and feels large. But because the soft head is so compressible it may partly enter the brim, is not mobile, and may not on that account be recognised by the novice. On vaginal examination, a wide fluctuant area is felt over the sutures and fontanelles. If undiagnosed, labour will be obstructed. An inexperienced midwife may not detect hydrocephaly until a small fetus, presenting by the breech and born as far as the umbilicus, does not advance.

### *Management*

In vertex presentation craniotomy and application of Briggs forceps is performed during the first stage of labour. In breech presentation the head is perforated (craniotomy) through the occiput or roof of the mouth; crushing is not always necessary as the head collapses when the fluid escapes. A long metal catheter is sometimes inserted into the spinal canal through an incision or spina bifida and the fluid drained off. In a case at the Simpson Maternity Pavilion, 2·3 litres were withdrawn in this way.

Hydrocephaly may develop after birth, and if suspected by undue growth of the head, the occipito-frontal circumference should be measured daily, the normal increase being 1·25 cm per month. Widening of the lambdoidal and occipito-mastoid sutures is almost diagnostic: ventriculography may be employed for confirmation of the diagnosis. The eyes point downwards giving the 'setting sun' sign. Some hydrocephalic babies die, others live, but may be mentally sub-normal. Good results have been obtained by draining the excess cerebro-spinal fluid from the lateral ventricle of the brain into the right atrium of the heart by using a Holter or a Pudenz Heyer valve.

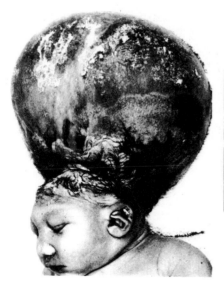

Fig. 33-16   Exencephalus acrania.

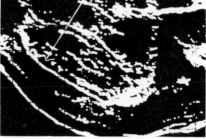

Fig. 33-17   Ultrasonogram of anencephalic fetus.

*Simpson   Memorial   Maternity   Pavilion, Edinburgh.*

### ANENCEPHALY

This is a severe form of arrested development; the vault of the skull and cerebrum being absent. The adrenal glands are atrophic. Frequently it is accompanied by an extensive spina bifida. Because there is transudation of fluid from the exposed meninges, polyhydramnios is usually present; this makes palpation difficult, but as the abdomen is usually X-rayed in cases of polyhydramnios the malformation is detected during pregnancy. Increased levels of maternal plasma alpha-fetoproteins and of alpha-fetoproteins in amniotic fluid have been found in cases of anencephaly at 16 weeks gestation.

Labour is induced prematurely, and the fetus commonly, but not invariably, presents by the face. The second stage may be somewhat prolonged, because the cervix must dilate further to allow passage of the shoulders, which are broad in comparison with the small head. Anencephalic fetuses live for only a few moments; 75 per cent are female.

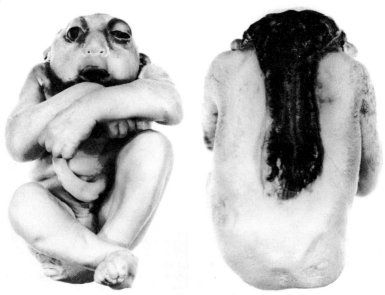

Anencephaly with spina bifida (*Myelomeningocele*).

Fig. 33-18  Anterior view.  Fig. 33-19  Posterior view showing extensive spina bifida.

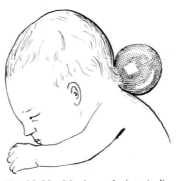

Fig. 33-20  Meningocele (*cervical*).

**The parents are advised** to attend a genetic clinic in a subsequent pregnancy for prenatal diagnosis and counselling.

### ENCEPHALOCELE: MENINGOCELE

These tumours, covered with meninges, usually protrude through the lambdoidal suture on the fetal skull. An encephalocele contains brain substance: it pulsates, is opaque, does not fluctuate, and usually has a pedicle. A large encephalocele may obstruct labour.

A meningocele contains cerebro-spinal fluid, is fluctuant, does not pulsate, and becomes tense when the baby cries. A large meningocele usually ruptures during delivery; small ones have been dealt with successfully by aspiration or other surgical means. The baby is nursed in the prone position. The sac should be covered with a non-adhering dressing or sterile gauze moistened with isotonic saline, pending the arrival of medical aid.

## SPINA BIFIDA

This fairly common defect is due to failure of the neural arches of the vertebrae to unite during embryonic life and permits the meninges, and sometimes the spinal cord to protrude through the gap. Several adjacent vertebrae may be involved. This condition may be suspected by the increase in alpha-fetoproteins in amniotic fluid obtained by amniocentesis at 14 to 18 weeks. The lesion has been defined by sonar at 16–19 weeks. Vitamin deficiency in early pregnancy is associated with spina bifida.

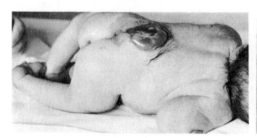

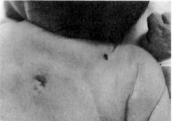

Fig. 33-21  Spina bifida. Note hair on skin surrounding tumour. The limbs are para-lysed.

Fig. 33-22   Very slight spina bifida; manif-est by dimpling of the skin.

3000 *cases occur in Britain every year*. The commonest form is recognised by the presence of a reddish mass, soft and fluctuant, in the sacro-lumbar region. More serious cases have exposed nerve tissue = myelomeningocele.

**The midwife should notify the doctor** isolate the baby, apply a non-adhering dressing (non-oily) kept moist with sterile isotonic saline solution maintained in position by a crepe bandage. Leg movement is reported. Some severe cases may not be suitable for surgery. Fifty per cent of babies develop hydrocephalus after operation.

**The parents need counselling** and can be advised to contact the local Spina Bifida Association, see also p. 597.

**Spina bifida occulta** may be manifest by mere dimpling of the skin or a patch of hair. The bony defect can be seen by radiography.

This abnormality, which may be unilateral or bilateral, occurs in about 3 per 2,000 babies, and is five times more common in the female. Frequently the hip joint is unstable, a condition that responds to splinting. The condition is more common in lands where babies are bound to a 'cradle board' with the thighs straight.

### BARLOW'S TEST

*This is a Modification of Ortolani's Test*

With the baby lying on a firm surface each leg with hip and knee flexed is held in one of the examiner's hands with the middle fingers over the greater trochanter and the thumb on the inner side of the thigh approximately opposite the lesser trochanter. With the thighs held in mid-abduction lifting with the middle finger will cause reduction of a dislocated hip, a movement that can be felt as a clunk. If no such 'clunk' occurs then the hip is not dislocated. In cases of doubt, steadying the pelvis with one hand while the doubtful hip is examined with the other hand makes the test more sensitive.

**Forced abduction is dangerous.** Some authorities consider that some tests are unreliable: many cases being missed, unless done by experts. Babies are usually examined at, 3–6 months to detect missed cases.

The midwife can apply double bulky napkins as an initial and temporary measure to abduct the hips.

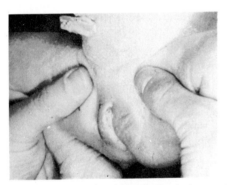 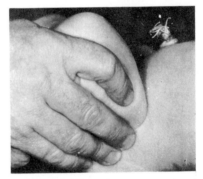

Fig. 33-23   Both thumbs applied to the inner aspects of the infant's thighs in front of the lesser trochanters.

Fig. 33-24   The middle fingers are placed over the greater trochanters.

Showing position of hands in carrying out Barlow's test for congenital dislocation of hip.

*Courtesy of Zimmer Orthopaedics Ltd., 176 Brompton Road, London, S.W.3*

### *Treatment*

A Vynide covered Duralumin splint, such as the Barlow, is applied at birth and worn constantly during the first 6 weeks of life to maintain 90 degrees flexion and full abduction: forced abduction is dangerous. The infant is seen at weekly intervals for adjustment of the splint.

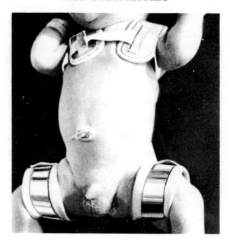

Fig. 33-25   Barlow splint in position.

*Courtesy of Zimmer Orthopaedics Ltd., 176 Brompton Road, London, S.W.3.*

## CLUB-FOOT

### TALIPES EQUINO VARUS

This deformity, in which the foot is bent downwards and inwards, may be unilateral or bilateral; the cause is not properly understood. There ought to be free movement of the normal foot in all directions and it should be possible to dorsiflex it until the small toe almost touches the leg.

### *Treatment*

Firm gentle stretching every few hours is commenced on the day of birth; the mother also being shown how to do this. The feet are maintained in the overcorrected position by the use of felt and adhesive strapping. The Denis Browne or the Bell Grice splint is usually applied. Manipulation and serial plaster of Paris casts are favoured in some centres. Complete correction is achieved in most cases before the age of 12 months.

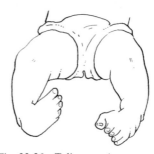

Fig. 33-26   Talipes equino varus.

### TALIPES CALCANEO-VALGUS

The foot is turned upwards and bent outwards—the opposite of talipes equino varus. This is a less severe type and some consider no treatment is necessary unless the deformity is excessive.

### ACHONDROPLASIA

In this rare condition the limbs are short due to failure in the ossification of the long bones during early fetal life. The body is of normal length. The majority of these babies survive and mental development is normal, but they remain permanently dwarfed.

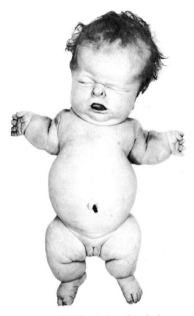

Fig. 33-27   Achondroplasia

## BIRTH MARKS

Most birth marks consist of an abnormal collection of small blood vessels. Small flat pinkish red areas, commonly seen on the eyelids and nape of the neck, disappear in a few weeks.

**Strawberry haemangioma,** are bright red in colour, slightly elevated and sharply defined. They appear during the first week of life, increase in size until six months and usually disappear before the 6th year. The spider naevus, a common vascular blemish, has a centre with blood vessels radiating from it and can be treated with a diathermy needle.

**Port wine stain** (or capillary haemangioma) is a deep purple discoloration, which is not raised and does not blanch on pressure, frequently seen on the face and sometimes extensive and very disfiguring. Cosmetic disguise is usually necessary for lesions on the face and good proprietary preparations are available.

**Pigmented naevi,** or moles, vary in size and may be covered with fine hair; the author having seen cases of melanomata in which the lesions were 10 to 12 cm in diameter. Some have a malignant tendency. Excision and radiotherapy are employed. No treatment is given for congenital naevi during the neonatal period.

## THE MENTALLY SUBNORMAL INFANT
### DOWN'S SYNDROME *(The Mongol)*

This is one of the few types of mental subnormality recognisable at birth, probably because of the striking resemblance they bear to each other. Mongols have an extra chromosome (trisomy 21)—47 instead of 46. The condition is associated with ageing of the maternal ovaries. Recent work suggests that 30 per cent are due to chromosomal errors in the father.

The incidence in age groups has been estimated as follows:

| | | | | |
|---|---|---|---|---|
| **Mothers under 30 years** | = | 1 – 1400 |
| ,, | 35–40 | ,, | = | 1 – 300 |
| ,, | 40–45 | ,, | = | 1 – 70 |
| ,, | over 45 | ,, | = | 1 – 30 |

Some recommend that all pregnant women over 35 years should be offered amniocentesis for Down's syndrome.

The head is small with a flat occiput; the upward slanting eyes, short upper lip and small mouth give the characteristic appearance which is said to resemble that of the Mongolian race. Rosy cheeks are present at birth, a feature which persists throughout life. The hands are short with crumpled palms: significant differences in the dermal configuration of finger, palm and sole patterns have been observed. A single palmar crease unbroken from side to side (the simian crease) is present; the great toe is widely separated from the other toes: the baby when held in the arms feels soft and hypotonic. Forty per cent have congenital cardiac lesions from which a number die in infancy.

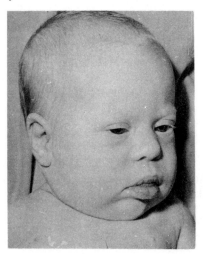

Fig. 33-28 Down's syndrome (the mongol).

*(Simpson Memorial Maternity Pavilion, Edinburgh).*

### DIAGNOSIS

A diagnosis of Down's syndrome should not be made until the facial appearance of both parents is studied. Should a skin biopsy be required for confirmation of the diagnosis, permission must be obtained in writing. A venous blood sample for chromosome study is preferable.

Mongolism occurring when the maternal age is under 30 is fully investigated. Some of these are translocation mongols who have only 46 chromosomes and this may recur in 30 per cent of cases. The parents are referred for genetic counselling.

In a subsequent pregnancy amniotic fluid can be withdrawn on abdominal amniocentesis at 14 to 16 weeks and the exfoliated skin cells examined microscopically. Therapeutic abortion may be considered if the fetus carries a translocation chromosome.

The midwife should neither tell the mother nor imply that the child is mentally subnormal. Some think it is better to allow the fact to dawn gradually on her, but that decision rests with the doctor, who may prefer to inform both parents together in hospital or at home after the first week and when the diagnosis is certain. Parents confuse the shock of 'knowing' with the time of the telling. Tact, consideration and kindliness are more important than the time, which is never right as far as the parents are concerned.

Mongol children learn to walk later than usual (2 to 3 years); their speech is usually poor: they are clean in their habits and happy children; some live to a ripe old age. The policy today is to keep as many of these children out of hospital as is possible; the family environment being considered best for every child. Much depends on the parents' wishes. Local government authorities are now providing day training centres for mentally handicapped children. Some can be gainfully employed as adults in industry at repetitive tasks in protected conditions.

#### THE MICROCEPHALIC INFANT

These infants have a small brain and miniature head of less than 28 cm occipito-frontal circumference at birth. The forehead is shallow and receding, the fontanelles small or closed. All babies whose heads are less than normal in size are not necessarily microcephalic even although mentally retarded. Spasticity of the limbs is often present. The condition is estimated to occur in about 1 in 15,000 births.

## THE MIDWIFE'S ROLE IN DEALING WITH THE PARENTS OF THE HANDICAPPED CHILD

The mother is likely to be profoundly distressed if her baby has some physical deformity or mental subnormality and may question the midwife regarding: the cause; whether she or her husband is to blame; whether the condition could have been prevented.

**Both parents should be assured** that they are not blameworthy and that the causes are not fully understood. Any further information or explanation will be given by the doctor in charge.

**Midwives should give emotional support** and help the mother to accept the situation. She should also assure her regarding facilities available and give counsel re the need for mothering, training, and education. It does not require much imagination to understand the mother's feelings and to appreciate the bitter disappointment both parents must face. The woman needs mental comfort and assurance. On no account should the midwife register surprise or exhibit disapproval of the mother's immediate reaction which may, particularly in young mothers, be one of self-pity or rejection of the infant. Having recovered from the initial shock the majority of parents resolve to do what is best for their child and to give him the loving care he will need. In fact some are overprotective. Parents need guidance in day to day management. Their attitude and co-operation affect the child's progress. They also need hope and encouragement to enable them to cope with continuing doubts and difficulties.

### Facilities Available

**Mothers should be told of the excellent results achieved by surgeons** in dealing with physical deformities, remedial and cosmetic. Appliances are provided to correct disabilities and, when necessary, to replace undeveloped limbs. To further surgical correction and enable the child to lead a happy independent life physiotherapists, speech and occupational therapists are available. Day and residential training centres are provided for children severely handicapped (physically and mentally). The help of social workers should be elicited in order that arrangements for contact with existing associations and agencies can be made.

**The attendance allowance** is tax free for children over the age of two who are severely disabled, physically or mentally. The rate varies, depending on the amount of care needed and whether during the day or night. See Leaflet N1 205.

**The mobility allowance,** is payable for children over 5 years who are unable to walk. It is taxable.

**Parent clubs,** at which experience in overcoming problems in home management of the child can be shared: give the mother help and fellowship in what can be a most distressing situation. The child must be provided with special opportunities for development that come naturally to the active normal child.

# COT DEATHS

## *Infant Sudden Death Syndrome*

This term is applied when babies who have been apparently well are found dead in their cots. The incidence is higher under poor social conditions, at about 1 to 3 months of age and during the winter months. It has been found that respiratory tract infection is the commonest cause. Inexperienced mothers may think their infants have only a 'cold'. They should be told that babies are nose breathers and if the nasal mucosa is swollen due to infection the baby does not know to breathe through his mouth and suffocation ensues. At post-mortem examinations the following respiratory conditions are found: viral pneumonia, congestion and oedema of the lungs, bronchitis. Gastro-enteritis is another cause; the baby is not given sufficient fluid and becomes dehydrated. Vomiting may occur as the terminal phase of anoxia. Cot deaths are rare in breast-fed infants. The young baby should be laid on his side, never on his back. During the first year of life babies should sleep in the mother's bedroom at night: if they have a 'cold' the room should be warm and the nostrils kept as clear as possible.

The coroner is notified in every case of sudden unexpected death: an inquest is held and the police may visit the home. This procedure is very disturbing to the grieving parents who may be distressed still further if they think they are being suspected of neglect. They are in need of support and should be assured that they are not to blame.

### NARCOTIC WITHDRAWAL SIGNS IN THE NEONATE

Babies of mothers addicted to heroin or other opiates will show withdrawal signs immediately or at any time during the first three days. Respiratory depression is usually manifest. The babies in 50 per cent of cases are light for date with tremors; irritability, hyperactivity, high-pitched cry, yawning, sneezing, vomiting, sweating excessive mucus secretion may occur. (Barbiturate withdrawal signs may appear during the second week.)

**Treatment.** Sedatives such as phenobarbitone 2 mg/kg i.m. six hourly for two weeks, given orally. During the next two weeks the drug is gradually withdrawn. Fluids are given freely.

#### Alcohol withdrawal (neonate)

**Signs** are similar to those of narcotic drug withdrawal: mental retardation, joint defects and cardiac abnormalities may be present.

**Treatment** is by the administration of phenobarbitone.

## BIRTH INJURIES

State how a midwife would prevent; recognise; treat (*until the doctor's arrival*) a fractured humerus.

What is the cause of a sternomastoid haematoma? How would you recognise facial paralysis? Describe how a midwife might cause Erb's paralysis. What are the signs?

Explain briefly, why intracranial injury is liable to occur in the following circumstances and state how the midwife could try to avoid this: the preterm baby; breech delivery; face to pubes delivery; rigid pelvic floor.

What do you understand by the following: diminished sucking and swallowing reflex; grunting expirations; apnoeic episodes?

What is: moulding; greenstick fracture; Erb's paralysis; duodenal atresia? Where is the: falx cerebri; brachial plexus; pericranium; tentorium cerebelli; sternomastoid muscle; vein of Galen?

**C.M.B.(Scot.) 30-min question.** What is a caput succedaneum? How is it formed and from what other swellings should it be differentiated?

**C.M.B.(Scot.) 30-min question.** What swellings may be found on a baby's head within a few days of birth? How would you differentiate and treat the condition?

**C.M.B.(Scot.)** What are the types of intracranial injury in the newborn? How is intracranial injury suspected and diagnosed? What are the principles of management of a baby with intracranial injury?

**C.M.B.(Scot.)** What signs would make you suspect that a baby had sustained intracranial injury. What is the investigation and nursing care of this baby.

**C.M.B.(Eng.)** Describe the common forms of birth injury to the baby. How may these be prevented and their dangers minimised?

## CONGENITAL ABNORMALITIES

**What precautions are taken when** transferring a baby with oesophageal atresia to hospital?

**How would you suspect hydrocephaly:** on abdominal palpation; during delivery; during first 2 weeks of life?

What advice would you give during a talk to expectant mothers on prevention of congenital abnormalities?

In what way can the midwife give emotional support to the parents of a severely handicapped baby?

A mother asks you whether she should keep her mongol baby at home: what would you say?

What are the midwife's duties during transportation of a baby who has: exomphalos; spina bifida? Why is it advisable for pregnant women over 35 years to have amniocentesis?

**Differentiate between** oesophageal and duodenal atresia; meningocele and encephalocele; exomphalos and umbilical hernia; hydrocephaly and anencephaly; talipes equino varus and talipes calcaneo valgus; amelia and phocomelia. How would you feed a baby at term with a cleft palate? What assurance could you give the mother.

**For what reasons are the following appliances used:** Denis Browne's splint; Barlow's splint; dental plates; Pudenz Heyer valve. Radio-opaque catheter.

**C.M.B.(Eng.) 30-min. question.** Give an account of the abnormalities of the alimentary tract of a baby which may reveal themselves in the first seven days of life.

**Council.(N. Ire.) 30-min question.** Discuss the care of an infant who becomes cyanosed and breathless during its first feed. What important causes must be excluded?

**Council.(N. Ire.) 30-min question.** A newborn infant is thought to be a mongol. What are the clinical features which may be present, and what is the basic cause of the condition?

**Council.(N. Ire.) 30-min question.** Which congenital abnormalities should be diagnosed in the first week of life? Describe briefly the treatment of any two of these.

**C.M.B.(Scot.** What examination of the newborn should a midwife make to detect congenital abnormalities?

**C.M.B.(Scot.)** What are the causes of convulsions in the neonatal period? Describe the investigations appropriate to this condition.

**C.M.B.(Scot.)** How are the following conditions in the newborn baby diagnosed: hydrocephalus, cleft palate, congenital dislocation of the hip, myelomeningocele.

**C.M.B.(Eng.)** What help is available to the mother who has given birth to a baby with hydrocephalus and spina bifida?

**C.M.B.(Scot.)** How are the following abnormalities of the baby detected and managed: (*a*) Congenital dislocation of the hip (*b*) Oesphageal atresia (*c*) Imperforate anus (*d*) Down's syndrome.

## C.M.B. (Short) Questions

**Eng.:** Cephalhaematoma. **N. Ire.:** Hydrocephalus. **Eng.:** Down's syndrome. **N. Ire.:** Cleft palate. **N. Ire.:** Anal atresia. **Eng.:** Oesophageal atresia. **Eng.:** Congenital dislocation of hip. **Eng.:** Hypospadias. **N. Ire.:** Meningomyelocele. **Eng.:** Tracheo-oesophageal fistula in the newborn. **N. Ire.:** Talipes equino varus. **Eng.:** Imperforate anus. **N. Ire.:** Exomphalos. **Scot.:** Cot deaths. **Eng.:** Tentorium cerebelli. **Eng.:** Clinical diagnosis of oesophageal atresia. **Scot.:** Intraventricular haemorrhage. **Eng.:** Cerebral irritation in the newborn. **N. Ire.:** Facial palsy. **Eng.:** Signs of cerebral trauma in the newborn. **Eng.:** The tentorium cerebelli. **Scot.:** Signs of intracranial injury. **Scot.:** Clinical features of intracranial haemorrhage in the newborn.

# 34

# Obstetric Operations

*Induction of labour, by i.v. syntocinon drip, prostaglandin E. Acceleration of labour. Version. Episiotomy, types, by midwives, analgesia for, suturing of. Forceps delivery. Avoiding errors in theatre. Anaesthetic requirements. Mendelson's syndrome. Epidural analgesia; observation, nursing care, 'topping up' by midwives. Caesarean section; midwives' duties, post-operative care.*

## INDUCTION OF LABOUR

There are numerous circumstances in which continuation of the pregnancy would exacerbate maternal complications, diminish fetal wellbeing and endanger fetal life.

### INDICATIONS FOR INDUCTION

(1) **Postmaturity** (7 or more days beyond term). Recent trends to allow pregnancy to continue for 14 days beyond term are now being reconsidered in the effort to reduce the perinatal mortality rate.

(2) **Pre-eclampsia.** The time of induction will depend on the severity of the condition. When severe, with proteinuria, induction at 34 weeks may be desirable if fetal lung maturity is adequate. Maternal and fetal wellbeing are both considered. Caesarean section might be necessary. The combination of postmaturity and pre-eclampsia is lethal for the fetus.

(3) **Diabetes** is a known cause of fetal death in late pregnancy so induction (or Caesarean section) is usually performed after 37 completed weeks of gestation.

(4) **Evidence of diminished fetal wellbeing** or growth, e.g. urinary oestriol secretion reduced to 11–18 micromoles serial ultrasonic bi-parietal cephalometry showing less than 1·1 mm weekly growth after 34 weeks: poor respiratory effort and sluggish movements detected by the sonar real-time scanner: abnormal fetal heart rate pattern on the electrocardiograph: adverse response to oxytocin challenge (fetal stress) test (see p. 108). Low kick count.

(5) **Placental abruption.** Puncture of membranes to drain off amniotic fluid is the recognised treatment: labour is thereby induced.

(6) **Rh incompatibility** is a less frequent indication since immunisation can now be prevented.

(7) **Other conditions are taken into consideration** such as: the older primigravida (over 30 years), bad obstetric history including perinatal deaths, gross fetal abnormality, fetal death.

**Caesarean section may be considered** as a less traumatic means of delivery. For the fetus at high risk a decision has to be made as to whether a compromised fetus can withstand the anoxic stress of labour.

**The maturity of the fetus** is of cardinal importance and whether there is sufficient pulmonary surfactant to avoid the risk of idiopathic respiratory distress syndrome. The lecithin sphingomyelin ratio in amniotic fluid will determine this: if low a course of betamethasone may be given to the mother to stimulate the production of surfactant in the fetal lungs.

**Inductions for non-medical reasons** are now less frequently performed since obstetricians question the benefits that have accrued from such inductions. Some expectant mothers are vocal in their disapproval of interference with normal labour.

**Cephalo-pelvic disproportion, malpresentation.** Caution should be observed when a previous Caesarean scar is present and particularly when the woman is under epidural analgesia. The uterus of the multiparous woman may rupture very readily.

**Buccal pitocin is now condemned as** a means of inducing labour. When tablets of pitocin citrate are placed between gum and cheek, absorption cannot be adequately controlled: tonic contractions may occur. A number of cases of uterine rupture have been recorded.

## The Successful Initiation of Labour Depends on:

(1) **The state of the cervix:** (see Bishop's score below) when soft, being taken up, and dilating the prognosis is good.

(2) **The period of gestation:** the nearer to term the better.

(3) **Level of the fetal head:** when 3/5ths of head or less is palpable at the pelvic brim, success is more likely.

(4) **Sensitivity of the uterus:** the uterus that responds readily to massage or to the oxytocin challenge (fetal stress) (p. 108) is more favourable.

### The Ripeness of the Cervix

This can be quantified by using Bishop's cervical scoring system, having first confirmed the expected date of delivery and maturity of the fetus.

| Inducibility Features | Score | | | |
|---|---|---|---|---|
| | 0 | 1 | 2 | 3 |
| **Dilatation** of cervix in cm. | closed | 1–2 cm | 3–4 cm | 5 cm |
| **Consistency** of cervix | firm | medium | soft | |
| **Position** of cervix | posterior | midline | anterior | |
| **Effacement** of cervix, percentage 0–30: 40–50 | 0–30 | 40–50 | 60–70 | 80 |
| **Station** In cm above or below the ischial spines −3: −2: −1: +1: +2 | −3 | −2 | −1 | +1 +2 |

| **BISHOP'S PRE INDUCTION CERVICAL SCORE SYSTEM** |
|---|

**Favourable induction features** are a score of 5 to 13
**Unfavourable induction features** are a score of 0 to 4

## Intravaginal Prostaglandin $E_2$

**This substance has proved to be effective** in ripening the cervix prior to formal induction of labour by i.v. Syntocinon. Prostaglandin in tylose, a viscous gel, is introduced into the extra amniotic space or the posterior vaginal fornix by a Nelaton urinary catheter attached to a syringe containing the gel. If ripening of the cervix occurs overnight, an induction pessary of Prostaglandin $E_2$ is introduced into the vagina or an i.v. oxytocin infusion started. Should the fetus be dead or seriously malformed the membranes need not be punctured when Prostaglandin $E_2$ is used.

### PUNCTURE OF MEMBRANES

This is the most certain method of inducing preterm labour usually done in conjunction with Prostaglandin to ripen the cervix followed by Syntocinon i.v. drip. In cases when placental dysfunction may be present, it is an advantage to see whether the amniotic fluid is meconium stained or not. The opportunity is taken to apply a scalp electrode to monitor the fetal heart rate pattern.

*Method*

The bladder is emptied. A sedative may be given if necessary for an apprehensive primigravida. The patient is placed in the lithotomy position, vulva cleansed, antiseptic precautions taken.

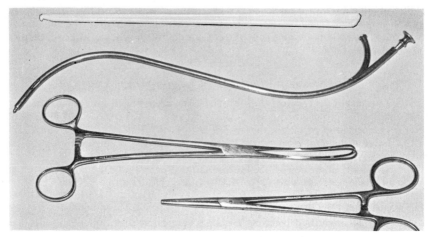

Fig. 34-1    Instruments to puncture the membranes. Amniotomy hook, Drew Smythe catheter, Goodwin's amniotomy forceps, Kochers forceps.

**Induction pack.** Lithotomy sheet, towel 90 × 90 cm: 2 sheets sterifield paper: amniotomy forceps: Goodwin's, Stiles or a disposable amniotomy hook.

Obstetric cream, Hibitane 1–2,000. Polythene sheet: cap, mask, gloves.

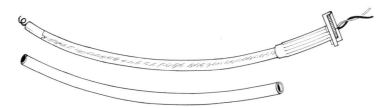

Fig. 34-2    Spiral scalp electrode to record the fetal heart beat. Can be applied to fetal scalp when the cervix is one cm dilated. Application is accomplished by a screwing movement, using the special introducer: not to be applied over a suture or fontanelle. The fetal heart rate is displayed on the panel meter of a cardiotocograph.

## OXYTOCIN I.V. INFUSION (SYNTOCINON)

**To induce labour.**

The Syntocinon i.v. infusion tends to ripen the cervix but not as effectively as is done by Prostaglandin $E_2$, which may be used prior to Syntocinon induction.

### *Technique of Administration*

Lie, presentation, fetal heart rate are checked: cephalo-pelvic disproportion excluded. An enema is given. Prior to starting the drip a careful vaginal examination is made regarding the dilatation and consistency of the cervix: the membranes usually being punctured at this time.

**A drug additive label is attached** to the bottle containing Syntocinon, with the signatures of those who have checked and added the Syntocinon. The two bottle technique is commonly employed in order that the Syntocinon drip may be started and stopped as required and the vein kept patent. This technique also permits adequate hydration of the patient by giving glucose 5 per cent 4 to 6 hourly. If ketonuria develops glucose 10 per cent can be given. The two bottles of glucose 5 per cent are connected by separate 'giving sets' via a four-way disposable tap to the infusion cannula.

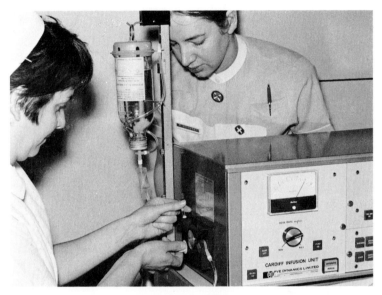

Fig. 34.3   Cardiff Infusion Unit. Sister is connecting the 17·8 cm length of sterile translucent silicone rubber tubing to the infusion bottle containing 500 ml glucose solution 5 per cent with 10 units oxytocin and to the rotary pump. The dose rate can be regulated in accordance with the strength and frequency of the uterine contractions. If desired, the dose rate is doubled every 15 minutes starting with a very low dose. Alarm conditions and safety monitors are incorporated. A catheter inserted through the cervix records amniotic fluid pressure. The alarm 'sounds' when the pressure is too high.

*Photographed at Royal Maternity Hospital, Rottenrow, Glasgow.*
*Courtesy of Pye Dynamics Ltd., Bushey Watford, Hertfordshire.*

### Electronic systems used

To attain precision in the administration of Syntocinon, various electronic systems are used.

**The Tekmar IVAC** apparatus continuously monitors drip rates. The IVAC 400 pumps at rates from 1 drop/min upwards.

**The Palmer syringe pump** is used by some when small amounts of fluid (at a slow rate) are being administered, as in pre-eclampsia.

**The 'Pye Dynamics'** automatic infusion system MP40 is used in conjunction with a standard fetal monitor and the rate of the infusion is programmed to increase until the uterine contractions are established at a safe level.

**The Cardiff Infusion System** is utilised in the Pye Dynamics induction and monitoring system type MM2, which operates on an automated titration method. It is usual to begin with 10 units of Syntocinon in 500 ml glucose 5 per cent; the flow delivers one milliunit Syntocinon per minute and is automatically doubled every 12·5 minutes to a maximum of 32 milliunits per minute. The Cardiff Syntocinon infusion rate is controlled by amniotic pressure which is monitored through a catheter in the amniotic sac via a transducer on the machine controlling the pump. When contractions of 45 to 50 seconds at 2 to 3 minute intervals are achieved, the switch is set to 'manual' and the dose rate is maintained (not doubled). If the contractions are too strong the dose rate can be reduced. Various safety devices and alarms are incorporated within the Cardiff unit. When contractions reach 32 mm Hg every 2·5 minutes, the dose of Syntocinon is not increased.

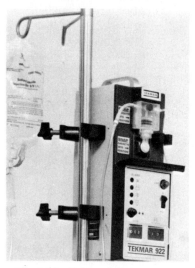

Fig. 34-4    Tekmar infusion pump.

### DOSAGE OF SYNTOCINON IN MILLIUNITS

Milliunits of Syntocinon per minute are quoted as a means of stating the exact amount of Syntocinon received by the patient. Whatever the concentration of Syntocinon used, milliunits are the one quantitative measurement that can be utilised whether the infusion is administered by 'giving set', manually adjusted fixed rate set, syringe pump or Cardiff titration infusion system.

### One unit of Syntocinon equals 1000 milliunits

If 2 units Syntocinon are added to 500 ml glucose 5 per cent

1 ml of the solution will contain $\dfrac{2,000}{500} =$ 4 milliunits Syntocinon

2 ml of the solution will contain $\dfrac{2,000}{250} =$ 8 milliunits Syntocinon

4 ml of the solution will contain $\dfrac{2,000}{125} =$ 16 milliunits Syntocinon

| | 1 ml/min | 2 ml/min | 4 ml/min |
|---|---|---|---|
| | | **Milliunits** | |
| 2 units Syntocinon in 500 ml glucose 5% | 4 | 8 | 16 |
| 4 units Syntocinon in 500 ml glucose 5% | 8 | 16 | 32 |
| 8 units Syntocinon in 500 ml glucose 5% | 16 | 32 | 64 |
| 10 units Syntocinon in 500 ml glucose 5% | 20 | 40 | 80 |

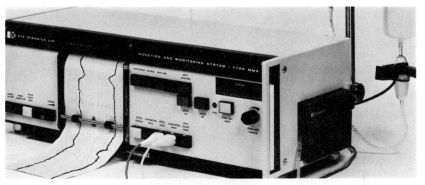

Fig. 34-5  Induction and monitoring system type MM2. Monitors and displays fetal heart rates and intrauterine contraction pressures. Administers synthetic oxytocin at accurately controlled rates. The infusion can be controlled manually if so required.

*Courtesy of Pye Dynamics Ltd.*

*To induce labour a typical regime would be:*

Two units of Syntocinon are mixed thoroughly with 500 ml glucose 5 per cent. A polythene cannula is introduced into the vein and the infusion given at 15 drops/min delivering 4 milliunits/min increasing to 30 drops in 20 minutes delivering 8 milliunits/min and to 60 drops in a further 20 minutes delivering 16 milliunits/min.

**If contractions do not start** a fresh bottle of glucose 5 per cent with 8 units of Syntocinon is prepared and the rate of flow started at 15 drops/min delivering 16 milliunits/min: increasing in 20 minutes to 30 drops delivering 32 milliunits/min: increasing in 20 minutes to 60 drops/min delivering 64 milliunits/min. When contractions are satisfactory neither units nor rate flow of Syntocinon are increased any further. Syntocinon may have to be decreased.

**If the uterus does not contract satisfactorily** with 8 units Syntocinon delivering 64 milliunits/min the doctor will reassess the situation. If the head has failed to engage, Caesarean section may be contemplated.

### INDICATIONS FOR STOPPING THE DRIP

**Strong contractions** lasting over 60 seconds and occurring oftener than every 2 minutes.

**Tumultuous or tonic contractions** with no adequate relaxation between them.

**Fetal distress,** e.g. slowing of the fetal heart, base line irregularity particularly in association with meconium stained amniotic fluid.

**Deterioration in the woman's condition,** e.g. severe hypertension.

These indications should be reported to the doctor in their incipient stages and the tap is switched to the bottle without Syntocinon.

## NURSING CARE

The induction procedure should be explained to the woman in simple reassuring terms, giving 'reasons why' and stressing the advantages. To counteract the objection currently expressed by some mothers that induction is 'unwarranted interference', midwives should persuade their patients that induction is a humane procedure, necessary and beneficial to mother and child.

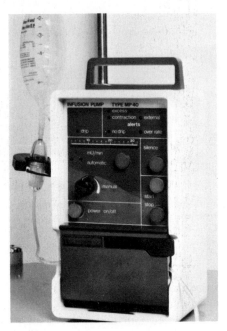

Fig. 34-6  Pye Dynamics infusion pump MP40. Can be used in conjunction with Pye Dynamics fetal monitor MM2 or most cardiotocographs on the market. The dose rate is programmed to increase progressively until strong contractions are established or until the dose rate reaches 32 milliunits per minute.

**Electronic monitors are used to** extend the midwife's powers of observation and enhance the supervision she gives but the woman should not gain the impression that she is receiving less attention than the electronic monitors.

**Supervision must be diligently carried out** and findings recorded. But recording is not enough: the doctor must be notified when early signs of impending complications arise.

### Pain relief

The patient decides when pain is becoming severe, usually when labour is established with contractions every 5 minutes and about one hour after the infusion is started. Oxytocin contractions are said to be more painful than those of spontaneous labour so pethidine 150 mg with promethazine (Phenergan) 25 mg is commonly prescribed if epidural analgesia is not being administered. Pain relief permits the woman to obtain the essential rest and sleep.

### Control of haemorrhage

After the baby is delivered, the drip is speeded up at the concentration then in use. When the placenta is expelled complete, and the uterus is contracting firmly, the drip rate is reduced gradually over a period of 30 minutes. If the uterus remains retracted, the tap is switched to the glucose drip and run for 30 minutes. Only then, if everything is satisfactory, should the drip be dismantled.

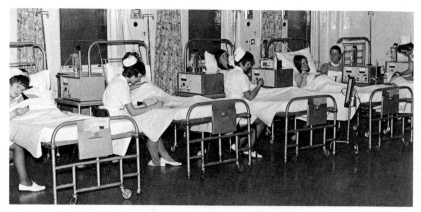

Fig. 34-7    Five Cardiff infusion units in use. Midwives assessing the tone of the uterus during and between contractions.

*Photographed at Royal Maternity Hospital, Rottenrow, Glasgow.*
*Courtesy of Pye Dynamics Ltd., Bushey, Watford, Hertfordshire.*

**OBSERVATION**

### Rate of flow

The drip must be started cautiously and to avoid uterine spasm the correct dosage strictly adhered to.

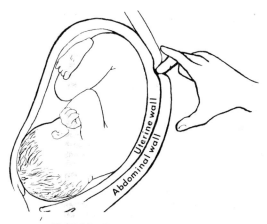

Fig. 34-8    Testing uterine tonus.

### Uterine contractions

Slight hardening of the uterus may be felt on palpation within 10 minutes. Constant supervision is essential until the maximal dose necessary is reached. Once contractions are adequate, Syntocinon is not increased either in concentration or flow rate. The time, duration and strength of the contractions are entered on the partogram: if no contractions occur that fact is recorded every half hour. Midwives should use 'finger tip' palpation to test the tonus of the uterus during and between contractions, particularly when no electronic uterine monitor is available. Tonic contractions are a danger that must constantly be kept in mind.

### Fetal heart rate

This is recorded on the partogram every 15 minutes. Continuous FH monitoring is carried out electronically on all 'high risk' cases and also during epidural analgesia: a scalp electrode being applied at amniotomy. Should signs of fetal distress be manifest the tap should be switched to the bottle with no Syntocinon and medical aid sought.

### Progress

This is noted by abdominal palpation of the descent of the fetal head and vaginal examination of cervical dilatation.

### Maternal condition.

*The blood pressure* is assessed every hour.

*The pulse* is taken at frequent intervals and recorded every half hour.

*The temperature* is taken every 4 hours and if raised an endocervical swab is obtained and an antibiotic administered.

*The urine* is measured and examined with Labstix reagent strips. Ketoacidosis must be averted or treated. More urine is passed when fluid is administered intravenously so the bladder should be emptied every 2 hours.

*A fluid balance chart is kept.* Dehydration should be avoided and the i.v. glucose solution will help to prevent this. The glucose will also provide some of the necessary calories.

**Prolapse of cord may occur during induced labour** and this should be kept in mind and dealt with. Prolapse of cord is predisposed to when the presenting part is high at the time of puncturing the membranes; a situation frowned on in most centres.

## PROSTAGLANDIN E$_2$

### TO RIPEN THE CERVIX. TO INDUCE LABOUR

Prostaglandin E$_2$ has been administered to induce labour by various routes: the extra amniotic and the intravaginal currently seem to be used in preference to the intravenous and oral routes.

**Intravenously administered,** PGE$_2$ may produce temporary pyrexia, gastro-intestinal side effects and erythema at the site of the injection.

**The oral route** causes a prolonged induction-delivery interval as well as nausea, vomiting and diarrhoea.

Whether the cervix is ripe or not has an important influence on induced labour: cervical effacement usually begins after 36 weeks' gestation.

Accurate assessment of fetal gestational age and pulmonary maturity is made prior to induction in order to avoid the risk of idiopathic respiratory distress syndrome.

### RIPENING THE CERVIX WITH PGE$_2$

**When Bishop's cervical induction score is unfavourable,** i.e. 0–4, PGE$_2$ administered intravaginally is an effective ripening agent to efface and dilate the cervix. Some women will go into labour during the ripening process: if not a repeat dose of PGE$_2$ will be necessary to induce labour.

*The woman empties her bladder:* an enema having been given on admission for induction.

(a) **An extra amniotic injection of viscous gel** containing PGE$_2$ is given during the evening prior to the formal induction. A Nelaton catheter attached to a syringe containing the gel is introduced into the extra amniotic space, i.e. between the fetal membranes and the posterior wall of the lower uterine segment. A solution of PGE$_2$ can also be administered by the extra amniotic route, using a Foley catheter and 'giving set' with 500 ml isotonic saline containing 5 mg PGE$_2$. The Cardiff pump may be used.

(b) **Intravaginal instillation.** The viscous gel containing PGE$_2$ is introduced via a syringe with a Nelaton catheter 16 FG: the tip being placed in the posterior vaginal fornix. The woman remains recumbent for 15 minutes.

(c) **A vaginal pessary** containing PGE$_2$ is introduced into the posterior vaginal fornix—some have used the tablets intended for oral administration. Insertion of the pessary is easy: only a sterile glove and obstetric jelly being required. If the uterine contractions become tumultuous or occur too rapidly, the pessary can be removed quickly.

### INDUCTION OF LABOUR BY PGE$_2$

When the cervix is effaced (softened, shortened, dilated) whether spontaneously or by Prostaglandin E$_2$. PGE$_2$ is administered for ripening. See (a), (b), (c). As soon as painful uterine contractions occur and the cervix is 2 cm dilated, the membranes may be punctured. This is advisable in order that an electrode can be attached to the fetal scalp to monitor the FH rate pattern.

The contractions may be erratic at first but a pattern of strong, regular contractions which resemble those of spontaneous labour develops. Hypertonic uterine contractions may occur if the dose of PGE$_2$ is too big or speeded up too rapidly.

A close watch must be kept on uterine activity. As well as using electronic monitors, the midwife should use finger tip palpation to assess uterine tonus. If contractions are too frequent or hypertonic the administration should be stopped, pessary or gel removed.

**Nursing care,** observation, pain relief, electronic monitoring, and recording, are similar to what has been outlined for Syntocinon i.v. drip (page 602). Fetal status and uterine activity must be diligently assessed and recorded throughout labour.

**Note**

**Prostaglandin E$_2$ must not be speeded up during the third stage** nor is it administered to treat postpartum haemorrhage. To do so would be dangerous.

When gross fetal abnormality is present or the fetus is dead, prostaglandin E$_2$ is particularly useful to induce labour. Because it is not necessary to puncture the membranes with PGE$_2$, the risk of sepsis in such cases is reduced.

**Contra-indications**

(a) **If placental function is seriously impaired,** Caesarean section is preferred.
(b) **The grande multipara** because of the possibility of uterine rupture.
(c) **Previous Caesarean section** because of the risk of a weak scar rupturing.
(d) **Cephalo-pelvic disproportion** or any condition that could obstruct labour.

# VERSION

The term 'version' is applied when an alteration in the lie of the fetus *in utero* is brought about or the location of its upper and lower poles reversed. It may occur spontaneously or by manipulation. The term 'cephalic version' is used when the head of the fetus is made to present, and 'podalic version' when the breech is made to present.

## EXTERNAL VERSION

External version is carried out by abdominal manipulation. It is usually done to rectify a breech or shoulder presentation in the latter part of pregnancy, preferably between the 32nd and 36th week, or at the beginning of labour if the membranes are intact. Version is performed by the doctor. A midwife should not attempt external version during pregnancy, but would be justified in doing so for shoulder presentation at the onset of labour or in the second twin if medical aid was not immediately obtainable.

### Contra-indications

Previous Caesarean section to avoid scar rupture: ante-partum haemorrhage to avert further placental separation: ruptured membranes: Rh negative woman to prevent transplacental bleeding: severe hypertension to avoid causing placental abruption: twin pregnancy.

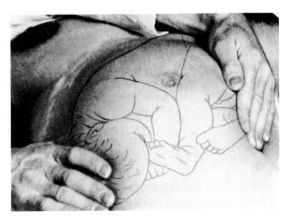

Fig. 34-9   External cephalic version. Head in right iliac fosa.

### *Method*

The woman should be on a table or bed, the head of which can be lowered quickly: her bladder having been emptied. Most authorities do not employ anaesthesia, because they consider the force that might be used on an unconscious woman may be greater than is in the interest of mother or child. The important factor in version is to get the fetus flexed into a ball so that it can be turned more readily, and to ensure that a well-flexed head or the breech will present. The head and back should be located and the fetus turned by using steady pressure, making it follow its nose if possible; otherwise the head may extend, resulting in a face or brow presentation.

**Mental and physical relaxation should be attained,** and it is a good idea to divert the woman's attention by engaging her in conversation during the manoeuvre. She is more likely to tighten her abdominal muscles if she is told what is being done, or why.

**Warm hands and smooth gentle manipulation** are essential. Partial flexion of the patient's thighs will aid relaxation of her abdominal muscles.

It is usual to find some alteration in the fetal heart beat pattern for a few minutes so the woman should remain in the recumbent position, under observation for three or four hours, and if there is no vaginal bleeding, uterine contractions or amniotic fluid draining she is allowed to get up. A light meal should be given before she is discharged under the care of a relative or friend. To have the presentation checked, the woman is asked to report back in one week. An unstable lie is investigated further: if version fails radiological assessment of the pelvis may be considered.

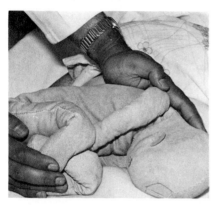 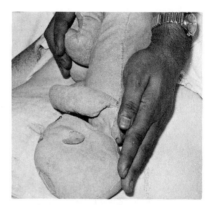

Fig. 34-10, 34-11    External version shoulder to vertex presentation.

### THE MIDWIFE'S DUTY

The X-ray films should be at hand, also a fetal stethoscope. The woman should empty her bladder. Some obstetricians want the foot of the bed raised 60 cm on blocks for half an hour prior to version, to disengage the breech from the pelvic brim. Talcum powder is sprinkled on the skin to reduce friction.

*Internal and bipolar version are described under emergency obstetric operations by midwives in developing countries (p. 649).*

# EPISIOTOMY

The making of an incision into the perineum to enlarge the vaginal orifice is known as an episiotomy. Such an incision is directed away from the anus to avoid a third-degree tear: the clean cut is more easily repaired and heals better than a ragged laceration.

### INDICATIONS FOR EPISIOTOMY

**Delay** due to: rigid perineum; disproportion between fetus and vaginal orifice.
**Fetal distress,** prolapsed cord in second stage. To hasten the birth of the baby.
**To facilitate vaginal or intra-uterine manipulation,** e.g. forceps: breech delivery.
**Preterm baby** under 2·2 kg to avoid intracranial damage.

### ADVANTAGES

**Fetal acidosis and hypoxia are reduced.**
**Overstretching of the pelvic floor is lessened:** a well sutured perineum provides greater support than a lax perineum.
**Bruising of the urethra is avoided.**
**In severe pre-eclampsia or cardiac disease** to reduce the effort bearing down entails.

**A previous third degree tear** which may occur again because of the scar tissue which does not stretch well is prevented.

## TYPES OF EPISIOTOMY

### (1) Medio-lateral (*Recommended for midwives*)

The incision is begun in the centre of the fourchette and directed postero-laterally, usually to the woman's right. It should be not more than 3 cm long and is directed, diagonally in a straight line which runs 2·5 cm distant from the anus. If the anus is considered to be 6 on the clock, the incision would be directed to 7 o'clock.

### (2) Median

The incision, begun in the centre of the fourchette, is directed posteriorly for approximately 2·5 cm in the midline of the perineum. It is favoured by, and is most successful in the hands of, the experienced obstetrician who will have absolute control of the fetal head: otherwise there is a risk that the incision will be extended during delivery and produce a third-degree tear. When vaginal manipulation is necessary or the baby large, the median incision does not provide as much space as the medio-lateral incision. The advantages are (*a*) less bleeding, (*b*) more easily and successfully repaired, (*c*) greater subsequent comfort for the woman.

### (3) J-shaped

The incision is begun in the centre of the fourchette and directed posteriorly in the mid-line for about 2 cm and then directed outwards towards 7 on the clock to avoid the anus. The suturing of this incision is difficult: shearing of the tissues occurs: the repaired wound tends to be puckered.

### (4) Lateral

This incision is begun one or more cm distant from the centre of the fourchette and is condemned. Bartholin's duct may be severed: the levator ani muscle is weakened, bleeding is more profuse: suturing is more difficult and the woman experiences subsequent discomfort.

## EPISIOTOMY BY MIDWIVES

### C.M.B. quotation

'The necessity for the performance of episiotomy may become apparent late in labour when immediate action is required. Unless medical aid is immediately available the operation should be performed by the midwife, after infiltration of the perineum with local analgesic when time permits.'

### LOCAL ANALGESIA FOR EPISIOTOMY

'A practising midwife should have available a supply of a local analgesic when in attendance on a woman in labour.' '10 ml of an 0·5 per cent solution or 5 ml of a one per cent solution of lignocaine or similar agent should be sufficient to infiltrate the perineum.'

Suture of the perineum should normally be referred to a registered medical practitioner.

Modern local analgesics are relatively safe. Lignocaine (Xylocaine) is safe and efficient: it takes effect rapidly (1 or 2 minutes).

### Toxic reactions

All analgesic drugs are potentially toxic. The midwife need not be unduly apprehensive: when adequately informed she will avoid such reactions: should they be caused inadvertently she will recognise and treat them promptly.

(1) **If the analgesic is injected into a blood vessel** the concentration in the blood stream could be dangerously high. Precautions must be taken prior to injection by withdrawing the piston and if no blood appears the needle has not entered a blood vessel: the injection should then be given while slowly withdrawing the needle.

(2) **Giving too high a concentration** of the drug or an excessive amount of a suitable concentration. The Central Midwives Boards have limited the concentration and the amount to be given by midwives, i.e. 10 ml of an 0·5 per cent solution, or 5 ml of a 1 per cent solution. Both injections contain the same amount of lignocaine. Midwives will no doubt, for additional safety, carry and use one strength of solution.

### Toxic signs

Tinnitus: drowsiness: twitching of face and limbs: tingling in area of mouth: convulsions: respiratory depression: circulatory collapse.

### *Treatment*

**Clear airway: lower head and raise legs: give oxygen.** Send urgently for the anaesthetist and anaesthetic machine.

#### INJECTION OF LOCAL ANALGESIC

10 ml sterile syringe with no metal fittings. Ampoule 0·5 per cent lignocaine, needle 3·75 cm 21 g. Sterifield paper 60 cm. 5 gauze swabs.

(*a*) The lithotomy or dorsal position is adopted in hospital: at home the dorsal with hips elevated on a firm pad.

(*b*) Vulva swabbed with Hibitane, 1 in 2,000. Explanation and assurance are given as necessary.

During the interval between contractions the first two fingers of the gloved left hand are inserted into the vagina, between the perineum and the fetal scalp, to ensure that the drug is not inadvertently injected into the fetus.

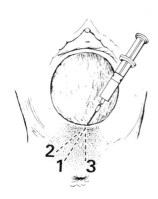

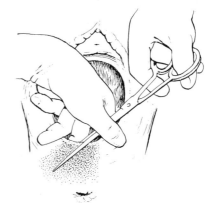

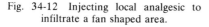

Fig. 34-12 Injecting local analgesic to infiltrate a fan shaped area.

Fig. 34-13 Making episiotomy; fingers protecting the fetus.

The needle is introduced in the midline of the inner edge of the fourchette and directed subcutaneously for a distance of 3 cm, usually to the woman's right side, along the line the episiotomy will follow, which should be 2·5 cm distant from the anal sphincter. Having introduced the needle for 3 cm and prior to injecting lignocaine the piston of the syringe is withdrawn and, if no blood appears in the barrel, a blood vessel has not been entered so 3 ml of lignocaine are injected while the needle is slowly withdrawn. Giving the injection while the needle is moving ensures that the drug does not enter a vein. (Some inject 0·5 ml of analgesic as the needle is being inserted.)

Without removing the needle, redirect it so that the tip will be 1 cm from the tip of the first injection, pull back piston and if no blood appears inject, while slowly withdrawing the needle, a further 3 ml of analgesic. Redirect the needle on the other side of the first injection and proceed as previously to inject the last 3 ml of analgesic. The three injections will infiltrate over a fan-shaped area and the incision is made down the centre.

(Midwives not permitted to administer a local analgesic could use inhalational analgesia, e.g. Entonox, or methoxyflurane (Penthrane) which will relieve, but not abolish, the pain of incision.)

### Making the incision

The scar of a previous episiotomy should be avoided; because it does not heal well but the incision can be made alongside the old scar. The length of the incision made by midwives would be not more than 3 cm on the stretched perineum.

In hospital the dorsal or lithotomy position is convenient: on district the dorsal position with the hips elevated on a firm pad. The left lateral position is not recommended because the scissors may slip sideways and incise the labium.

After injecting the local analgesic and waiting for one or more minutes, two fingers are inserted between the perineum and the fetal scalp to protect it from injury by the scissors. During a uterine contraction would be a suitable time as it is easier to gauge the required length of the incision when the perineum is on the stretch. One deliberate cut should be made beginning in the centre of the fourchette (edge of the perineum) 3 cm in length and directed 2·5 cm away from the anus. A tentative series of small snips will result in a ragged incision which is difficult to suture and slow to unite. The episiotomy ought to be adequate to remove any resistance to the fetal head. Mayo straight, blunt pointed, scissors 17·5 cm are commonly used. They must be sharpened at frequent intervals: blunt scissors bruise the perineum.

#### SUGGESTIONS FOR EPISIOTOMY BY MIDWIVES

There are so many different opinions regarding the various aspects of episiotomy that no one method will be acceptable to all midwives. The preferences of the medical practitioners who are likely to be called to repair the incisions should be known and respected.

### Timing the incision

Judgment is needed, for the episiotomy must be made neither too soon nor too late: the head should be well down on the perineum, low enough to keep it stretched. Some consider that 4 to 5 cm of scalp should be showing but the bulging thinned perineum is probably a better criterion. In breech presentation the posterior buttock would be distending the perineum. If made too soon bleeding will be profuse from the thick vascular tissue: if the descending head has not displaced the levator ani muscle it will be damaged. If made too late the supports of the neck of the bladder are weakened, the pelvic floor overstretched: bruised tissues do not heal well: mother and fetus are subjected to unnecessary stress and the purpose of the episiotomy is defeated.

### Bleeding from the episiotomy

Bleeding always occurs to some extent but it can be profuse when the incision is made too soon and the perineum is thick. The pressure exerted by the fetal head usually controls any bleeding: if not, direct pressure using a gauze swab can be applied. Should bleeding continue after the birth of the baby, which is not controllable by firm pressure with a folded vulval pad, two Spencer Wells forceps should be applied to the bleeding vessels. The episiotomy should be repaired as soon as possible; union of tissues is better, with less risk of sepsis and a broken down wound; nor should the woman be subjected to the prolonged apprehension of 'stitches'.

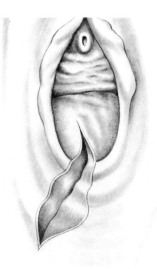 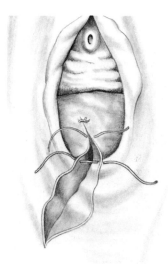

Fig. 34-14  Episiotomy wound.      Fig. 34-15  First suture inserted in apex of wound.

## HINTS FOR MIDWIVES ON SUTURING THE EPISIOTOMY

C.M.B. Memo England. 'Midwives who have been taught to suture the perineum and are judged to be competent may be authorised by the doctor to carry out this procedure. The final responsibility rests with the doctor.'

The local analgesic given for making the episiotomy should be effective for one hour. Early suturing is recommended.

The area is cleansed with antiseptic solution and blood clot removed from the vagina. Oozing from the uterus may obscure the field and, if so, a taped vaginal tampon or a small taped vaginal pack should be inserted into the vault of the vagina and recorded on the chart (subsequent removal of the pad is, of course, mandatory). A good light is essential. Some attach an Allis's tissue forceps on either side of the incision at the junction of perineal skin and vaginal epithelium, to facilitate adequate inspection of the wound in depth and, when suturing, to provide an aid to the accurate apposition of the incised edges of the fourchette. The full extent of the laceration is determined, including that the anal sphincter is intact.

An episiotomy, which is comparable with the wound of a second degree tear, must be repaired in three layers—

**Vaginal wound:** (*a*) deep and superficial tissues, (*b*) vaginal mucosa.

**Pelvic floor muscles and perineal body.**

**Perineal skin** and subcutaneous tissue.

It is most important that the first stitch inserted is at the apex of the incision, the upper limit of the wound in the posterior vaginal wall. Some use three or four interrupted sutures of chromic catgut No. 1/0 on a round-bodied Mayo needle No. 2 for the deep tissues or Ethicon eyeless needled chromic suture W 759. Some use, for vagina and muscle layers, Dexon atraumatic 40 mm round bodied needle: for skin No. 0 atraumatic 37 mm diamond taper needle. If the deep structures are not properly sutured, lochial discharge may collect in the dead space and decompose; the epithelium breaks down exposing a gaping infected area. To avoid injury to the rectum while inserting the deep sutures the forefinger of the left hand placed in the vagina can press the rectum downwards. Superficial sutures in the vaginal mucosa must be close enough (0·5 cm) to prevent blood seeping into the deep tissues and forming a haematoma. Some authorities use a continuous suture to ensure against this, but too many stitches may cause puckering and shortening of the posterior vaginal wall.

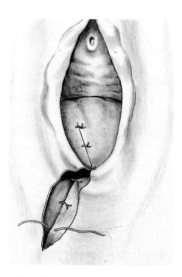

Fig. 34-16  Deep sutures inserted.

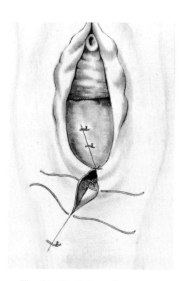

Fig. 34-17  External sutures.

### EXTERNAL SUTURES

The future integrity of the pelvic floor depends on good union achieved by suturing the wound layer by layer: the muscles must be united, the perineal body reconstructed. Merely suturing the skin of the perineum is futile: the wound must be sutured in its entire depth with interrupted sutures.

The skin and subcutaneous tissues are carefully apposed and united with interrupted Mersilk sutures No. 1 inserted not less than 0·5 cm from the edge of the incision, otherwise when oedema occurs they may cut out. Ethicon W 562 on a curved cutting needle may be used. Allis's forceps previously applied facilitate good alignment of the perineal skin and vaginal epithelium at the fourchette. The edges of the incision should merely meet and must on no account be tied tightly or the wound is likely to break down. Chromic catgut No. 0 or 2/0 or Dexon with a half circle cutting needle No. 7 is favoured by some. At the end of the procedure it would be a wise precaution to insert the gloved finger into the rectum in case a suture has been extended beyond the intended limit.

All perineal lacerations should be sutured and this the doctor will do as soon as possible. A good light is essential. Some insert subcuticular sutures which are not interrupted: they are successful in the majority of cases but if sepsis or a haematoma occurs the wound may break down. A general anaesthetic is necessary for the repair of a third degree tear.

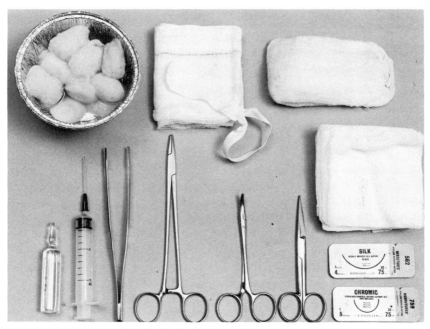

Fig. 34-18    Perineal suture requirements.

*Aberdeen Maternity Hospital.*

**LINEN AND DRESSINGS**

1 Gown; cap; mask; gloves; hand towel.
2 towels 90 cm
1 taped tampon
10 gauze swabs
20 wool mops
1 perineal pad

1 5 metric chromic catgut with
  eyeless round bodied needle
  40 mm Ethicon W759
1 needle 219

**INSTRUMENTS**

1 dissecting forceps toothed
1 Mayo needle holder
1 Spencer Well's artery forceps
1 Mayo scissors

**SUTURES AND NEEDLES**

1 4 metric mersilk with eyeless
  cutting needle
  60 mm Ethicon 562
1 10 ml ampoule Lignocaine 1 per cent.
1 10 ml syringe

# DELIVERY OF THE FETUS BY FORCEPS

*The procedure is explained for midwives in developing countries (on page 642).*

Obstetric forceps consists of two blades, with a cephalic curve that accommodates the fetal head and a pelvic curve which conforms to the curve of the pelvic canal.

## Low forceps

In this case the largest presenting skull diameter is below the level of the ischial spines and the head distending the perineum; the more common indication being delay, physical or emotional fatigue. Haig Ferguson's, or Wrigley's forceps are suitable for this purpose.

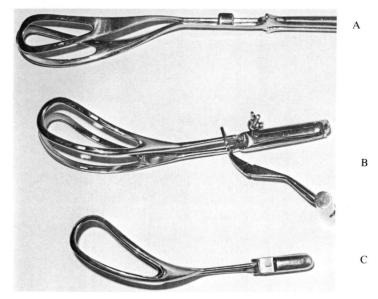

Fig. 34-19   Obstetric forceps.
A. Kielland's. B. Haig Ferguson's. C. Wrigley's.

## Mid-forceps

In this case the head is engaged; the presenting part (not only the caput) is at the level of the ischial spines; the most common indications being delay due to deep transverse arrest, occipito-posterior position of the vertex and for fetal distress. Haig Ferguson's and Barnes Neville's forceps are generally used in Great Britain.

## Kielland's forceps

These are straight and have a sliding lock. They are admirably suited for rotation of the fetal head in cases of deep transverse arrest or occipito-posterior position.

### INDICATIONS FOR FORCEPS

Forceps are applied during the second stage only. Although it is not within the midwife's province to decide when forceps should be applied, she must be aware of the various indications for their use, in order that she may notify the doctor in time and have the necessary equipment at hand. (A paediatrician is present in hospital.)

### Delay in the second stage due to

Hypotonic uterine action.      Deep transverse arrest.
Minor degrees of outlet contraction.      Persistent occipito-posterior position.

## Maternal complications

In cases of severe pre-eclampsia and eclampsia, to eliminate strenuous pushing, which raises the blood pressure and is apt to provoke fits.

Ketoacidosis, incipient or established. Preterm labour

In the more serious degrees of cardiac disease or advanced pulmonary tuberculosis, forceps are usually applied.

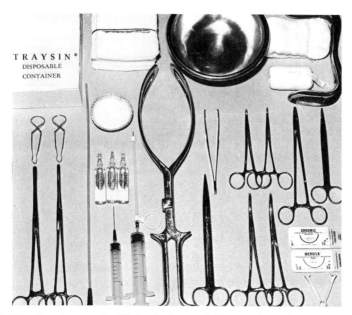

Fig. 34-20   Requirements for Kielland's forceps delivery under pudendal nerve block.

*Simpson Memorial Pavilion, Edinburgh.*

### SUTURES AND NEEDLES
One 5 metre chromic catgut with
  eyeless round bodied needle
  45 mm Ethicon W727

One 3·5 metric Mersilk with
  eyeless needle
  50 mm Ethicon W552

### LINEN
1 gown; lithotomy sheet; leggings;
  baby wrap.

### DRESSINGS
10 gauze swabs; 20 wool swabs
2 anal pads
1 vaginal tampon

### SEPARATELY WRAPPED
gloves; cap; mask; mucus extractors.
1 large metal basin for Savlon 1–100
1 measuring jug 1200 ml

### INSTRUMENTS
2 prs. sponge holding forceps
2 towel clips
1 disposable catheter 14 FG
1 10 ml syringe 21 needle
1 20 ml syringe with pudendal
  needle and guide
3 10 ml ampoules lignocaine 1 per
  cent plain
1 pr. Kielland's forceps
1 pr. Mayo scissors 21 cm straight
2 prs. Mayo forceps 18 cm for cord
1 pr. toothed dissecting forceps
2 prs. Spencer Well's 14 cm forceps
1 needle holder
1 pr. Mayo scissors 17 cm
1 disposable container for urine
1 foil gallipot with obstetric cream
1 Sim's speculum
1 Hollister cord clamp
1 bowl for placenta

**Fetal complications**

Fetal distress.       To control the aftercoming head in
Prolapse of cord during second stage. breech presentation.

*The Midwife's Duties*

The signed permission slip for operation and anaesthesia is attached to the patient's chart.

Requirements for catheterisation, episiotomy and perineal suture are at hand.

Equipment must be in readiness to treat an asphyxiated baby, control postpartum haemorrhage and combat shock.

The woman is usually delivered in the lithotomy position, and both legs must be raised and lowered simultaneously to prevent injury to the sacro-iliac joints.

To avoid trauma of leg veins, care is taken by padding leg rests and preventing undue pressure by stirrup-rods.

The midwife washes pubes, groins and thighs with a perineal pad. A polythene sheet is placed under the buttocks to direct fluid into the bucket.

The doctor swabs the vulva and passes the catheter. A sterile towel is placed under the buttocks, lithotomy leggings and perineal towel are arranged in position.

The senior midwife listens to the fetal heart and notifies the doctor when the uterus contracts if a cardiotocograph is not available.

Resuscitation equipment for the baby should be in readiness. Vitamin $K_1$ (Konakion) is usually administered.

# SAFEGUARDS AGAINST ERRORS IN OPERATING THEATRE

### 1. To avoid operating on wrong patient

**An identity disc or band** should be attached to the patient's wrist by the ward sister and checked with the operation list by the theatre sister. Name, initials, hospital number and nature of operation should be stated.

**The correct case notes, X-ray films,** and signed 'consent to operation and anaesthetic' form should accompany the patient. The obstetrician identifies the patient.

**Pre-operative medication ordered and given should be recorded** on the chart. This is checked by the anaesthetist.

**For the baby an identity wrist-band** should be prepared and applied in the theatre.

### 2. To avoid leaving any foreign body within the operative area

**An efficient system of counting and checking swabs, packs, instruments, needles,** should be set out in writing and observed in practice. Swabs to be used within the body must be white and contain a radio-opaque substance. (Raytec swabs are available). Such swabs must not be used as dressings. Swabs should be in bundles of five (that number is recommended for universal use) and counted by the 'scrubbed' nurse and the 'unscrubbed' nurse together before the operation begins. Swabs used in theatre for purposes other than within the body, e.g. by anaesthetist or paediatrician, or for cleansing the skin, should have a distinctive colour (usually green) and should also have radio-opaque material incorporated in the meshes.

The 'unscrubbed' nurse accounts for swabs discarded from the field of operation. A rack with hooks arranged in rows of five facilitates this.

**The obstetrician is responsible that all swabs are removed** from within the wound before closure of the incision. He will ascertain that the swab count is correct; 'scrubbed' and 'unscrubbed' nurses having accounted for recovery of the number of swabs issued.

The number of instruments and needles used at each operation should be known. The 'scrubbed' nurse counts haemostats and needles prior to starting the operation and accounts for them before the wound is closed.

The number of non-absorbable sutures inserted should be recorded on the chart and checked when they are removed.

**Vaginal tampons or packs are removed by the obstetrician.** If left intentionally, the size, number and time of removal should be recorded on the chart. The ward sister is responsible for their removal at the time stated.

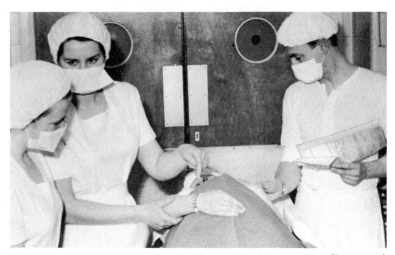

Fig. 34-21 Anaesthetist verifying identity of patient, medication, case notes. Sister stressing to student midwife the importance of checking identity wristband.

*Aberdeen Maternity Hospital.*

## ANAESTHETIC REQUIREMENTS

The trolley for general anaesthesia must always be in readiness with cylinders of nitrous oxide (more rarely halothane, cyclopropane) and other gases; oxygen cylinders must be checked and suction apparatus in readiness.

Intubation packs should be at hand with the necessary equipment for the induction of general anaesthesia.

Atropine and Scopolamine should be available for intravenous use. Sodium thiopentone (Pentothal) and suxamethonium (Scoline), one of the shorter-acting muscle relaxants, may be administered.

**Pre-oxygenation.** Prior to the induction of a general anaesthetic the patient is given oxygen for 3 minutes.

### The following may be required

Stomach tube and Brunswick disposable syringe 50 ml with catheter nozzle; vomit bowl; swab holders; green gauze swabs. Airways; mouth gags; laryngoscope; endotracheal tubes; sphygmomanometer; bin-aural and fetal stethoscopes; oscillo-tonometer: Mitchell cuff inflator.

Digoxin; hydrocortisone.

Vasopressor substances such as ephedrine.

## MIDWIVES' DUTIES

The midwife keeps the equipment clean, trolleys tidy and provides an adequate supply of sterile syringes, needles, drugs and other necessary requirements. She stays with the woman from the time she is brought into the anaesthetic room until she is transferred to the theatre. Absolute quietness should prevail and talking should be a mere whisper; the patient should not hear the rattling of instruments. One midwife should be delegated to assist the anaesthetist as required, preparing injections and ensuring that the patient's arms do not slip off the table.

### DANGERS OF INHALATION OF GASTRIC CONTENTS

The stomach contents are highly acid and the anaesthetist endeavours to avoid inhalation of regurgitated fluid or food. Some pass a large stomach tube, 20 FG and empty the stomach by suction or syphonage. A cuffed endotracheal tube is inserted by the anaesthetist to ensure a clear airway.

**Cricoid pressure** (Sellick's manoeuvre) is applied to compress the oesophagus and prevent regurgitation while the anaesthetic is being induced but is not used to stop active vomiting. The first two fingers are placed on one side of the cricoid cartilage, the thumb on the other side and backward pressure is applied to compress the oesophagus between the cricoid cartilage and the bodies of the vertebrae behind.

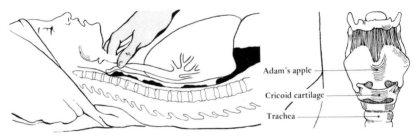

Adam's apple

Cricoid cartilage

Trachea

Fig. 34-22  Cricoid pressure, applied while anaesthetic is being induced, to prevent regurgitation.

A tilting table or labour ward bed, e.g. Steel's, which is controlled by the anaesthetist who can rapidly lower or raise the head, has proved to be invaluable.

Suction apparatus, instantly ready, is imperative.

### MENDELSON'S SYNDROME

*(Pulmonary Acid Aspiration Syndrome)*

This significant cause of obstetric anaesthetic deaths is due to the inhalation of vomited or regurgitated gastric juice. It can occur even when no food has been partaken for many hours: the acid gastric juice being highly irritant to the bronchial tree and lungs produces bronchospasm, dyspnoea, cyanosis and pulmonary oedema. Death may ensue in hours or days.

**Prophylactic treatment** consists in giving 15 ml mist. magnesium trisilicate every two hours during labour and less than 30 minutes prior to a general anaesthetic or operative procedure to reduce the acidity of the stomach contents.

**Active treatment.** The bed is lowered at the head, airway cleared by suction: oxygen given: intermittent positive pressure ventilation may be necessary. Steroids and aminophylline are administered for the relief of bronchospasm: glucose is given intravenously: antibiotics are usually prescribed. Ergometrine is not administered.

## INTRAVENOUS ANAESTHESIA

Sodium thiopentone (Pentothal) is given intravenously to induce anaesthesia.

No food should be taken for six hours prior to giving sodium thiopentone (Pentothal), because the barbiturates may cause the cardiac sphincter of the stomach to relax and the presence of vomitus in the pharynx may induce laryngeal spasm. Moreover vomitus may be inhaled and cause a degree of cyanosis which may be lethal to the fetus *in utero*, and may result in the death of the mother from asphyxia.

### Requirements for intravenous anaesthesia

Ampoule sodium thiopentone, 0·5 g.
Ampoule of 20 ml distilled water to make 2·5 per cent solution.
Rubber velcro arm band.
Green swabs (5); dressing towels.
Cap, mask.
Filling cannula.
Hypodermic needles, sizes 21 and 23 gauge.
Venflon i.v. cannula.
20 ml syringe, eccentric nozzle.
2 ml syringe, central nozzle.
Thiomersil 1 per cent for skin preparation.

### SPINAL ANAESTHESIA

This procedure is being used more frequently in Britain for caesarean section and forceps delivery. To avoid the severe hypotension which may occur, one litre of Hartmann's solution is administered to load the circulation prior to and during induction of spinal anaesthesia.

### REQUIREMENTS

2 ml syringe and needle to raise skin weal; Luer-lok 5 ml syringe.

Rowbottom's introducer, fine spinal needles with stilettes.

Ampoules of lignocaine (Xylocaine) 0·25 per cent with adrenaline 1–400,000. Ampoules of ephedrine. Cap, mask. Thiomersil 1 per cent.

The equipment including ampoules of local anaesthetic must be autoclaved before use.

# EPIDURAL ANALGESIA

This procedure is utilised to provide continuous analgesia which in 95 per cent of cases abolishes the pain of labour. The woman is consulted in advance: the anaesthetist offering to give her epidural analgesia, but if she is unwilling her wishes are respected. If she accepts, the procedure is explained to her in simple terms.

### INDICATIONS AND ADVANTAGES

**The painless labour** is more satisfying and serene.

**The improved placental circulation** is beneficient to the fetus, particularly when at 'high risk'. Fetal metabolic acidosis is reduced during the second stage.

**Less intracranial injury** occurs to the preterm infant because the pelvic floor is relaxed.

**There is no need for giving the mother narcotic** or analgesic drugs that may have a detrimental effect on the fetus. (Bupivacaine does not harm the fetus.)

**Pre-eclampsia.** The hypotensive effect of the epidural drug, e.g. bupivacaine (Marcain) 0·5 per cent, combined with the absence of pain, helps to prevent eclampsia. An anti-convulsant drug such as chlormethiazole, can also be administered.

**Twin delivery.** Any necessary manipulation is more easily accomplished. The perinatal mortality is reduced.

**Breech delivery.** Premature bearing down is prevented. Although the woman feels no urge to 'push' during the second stage, she still has the power to 'push' when asked to do so. The relaxed pelvic floor facilitates any manoeuvres to assist the birth.

**Caesarean section.** The anaesthetist will discuss in advance whether the woman prefers a local or a general anaesthetic. Some prefer to be conscious and aware of the birth of the baby. During the operation the woman is positioned in a left half lateral tilt to avoid vena caval compression and the ensuing hypotension.

**Epidural analgesia is safer** than general anaesthesia and particularly so in cases of cardiac or respiratory disease.

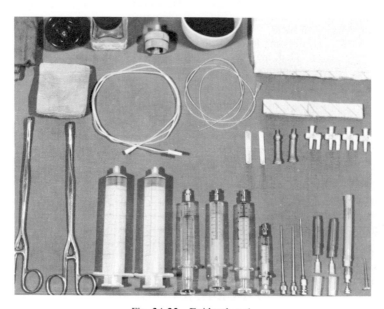

Fig. 34-23   Epidural pack.

*Aberdeen Maternity Hospital.*

| | |
|---|---|
| 1 gallipot for iodine. | 2 hypo needles No. 17. |
| 2 sponge holding forceps. | 1 Tuohy needle. |
| 10 green gauze swabs. | 1 Sise introducer. |
| 1 lumbar puncture towel. | 1 Portex epidural cannula. |
| 2 disposable syringes 50 ml. | 1 × 160 cm manometer tubing. |
| 3 glass syringes 10 ml Luer-lok tip. | 4 stop-cocks 3 way. |
| 1 glass syringe 2 ml Luer-lok tip. | 2 MacIntosh balloons, Luer adaptors. |
| 1 filling cannula. 1 spinal needle. | 1 polythene bag 20 × 60 cm and tape. |

Sterilised separately.

60 ml bupivacaine (Marcain) 0·5 per cent.   Cap, mask, gown, gloves.   1 Millipore bacterial filter.
0·5 and 1 per cent lignocaine.

### CONTRA–INDICATIONS

Refusal of consent by the patient. Sepsis at site of injection. Grande multipara. Lack of expert personnel. Patient on anti-coagulant therapy. Neurological disease.

## *Precautionary Measures Prior to Epidural Block*

### STRICT ASEPTIC TECHNIQUE

This is mandatory because of the serious results should infection of spinal tissues occur. The operator 'scrubs up' and wears mask, gown and gloves; sterile drapes are used. Single dose ampoules of the analgesic drug are recommended; they must be autoclaved once only in case the high pressure produces minute cracks in the glass.

*The following should be provided and set out for urgent immediate use:*

### RESUSCITATIVE REQUIREMENTS

(a) **Vasopressor drugs** such as ephedrine 15–30 mg.

(b) **Pharyngeal suction apparatus.**

(c) **Positive pressure oxygenation apparatus** is placed at the head of the bed.

(d) **Blood volume expanders** such as glucose 5 per cent or Macrodex.

**The woman should be lying on a tilting (head lowering) bed.**

**To facilitate immediate i.v. therapy,** a plastic cannula (Venflon) should be inserted into a convenient vein in the back of the hand so that i.v. drugs or fluids may be administered immediately should the need arise.

**The bladder should be emptied** by micturition prior to the first and each subsequent injection.

**An i.v. oxytocin drip is usually begun** before the epidural block is started.

Some anaesthetists prefer an elective epidural: the catheter being inserted into the epidural space before labour is painful and while the woman is relatively quiescent. Effective doses are administered when she considers labour to be uncomfortably painful.

**The first epidural injection** is usually given when labour is established; a preliminary test dose of bupivacaine (Marcain) 0·5 or 0·25 per cent 2 ml being administered. This precaution would indicate by paraesthesia or weakness in the lower limbs within 5 or 10 minutes that the injection had inadvertently entered the spinal subarachnoid space. Because of this risk the resuscitative requirements must be set out beside the tilting bed; a Venflon i.v. cannula having been inserted in every case.

## EPIDURAL BLOCK PROCEDURE

While receiving the injection, the woman lies on her side with her back at the edge of the bed. To separate the vertebrae she flexes her back, bringing her knees as near to her chin as her distended abdomen will allow. Her back is painted with 2 per cent iodine and wiped with chlorhexidine in spirit.

**Lignocaine 1 per cent is injected** for subcutaneous analgesia. A Tuohy needle 16 G is inserted, via the lumbar 3–4 intervertebral space, into the epidural space and a fine polyvinyl catheter introduced through the bore of the Tuohy needle and left *in situ* for 'topping up'. The site of the catheter insertion is covered with gauze swabs and sealed off with sleek occlusive strapping to prevent contamination with amniotic fluid and other substances. The catheter is taped up the woman's back and covered with sleek.

**A millipore bacterial filter** is attached to the end of the cannula to prevent contamination of the drug as it is being injected. The filter remains in position as long as the epidural drug is being administered. 'Top up doses' are injected with a sterile 10 ml glass syringe.

Some authorities prefer to have a reservoir of local analgesic attached to the epidural cannula in the form of preloaded syringes in a sterile sealed transparent plastic bag.

### HYPOTENSION

**A significant fall in blood pressure may occur** soon after the local analgesic has been injected. The effect of the drug, in conjunction with the supine position, the pressure of the large gravid uterus, i.e. vena caval compression, results in hypotension. The collateral circulation is unable to deal with the impeded blood flow because the epidural drug negates this. Due to reduction in the placental circulation, maternal hypotension, (a systolic pressure of or below 100 mm Hg) can be lethal to the fetus.

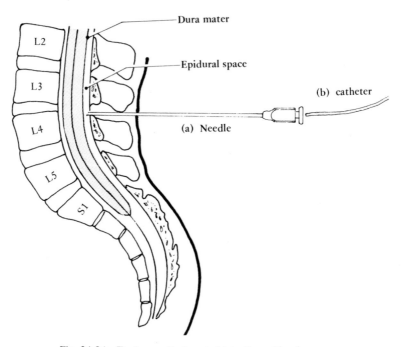

Fig. 34-24   Tuohy needle inserted into the epidural space.

**Prophylaxis**

The woman could be placed in the supine position prior to the epidural to test whether her collateral circulation can deal with any reduction in blood flow caused by vena caval compression.

**During labour she should lie on one or other side;** a foam rubber wedge being useful to maintain a lateral tilt.

**Dehydration must be avoided** or combated as this will cause hypotension.

**Drugs having a hypotensive action, such as promazine** (Sparine), **should not be given** to the woman in labour who will have, or is having, epidural analgesia.

## Prophylactic Assessment of Blood Pressure

This is one of the most important duties carried out by the midwife because hypotension can be lethal to mother and fetus.

To detect hypotension the blood pressure, having been recorded prior to the epidural, must be taken every 5 minutes for 30 minutes following the first and each subsequent injection, and every 30 minutes thereafter. The sphygmomanometer cuff is left *in situ* for the frequent readings that are essential.

### Signs and symptoms of hypotension.

The woman looks pale, feels faint and dizzy; she complains of nausea and cold perspiration. Tachycardia followed by bradycardia occurs. The doctor is notified if the systolic pressure falls to 100 mm Hg or a fall of over 10 mm Hg occurs.

#### TREATMENT OF HYPOTENSION

**The patient is turned on her left side immediately.** The foot of the bed is heightened or her legs may be raised. This usually succeeds but if hypotension persists 0·5 to 1 litre of a blood volume expander such as glucose, 5 per cent, or Macrodex is given. Very rarely is it necessary to inject a vasopressor drug such as ephedrine via the venflon cannula in the hand vein. When a vasopressor drug is given ergometrine or Syntometrine should not be administered to control third stage haemorrhage or severe headache may ensue: Syntocinon is preferred.

#### NURSING CARE DURING EPIDURAL ANALGESIA

**Emotional support with much assurance should be given** to the woman and the various procedures ought to be explained in terms she will comprehend. For fetal and maternal safety, diligent, intelligent supervision is even more important, than in labour without epidural analgesia.

**The midwife must be aware of the effects of epidural analgesia** and the untoward conditions such as hypotension that may arise: she must also be competent to cope with these pending the arrival of the anaesthetist.

**The woman is not allowed out of bed** because any hypotension would cause her to faint. Although she can move her legs there is some loss of sensory and motor function: heat and swelling of the legs and numbness of the buttocks may be present.

**To avoid the vena caval compression syndrome** she should not lie on her back: her position should be changed from side to side every hour or so; a foam rubber wedge being useful to maintain a lateral tilt. Pressure areas need attention; fresh linen will help to keep her back clean and dry.

#### PROGRESS OF LABOUR

The first stage usually proceeds quickly because of the woman's relaxed state. Because labour is silent the midwife will have to assess progress by meticulous observation.

### Uterine contractions

The woman is not aware when uterine contractions occur and although they may be recorded electronically, the midwife should also palpate the degree of uterine tonus with her finger tips. She notes the length, strength and frequency of the contractions. When oxytocin is being administered to induce or accelerate labour, there is an increased risk of hypertonic uterine action. Signs of impending rupture are masked, so constant vigilance is essential.

### The fetal heart

Constant electronic monitoring of the fetal heart beat is usually carried out: a scalp electrode commonly being used; otherwise the midwife auscultates and records the FH before and after each epidural injection and every ensuing 15 minutes. Tachycardia, bradycardia or an irregular fetal heart beat may be due to maternal hypotension.

### Attention to the bladder.

The woman is required to empty her bladder prior to the first and every subsequent epidural injection. She is not aware of a full bladder so the midwife is responsible for recognising this by abdominal palpation and percussion. The midwife must ensure that the bladder is emptied prior to each 'top up', or two-hourly. Instruction regarding micturition should be given for although the woman is not aware of the presence of urine in the bladder, she still retains the ability to pass urine. The urine is measured and examined for protein and ketones.

**Fluid balance** maintenance and dietary restrictions are similar to those in normal labour. Dehydration causes hypotension so it is usual to administer glucose sol. i.v. prior to giving the epidural block.

**Magnesium trisilicate** 15 ml is given orally every two hours to reduce gastric acidity.

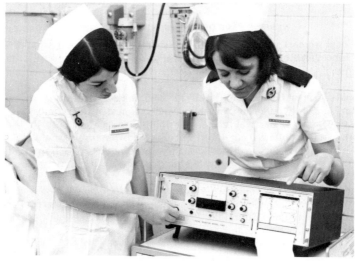

Fig. 34-25   Auditory and visual fetal heart monitoring by Sonicaid FM2. Labour ward sister showing student midwife how to check that the auditory recording coincides with the visual tracing.

*Aberdeen Maternity Hospital.*

### Vaginal examinations

During labour with or without epidural analgesia, it is now common practice to make vaginal examinations more frequently and particularly since recording the salient features of labour by partogram has been introduced. Some anaesthetists recommend making a vaginal examination prior to the first injection and each 'top up'; others do not consider this to be necessary. A vaginal examination gives valuable information regarding the progress of labour under epidural analgesia, which is appreciated by midwives, i.e.

(a) **Dilatation of the cervix** reliably indicates how far the first stage has advanced and that the second stage is imminent or in progress.

(b) **Descent of the head** can be assessed when it is no longer palpable abdominally.

(c) **That internal rotation is being or has been accomplished** in cases of posterior vertex position.

(d) **The presence of deep transverse arrest,** a situation associated with epidural analgesia, is detected.

(e) **Onset of the second stage** can be anticipated when it is no longer possible to palpate the head abdominally. Seeing the caput at the height of a contraction is a probable sign. A vaginal examination will disclose whether the second stage is in progress.

**To avoid making too many vaginal examinations,** the method used by midwives (shown in Fig. 34-26) is helpful. The middle finger is pressed inwards between the coccyx and anus. Tenseness is detected and usually indicates that the head is pressing on the pelvic floor and the second stage is in progress. Later the hard head can be felt.

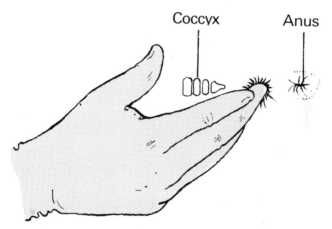

Fig. 34-26   Pressure applied between coccyx and anus detects tenseness indicating that the head is on the pelvic floor and the second stage is in progress.

### MANAGEMENT OF THE SECOND STAGE

The second stage is sometimes 20 or 30 minutes longer than normal because of delayed internal rotation particularly in posterior vertex positions.

**The woman does not experience the expulsive type of uterine contraction** and has no inclination to 'push' but she can be advised how to and encouraged to do so. When the head is visible during a contraction 'pushing' is advocated. By abdominal palpation the midwife detects the onset of a uterine contraction and urges the woman to 'push': this she can do effectively when taught how to use her expulsive efforts.

**If spontaneous delivery is anticipated** the woman should lie flat on her left side because the analgesic drug tends to flow up or down within the epidural space depending on whether the woman lies flat or is propped up.

**When forceps are likely to be required** the woman is propped up on her left side by foam rubber wedges. The analgesic drug flows downwards and anaesthetises the pelvic floor.

### 'TOPPING UP' BY MIDWIVES

'Topping up' describes the administration of subsequent doses of the analgesic drug to achieve continuous epidural analgesia. The doctor gives the preliminary test dose and the first injection. Responsibility for 'topping up' rests with the doctor.

**The Central Midwives Board (Eng.)** sanction experienced midwives to undertake the 'topping up' procedure provided the following safeguards are observed.

'That the ultimate responsibility has been stated to rest with the doctor: written instructions regarding the dose are given by the doctor in writing and that the dose being given is checked by one other person: that instructions regarding posture of the patient at the time of injection, observation of blood pressure and measures to be taken in the event of any side effect be given by the doctor. The midwife should have been thoroughly instructed in the technique so that the doctor concerned is satisfied as to her ability.'

The Central Midwives Board (Scot.) sanction midwives to undertake 'topping up' under the safeguards outlined above but only in maternity hospitals that have been approved for the purpose.

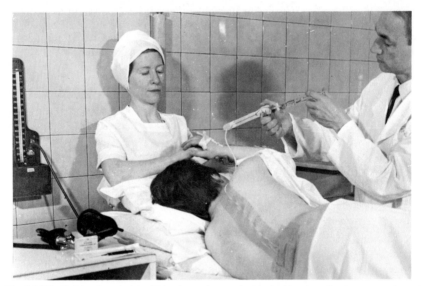

Fig. 34-27    Epidural analgesia. 'Topping up' a continuous epidural analgesic; repeat dose of local analgesic being injected through a millipore bacterial filter.

*Aberdeen Maternity Hospital.*

'Topping up' injections may be needed every 2 hours and ought to be given without delay as soon as the woman is aware of uterine discomfort. In cases of pre-eclampsia a rise in blood pressure could indicate the need for 'topping up'. The usual number of additional injections is 5: the anaesthetist will state the number that may be given without consulting him.

**Toxic reaction to the drug is rare** with bupivacaine (Marcain) but this should be kept in mind if an undue number of 'topping up' injections are made. Great care and caution are mandatory.

### Procedure for 'Topping Up'

**The woman empties her bladder.**

**A vaginal examination is made when necessary to** assess cervical dilatation, (see p. 281).

Blood pressure estimated, pulse taken and fetal heart rate monitored before giving each dose.

**Strict aseptic precautions are observed.**

**The drug is checked and injected** slowly.

**Following the injection the blood pressure is taken** as previously described. Uterine discomfort may continue for 10 minutes. (See also nursing care p. 627.)

**Removal of the epidural catheter by midwives is sanctioned by the Central Midwives Board (Eng.)** when analgesia is no longer required, provided the midwives concerned have been properly trained and are individually competent. The tip of the catheter should be examined to ensure that it is complete and this fact recorded.

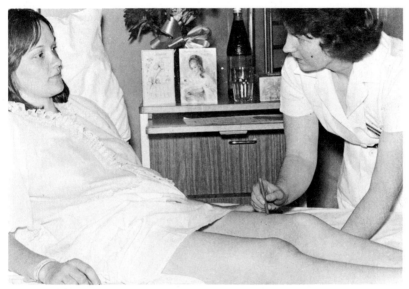

Fig. 34-28   Physiotherapist testing postnatal sensory and motor function of lower limbs.
*Royal Maternity Hospital, Rottenrow, Glasgow.*

### POSTNATAL ASSESSMENT

**Appraisal of sensory and motor leg function** is carried out 6 to 8 hours after delivery. Muscle control of the legs has usually returned in 3 or 4 hours, but the woman is not allowed out of bed until the leg muscles have recovered sufficiently for weight bearing. Diminished sensation is elicited by gentle pricking.

**The headache that occasionally occurs** is not due to the epidural per se but to accidental puncture of the dura mater. The woman with headache ought to lie flat for at least 24 hours; fluids should be taken freely and straining at stool avoided: the usual analgesic drugs being prescribed to relieve pain. In severe cases epidural infusion of Hartmann's solution at one ml/minute for 24 hours gives relief. Should the headache persist for several days, 10 ml of the patient's blood (dural blood patching) may be injected, near the puncture site, into the epidural space.

**Backache which may be troublesome** responds to analgesic drugs such as paracetamol.

**Difficulty in micturition** is usually overcome when the woman is allowed out of bed.

## CAESAREAN SECTION

The operation to remove the fetus through an incision in the abdominal wall and uterus is known as 'hysterotomy', and when performed after the 28th week of pregnancy the term 'Caesarean section' is used. It was first employed in Roman times to remove the child after the death of the mother.

**MAIN INDICATIONS**

| | |
|---|---|
| **Contracted pelvis** | **Disordered uterine action** |
| **Cephalo-pelvic disproportion** | **Severe pre-eclampsia** |
| **Placenta praevia   Abruptio placentae** | **Diabetes   Prolapse of cord** |
| **Failed induction   Fetal distress** | **Previous Caesarean section** |

Other factors are also taken into consideration, such as bad obstetric history, the older primigravida, fetal wellbeing. The tendency to treat breech, shoulder and posterior face presentations by Caesarean section in the interest of the fetus is increasing. Some authorities advocate radiological examination prior to Caesarean section to exclude fetal abnormalities.

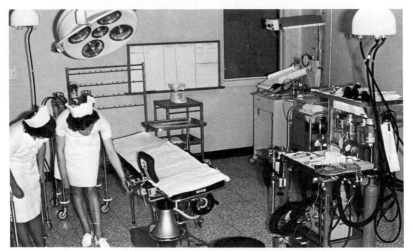

Fig. 34-29   Caesarean theatre. Sister demonstrating Thackray table with lateral tilt.
*Forthpark Maternity Hospital, Kirkcaldy, Scotland.*

**BRIEF DESCRIPTION OF CAESAREAN SECTION**

### Elective Caesarean section

This is one which is planned because the need is apparent prior to labour. The woman is admitted to hospital after the 38th week for one or two days before the operation, which is usually performed on the approximate day of delivery or sooner if the membranes rupture.

### Lower segment Caesarean section

The abdomen is opened through a vertical paramedian or midline incision, just above the upper border of the symphysis pubis to 2·5 cm below the umbilicus. The Pfannenstiel incision which is transverse is preferred by some because it heals well and with good cosmetic result. The peritoneum is incised transversely at the utero-vesical junction, where it is loosely attached, and the bladder gently pushed down. The lower segment is incised transversely. It may be necessary to use one or two blades of obstetric forceps to extract the head. The mouth is cleared of mucus, the body extracted and the baby held upside down for a few seconds. The cord is clamped and cut: the placenta delivered. The edges of the uterine wound are defined with Green-Armytage or Allis's forceps and sutured with catgut in three layers. The abdomen is closed in the usual manner.

## Classical Caesarean section

A paramedian incision is made 16 cm long and extending slightly above the umbilicus: the uterine incision is also longitudinal, and involves the upper segment. The classical section is utilised when the fetus lies transversely or a placenta praevia is anterior. The membranes are pierced, the child and placenta extracted. The contractions of the upper segment during the post-operative period militate against good healing of the uterine scar, and rupture takes place during a subsequent pregnancy in about 4 per cent of cases.

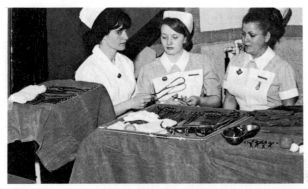

Fig. 34-30    Pre-set trays for Caesarean section. Labour ward sister giving clinical instruction using non-sterile equipment.

*Simpson Memorial Maternity Pavilion, Edinburgh.*

### PRE–OPERATIVE PREPARATION

Routine examination of blood and urine is carried out, with the exception of certain tests previously made on booked patients. Blood is sent for cross-matching: 2 units are available prior to operation for checking by the anaesthetist. The abdominal wall and vulva are shaved. On the previous day skin and bowel preparation are similar to what is given for any abdominal operation.

**The anaesthetist discusses** with the patient whether her choice is epidural, spinal or general anaesthesia.

**The physiotherapist** will demonstrate deep breathing and leg exercises.

## A sedative is administered

To ensure sound sleep during the night no food or fluid is given for 6 hours prior to operation. Premedication does not include a narcotic drug because of the depressant effect on the fetal respiratory centre.

Mist. mag. trisilicate, 15 ml. is given within half an hour prior to Caesarean section.

The patient, her charts, permission slip and X-ray films are taken to the anaesthetic room: an identification band having been applied to her wrist. A catheter is introduced and the bladder emptied: the urine drains into a plastic bag or perineal pad throughout the operation.

## SET-UP OF THEATRE FOR CAESAREAN SECTION

The set-up required is very similar to what is needed for an abdominal section, with the addition of midwifery forceps, hypodermic syringes, ergometrine, Syntometrine, Syntocinon and requirements for reception and resuscitation of the baby.

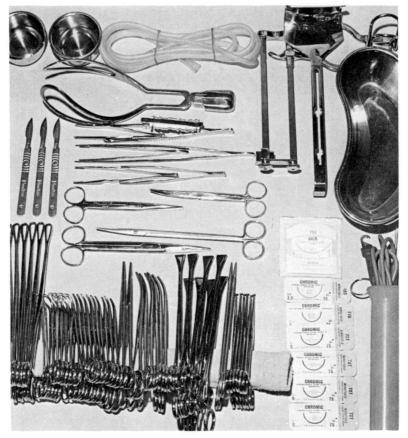

Fig. 34-31   Instruments for Caesarean section.
*Simpson Memorial Maternity Pavilion, Edinburgh.*

## Instruments

6 sponge forceps
6 towel clips
10 Crile's artery forceps
2 Kocher's artery forceps straight
6 Mayo artery forceps curved
8 Green Armytage forceps
6 Allis tissue forceps
3 scalpel handles and blades No. 23
2 Mayo scissors straight 17 and 19 cm

2 Mayo scissors curved 19 and 23 cm
2 toothed dissecting forceps 15 and 18 cm
2 non-toothed dissecting forceps 18 and 25 cm
2 Mayo needle holders
Suction nozzle and tubing
1 pr. Wrigley's forceps
1 Balfour self retaining retractor
Michel clips and inserting forceps
2 gallipots
1 dish for placenta
1 diathermy pencil, cable and quiver

## ADDITIONAL PACKS

(a) For removal of previous scar:
    1 Bard Parker handle and blade;
    2 dissecting forceps; 1 pair scissors

(b) 2 ml syringes and needles 21 g
(c) Disposable catheters, gloves

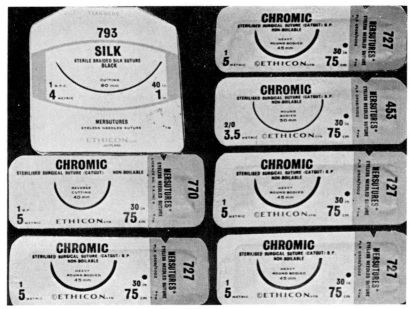

Fig. 34-32

## Sutures

For 3 layers sutures in uterus

3 × 5 metric catgut with eyeless round bodied needle 45 mm Ethicon W 727

1 for peritoneum: 5 metric chromic catgut with eyeless round bodied needle 45 mm Ethicon W 727

1 for rectus sheath: 5 metric chromic catgut with eyeless reverse cutting needle 40 mm Ethicon W 770

1 for fat (if required) 3·5 metric chromic catgut with eyeless round bodied needle 50 mm Ethicon 453

2 for skin: 4 metric mersilk with cutting hand needle 90 Ethicon W 793

Alternating Michel clips and synthetic sutures, e.g. 2 metric Prolene mono-filament polypropylene with eyeless straight cutting needle 60 mm. Two beads and 2 collars for each end of continuous suture, Ethicon W 630

or 2 metric Ethibond braided polyester suture with eyeless straight cutting needle 75 mm Ethicon W 996

or 3 metric Dexon braided polyglycolic acid with eyeless straight needle 60 mm Davis and Geck 7908–51

## PACKS FOR CAESAREAN SECTION

### Linen and Dressing Pack

4 foam sponges
1 Laparotomy sheet
7 drapes 1 metre
1 Mayo table cover
4 packets × 5 Raytec swabs 10 × 10 cm

1 moisture repellent cotton square, 90 × 100 cm
5 packets × 5 Raytec abdominal swabs, 30 cm with tapes
1 perineal pad

### PACK

4 sets of gown, cap, mask, hand towel

### BOWL PACKS

Two 2-basin, one 1-basin for hand lotion

### BABY PACK

1 cellular cotton baby blanket; 1 Turkish towel wrap; 5 green gauze swabs
2 mucus extractors; 2 rubber bands on Spencer Wells forceps to ligate cord, or Hollister clamp
1 × 10 ml syringe to extract gastric fluid and oesophageal tube 14 FG if necessary

## MISCELLANEOUS

1000 ml of crossmatched blood in readiness. A drip of Hartmann's solution is set up at the beginning of the operation and this facilitates the giving of blood or oxytocin should the need arise. To women 'at risk' of deep vein thrombosis some give Macrodex, 0·5 litre i.v., during and following operation.

Oxytocic and other drugs with the requisite syringes are on the anaesthetist's tray. Digoxin, hydrocortisone, should be at hand.

Thiomersil, one per cent, for skin. Redivac drain introducer tubing and bottle. Adhesive plaster. Elastoplast Airstrip dressing or Steristrip skin closure. Spray, with polybactrin.

### MIDWIVES' DUTIES DURING CAESAREAN SECTION

The 'scrubbed' midwife counts the swabs in the presence of the 'non-scrubbed' midwife. The anaesthetised patient is brought in and the 'non-scrubbed' nurse auscultates the fetal heart, and applies pressure on the suprapubic region to empty, the bladder. The patient will be placed in a half lateral tilt on her left side supported by a sponge rubber wedge to prevent vena caval occlusion.

The 'scrubbed' midwife hands to the obstetrician a holder with swab or polyester foam cube soaked in Thiomersil 1 per cent. Places moisture repellent cotton or surgical sheet over patient's thighs; hands four towel clips and drapes to surround incision area. Helps to apply laparotomy sheet.

### Skin incision

Places instrument table over thighs. Hands scalpel and taped swab; places kidney-basin on table to receive discarded scalpel. Places dissecting forceps, scissors and Crile's forceps on table. Hands short lengths of catgut to ligate vessels if diathermy is not being used.

### Peritoneal incision

Lays two artery forceps, two Allis's tissue forceps, clean scalpel and scissors on table. Some use a dry pack others prefer a wet pack with forceps attached to the tape to pack off intestines. Hands abdominal retractor.

### Uterine incision

Places clean scalpel, dissecting forceps and curved scissors on table. Gives dry, taped swab for mopping wound. Places obstetric forceps on table in readiness. Hands suction-nozzle as membranes of the fetal sac are being punctured.

### Extraction of baby

Clears all instruments from the table on which the baby will be laid. The obstetrician will hold the baby upside down to facilitate pulmonary drainage: the baby is then laid at a lower level than the placenta in utero to allow some placental transfusion. Time of birth noted. Mechanical suction to clear the airway may be used. Hands swabs to wipe nose and mouth, two Mayo forceps and scissors for cord. The anaesthetist gives ergometrine or Syntocinon intravenously as the baby's body is being extracted but if the patient is pre-eclamptic Syntocinon is given intramuscularly. The infant wrapped in a cellular cotton blanket is taken by the paediatrician to the recovery room for resuscitation and examination.

Hands basin for placenta and Mayo forceps to detach membranes. Hands six Green-Armytage forceps to pick up edges of wound.

#### SUTURING PROCEDURE

**Suture of Uterus.** Places clean towel on instrument table with needle holders and dissecting forceps. Hands catgut and round bodied needle on needle holder for 3 layers of sutures, Ethicon W 727. Hands taped swab to mop uterine wound.

**Swabs, needles and instruments are now counted** and checked by the 'scrubbed' and 'non scrubbed' midwives: abdominal pack removed. The total counted must be confirmed as correct by the obstetrician before proceeding.

**Suture of peritoneum.** Hands 4 Allis forceps and a round bodied needle with Ethicon W727 on needle holder. Obstetrician wipes wound with dry taped swab.

**Suture of fascia.** Ethicon W770 on a reverse cutting needle.

**Suture of fat.** (Subcutaneous tissue) Ethicon W453.

A Redivac drain may be inserted when there is a Pfannenstiel incision.

**Suture of skin.** Hands 4 Allis forceps, Michel clips with holder and inserter or Mersilk Ethicon W743. Obstetrician wipes wound, applies Steripad dressing; removes abdominal drapes, expresses clots from the uterus; removes catheter. The vulva is swabbed and a pad placed in position.

## IMMEDIATE CARE OF THE BABY

A Resuscitaire with suction, oxygen, drugs, laryngoscope, endotracheal tubes, blood sample tubes, ampoules of sodium bicarbonate 8·4 per cent and glucose 10 per cent should be provided; cord ligatures, elastic bands or clamps, 10-ml syringe and catheter. Naloxone neonatal (Narcan) 0·01 mg/kg and vitamin $K_1$ (Konakion) 1 mg. Newborn baby chart. Means of identification.

Some use a 14 FG disposable catheter and 10-ml syringe to aspirate the gastric fluid and prevent regurgitation and inhalation of the stomach contents. Caesarean babies tend to become limp within a few moments, even when they have cried vigorously at birth; adequate pulmonary drainage, oxygen and warmth are usually sufficient to restore the infant's colour and muscle tone.

The cord is ligatured; means of identification applied, sex and time of birth recorded and the baby transferred to the nursery in a portable heated incubator or cot. Prior to transfer, if epidural or spinal analgesia was used, the mother is allowed to hold her baby.

## POST-OPERATIVE CARE

The patient remains in the intensive care unit with an i.v. drip of glucose, 5 per cent, running: Macrodex being used if the woman is over 25 years of age.

She is placed on her side, with a pillow behind her shoulders until conscious.

The midwife records the pulse every 15 minutes for at least three hours, and watches for any sign of wound or vaginal haemorrhage. As soon as consciousness is regained a sedative such as papaveretum (Omnopon), 20 mg, is administered, the midwife remaining with the patient until the drug has taken effect. The blood pressure is taken on return to the ward and every two hours: if shocked or having blood, every half-hour for three hours, then four-hourly for 24 hours.

**During the evening.** The patient is sponged, vulva swabbed, mouth and back attended to. Intravenous fluids are usually administered until bowel sounds return. Papaveretum (Omnopon), 20 mg, is administered and to ensure a comfortable night it is repeated at midnight and at 04.00 hours if necessary. The woman may not void urine on the day of operation as she is taking very little fluid and it may be 24 hours before a catheter need be passed unless she is very uncomfortable.

Temperature, pulse and respirations are recorded every four hours. The patient is turned on alternate sides every two hours.

**Second day.** Papaveretum, 20 mg, is given six-hourly. Vulval swabbing is carried out and a daily sponge bath given. The physiotherapist inaugurates deep breathing and leg exercises. If the patient is in good condition, she is allowed out of bed to take a few steps. The legs are examined, groins palpated for tenderness every day.

**Third day.** Promethazine (Phenergan) or Ponstan may be given instead of papaveretum.

A laxative, such as Senokot is given; a prepacked enema or a Dulcolax suppository may be necessary if the bowels do not move. Some allow patients to have a shower (using a mobile hand spray.)

Alternative clips or sutures are removed on the fifth or sixth day, the remainder on the eighth day; Mersilk on the ninth day. The woman is discharged on the 10th to 12th day. The Health Visitor is notified and help in the home arranged for if necessary.

## SUBSEQUENT PREGNANCIES

All women having had Caesarean sections ought to be booked for hospital confinement and admitted prior to the expected date of delivery. Under no circumstances should any subsequent confinement be booked to take place at home. The woman should be instructed to report any abdominal pain during the last month and to come to hospital at once should any sign of labour occur. In Britain vaginal delivery is permitted if the previous indication is absent. Signs of imminent scar rupture may be masked under epidural analgesia. Vigilant observation is essential.

## QUESTIONS FOR REVISION

**Induction of labour**

Give 4 reasons why labour may be induced. What do you mean by induction delivery interval? Describe in not more than 10 lines: observation of a woman having puncture of membranes and oxytocin drip. What are the dangers in giving an intravenous oxytocin drip? Mention the observations you would make when giving it. State what you would set out in readiness for surgical induction of labour. What do you understand by the automatic oxytocin titration method of induction? For what reasons would you stop the drip?

**C.M.B.(Scot.) 30-min question.** Give an account of (a) the indications, and (b) the methods available, for the induction of labour.

**(N. Ire.) 30-min question.** What are the main indications for induction of labour? What are the responsibilities of the midwife in: (a) induction of labour by oxytocin 'drip'; (b) surgical induction of labour?

**C.M.B.(Eng.) 30-min question.** What are the indications for induction of labour? Discuss the methods that may be used, and complications that may arise.

**C.M.B.(Scot.) 30-min question.** Describe (a) the nursing care of and (b) the observations on a patient who is having labour induced by oxytocin. What dangers are associated with this procedure?

**Acceleration of labour**

Under what circumstances is labour accelerated by oxytocin drip? What do you observe on abdominal examination? How often is a vaginal examination made and why?

**Version**

Describe the procedure. Define the following types of version: external; cephalic. Under what circumstances would a midwife be justified in performing external version?

**C.M.B.(Scot.) 30-min question.** Define fetal lie. What are the possible causes of unstable lie? What is the management of a patient who is discovered to have an unstable lie during the last four weeks of pregnancy?

**Episiotomy**

**Differentiate between** a median, medio-lateral and J-shaped episiotomy and state advantages and disadvantages of each. What are the C.M.B. rules regarding: (a) making an episiotomy; (b) administering a local analgesic? What are the toxic reactions of local analgesics? How could these be averted?

**C.M.B.(Scot.) 30-min question.** Outline the anatomy of the perineal body. Describe the technique of making an episiotomy. During the postnatal period what observations should the midwife make on the perineum following an episiotomy.

**C.M.B.(Eng.) 30-min question.** What are the indications for episiotomy? When should a midwife undertake this procedure? Describe the technique employed.

**(N. Ire.) 30-min question.** What are the indications for episiotomy? Describe in detail the method you would employ in performing this operation, and indicate the precautions you would take.

**Why:** (a) should the piston of the syringe be withdrawn prior to injecting the local analgesic? (b) is injecting the drug while the needle is being withdrawn a wise precautionary measure? (c) should be from the lateral border of the anus? How would you control bleeding from the incision?

**Forceps delivery**

**(N. Ire.) 30-min question.** Enumerate the articles set out for a forceps delivery, mentioning the purpose of each one.

**(N. Ire.) 30-min question.** What are the indications for forceps delivery? Describe, in detail, the preparations necessary for such a delivery.

**Caesarean section**

Describe the immediate pre-operative care of the patient. What are the duties of the 'non-scrubbed' nurse? Why should swabs be in packs of 5? Why is Macrodex given during and after Caesarean section? How would you prepare to receive the baby in the theatre? Outline the post-operative care during the first three days.

**(N. Ire.) 30-min question.** How would you nurse a mother during the first two weeks following a Caesarean section?

**C.M.B.(Scot.) 30-min question.** List the indications for Caesarean section. What are the duties of a midwife before, during and immediately following this operation?

**C.M.B.(Scot.) 30-min question.** Describe the management of a patient delivered by Caesarean section for abruptio placentae.

## EPIDURAL ANALGESIA

Why is the bladder emptied prior to each injection of epidural analgesic? How often is the blood pressure taken after injection? Why must the uterine contractions be carefully noted by the midwife? What would you do, in the absence of the anaesthetist, for hypotension? What precautions must be taken by midwives who are sanctioned to maintain epidural block, i.e. 'topping up'?

How can a midwife help to facilitate spontaneous delivery under epidural analgesia?

For what reasons are the following used: Venflon cannula, Tuohy needle, millipore bacterial filter?

Differentiate between: Anaesthesia and analgesia; spinal and epidural analgesia; pudendal and epidural block.

## C.M.B. Short Examination Questions

**Eng.:** Give the indications for performing an episiotomy. **Eng.:** Give indications for induction of labour. **Eng.:** Syntocinon infusion for induction of labour. **Scot.:** External version. **Eng.:** External cephalic version and its dangers. **Eng.:** What are the hazards of general anaesthesia in labour? **Eng.:** Mendelson's syndrome. **Eng.:** Episiotomy. **Scot.:** Epidural anaesthesia. **Eng.:** Give care of a baby after a difficult forceps delivery. **Eng.:** Pulmonary acid aspiration syndrome. **Scot.:** Oxytocin infusion. **Eng.:** Epidural analgesia.

# 35
# Some Emergency and other Procedures undertaken by Midwives
### (IN REMOTE AREAS OF DEVELOPING COUNTRIES)

*Intravenous injection: Application of forceps: Malmström vacuum extractor: Pudendal nerve block: Internal version: Shoulder dystocia: Embryotomy: Symphysiotomy.*

It would seem reasonable that qualified midwives assigned to practise in remote areas of developing countries, sometimes 300 miles distant from medical assistance, should be given post-registration instruction and experience to equip them to cope with some of the obstetric emergencies they may encounter.

**Permission must be obtained from their employing authority** and National Statutory Body prior to undertaking operative procedures outside their province as midwives.

Much of the midwife's work consists in dealing with everyday normal situations. Although use is being made of biochemical tests, ultrasonic scans and electronic equipment, the skill and judgment of the well qualified midwife should not be underestimated. She can do much to improve the quality of maternal and fetal life as well as dealing with emergencies to save life.

### Screening by midwives

Many of the traditional diagnostic procedures carried out by midwives can be classified as screening methods, e.g. careful history taking; blood and urine testing; abdominal and vaginal examinations; diligent observation. These skills must be fostered. Personal supervision and management when linked with sound judgment can provide a satisfactory standard of obstetric care.

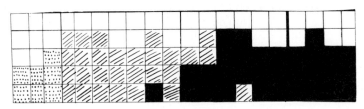

*The partogram*
When uterine contractions are recorded in graphic form, deviations from normal are detected early (each block = 12 minutes).

### PREVENTION OF EMERGENCIES

It is just as important for midwives to know how to prevent and anticipate emergencies as how to treat them: may obstetric disasters could be avoided. Some women are debilitated by diseases such as malaria, tuberculosis, and dysentery; their physical stamina is undermined by infestations and malnutrition; taboos and fasting days deprive them of protein foods. Profound anaemia is common and this grossly increases the hazards of repeated childbearing: so the midwife should be provided with the equipment for assessing the haemoglobin level and permitted to prescribe iron and folic acid preparations.

**Obstetric complications are always exaggerated** when prenatal supervision is neither available nor acceptable and when the attendant during labour is incompetent or negligent.

It is understandable that prolonged labour will still occur where it is traditional for native women not to seek skilled help until labour has lasted for 3 days or the placenta is retained for 24 hours. Untrained midwives should be taught the commendable maxim that **'The sun should not set twice on the woman in labour'**.

### INTRAVENOUS INJECTION

N.B. When treating a collapsed woman with postpartum haemorrhage her veins may be difficult to penetrate and valuable time is lost. It may be quicker to give Syntometrine intramuscularly.

### *Technique*

Velcro or soft rubber tubing is applied to the extended arm tightly enough to distend the veins without obliterating the arterial pulse (at the wrist). Clasping and unclasping the fist helps to make the veins stand out.

The syringe should rest closely on the forearm so that if the woman moves her arm the relation of needle to vein will not be disturbed. A 23 g needle is the smallest suitable size.

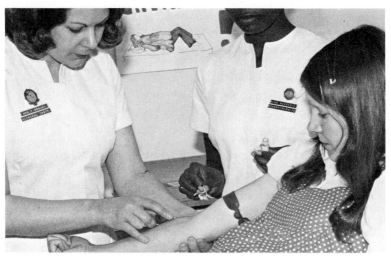

Fig. 35-1 Midwife taking blood at prenatal clinic.
*Maternity Hospital, Stirling.*

#### INSERTION OF THE NEEDLE

The skin is cleansed: air expelled from the syringe. Penetration of the skin is made with the needle almost parallel to the vein, bevel downwards; while doing so the vein is steadied in position by stretching the skin that lies over it with the thumb of the left hand which is grasping the patient's arm below the elbow. The needle is advanced alongside the vein for about 1/8th inch (3 mm) before being inclined sufficiently to be introduced into it. This minimises the risk of penetrating both walls of the vein. A slight sensation of 'give' is detected as the vein is entered.

Successful penetration of the vein is confirmed by raising the syringe and needle slightly with the right hand and gently withdrawing the plunger with the left, when dark venous blood will be aspirated into the syringe.

**No injection is made unless blood appears in the syringe.** The venous circulation is restored by releasing the tourniquet. Pressure on the plunger by the thumb of the left hand is applied to give the injection. It should be noted that the grip of the syringe by the right hand remains unaltered throughout the procedure.

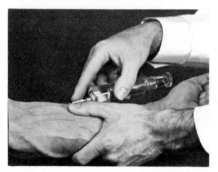 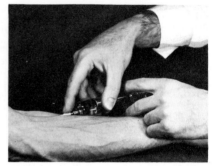

Fig. 35-2   Inserting the needle intravenously.   Fig. 35-3   Injecting the drug intravenously.

## FORCEPS DELIVERY BY MIDWIVES
*(In Developing Countries)*

**Prior to any operative procedure on a woman in prolonged labour** ketoacidosis must be rectified, so 500 ml of 10 per cent glucose or glucose and Ringer's lactate should be administered intravenously.

### Conditions that should be fulfilled

(a) **Thorough abdominal and vaginal examinations should be made:** presentation, position, station and flexion of the head being important.

(b) **The cervix should be fully dilated:** an incompletely dilated cervix may be stimulated to contract by the application of forceps and hinder extraction of the head: laceration of the cervix may extend into the lower uterine segment producing profuse haemorrhage and shock, sometimes rupture of the uterus.

(c) **The station of the head,** not merely the caput, should be at or below the level of the ischial spines.

(d) **The membranes ought to be ruptured.** The sagittal suture should be in the antero-posterior diameter of the pelvic cavity: if not, the head must be rotated manually one or two eighths of a circle, i.e. from LOA or LOL to antero-posterior. If the occiput is persistently posterior it may be easier for the midwife to deliver the baby face to pubes than to attempt rotation. The forceps must not be used to rotate the head; doing so may injure the vagina and urethral sphincter.

### APPLICATION OF FORCEPS
#### (FOR INDICATIONS SEE p. 618)

The midwife would be well advised to rehearse the application of forceps using doll and pelvis. Haig Ferguson's forceps minus the axis traction handle are suitable for use by midwives.

The woman is in the lithotomy position; the midwife seated facing her. (If the woman is on the floor her buttocks should be raised on a firm pillow or folded blanket: instruments on a tray beside the midwife.) Thighs are washed, vulva swabbed, catheter passed, local analgesic administered for pudendal nerve block (see p. 648) or infiltration of the vulval ring and of perineum for episiotomy.

### Selecting the left blade

This blade is inserted first. The blades are articulated, lubricated and held horizontally with the tip pointing to the vulva. The left blade is on the midwife's right: the handle of the left blade is on her left.

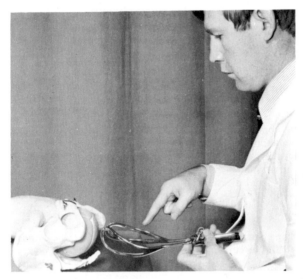

Fig. 35-4   Selecting the blade to be inserted first. The one which will lie on the left side of the woman's pelvis, the handle of which is to the left in the operator's hand: the lower blade.

*Aberdeen Maternity Hospital.*

**Inserting the left blade.** Two or more fingers of the right hand are inserted along the maternal left side of the vagina, their palmar surface in contact with the baby's head, the back of the hand retracting the perineum to the patient's left posteriorly.

The midwife, with her left hand, holds the left blade lightly like a pencil and almost vertically (see Fig. 35-5): the blade being inserted with the convex (outer rounded) part in apposition with the palmar surface of the fingers of the right hand in the vagina; the tip of the blade being maintained in contact with the baby's head. The handle is then depressed and swept gently in an arc, curving towards the mother's right thigh until it reaches the horizontal position. This manoeuvre brings the left blade alongside the head in the mento-vertical line. The fenestra (window) of the blade lies over the parietal eminence; the tip guided by the fingers of the right hand rests on the cheek.

**To insert the right blade** the procedure is similar, but opposite hands and sides of the vagina are involved. The fingers of the left hand are introduced along the maternal right side of the vagina, the hand retracts the perineum and also depresses the handle of the left blade already inserted, and maintains it in position. The right blade held in the midwife's right hand is inserted and kept in contact with the fetal skull, the handle depressed and swung in an arc towards the mother's left thigh. The two blades should lock easily if a proper cephalic grip has been obtained: if they do not lock readily both blades are gently manipulated with a sliding movement until they lie parallel: the ear can be felt within the fenestra of the blade. The handles may have to be pressed downwards (posteriorly) and the blades inserted somewhat further until the tips lie over the cheeks. Force must not be used.

### Wrong application

If the handles remain apart or will not lock, the forceps must be removed, the position of the head reassessed and the forceps reapplied. Difficulty may occur if the blades are applied obliquely, i.e. one partly over the face, the other over the occiput instead of a true side to side position: oblique application will cause the blades to slip off and may also inflict intracranial injury. Incomplete forward rotation of the head may be the cause of wrong application.

### *The Principle of Direction in Traction*

The direction of pull is altered as the head descends to coincide with the curve of the birth canal.

The midwife must understand the differences in direction of pull which depend on whether the application of forceps is mid-cavity or low. When the head is in mid-cavity (woman in dorsal position) the direction of pull is outwards towards the midwife. When the head is at the outlet the direction of pull is inclined slightly upwards. As the occiput escapes under the apex of the pubic arch crowning takes place, the head begins to extend so the pull is upwards to allow the face to sweep over the perineum.

### TRACTION

Before applying traction the midwife ascertains that the cervix is not being nipped between the forceps blade and the fetal head. Traction should be applied during a uterine contraction to obtain the advantage of the expulsive power of the uterus. A tentative pull is made: if the forceps do not slip and some advance of the head occurs, the midwife may proceed. Should no advance take place further investigation of the situation is necessary: the occiput may be posterior, the pelvic outlet may be contracted. Periods of traction should not exceed 15 seconds and to enable the fetus to recover from the effect of pressure on the skull the lock on the handles should be loosened between contractions: the fetal heart being auscultated during this resting phase. Excessive force should not be used, neither should leverage by the forceps be applied or fracture of the pubic bone may occur.

Prolonged and forceful traction can cause intracranial injury and hypoxia.

**An episiotomy is made** when the head distends the perineum; doing so too soon will give rise to free bleeding. After the head is properly crowned and ready for active extension the forceps are removed.

The baby may need resuscitation. To control intracranial haemorrhage he should be given vitamin $K_1$ (Konakion) 1 mg intramuscularly.

## MALMSTRÖM VACUUM EXTRACTOR *(ventouse)*

### *For Midwives in Developing Countries*

This apparatus is used to aid extraction of the fetus by a suction cup applied to the scalp: four sizes are available—30, 40, 50, 60 mm. The larger the cup the greater the suction area, thereby increasing the extractive force that can be applied. Connected to the cup is strong rubber tubing containing a metal chain that terminates in a traction handle: the rubber tubing extends through the handle and enters a glass container fitted with a pressure gauge. Leaving the glass container is a short piece of rubber tubing to which the electric or hand pump, that extracts the air and produces the vacuum, is attached.

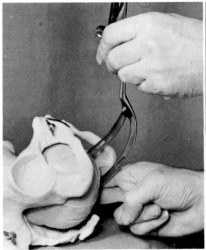

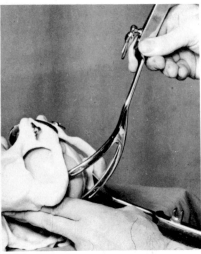

Fig. 35-5 Left blade inserted first. Two fingers of right hand are placed along the left side of the vagina.

Fig. 35-6 Right blade being inserted. Two fingers of left hand are placed along the right side of the vagina.

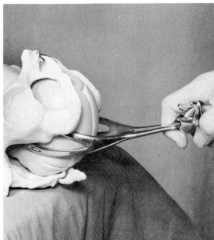

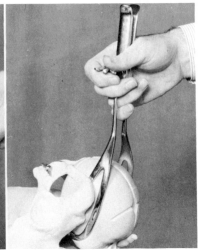

Fig. 35-7 When head is low, the direction of pull is outward, towards the midwife.

Fig. 35-8 When crowning occurs, the direction of pull is upwards to extend the head so that the face can sweep the perineum.

*Aberdeen Maternity Hospital.*

### Indications for using the vacuum extractor

Delay towards the end of the first stage. Delay during the second stage. Delay with the second twin. Deep transverse arrest of the head. To rotate the head in occipito-posterior position of the vertex.

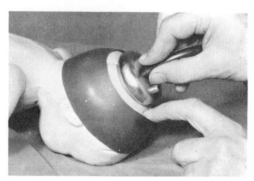

Fig. 35-9   Demonstration of application of ventouse cup. Half of rubber ball denoting the cervix. Cup applied to posterior area of head.

## THE PROCEDURE

**An abdominal examination is carried out** to determine presentation and position. The head should be engaged. Requirements are similar as for forceps. Analgesia is produced usually by local infiltration of the pelvic floor. Preparations are made for episiotomy and resuscitation of the infant. The vacuum extractor is set up.

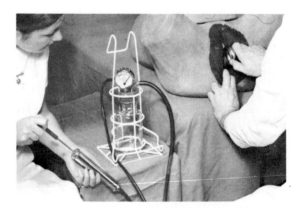

Fig. 35-10   Hand pump being used to create vacuum; doctor inserting cup.

*Aberdeen Maternity Hospital.*

**The woman is in the lithotomy position:** thighs are washed, vulva swabbed catheter passed and a vaginal examination made, membranes punctured if intact. The cervix need not be fully dilated. When the head is at the level of the ischial spines a pudendal nerve block with lignocaine, 0·5 per cent, is made. If the head is on the perineum infiltration of the vulval ring and perineum with lignocaine, 0·5 per cent, may suffice.

**Introducing the cup**

The cup is dipped in sterile water and inserted into the vagina sideways. Obstetric cream should not be used as it may interfere with the airtight fit of the cup and prevent adequate vacuum pressure from being created. The cup is attached to the posterior area of the head to increase flexion, avoiding the posterior fontanelle.

While holding the cup firmly applied to the head, sufficient suction is created by pumping to make the cup self-adherent. Pumping is continued until the vacuum pressure registered on the gauge is $0 \cdot 2$ kg/cm$^2$ then 90 seconds are allowed for each $0 \cdot 1$ kg/cm$^2$ until in about 10 minutes the pressure reaches not more than $0 \cdot 8$ kg/cm.$^2$ The scalp is sucked into the cup and a caput succedaneum or 'chignon', is thus produced. After each individual increase in pressure from $0 \cdot 2$ to $0 \cdot 8$ kg/cm$^2$—about every 90 seconds—the midwife checks that the vaginal wall or cervical rim has not inadvertently been sucked into the cup. The fetal heart is auscultated after each increase in pressure and each uterine contraction. When a vacuum pressure of $0 \cdot 8$ kg/cm$^2$ is registered traction is applied. N.B. cm$^2$ is a square centimetre.

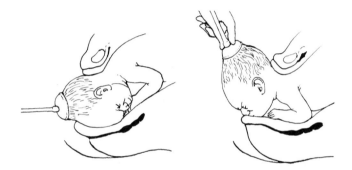

Fig. 35-11&35-12   Note alteration in direction of pull as head sweeps the perineum.

## TRACTION

This is employed only during uterine contractions, never between them; the patient assists by pushing. At the beginning of a contraction the pull is made gently, increasing the extractive force and exerting about half the amount of power applied when forceps are used. Two fingers of the left hand press the cup on to the head and direct the fetal head backwards on to the sacral area: they also feel for descent of the head. The direction of pull must be at right angles to the cup: any deviation from this will detach it at one side, air will be sucked into the cup which will come off. Progress should be obvious with traction during one or two contractions. The direction of pull is altered as the head descends to conform with the curved birth canal as in forceps delivery (p. 644). When the head is crowning the direction of pull is upwards, almost vertical.

**An episiotomy is made** if necessary when crowning of the head takes place. After delivery of the head the vacuum is reduced by opening the screw-release valve: the cup is then detached.

**If no advance is made** during four contractions no further attempts are made: the question of disproportion must be considered and forceps may have to be applied.

**Should the cup become detached** this is probably due to pulling in the wrong direction or by using too much force, so the vacuum must be created again, and if the 'chignon' is large and bruised another area of the scalp is used. Repeated application traumatises the scalp and may cause it to slough. In prolonged labour the scalp may be oedematous and traction detaches it from the bony structure giving a misleading impression of descent.

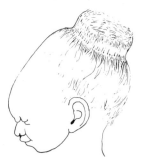

Fig. 35-13 'Chigon'.

# PUDENDAL NERVE BLOCK

*For Midwives in Developing Countries*

**Blocking the two pudendal nerves** with lignocaine, 0·5 per cent, anaesthetises the lower vagina, vulva, anterior area of the pelvic floor and perineum. It does not reduce the pain of uterine contractions. In addition the posterior area of the perineum should also be infiltrated with 0·5 per cent lignocaine.

The pudendal nerve emerges from the lower border of the sacro-sciatic foramen, runs alongside the ischial spine and after coming from behind the tip of the ischial spine it runs medially (towards the mid-line). The pudendal nerve and the pudendal artery run parallel to each other on the outer border and alongside of the ischial spine. Great care must be exercised on that account to make certain that the needle has not penetrated the pudendal artery. The piston of the syringe is withdrawn before injecting the lignocaine and if blood is present the needle is withdrawn, reinserted and the test done again. The block is made before the head is below the ischial spines.

### Requirements

Pudendal needle 20 gauge with guide; 20 ml syringe. For infiltration of the perineum a needle 21 gauge, 3·5 cm.

Lignocaine, 0·5 per cent.

| | |
|---|---|
| For left pudendal nerve | 15 ml lignocaine, 0·5 per cent |
| For right pudendal nerve | 15 ml lignocaine, 0·5 per cent |
| For perineum | 10 ml lignocaine, 0·5 per cent |
| Total | 40 ml lignocaine, 0·5 per cent |

Some prefer lignocaine, 1 per cent. The amount administered would be reduced by half: the total given, 20 ml.

The drug takes effect in 3 minutes and lasts for 30 minutes.

## PROCEDURE

Having checked the fetal heart rate the woman is placed in the lithotomy position or her buttocks raised on a firm pillow or folded blanket. Vaginally, full dilatation of the cervix and station of the head are verified. The ischial spines are located with the first and second fingers of the left hand: feeling the sacrospinous ligament as a firm ridge leading to the ischial spine is an aid to identification. The two fingers in the vagina are slightly withdrawn and the guide containing the partly withdrawn pudendal needle is laid in the furrow between the two fingers and directed to a point just below the tip of the ischial spine. The needle is pushed through the guide and penetrates the vaginal mucosa for one cm posterior to the tip of the spine.

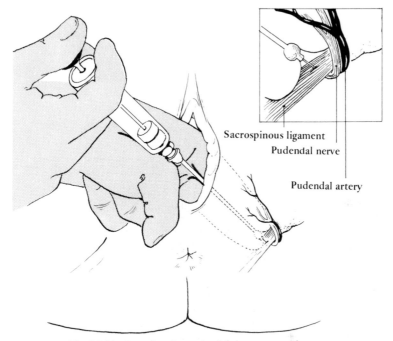

Sacrospinous ligament
Pudendal nerve

Pudendal artery

Fig. 35-14   Locating the pudendal nerve per vaginam.

**Before injecting the lignocaine the piston is withdrawn** and if no blood appears, about 5 ml of lignocaine, 0·5 per cent, is injected. The needle is then introduced lateral to the ischial spine and the test for blood again made: if none appears 5 ml lignocaine is injected. The needle is then introduced antero-laterally with the same precautions to ensure against introducing the drug into the blood stream. The procedure is repeated on the other pudendal nerve, thus infiltrating a wide area surrounding both nerves. Finally 10 ml lignocaine, 0·5 per cent, is administered into the posterior area of the perineum.

### INFILTRATION OF THE VULVAL RING

If the head is too low or the midwife is apprehensive in performing pudendal nerve block the lower vagina, vulva and perineum can be infiltrated with 10 ml lignocaine, 0·5 per cent. Entonox could be administered as a supplement.

## INTERNAL VERSION

### *For Midwives in Developing Countries*

This procedure involves inserting the whole hand into the uterus when the cervix has dilated sufficiently to permit this. Some obstetricians consider that in modern obstetric practice transverse lie of the second twin, that cannot be rectified by external version, is the only indication for internal version because of the grave risk of uterine rupture. Transverse lie during labour is the most likely indication, but internal version should not be attempted when labour is prolonged because the lower uterine segment will be overstretched, thin and liable to rupture. The danger is increased if the amniotic fluid has drained away and the uterus is retracted closely on the fetus. If the shoulder is impacted and the arm prolapsed no type of version should be attempted.

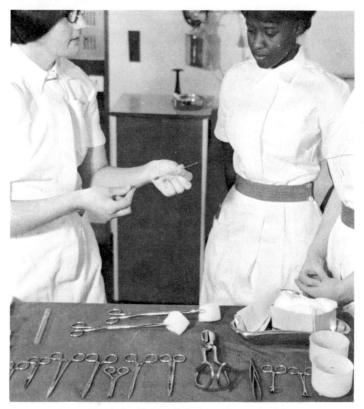

Fig. 35-15   Set up for forceps delivery under pudendal nerve block.

*Bellshill Maternity Hospital, Lanarkshire.*

## Method

A careful abdominal examination is made to locate the head, back and breech. General anaesthesia is a great advantage in relaxing the uterus and abdominal wall. If this is not available, an inhalational analgesic such as Entonox would be helpful.

Between contractions the midwife inserts her hand with palm facing the fetal abdomen, locates and differentiates a foot: the external hand pushing on the fundus to bring the breech within reach. The foot is drawn through cervix and vulva until the popliteal space is visible to make sure that the longitudinal lie will be maintained until the cervix is fully dilated. The hand on the abdomen then pushes the head upwards towards the fundus. Manipulations must cease during a uterine contraction.

## BI-POLAR VERSION *(rarely used)*

Bi-polar version is only performed nowadays in remote areas of developing countries; shoulder presentation being the most likely indication. This manoeuvre is a combination of internal and external manipulation carried out during labour before engagement of the presenting part or rupture of the membranes and when the cervix is not sufficiently dilated to admit the hand. Bi-polar version is only possible when there is ample amniotic fluid and should not be attempted when labour is prolonged. It is difficult to perform. Bi-polar version is always podalic: the whole hand is introduced into the vagina and two fingers, passed through the os, displace the shoulder. The external hand applies steady pressure abdominally over the breech and moves it down into the lower pole of the uterus: the membranes are then punctured and a foot brought through the cervix.

### IMPACTED SHOULDER PRESENTATION

The arm is likely to be prolapsed and the fetus dead. In the absence of medical aid and the likelihood of Caesarean section the midwife should sedate the woman heavily with the suitable drugs in her possession to damp down uterine activity. Decapitation may be necessary. Internal version is too dangerous to attempt and would inevitably cause uterine rupture.

## SHOULDER DYSTOCIA

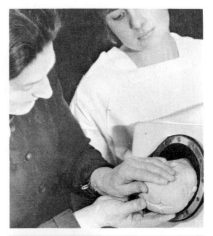

Fig. 35-16 To prevent shoulder dystocia when delivering a normal vertex presentation the midwife must avoid delivering the shoulders until they have rotated internally into the antero-posterior diameter of the outlet. This will be evident by external rotation of the head which occurs after restitution. With restitution the shoulders are still in the oblique diameter of the outlet. When the head has rotated externally the midwife uses downward traction.

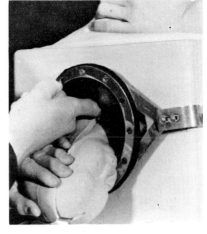

Fig. 35-17 When dystocia is present an episiotomy is made. If the shoulders are not in the antero-posterior diameter, hook two fingers into the anterior axilla, rotate the shoulder forwards and apply judicious traction to the head downwards and backwards. Should this fail, as it may do with a very large baby or when the anterior shoulder is caught on the pubic bone, an assistant tries to dislodge the anterior shoulder abdominally by pushing it towards the mid-line. At the same time an attempt is made to push the anterior shoulder forwards vaginally. Judicious traction is then applied to the head in a downward backward direction. (The neck must not be twisted.)

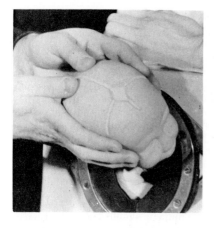

Fig. 35-18   If this fails to bring down the anterior shoulder, deliver the posterior shoulder by drawing the head in an upward curving direction while the assistant uses suprapubic pressure on the anterior shoulder. The lithotomy position or raising the buttocks on a firm pillow and an episiotomy will facilitate matters.

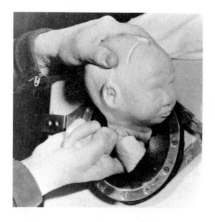

Fig. 35-19   Four fingers are inserted behind the posterior shoulder and an attempt is made to push it into the hollow of the sacrum. If this causes the anterior shoulder to be dislodged it can then be rotated forwards. Further traction can be applied by placing the fingers in the axilla of the posterior arm and if this does not succeed an attempt is made to rotate the shoulders and make the posterior shoulder anterior.

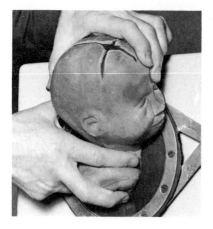

Fig. 35-20   As a last resort the whole hand is inserted into the hollow of the sacrum, two fingers splint the humerus of the posterior arm, flex the elbow, sweep the forearm over the chest and bring the hand out—a very difficult manoeuvre. If the fetus dies, cleidotomy may have to be performed, i.e. the clavicles are cut with embryotomy scissors.

# RESUSCITATION OF THE NEONATE

(see also p. 546)

The midwife should be competent in resuscitating the asphyxiated baby including intubation and administering oxygen, if available.

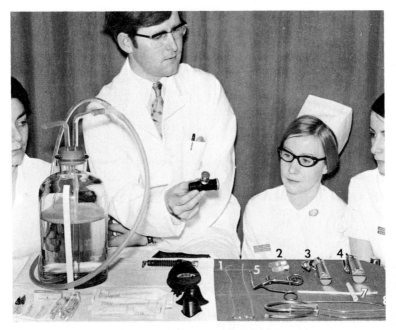

Fig. 35-21    Resuscitation without a Resuscitaire suitable for remote areas. Paediatrician giving clinical demonstration to student midwives.

**Left-hand Side of Trolley (Unsterile)**

Winchester with hibitane and water solution to act as water manometer if no Resuscitaire is available.
Ampoules frusemide, lanoxin, naloxone neonatal (Narcan), sodium bicarbonate, 8·4 per cent, glucose, 20 per cent.
Assorted sizes disposable needles. Assorted sizes disposable syringes.
Antistatic ventilation bag with blow-off valves (paediatrician demonstrating valve).
Rendell-Baker mask (2 sizes).

**Right-hand Side of Trolley (Sterile)**

Disposable Warne or Portex nasal catheters—size FG 4·5 or FG 6.
Protex Guedel airways—sizes 00 and 000.
Baby laryngoscopes (with sterilised blades). Magill endotracheal forceps.
'Y' connections for endotracheal tubes—sizes 00 and 0. Introducer for endotracheal tubes.
Disposable mucus extractor. Disposable Warne neonatal endotracheal tubes—FG 14, 12 or 10.
*Maternity Hospital, Stirling.*

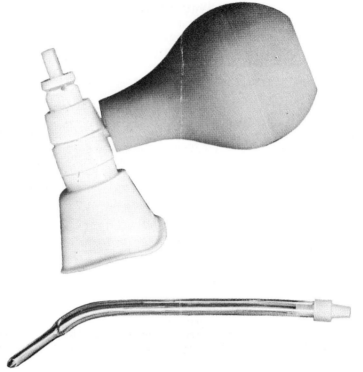

Fig. 35-22 Blease Samson neonatal resuscitator. It can be used with mask or endotracheal tube. The pharynx and nostrils must be cleared first: the lower jaw held up.

*Blease Medical Equipment Ltd, Deansway, Chesham, Bucks.*

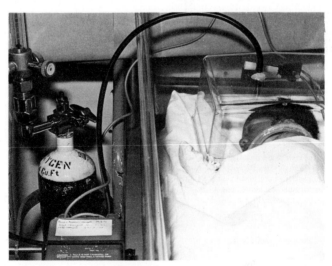

Fig. 35-23 Head box for oxygen concentration (home-made, cost 75 pence). IMI oxygen analyser in use. If no analyser is available sufficient oxygen should be given to maintain the baby's pink colour: one litre.

# EMBRYOTOMY

*For Midwives in Remote Areas of Developing Countries*

All operative procedures involving 'cutting into' and destruction of the fetus to diminish its bulk are included under the term 'embryotomy'.

*The four operations are:*

### Craniotomy, Cleidotomy, Decapitation, Evisceration

They are usually, but not invariably, carried out on the dead fetus, in order to terminate labour which will be or has obstructed. The need for embryotomy should not arise except in cases of hydrocephaly or other gross fetal malformation, for, with good prenatal care, conditions liable to obstruct labour can be diagnosed during pregnancy. With competent supervision during labour, factors which cause obstruction can be detected and rectified early, or dealt with by lower segment Caesarean section.

## CRANIOTOMY

The indications are hydrocephaly, large baby, contracted pelvis, impacted brow and face presentations.

Dehydration and ketoacidosis are rectified if present: cross-marched blood should be available; catheter passed; episiotomy made.

### Instruments

Skull perforator (Oldham or Simpson); obstetric forceps. A blunt hook and crotchet may be required to extract the aftercoming head of the breech. The 'set up' is similar to that described for forceps delivery. *(The use of the cranioclast and cephalotribe is no longer advocated.)*

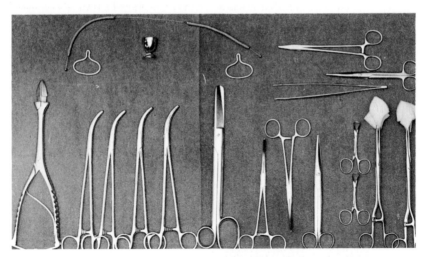

Fig. 35-24   Instruments for embryotomy.

| | |
|---|---|
| 2 sponge holders; 2 towel clips. | 1 needle holder. 1 Mayo scissors 15 cm. |
| 1 Mayo scissors 20 cm. | 1 dissecting forceps. 1 Simpson perforator. |
| 2 Mayo forceps; 4 Briggs forceps. | 1 Blond Heidler decapitating wire saw. |
| 1 embryotomy scissors. | |

*Simpson Memorial Maternity Pavilion, Edinburgh.*

## Method

After making an episiotomy midwifery forceps are applied to steady the head during perforation. The point of the perforator, which should be sharp and kept under control so that it does not slip off the skull and lacerate maternal tissues, is inserted. The point of insertion in a vertex presentation would be the parietal bone; in a face the orbit or roof of mouth; in the aftercoming head of the breech presentation, the sub-occipital region or behind the ear. Having perforated the skull the blades of the perforator are opened to make a cruciform incision in the skull bone; then closed and passed into the cranium, opened widely and rotated to fragment the brain tissue; the perforator is withdrawn. Traction on the obstetric forceps is applied to extract the head.

If unsuccessful or if the cervix is not fully dilated 4 pairs of Briggs forceps (which resemble but are larger than curved Mayo forceps) are attached to the edges of the perforated bone, a bandage is threaded through the handles and a one kg weight attached and allowed to hang over the foot of the bed. This method facilitates dilatation of the cervix and accomplishes extraction slowly.

## CLEIDOTOMY

This operation consists in the cutting of one or both clavicles, to reduce the width of the shoulders in cases such as a contracted pelvis, an excessively large baby or shoulder dystocia, with a dead baby. Embryotomy scissors are used.

## DECAPITATION

Decapitation, as the name implies, is severing of the head from the trunk; the indications being: an **impacted shoulder** presentation; **locked twins; double-headed monster.**

This operation would be necessary for a neglected shoulder presentation; one that had become impacted. If an obstetrician was available Caesarean section would be done, otherwise to avoid uterine rupture or to terminate a dangerously long labour, decapitation would be necessary. On no account should version be attempted for neglected shoulder presentation by the midwife. Because of excessive retraction of the upper segment this would be difficult to do. The extreme thinning and overstretching of the lower uterine segment, by the fetus lying transversely, creates the risk of ruptured uterus.

### Instruments

Blond Heidler decapitator; or sharp and serrated decapitation hooks; embryotomy blunt pointed-scissors; blunt hook and crotchet; heavy volsellum forceps.

### Procedure

Prior to the general anaesthetic and operation, dehydration and ketosis must be combated by an intravenous infusion of 10 per cent glucose. A catheter is passed, to ensure that the bladder is empty. After a liberal episiotomy is made traction is applied to the arm to bring the neck within reach.

**The Blond Heidler wire saw,** the best decapitating instrument, is used. After the thimble introducer is attached to one end of the saw it is passed round the baby's neck and a handle attached to each end of the wire. By pulling on each handle alternately the sawing movement severs the neck: the body being delivered by traction on the arm. Great care must be exercised to avoid lacerating the bladder and vaginal tissues with the spikes of bone at the point of severance.

**The detached head is fixed** at the pelvic brim by suprapubic pressure. Vaginally a finger is inserted into the mouth or foramen magnum, aided by the use of a crochet or heavy volsellum forceps. Obstetric forceps can be applied to the head which may have to be perforated if difficulty is encountered.

**A sharp decapitating hook can be used** if the wire saw is not available. The hook is passed along the palmar surface of the fingers of the midwife's left hand, over the baby's shoulder and round the neck. The hook is manipulated until a firm grasp of the neck is obtained; backward and forward movement of the handle will cause the blade to sever the neck. Embryotomy scissors could be used to complete the decapitation.

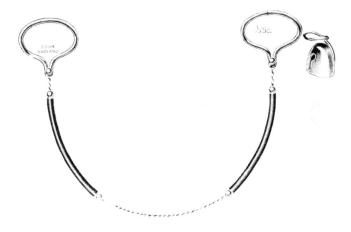

Fig. 35-25   Blond Heidler wire saw decapitator.

*By courtesy of Down Bros. and Mayer and Phelps Ltd., Mitcham, Surrey.*

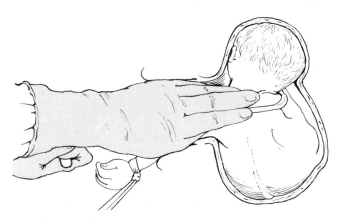

Fig. 35-26   Jardine's decapitation hook is passed round neck of fetus. Traction on arm by an assistant brings the neck within reach and fixes the head and trunk.

## EVISCERATION

The operation consists in incising the fetal abdomen with embryotomy (or long) scissors for the removal of the contents of the abdominal cavity. This may be necessary because of excessive distension by fetal ascites or a tumour in the fetal abdomen obstructing labour. Occasionally evisceration is carried out in cases of impacted shoulder presentation to reduce fetal bulk when the neck is inaccessible for decapitation.

## SYMPHYSIOTOMY

**This operation is employed in some African countries** where the women are unlikely to return for a repeat Caesarean section. It is mainly done in the primigravid woman with a minor degree of cephalo-pelvic disproportion which is causing delay toward the end of the first stage; the cervix being almost fully dilated. Rarely is it done for prolonged or obstructed labour.

The pubic area is shaved, cleansed thoroughly and infiltrated with 10 ml one per cent lignocaine: also the perineum for an episiotomy. To protect the urethra, a firm catheter inserted to empty the bladder is left in position and held to one side by a finger in the vagina during the incision. Two midwives support and abduct the legs during the operation.

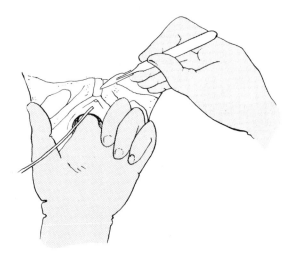

Fig. 35-27   Symphysiotomy. Fibrocartilage of the symphysis pubis being incised.

**The fibro-cartilage is incised over the centre of the symphysis pubis.** As a rule the ventouse vacuum extractor is applied to facilitate vaginal delivery. An extensive episiotomy is usually made so that the fetal head will not exert too much pressure on the urethra and bladder.

Applying broad strips of elastoplast round the pelvis gives support; with a towel pinned round the knees and the woman lying on her side. Antibiotics are usually prescribed. A self retaining catheter remains in position for 4 or 5 days and the woman is allowed up on the 6th day. Following symphysiotomy, some women suffer permanent backache; others have difficulty in walking.

---

## QUESTIONS FOR REVISION

What can the midwife do to prevent debilitating diseases in potential mothers and pregnant women? Name six such diseases. Elaborate on the phrase 'The sun should not set twice on the woman in labour'. Explain how by proficient abdominal examination causes of obstructed labour would have been detected.

Why is it important that (a) ketoacidosis is corrected prior to operative procedures. (b) the bladder is empty prior to vaginal operative procedures. (c) the midwife is aware of causes of rupture of uterus?

### INTRAVENOUS INJECTION

How do you avoid penetrating both walls of the vein? Why should blood be withdrawn prior to injection?

### FORCEPS

For what reasons is a comprehensive vaginal examination made prior to application of forceps? Differentiate between: mid and low forceps, and describe the direction of traction in each case. Which blade is inserted first?........................ In which maternal side of the vagina is it inserted?........................ The fenestra lies over the........................ Each period of traction should not exceed........................

### MALMSTRÖM EXTRACTOR

Give 4 indications for its use. Which analgesic would a midwife administer during the procedure? What should be determined abdominally and vaginally before applying the extractor? Why is the cup not lubricated with any emollient substance? What is the direction of pull? What is the cause of the cup being detached?

During how many contractions may traction be applied? The term for the large caput is........................? What are the dangers to the fetus?

### INTERNAL VERSION

Differentiate between external, internal, bi-polar, cephalic and podalic version. In which circumstances would it be dangerous to attempt internal version? What is the main danger? Describe the procedure in detail.

### SHOULDER DYSTOCIA

Explain how knowledge of the mechanism of labour enables the midwife to avoid shoulder dystocia in babies of average size. Describe how you would deal with the situation in a vertex L.O.A.

### EMBRYOTOMY

Define the term. Why is embryotomy seldom necessary today?

Give indications for craniotomy and name the outstanding one. How would you avoid injury to the bladder when inserting the perforator? Which instruments could be applied and a weight attached if the cervix was not fully dilated? Write 5 lines on cleidotomy.

Give 2 indications for decapitation. Which is the best decapitating instrument? Why is there grave danger of injury to the bladder? How can the midwife try to avert this? How is the decapitated head extracted? Describe how you would use a sharp decapitating hook?

For what reasons are the following instruments used? Simpson's perforator; Briggs forceps; embryotomy scissors; Blond Heidler wire saw; crotchet.

Define the terms craniotomy, decapitation, cleidotomy, evisceration.

### SYMPHYSIOTOMY

At what stage of labour is symphysiotomy performed? Where is the incision made? How is injury to the urethra avoided?

# 36
# Aids to Diagnosis in Obstetrics

*Radiology. Ultrasonography. Blood tests. Urine analysis*

Radiology is one of the aids to diagnosis in obstetrics, used mainly to supplement and confirm findings which have been made on clinical examination during pregnancy.

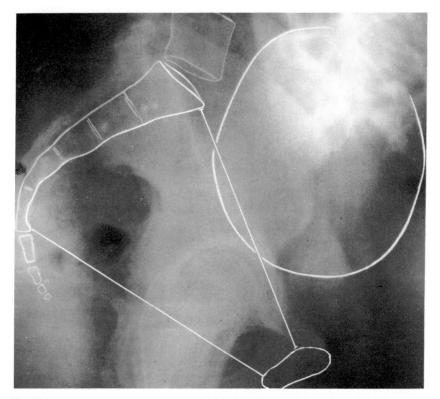

Fig. 36-1   Lateral radiograph (retouched), showing the antero-posterior diameters of the brim and outlet.

### RADIATION HAZARDS

Certain risks may be involved in the use of radiography, but these must be balanced against the advantages in the saving of maternal and infant life.

An increased mutation rate in the germ cells of mother and child may affect future generations by causing congenital disease and abnormalities.

Attempts to prevent these dangers are being made by the use of modern radiological techniques; shielding of fetal and maternal gonads, shorter exposures, smaller doses and shorter wave lengths.

**The 10 day rule.** During the childbearing years X-ray examination of abdomen, pelvis or hips should be made during the 10 days following the last menstrual period to avoid the possibility of pregnancy having occurred.

## PELVIC SIZE AND SHAPE

Radiography to determine pelvic size and shape might be indicated (*after the 32nd week*) in the following circumstances:

When there is a history of injury or disease of the pelvis or spine, or of a previous difficult delivery.

In cases of limp or deformity, cephalo-pelvic disproportion, persistent breech or shoulder presentation.

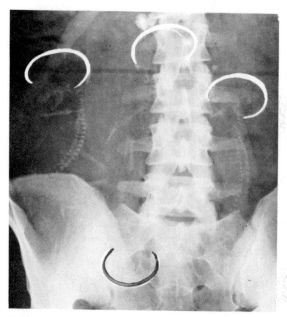

Fig. 36-2   Quadruplets (retouched). All four babies survived and were discharged weighing over 2·5 kg. The mother had two sets of twins, aged 6 and 2 years.

*Aberdeen Maternity Hospital.*

### FETAL ABNORMALITIES

Malformations, such as anencephaly and hydrocephaly, achondroplasia, conjoined twins, spina bifida, may be diagnosed.

### UTERINE RADIOGRAPHY

**Localisation of placenta.** By soft tissue X-ray it is possible in about 90 per cent of cases to diagnose placenta praevia by the absence of placental shadow in the upper uterine segment.

**In cases of infertility,** opaque substances injected into the uterus and Fallopian tubes (hystero-salpingogram) produce a shadow on an X-ray film which demonstrates the patency or non-patency of the tubes.

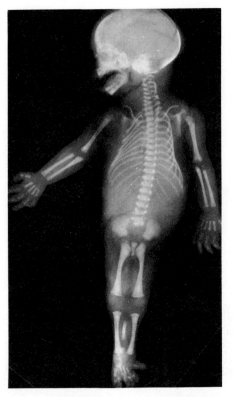

Fig. 36-3 Sympodia (mermaid-like fetus). The lower limbs are fused to form a tail-like structure with one foot, eight toes; no uterus, external genitalia, urethral or anal orifices; no sex identified; weight 1·5 kg; stillborn. The fetus was the second of dizygotic (binovular) twins; the first, born alive, weighed 3·4 kg.

*Maternity Hospital, Motherwell.*

## ULTRASONOGRAPHY IN OBSTETRICS

Ultrasonography is a means of diagnosing the presence, size and position of a mass from the sound echo evoked by the density of the mass. In the 1914-1918 war ultrasound was used in submarine warfare (known as Asdic). If the presence of a submarine was suspected, a beam of ultrasonic energy was projected and the echo received would depend on the resistance of the mass, e.g. a rock, shoal of fish or a submarine. Ultrasound was first employed in obstetrics by Professor Ian Donald, Queen Mother's Hospital, Glasgow, and is now a successful diagnostic technique with none of the radiation hazards of radiography.

### PROCEDURE

The woman lies on a couch and a probe connected to the ultrasonic machine is 'run over' her abdomen which has been smeared with KY jelly to obtain acoustic coupling.

The ultrasonic diagnostic machine transmits a beam of ultrasonic energy (sound waves far above the range of human hearing) generated by an electric current causing a small crystal in the probe to vibrate. When this beam strikes the junction between objects of different densities, fetal limbs, fluid, skull or placenta the returning echoes are amplified and displayed on a cathode ray tube as dots of light and may be recorded with a polaroid camera. The image so produced is an ultrasonogram, an echo picture. The examination takes only a few minutes, the results are immediately available.

The A scan is a one-dimension picture useful when measuring a diameter as in fetal cephalometry. The B scan gives a composite two-dimensional picture.

### REAL-TIME ULTRASOUND SCANNER

**System 85 Diagnostic Sonar** is a portable piece of up-to-date ultrasonic equipment, easy to operate and is being used in prenatal clinics and wards. Midwives have in some centres been trained to use the real-time scanner to assess gestational age, exclude twin pregnancies, to elucidate doubtful presentations: serial measurements of the bi-parietal diameter to assess fetal growth are less accurate.

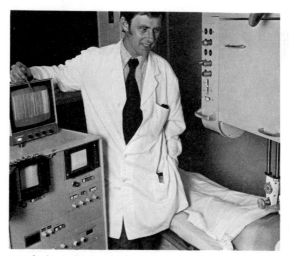

Fig. 36-4    Ultrasonologist explaining the findings on an ultrasonic scan to expectant mother.
*Queen Mother's Hospital, Glasgow.*

A static scanner utilises one single transducer in the probe placed on the abdomen to transmit and receive ultrasound pulses. In the real-time scanner the probe is large and consists of a series of transducers which 'fire' in sequence so rapidly that a 'moving' picture is produced, e.g. random limb movements, heart beat, breathing, sucking, hiccups. The real-time scanner produces images in 10 distinct shades of grey, that gives a most impressive picture.

**The full bladder technique** is used to raise the uterus out of the pelvis and displace loops of intestine: the patient being asked to drink 600 ml of fluid 1½ hours prior to the examination. A bladder containing urine shows up as a well defined black area and is an aid to delineating the gestation sac in early pregnancy and in defining fetal parts and placenta later.

## ULTRASOUND AS A DIAGNOSTIC AID

**Diagnosis of pregnancy.** A gestational sac has been seen as early as 5 weeks' amenorrhoea. The fetal heart beat is visible on the real time scanner at 7 weeks. Change in the shape of the uterus is manifest.

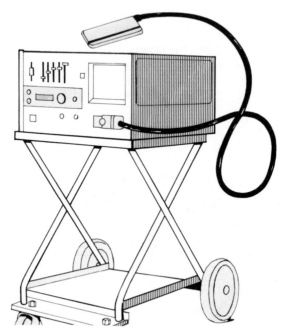

Fig. 36-5    Portable real-time ultrasound scanner.

**Gestational age.** Crown-rump measurement can be estimated at 6–12 weeks. Random fetal movements are obvious at 9 weeks. The bi-parietal diameter can be measured at 9–10 weeks.

**Abortion:** a blighted ovum has a blotchy speckled appearance with an imperfect ring. From 7 weeks the fetus can be seen within the gestation sac and fetal heart movement observed on the real time scanner. An incomplete abortion would show white echoes in the uterine cavity which are retained products of conception.

**Hydatidiform mole** shows a speckled area: no fetal heart sounds or movement are evident.

**Twins** are diagnosed at 8 weeks by the identification of 2 fetal sacs. Two fetal heads are seen at 15–17 weeks.

**Prior to amniocentesis.** Localisation of the placenta immediately prior to amniocentesis will minimise the risk of transplacental bleeding and the subsequent production of antibodies in cases of Rh incompatibility.

**Antepartum haemorrhage.** The placenta is localised in all cases of antepartum haemorrhage to confirm or exclude the diagnosis of placenta praevia.

**Polyhydramnios** is shown by large clear areas of fluid: blobs which appear to be floating in the fluid are limbs.

**Fetal abnormalities.** Spina bifida has been detected at 16–20 weeks, hydrocephalus at about 20 weeks, anencephalus at 15–17 weeks. Some use sonar prior to Caesarean section to rule out fetal abnormality.

**Fetal growth.** Gestational age must first be established; crown rump measurement being accurate. The bi-parietal diameter can be estimated at 9 to 10 weeks. After 30 weeks serial scans are made every 2 weeks to observe growth rate. Some estimate fetal girth measurement.

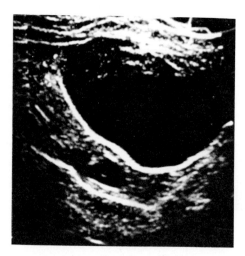

Fig. 36-6
Small for dates gestational sac. 9 weeks amenorrhoea. 7 weeks sac. Bladder full to provide a well-defined area to aid locating the fetal sac.

*Courtesy of Western Infirmary, Glasgow.*

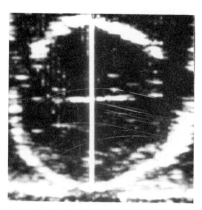

Fig. 36-7   Bi-parietal fetal cephalogram.

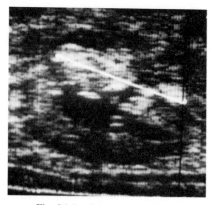

Fig. 36-8   Crown rump fetal length.

**Malpresentation.** Breech and shoulder presentation are most commonly diagnosed.

**Integrity of a previous Caesarean scar.**

**The detection of retained products of conception post partum.**

## THE ULTRASONIC FETAL PULSE DETECTOR

*Ultrasound Cardioscope*

**The Sonicaid and the Doptone,** portable battery run machines, are in common use today. By utilising ultrasound and the Doppler effect, fetal heart sounds can be heard. KY jelly is smeared on to the skin before the transducer is applied in order to obtain good acoustic coupling.

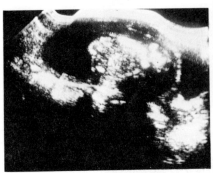
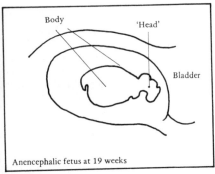

Anencephalic fetus at 19 weeks

Fig. 36-9

*The Apparatus is employed as follows:*

**To detect the presence of a living fetus:** (*a*) pregnancy diagnosis (from 12 weeks); (*b*) threatened abortion; (*c*) missed abortion; (*d*) hydatidiform mole; (*e*) intrauterine death.

**To confirm the diagnosis of thrombosis in** major leg veins above popliteal level. If the vein is occluded by a thrombus no blood flow is detected.

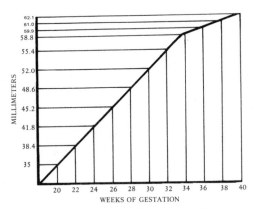

Fig. 36-10   Growth of biparietal diameter at 2 week intervals.

## BLOOD TESTS

### Grouping

Blood of different individuals belongs to one of four groups, classified under the ABO system. The patient should be given blood of her own particular group if possible, but in an acute emergency, when there are neither facilities nor time for ascertaining this, Group O blood, being compatible with all four groups, may be given.

### Direct cross-matching

As an additional precaution against giving incompatible blood, the serum from the recipient's clotted blood is mixed with blood from the 'pilot tube' which is attached to the bottle of donor blood. If agglutination of red cells is manifest, the donor blood is not compatible.

### Rh factor grouping

The Rh factor of every pregnant woman should be ascertained early in pregnancy because of the grave risks in giving Rh positive blood to an Rh negative woman. In an emergency Rh negative Group O blood is given.

**Rh antibodies.** Tests for the presence of antibodies are carried out on Rh negative women: Coombs' indirect anti-globulin test (I.A.G.T.). Coombs' direct anti-globulin test (D.A.G.T.) is used when examining the baby's blood if haemolytic disease is suspected.

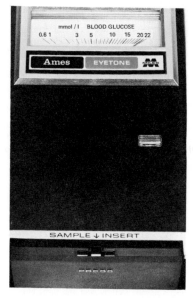

Fig. 36-11 Dextrostix reflectance meter. Provides immediate quantitative blood glucose determinations. (See p. 668)

*Courtesy of Ames Company.*

**Glucose** (*see p. 123*).
**Haemoglobin** (*see p. 123*).
**Rubella antibodies** (*see p. 215*).
**Syphilis** (*see p. 221*).
**Plasma oestriol** (*see p. 109*).
**Alpha-feto-proteins** at 18 weeks 50–150 micrograms/.l (*see p. 109*).
**Placental lactogen** after 34 weeks 4–5 mg/l or micrograms/.l (*see p. 109*).

## DEXTROSTIX GLUCOSE SCREENING TEST

**With Dextrostix Reagent Strips** glucose levels in whole blood can be estimated in one minute.

The midwife carries out this test in babies suspected of hypoglycaemia within one hour of birth and if low, before feeds for 72 hours. The risk of hypoglycaemia is even greater on the second day. Blood is obtained by heel prick. The foot should be warm; the heel cleansed with Hibitane, 0·5 per cent, in spirit 70 per cent and dried. With a sterile disposable lancet a puncture 2 mm deep is made parallel to the sole, avoiding bone. One large drop of blood is allowed to drip on to the reagent area and after exactly 60 seconds it is washed off using a squeezy bottle (not under the water tap). The strip area is compared with the colour chart according to instructions on the bottle. If the result is under 1·1 mmol/l, the doctor does a blood glucose estimation. For photograph of method see Fig. 31-1.

### BLOOD REQUIRED FOR LABORATORY TESTS

| Test | Test Tube | Amount of Blood | Normal Result |
|------|-----------|-----------------|---------------|
| Rh factor ⎫<br>ABO group ⎭ | Plain | 5 ml | |
| Antibodies | Plain | 10 ml | |
| Serum bilirubin | Plain | 3 ml | below 17 micromols/l |
| Coombs' | Plain | 5 ml | |
| Blood urea | Lithium heparin | 3 ml | 3–7 mmol/l |
| Fasting blood glucose | Oxalated fluoride | 2 ml | 4–5 mmol/l |
| Erythrocyte sedimentation rate (E.S.R.) | Sequestrene | 5 ml | From 2 to 5 mm in first hour |
| Blood culture | Bacteriological broth, 50 ml | 5 ml | |
| White cell count | Sequestrene | 2·5 ml | 5,000 to 10,000 |
| Red cell count | Sequestrene | 2·5 ml | 5,000,000 |
| Coagulation time | Plain | 1 ml | 5 to 8 minutes |
| Prothrombin time | Sodium citrate or sodium oxalate | 2·5 ml | |
| Haemoglobin | Sequestrene | 2·5 ml | 14·8 g/dl |
| Plasma fibrinogen | Sodium citrate | 5 ml | 2–4 g/l |

## URINE ANALYSIS *(In Pregnancy)*

**Note the appearance.** Crystal clear urine may contain protein; blood gives a red or dark brown colour; bile produces a greenish-gold or greenish-brown colour.

**Odour.** An offensive odour may be due to pus; an odour of stale fish is associated with an *E. coli* infection. A fruity odour, or one of violets, is due to ketones.

**Reaction.** Freshly voided urine is usually slightly acid and turns blue litmus-paper red; alkaline urine turns red litmus paper blue.

**The specific gravity** normally ranges from 1010 to 1025.

## PROTEINURIA

Proteinuria may be present in the following conditions in obstetrics: pre-eclampsia, eclampsia, serious hyperemesis, chronic nephritis and pyelonephritis. A trace is also found in urine which contains blood, pus, vaginal discharge or amniotic fluid.

### *Tests for Protein*

**ALBUSTIX REAGENT STRIPS** test for protein. If positive, further tests are made.
**URISTIX REAGENT STRIPS** detect proteinuria and glycosuria simultaneously.

**THE SALICYL SULPHONIC ACID TEST**

This is a cold test which is rapid and sensitive. With a pipette add a few drops of 20 per cent salicyl sulphonic acid to half a test tube of urine, and a turbid streak will appear if protein is presesnt. If the urine is alkaline, a few extra drops of salicyl sulphonic acid are needed.

**ESBACH'S QUANTITATIVE TEST FOR PROTEIN**

The vulva is swabbed with water and a midstream specimen of urine obtained.

The urine must be filtered unless clear, and acidified if alkaline. If the specific gravity is over 1010 the urine must be diluted with an equal volume of water, because the protein precipitate does not settle properly if the specific gravity is over 1010.

The graduated tube is filled to the mark 'U' with urine and to the mark 'R' with reagent. The tube is stoppered, then inverted two or three times without shaking and allowed to stand undisturbed for 24 hours. The height of the precipitate in the tube is read and recorded in grammes per litre, the result being doubled if the urine is diluted.

The patient's name, time when set up, and whether the urine is diluted must be clearly marked.

**BIURET TEST**

This test is more accurate than the Esbach test. To a 24-hour speciment of urine Biuret reagent is added and the urine forms a deep blue colour. Photoelectric cells assess the degree of light in the colour from which is calculated the amount of protein in the urine.

## GLYCOSURIA

A trace of glucose is found in the urine of about 10 per cent of pregnant women, and when diabetes is present.

**CLINITEST REAGENT TABLETS** estimate glucose in urine.

**DIASTIX REAGENT STRIPS** are specific for glucose.

**URISTIX REAGENT STRIPS** now commonly used to detect glucose and protein simultaneously. If glucose is detected by Clinistix or Uristix reagent strips Clinitest tablets are used to estimate quantitatively.

**MULTISTIX REAGENT STRIPS** test simultaneously for pH, protein, glucose, ketones, bilirubin, blood, urobilinogen.

## KETONURIA (Acetonuria)

Ketones are found in the urine of obstetric patients who are diabetic or when the carbohydrate intake is diminished, such as in hyperemesis gravidarum. During prolonged labour, with or without vomiting, acidosis will occur unless the carbohydrate intake is adequate.

**KETOSTIX REAGENT STRIPS** detect the presence of ketones.

## BLOOD IN THE URINE

In obstetric practice blood in the urine is most commonly due to vaginal bleeding. Very occasionally it may be due to nephritis and is then bright red; in cases of eclampsia the urine may be dark brownish-red, almost chocolate colour, due to the presence of blood in highly concentrated urine.

**HEMASTIX REAGENT STRIPS** test for blood in the urine.

## BILE IN THE URINE

Bile is found in the urine when jaundice is present, in cases such as severe hyperemesis gravidarum, and puerperal sepsis due to the *Clostridium welchii*.

**ICTOTEST REAGENT TABLETS** detect the presence of bilirubin in urine.

## URICULT

This dip slide system for urine culture is suitable for large scale screening. A slide with MacConkey's agar on one side, nutrient agar on the other is dipped into urine and placed in a plastic container incubated or kept at room temperature; sent for identification and sensitivity test. Used for asymptomatic bacteriuria.

---

# QUESTIONS FOR REVISION

**Urine analysis**

For what reason should urine (a) be acidified when examined for protein? (b) be diluted when setting up an Esbach test? Why do normal pregnant women have glycosuria? Which is the most reliable test for pus? Differentiate between Uricult, Uristix: Diastix, Ketostix, Multistix: Albustix.

**C.M.B.(Scot.) question.** What abnormal constituents are present in the urine in a case of (a) pre-eclampsia; (b) hyperemesis gravidarum; (c) pyelonephritis of pregnancy? Describe the tests for these.

**C.M.B.(N. Ireland) question.** Enumerate the abnormal constituents which may be found in the urine of a patient 28 weeks pregnant. Describe their significance.

**C.M.B(Scot.) question.** Discuss the importance of urine testing during pregnancy.

**Ultrasonography**

Pregnancy has been diagnosed by ultrasound as early as ........................................................................

Crown-rump measurement has assessed gestational age at ................................................................

Twins have been detected at ...................................................................................................................

Give 2 occasions when the placenta would be localised by ultrasound. ............................................

Name 3 fetal abnormalities that have been detected by sonar. .............................................................

Why is bi-parietal cephalometry carried out? ......................................................................................

# 37

# Confinement in the Home
*Preparation. Postnatal care.*

There are many instances when the midwife should not undertake the management of labour at home. In a number of cases some obstetrical or medical abnormality exists which necessitates supervision by specialists and the provision of facilities for operative procedure. Hospitalisation is then essential.

## WOMEN 'AT HIGH RISK'

Obstetric patients 'at high risk' can be detected by 'screening' during the prenatal period. Important points are: high parity, age, height; medical and obstetrical histories; findings in the present pregnancy; poor socio-economic conditions.

### Conditions in which home confinement is contra-indicated

*Either Mother or Baby is 'at high risk'*

| THE HOME | THE MOTHER | | THE BABY |
|---|---|---|---|
| | OBSTETRICAL | MEDICAL | |
| Overcrowding. | Cephalo-pelvic dis-proportion. | Cardiac disease. | History of previous stillbirths, neonatal deaths. |
| Infectious disease present. | Pre-eclampsia: eclampsia. Multiple pregnancy. Antepartum haemorrhage. | Tuberculosis. | or no living child. |
| Destitution. | Polyhydramnios. | Diabetes. Venereal disease. | Breech presentation. |
| Poor environmental conditions | Rh immunisation. Previous; Caesarean section, difficult forceps delivery; postpartum haemorrhage or adherent placenta. | Essential hypertension. Subfertility. | Gestation period less than 36 weeks. Rh haemolytic disease. Fetal abnormalities |
| | Primigravida over 30 yrs. Multipara 4 + Multipara over 35 yrs. | Anaemia. below 10 g/dl | Postmaturity. Small baby syndrome. |

## PREPARATION FOR CONFINEMENT

The midwife must visit the home before confinement to see whether it is suitable and to give the necessary advice. The mother should be told what to do, and what she should provide. It is a good plan to give her a leaflet of printed instructions.

*A midwife must, as soon as practicable, visit the patient and inquire into the suitability of the accommodation and of the equipment, and* **where these are not suitable she must notify the fact to the** Local Supervising Authority and to the patient's general practitioner.

**Some form of heating must be provided** by day and night in cold weather to prevent neonatal hypothermia.

The room should, of course, be clean, but there is little value in clean walls, fresh curtains and a scrubbed floor if the blankets and quilt are dirty. It is what the woman in bed comes in contact with that matters most. The carpet can be cleaned with a vacuum cleaner or washed with soap and water and protected with a piece of linoleum, canvas or mackintosh, but not paper which only gets ruffled. The thorough cleaning should be completed at least one month before the date of confinement, the mother obtaining assistance for this strenuous task. On no account should any sweeping or dusting be done when labour is in progress. Dirty surfaces can be wiped with a cloth wrung out of antiseptic lotion.

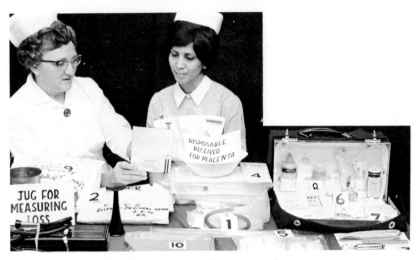

Fig. 37-1   Equipment for home confinement.

1. **Enema tubing and funnel;** KY Jelly: disposable enema; Dulcolax suppositories; disposable razor.
2. **Perineal repair pack:**—1 tinfoil tray; 1 scissors; 1 dissecting forceps; 1 needleholder; Ethicon foil packed eyeless needles and No 1 chromic sutures W 759 and Mersilk on cutting needle W 562; 1 perineal pad; 10 gauze swabs; 1 paper hand towel; 1 paper dressing-towel. (*All wrapped in disposable bag.*)
3. **T.P.R. chart; low reading thermometer; weighing scales; metric tape measure.**
4. **Pack for vulval toilet; Vaginal examination pack; Catheter pack.**
5. **Disposable mucus extractors.**
6. **Drugs.** Pethidine obtained on a midwives' Supply Order. Promazine (Sparine) (Eng.) and pentazocine (Fortral) (Eng.). Konakion, naloxone (Narcan neonatal), lignocaine 5 ml one per cent solution. Syntometrine, ergometrine, magnesium trisilicate.
7. **Syringes and needles, disposable.**
8. **Lotions:** Hibitane, Hibitane in spirit, obstetric cream, mediswabs.
9. **Delivery pack:**—2 tinfoil bowls; 2 cord forceps; 2 scissors (1 for episiotomy); 1 Spencer Wells forceps with elastic band for ligating cord or plastic cord clamp: 2 perineal pads; 3 paper dressing towels; cotton-wool balls; 1 gown; 1 turkish wrap (for baby); 1 disposable bowl for placenta. Forceps to puncture membranes, if necessary, packed separately. Jug for measuring blood loss.
10. **Plastic apron;** nail brush; torch; disposable gloves; Dispos-a-glove; Multistix for urine testing; Dextrostix reagent strips.

**Entonox,** Blease Samson neonatal resuscitator.

**Maternity set:**—0·5 kg cotton wool, 2 dozen perineal pads (wrapped separately), cord ligatures, dressings, powder, accouchement pad, polythene draw sheet.

*Simpson Memorial Maternity Pavilion, Edinburgh.*

**The bed** should be placed so that it is accessible from both sides and conveniently situated in regard to light. Two or three 25-cm boards under the mattress will remedy the sagging.

**The linen** to be used during confinement should be freshly laundered. Pieces of old folded sheeting are useful to lay under the patient and reduce the amount of 'washing'. Towels are needed to cover tables and jugs as well as for the hands.

**Two tables will be necessary;** a card table and a strong kitchen chair would do. The possibility of spoiling furniture should be kept in mind, and an inverted kitchen tray placed under jugs and kettles will prevent such damage.

**The midwife** supplies a maternity pack (see Fig. 37-1).

## Requirements provided by patient

### For the confinement

2 large basins: 1 for the mother, 1 for midwife's hands. 1 bed-pan. Plastic bag for soiled dressings.
2 kettles; 1 jug (1200 ml).
Plastic sheet, 2 × 1 metres.
Hibitane or other antiseptic.
2 old nightdresses for labour.

2 bath, 2 face towels: 2 face cloths.
2 firm uplift brassières. Sanitary belt.
1 new nailbrush, boiled and kept in jar of antiseptic solution.
Large pieces of clean, strong brown paper, or newspapers, to protect the mattress.
1 or 2 hot-water bottles with covers.

### For baby's immediate needs

A soft towel to wrap baby in when born. A baby bath or large wash-hand basin; soft bath towel and face towel. Face cloth, and one of different colour for buttocks; cake of good soap.

Bathing aprons, one plastic, and one made from a bath towel. Baby clothes. Safety pins.

Cot and bedding (a drawer can be used in an emergency). Stool or low chair.

*A full list of baby's requirements is given in the Parentcraft section.*

## Immediate preparations for labour

The woman will have been told what to do pending the midwife's arrival, i.e. she will see that the room is warm, boil two kettles and set one apart to cool and have the bed linen and baby clothes sought out.

The mattress is protected with layers of brown paper or newspaper, especially in the middle, and laid over these is the large plastic sheet.

If basins are not sterile and there are no means of boiling them, they can be scoured, rinsed, smeared with Hibitane and scalded by pouring boiling water over them.

The management of labour is similar to that in hospital. The placenta must be burned or arrangements made for its disposal by the midwife.

### POSTNATAL CARE

The midwife greets the woman by asking her how she feels, removes outdoor uniform, washes her hands and puts on cap and gown, some wear masks. While unwrapping bowls and preparing solutions she questions the woman about her well-being and the baby's behaviour.

Temperature, pulse, respirations are taken and recorded: breasts and nipples examined; fundus and bladder palpated; perineal pad inspected. The woman is questioned regarding her appetite, sleep, bowels. Kardex records may be continued after discharge from hospital. Any untoward signs and symptoms are reported to the doctor.

The mother is asked if the baby feeds well and is contented, and should be told to keep one napkin for inspection of stool every day. The baby is examined by the midwife daily and by the doctor (a) following birth and (b) prior to discharge, as in hospital: temperature taken with a low reading thermometer and recorded. The midwife watches the baby being fed once daily during the first few days.

Preparations are made to wash the woman's thighs, lower abdomen and buttocks, care being taken not to shake the blanket and disseminate dust and organisms. Breast, and swabbing technique are carried out as in hospital: a shower or tub bath is taken if available.

To avoid neonatal hypothermia the bedroom temperature should be maintained at 18·3° to 21·1°C. A wall thermometer is loaned if necessary.

If bottle fed, the baby should be properly established on a suitable formula and the mother instructed on how to make up the feeds and on the necessity for further supervision and advice at the child health clinic.

## ADVICE TO MOTHER

Any necessary instruction is given to the home-help regarding the comfort and care of the woman. Bowls are destroyed if disposable, otherwise wiped with Hibitane and scalded; her gown and cap wrapped in clean paper and laid in a drawer or cupboard. The cold sterile water-jug is filled with boiling water, all soiled dressings and papers are placed in a plastic bag and disposed of: the room is left tidy. The midwife should write her report before leaving the house, accurate records are essential.

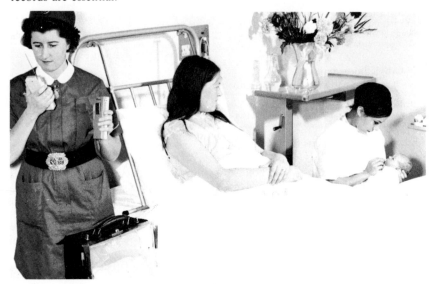

Fig. 37-2 Community midwife visiting patient in General Practitioner unit receives call by portable radio-telephone to go to a woman in labour. Student midwife attending to baby.

*Courtesy of Portsmouth Group Hospital Management Committee.*

The Guthrie test is carried out before the 14th day preferably on the 8th day (see p. 543).

**Family planning is discussed.**

Care of patients transferred from hospital within 48 hours is discussed on page 452.

**According to the Central Midwives Board,** a midwife must visit her patients daily for not less than 10 days after the end of labour, some midwives visit for 28 days. In England she is expected to, in Scotland she must visit morning and evening for the first three days. If a rise in temperature (or any other condition requiring close supervision), be found at the morning visit, an evening visit must be paid.

---

### QUESTIONS FOR REVISION

**C.M.B.(Eng.) 30-min. question.** Write not more than five lines on the importance of each of the following in deciding where a mother should have her third baby:

Her husband's occupation. Her past obstetric history.
Her age. Her blood group.

**C.M.B.(Eng.) short question.** What are the social criteria to be met in selection for home confinement?

**C.M.B.(Eng.) 30-min. question.** Why should you persuade a gravida-7, aged 36, who wants to have her baby at home, that she should be delivered in hospital?

# 38
# Infertility

*Investigation of both partners. Causes. Treatment. Ovulation-induction clinic*

Midwives should have some knowledge of the procedures carried out at infertility clinics in order to assure infertile women and encourage them to attend. They will also comprehend the patient's version of investigations made.

The majority of women become pregnant during the first year of marriage: unless contraception is practised they should be advised to seek advice after one year of infertility. Those who marry nearer the age of 40 than 20 are less likely to conceive and should seek advice after 6 months of infertility. About 7 per cent of marriages are infertile.

**The causes** of infertility may be gynaecological, endocrinological, medical, psychological, social or a combination of these. Investigations will cover all those fields so the woman may have to attend the clinic for some months. Because of the comprehensive investigations necessary some authorities check the husband early in the proceedings to find out whether he is fertile.

## INFERTILITY IN THE HUSBAND

In about 50 per cent of cases the husband is partially and in 15 per cent completely responsible for the infertile marriage. It is believed that 20 million sperms per ml of seminal fluid are sufficient for fertility: Huhner's test is carried out: the woman attends the clinic less than 12 hours after coitus; mucus is aspirated from the cervical canal and examined microscopically for active sperms; 60 per cent should be normal and active. If on seminal fluid analysis the husband is found to be sterile the wife need not be subjected to further detailed investigation.

## INVESTIGATION

A full history is obtained from both partners: age, occupation and whether this involves contact with certain metals and radio-active substances. The woman's family, medical and menstrual histories are taken: mumps, tuberculosis and pelvic infection being significant. The obstetric history is reviewed if the woman has previously aborted or given birth to a child. Her general development is noted, height, weight and blood pressure recorded, heart and lungs are examined. Excessive smoking, alcoholism and drug addiction may be contributory causes: advice is given *re* defective diet: obesity is corrected. Blood examination is carried out for ABO group, Hb, Rh factor, VDRL test for syphilis: urine analysis for protein and glucose. For conditions such as tuberculosis, diabetes, renal or venereal disease the woman is referred to a medical specialist. The vulva is inspected and a bimanual and speculum examination made to detect gross pelvic pathology. Discharge is collected for detection of gonorrhoea, trichomoniasis, candidiasis: any cervical infection is treated. A Papanicolaou smear is taken.

Investigations are made regarding the functional activity of the ovaries and Fallopian tubes to find out whether (*a*) ovulation is taking place, (*b*) there is any mechanical barrier to fertilisation.

### Is the woman ovulating?

An endometrial biopsy taken about the 22nd day of the menstrual cycle will show the secretory changes due to the action of the hormones of the corpus luteum which

675

can only be present following ovulation. The biopsy also shows whether the endometrium is healthy and contains sufficient glycogen for the successful embedding of a fertilised ovum. Regular menstruation is a suggestive but inconclusive sign that ovulation is taking place.

### Basal temperature recording (see Fig. 26-12)

A drop in body temperature followed by a rise occurs at the time of ovulation. The woman is asked to take and record her temperature over a series of menstrual cycles. By 'pin pointing' the time of ovulation plans can be made for coitus to take place when the ovum is available as it only lives unfertilised for 36 hours. For a healthy ovum, fertilisation should occur within 12 hours of ovulation.

### Endocrine imbalance

Insufficient gonadotrophic hormone inhibits the development of the Graafian follicle and reduces the likelihood of ovulation. Insufficiency of oestrogens may affect the cervical and vaginal secretions as well as reducing the contractions of the Fallopian tubes necessary for propulsion of the ovum and zygote.

### Is there any barrier to fertilisation?

It has been estimated that the cause of female infertility in 30 per cent of cases is in the Fallopian tubes which may be wholly or partly occluded due to previous infection; tubercular salpingitis is not rare.

The viscosity of the cervical mucus is tested by a consistometer around the time of ovulation to determine whether it is clear, thin and copious to provide a medium in which the sperms will survive.

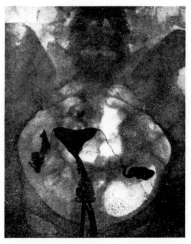

Fig. 38-1   Hystero-salpingography showing normal bilateral tubal patency.

**Hystero-salpingography** is performed in some cases by injecting an opaque dye (Urografin) into the uterus and tubes. The blocked or narrowed part of the tube is manifest on an X-ray film.

**Laparoscopy** is being used in preference to tubal insufflation to test the patency of the tubes, and if they are patent, aqueous methylene blue introduced through the cervix is seen traversing the tubes.

*Treatment*

The treatment of infertility is directed towards the alleviation or adjustment of whatever is preventing conception. Coitus is advised during the period of ovulation. Encouragement is essential and a relaxed outlook fostered: over-anxiety to conceive may by stimulating the sympathetic nervous system produce spasm in the Fallopian tubes. The fact that women who have given up hope of conception, and adopted a child, become pregnant is suggestive that the psychological aspect is a contributory one. About 40 per cent of women attending infertility clinics become pregnant.

## Ovulation-induction

Special ovulation-induction clinics are being established in maternity hospitals for the treatment of oligomenorrhoea and secondary amenorrhoea including cases of 'post pill' amenorrhoea. As well as the usual investigations assays of progesterone and oestradiol are made to assess ovarian function. To induce ovulation clomiphene (Clomid) or tamoxifen (Nolvadex) tablets are prescribed. If ovulation does not take place, human pituitary gonadotrophin (follicle stimulating) hormone Pergonal may be given by i.m. injection. When the plasma oestradiol rises to a level indicating the presence of a mature Graafian follicle an injection of human chorionic gonadotrophin is given to precipitate ovulation. When these 'fertility' drugs are prescribed careful assessment of pregnanediol excretion is made to avoid multiple pregnancy. In some cases failure of ovulation may be due to hyperprolactinaemia: treatment with bromocriptine (Parlodel) can control the prolactin levels and induce ovulation.

### ARTIFICIAL INSEMINATION

**Artificial insemination by donor** (AID) using the semen of a fertile donor is one solution to male subfertility. The woman must be potentially fertile, i.e. menstruating regularly and medically fit. Counselling is necessary to enable the husband to come to terms with his infertility and to ensure that he is willing to be the social father of the child. The donor should be of the same race as the couple with no history of a hereditary disease. His name is not revealed.

# 39
# Carcinoma of Cervix and Breast

*Cervical cytology. Treatment of carcinoma of cervix. Diagnosis of carcinoma of breast*

---

**Early cancer of the cervix is detected by cytology** (study of cell formation).

All epithelia desquamate their surface cells, and malignant epithelia do so more rapidly. The Papanicolaou cervical smear provides a means of detecting such malignant cells before any cancerous lesion of the cervix is clinically manifest. Ayres spatula is inserted into the os, placed against the cervix and rotated 360°—(a full circle) to scrape off surface cells from the region of the internal os. Should suspicious cells be found a cone biopsy is taken.

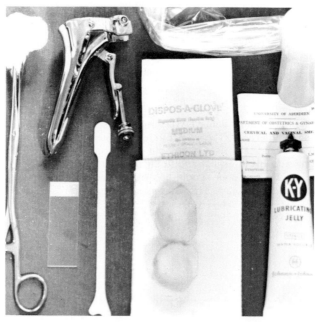

Fig. 39-1    Requirements for Papanicolaou cervical smear.

| | | |
|---|---|---|
| Sponge holder. | Glass slide. | 3 wool balls. |
| Vaginal speculum. | Dispos-a-glove. | Laboratory form. |
| Ayres spatula. | Tube of lubricant. | Disposal bag. |

Container for slide with alcohol and ether.

*Aberdeen Maternity Hospital.*

A cervical cytology service where a diligent search is made at gynaecological, prenatal, postnatal, 'well woman' family planning and infertility clinics, provides a means of accelerating the detection of early cancer of the cervix, which will result in a higher survival rate.

678

**Population screening.** Women 20 to 60 years of age should have a Papanicolaou test taken every 5 years. About 2 cases per 1000 women examined will be detected and at the pre-invasive stage cure is almost certain.

### SIGNS AND SYMPTOMS

Intermittent vaginal bleeding during pregnancy, not associated with abortion, moles or antepartum haemorrhage, and a watery discharge should give rise to suspicion. The usual sequence is vaginal discharge which is at first serous and later foul smelling, bleeding and pain in that order.

No time should be lost. Early cancer is curable. The patient is referred to her doctor, who will, in cases of suspected carcinoma, arrange for expert investigation. (*Late symptoms such as foul-smelling discharge and pain, are not usually seen by midwives in the course of their work, as in such cases the women do not become pregnant.*)

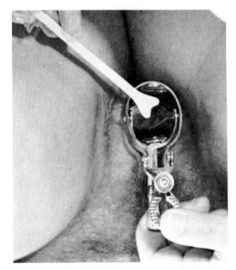

Fig. 39-2    Using Ayres spatula to take Papanicolaou smear.
*Aberdeen Maternity Hospital.*

### *Treatment*

In early pregnancy a radical hysterectomy (Wertheim) is performed followed by radiotherapy.

When diagnosed late in pregnancy, vaginal delivery is not permitted. After Caesarean section, hysterectomy is performed because of the danger of sepsis and metastases *via* the placental site. Radical hysterectomy is performed, if operable; if not, subtotal hysterectomy and radiotherapy are employed.

Radiotherapy is being used more frequently, either alone or in conjunction with radical surgery, in the treatment of invasive cervical cancer. The uterus is evacuated first.

**Carcinoma of the body of the uterus** is not found in association with pregnancy and tends to occur in women at the time of and following the menopause. Should the midwife's advice be asked about irregular or free bleeding at this period of life, the woman must be advised to see her doctor without delay.

# CARCINOMA OF THE BREAST

This serious condition is occasionally diagnosed during pregnancy or the puerperium. Any lump during pregnancy, or during the puerperium which persists for longer than one month should be investigated. The lump is painless in the early stages, and not usually movable; later there may be dimpling of the nipple.

Immediate investigation should be advocated by the midwife if her advice is asked for by a woman of any age regarding a lump in the breast. The woman should be told that it may be a simple tumour which, if dealt with promptly, will be prevented from becoming serious.

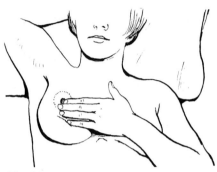

Fig. 39-3　Palpating with a smooth rotary movement using the 'flat' of the fingers the 4 quadrants of the breast to detect 'lumps'.

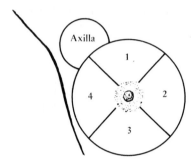

Fig. 39-4　The breast is divided into 4 imaginary quadrants and axilla, which is palpated following each menstrual period.

The nulliparous breast is more susceptible to cancer.

In Britain 18 000 new cases are diagnosed every year and 13 000 women died in 1974: 85 per cent of cases of breast carcinoma are suspected by the woman. The midwife should encourage her patients to examine their breasts systematically at monthly intervals. A thorough examination of the breasts by a specialist is at present the most effective means of detecting cancerous lesions. Discrete lumps are subjected to biopsy. In suspected cases mammography or the newer Xeroradiology which has fewer false positives, and thermography are carried out to assess the size of the lesion and to detect any tumour in the other breast. Thermography is infra-red scanning of the surface temperature and records the infra-red radiation emitted from the breast. Areas of thermal activity indicate further investigation. The frozen section technique is employed under general anaesthesia and, if positive, simple mastectomy is proceeded with. Radiotherapy is sometimes given.

---

## QUESTIONS FOR REVISION

Explain how a Papanicolaou cervical smear is taken. What advice would you give a woman who complained of: (*a*) bleeding at the time of the menopause; (*b*) a lump in the breast.

### Give the definitive word for:

Study of cell formation.　　　　A radical hysterectomy.
Infra-red scanning of breast surface temperature. Radiographic examination of the breast.

## *C.M.B. Short Questions*

Discuss the present arrangements for detecting early cancer of the cervix.
**Scot.:** Cervical cytology. **Eng.:** The cervical smear. **Eng.:** Facilities available for cervical cytology.

# 40
# Vital Statistics

*Registration and notification of births and stillbirths. Mortality rates; stillbirth, perinatal, neonatal, infant, maternal; causes and prevention. The bereaved parents. Immunisation of infants*

**Under the Registration of Births Act** information regarding a birth or stillbirth including weight of the baby must be given by one of the parents. The majority of parents fulfil this requirement of the law, but should they neglect to do so the duty falls on the occupier of the house or any person present at the birth, including the midwife.

In the case of an illegitimate child the information must be given by the mother. The child is registered under the mother's surname and can only be given the father's name if he attends personally with her or if the mother can produce proof of paternity. The father of an illegitimate child cannot register the birth in the absence of the mother.

### ENGLAND AND WALES

**The birth is registered within 42 days of birth** by the Registrar of the district in which the child is born (Local Government Regional Authority). A short certificate giving name, sex, date and place of birth is issued free at the time of registration: £2·00 later; a full copy at the time of registration costs £1·50, later the fee is £3·50.

### SCOTLAND

**The birth is registered within 21 days of birth** by the Registrar of the district in which the child is born (Local Government Regional Authority), or, if preferred, the district of the parent's home address, provided this is in Scotland. An abbreviated certificate is issued free; if obtained later £2·00. If the parents ask for a full certificate at the time of registration it will cost £1·50, if obtained later £3·50. Most parents ask for a full and an abbreviated certificate.

**For adoption** a full certificate is required; adoptive parents get a new certificate.

### THREE CLASSES CONCERNED WITH REGISTRATION

1. An infant born at any stage of pregnancy who breathes or shows other signs of life after complete expulsion from its mother is born alive. If such an infant dies after birth, both the birth and the death must be registered.

2. An infant who has issued forth from its mother after the 28th week of pregnancy and has not at any time after being completely expelled from its mother breathed or shown any other signs of life is a stillborn infant and must be registered.

3. The birth before the 28th week of pregnancy of an infant who did not breathe or show signs of life after complete expulsion from its mother is neither a live birth nor a stillbirth and need not be registered.

### NOTIFICATION OF BIRTHS AND STILLBIRTHS

The Notification of Births Acts (England) 1907 and (Scotland) 1915 amended by the Public Health Act 1936 and the National Health Service Act 1948 make it obligatory for the father of the child or any person in attendance on the mother at the time of birth to give notice in writing to the Chief Administrative Medical Officer of the Area Health Authority (Eng.) or Health Board (Scot.) of the area in

681

which the birth occurred within 36 hours under a penalty of £1·00. In England, for administrative convenience, notification may be channelled to the District Community Physician.

Area Health Authorities or Health Boards (Scot.) supply to doctors and midwives prepaid addressed envelopes together with the forms of notification of birth. The majority of births are notified by midwives.

The purpose of notification of births is that the Chief Administrative Medical Officer of the Health Board, Scotland, The Area Health Authority, England may arrange for the health visitor to call at the home as soon as the midwife ceases to visit or the woman returns home from hospital.

Doctor or midwife is required to record on the Notification of Birth's card the period of gestation any malformation discovered in the child whether live or stillborn (in order to compile statistical data and to provide the basis of various health records used by the A.H.A. or H.B. to ensure periodic recall for screening).

## STILLBIRTHS

The stillbirth rate is the number of stillbirths registered during the year per 1000 registered total (*live and still*) births in the year. During 1978, England, 8·3; Scotland, 8·0.

A stillbirth is (as defined on p. 681) a birth after the 28th week of pregnancy in which the baby does not breathe or show any other signs of life after being completely expelled from the mother. It is conceivable that in delivering a baby presenting by the breech the cord may be pulsating when the baby is born as far as the umbilicus, but if after delivering the head the baby does not breathe or show any other signs of life it is stillborn.

**Causes and prevention,** p. 685.

*Midwives' Duties Regarding Stillbirths (imposed by Statute)*

### (1) Certificate of stillbirth

When a Registered medical practitioner is present at the stillbirth or examines the stillborn baby, delivered or examined by the midwife, he will give the parent(s) a Certificate of Stillbirth which they will take to the Registrar of Birth Deaths and Marriages.

### (2) Registration of stillbirths (as for live births p. 681)

On receipt of the Certificate of Stillbirth the Registrar of Births, Deaths and Marriages will issue a certificate of Registration of Stillbirth.

### (3) Interment or cremation of a stillborn baby

**England** A still born infant may not be buried or cremated until a burial certificate (Certificate for Disposal of Stillbirth) has been obtained from the Registrar of Births, Deaths and Marriages or from the Coroner. The certificate of disposal must be taken to the undertaker in cases of private funeral or to the hospital if the parents wish the hospital to assume responsibility for disposal of the stillborn baby.

**Scotland** A stillborn baby may not be interred or cremated until the Certificate of Registration of Stillbirth issued by the Registrar of Births, Deaths and Marriages is transmitted directly, or by the undertaker, to the person having charge of the place of interment or cremation.

#### ARRANGEMENTS FOR DISPOSAL BY HOSPITAL

The Area Health Authority (Eng.) Health Board (Scot.) will arrange for and meet the cost of the disposal of stillborn babies. If arrangements are made privately the parents must meet the cost. No death grant is paid for a stillborn baby.

**(4) Notification of stillbirth** (as for live births, p. 681)

The Local Supervising Authority i.e. Regional Health Authority (sometimes delegated to the Area Health Authority (Eng.) or Health Board (Scot.)) must be notified in all cases of stillbirth whether or not a medical practitioner was present, using for the purpose the prescribed form.

## MATERNAL MORTALITY

The maternal mortality rate is the number of deaths registered during the year of women dying from causes attributed to pregnancy and childbirth per 1000 registered total (*live and still*) births in the year. During 1978 the maternal mortality rate was: England—0·13 per 1000, including abortions; Scotland—0·1 per 1000, including abortions.

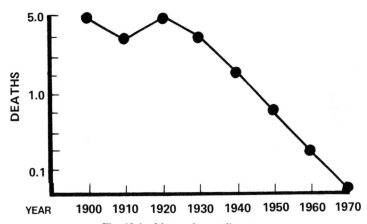

Fig. 40-1   Maternal mortality rate.

### The Prevention of Maternal Mortality

A maternal death is a tragedy. The childbearing woman is probably the most important person in the community, for the baby, husband and family all depend for their health and happiness on the mother's care. A maternal death also does harm indirectly by creating fear of childbirth in the minds of relatives and neighbours. Midwives must therefore do all in their power to prevent maternal deaths.

#### THE DECLINE IN MATERNAL MORTALITY

Childbirth is safer now than at any period in history. During this century until 1935 the maternal death rate had remained between 4 and 5 per 1000. Mortality is lowest in the second pregnancy, and rises steeply after the third.

### The following factors have contributed to the decline in maternal mortality:

1. Early recognition and improved treatment of pre-eclampsia. With preventive care and efficient management, eclampsia can now usually be averted.

2. The prophylactic use of Syntometrine. Improved methods of treating postabortum, antepartum and postpartum haemorrhages. The blood bank and 'flying squad' have done much to prevent loss of maternal life.

3. The introduction of antibiotics, has progressively lowered the number of deaths from sepsis.

4. Improved anaesthetic techniques and the skill of obstetric anaesthetists.

5. Closer co-operation with specialists in diabetes, renal and cardiac disease, haematology and chest conditions.

6. Advances in knowledge of blood coagulation disorders.

7. Improved standards in the Maternity Services including more intensive prenatal care and the greater willingness of women to take advantage of such care.

8. Earlier hospitalisation for complications of pregnancy and labour; better selection of cases for hospital confinement and more prenatal beds available.

9. Better social conditions, including nutrition, have improved health and physique; family planning has reduced the number of children a woman bears; fewer children now are born to overworked, malnourished multiparae.

10. Highlighting and screening women at risk and providing intensive care when needed.

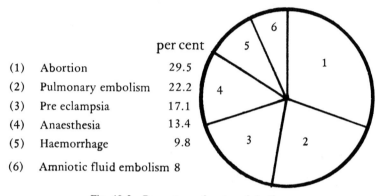

| | | per cent |
|---|---|---|
| (1) | Abortion | 29.5 |
| (2) | Pulmonary embolism | 22.2 |
| (3) | Pre eclampsia | 17.1 |
| (4) | Anaesthesia | 13.4 |
| (5) | Haemorrhage | 9.8 |
| (6) | Amniotic fluid embolism | 8 |

Fig. 40-2    Percentage of maternal deaths.

### *How the Midwife can help to Prevent Maternal Deaths*

1. By co-operating with all branches of the Health Service to ensure that the mother is receiving the necessary advice, health education, close supervision and care.

2. By maintaining high standards of prenatal, intranatal and postnatal care, paying special attention to the prevention of haemorrhage, sepsis and eclampsia.

## INFANT MORTALITY RATE

The infant mortality rate is the number of deaths registered during the year of infants dying under one year of age per 1000 registered live births in the year..

During 1978 the infant mortality rate was England, 13·0; Scotland, 13·0. These figures show a marked reduction from the rate of 140 to 150 which obtained at the beginning of this century.

### *Such an improvement may be attributed to two main factors:*

#### 1. PREVENTIVE MEDICINE

(*a*) Improvements in housing and environmental conditions, with a higher standard of living; immunisation of infants against infectious diseases; more rigid observance of methods to prevent cross-infection among babies in maternity and children's hospitals.

(*b*) Education of the public and their increased interest in nutrition, preparation for parenthood and the care of babies.

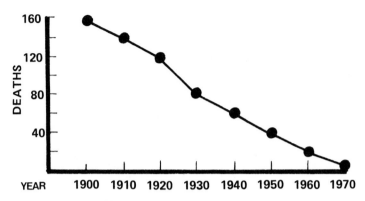

Fig. 40-3   Infant mortality rate.

### 2. MEDICAL ADVANCES

The appointment of paediatricians to supervise the health of all newborn babies; research into neonatal physiology. More effective methods of resuscitation; biochemical studies of the newborn. Increased knowledge in treating preterm and sick babies, especially the use of neonatal intensive care units, intravenous therapy, chemotherapeutic agents, anitbiotics and mechanical monitoring devices.

### NEONATAL MORTALITY RATE

The neonatal mortality rate is the number of deaths registered during the year of infants dying under the age of 1 month (28 days) per 1000 registered live births in the year. During 1978, England 9·7; Scotland, 9·00.

The neonatal mortality rate has great obstetrical significance, for the majority of these babies die during the first 48 hours of life.

A death grant of £9·00 under the National Insurance Scheme is paid on the death of a child under 3 years, if contribution conditions are fully satisfied.

### *The Prevention of Stillbirths and Neonatal Deaths*

Stillbirths and early neonatal deaths are very closely related, the same obstetrical causes giving rise to both. The midwife must therefore share the responsibility for a proportion of these deaths. Preventive medicine has played some part, in that the improved nutrition and health of childbearing women have resulted in more vigorous babies who can withstand the trauma of birth and survive the critical first few days of life. The midwife should ensure that the mothers under her care are having a nourishing diet and are taking the welfare foods made available by the State.

### PERINATAL MORTALITY RATE

This term is applied to stillbirths and to neonatal deaths during the first week of life per 1000 live and stillbirths in the year. During 1978, England, 15·5; Scotland, 15·0.

Medical and social factors have reduced perinatal deaths; babies born in hospital receive expert supervision during labour and subsequently. Midwives can help to reduce the perinatal mortality rate by promoting early prenatal care and the education of expectant mothers.

## Causes

### 1. LOW BIRTH WEIGHT

*Prevention is the best treatment and includes:*

(*a*) **Good prenatal care.** (i) Education of the mother regarding health, diet, rest; (ii) expert supervision; detection and management of conditions such as pre-eclampsia, antepartum haemorrhage, multiple pregnancy.

(*b*) **Good intranatal care.** Preterm and light for date babies do not stand up well to labour. Constant vigilance of the fetal condition during labour is essential. Episiotomy is performed when the baby is expected to weigh under 2·5 kg.

(*c*) **Intensive neonatal care.** This embraces efficient transport of the infant to hospital and expert nursing by midwives under the supervision of a paediatrician.

### 2. HYPOXIA

This is a high cause of stillbirth: anoxia being the terminal stage. Fetal heart monitoring, blood sampling and correction of acidosis save fetal lives. Respiratory distress syndrome may be avoided by testing the lecithin sphingomyelin ratio in the amniotic fluid to ensure pulmonary maturity prior to inducing labour.

### 3. ASPHYXIA

Asphyxia was a potent cause of perinatal deaths: intubation and improved resuscitative measures have reduced the number.

### 4. INTRACRANIAL INJURY

This serious condition can sometimes be averted by seeking medical assistance for delay during the second stage before fetal distress is manifest.

### 5. CONGENITAL MALFORMATIONS

Spina bifida can be detected at 14–16 weeks by finding raised alpha feto proteins in amniotic fluid. Pregnancy can be terminated. Anencephaly can be diagnosed by ultrasonic scanning at 16–20 weeks.

Cardiac, eye and ear defects due to the effect of rubella in the embryo can be prevented by immunisation of schoolgirls.

## Predisposing Causes of Perinatal Mortality

**Pre-eclampsia.** Early recognition and treatment will help to reduce the number of babies who are either stillborn or too puny to survive. By treating pre-eclampsia the serious condition of eclampsia with a high perinatal mortality rate can usually be prevented.

**Multiple pregnancy.** The death rate in the case of twins is almost three times as great as in single births. Some obstetricians encourage women pregnant with twins to take advantage of the opportunity to enter hospital for rest during the 30th to 36th week. Weekly prenatal visits are advisable to detect pre-eclampsia the incidence of which is higher in multiple pregnancy.

**Antepartum haemorrhage.** Early and more prolonged hospitalisation, expectant treatment, blood transfusion and Caesarean section will save many babies.

**Breech presentation.** The midwife should not undertake to deliver the woman at home, nevertheless, she must be qualified to deal competently with cases not

previously diagnosed. Caesarean section is employed more frequently in primigravid women.

**In the lower socio-economic groups.** The death rates are much higher. The
mothers tend to be younger and less well educated: poor home conditions including
infant hygiene cause gastro-intestinal and respiratory infections. Midwives should
intensify the teaching of these mothers.

## THE BEREAVED PARENTS

*(The role of the midwife)*

**Midwives have in the past comforted bereaved parents** in an intuitive fashion,
depending mainly on their sympathy, experience and maturity: more is expected of
them today. The midwife should have some understanding of the grieving process
and the emotional needs of bereaved parents as well as an awareness of how to give
them consolation, support and counsel.

If the pregnant woman is not aware that her fetus is dead, some authorities
consider that she should be told: if so, her husband ought to be present. Whether to
tell her before labour is a debatable point and the husband's advice should be
obtained. The pain and stress of labour will be more unbearable when added to the
anguish of being deprived of her child. Analgesics and narcotics should be
administered during labour in sufficient dosage to lessen physical and mental
suffering.

**The birth of a stillborn baby** or one who dies within a few days of birth may be the
first occasion on which either parent has been intimately associated with death.
Their response will depend on cultural traditions, intelligence, personality and
marital status. The immediate reaction may be numbness in the ability to think but
their stunned silence must not be interpreted as indifference: crying may not occur
until later.

**A kindly approach is of supreme importance;** the midwife's compassion will shine
through her words and actions and manifest her sympathetic understanding. Time
devoted to comforting and consoling the grieving mother will be recalled by her
with gratitude.

**The provision of some degree of privacy** is the first essential and a cup of tea in a
room providing a relaxed atmosphere will have a calming effect. It is advisable to
encourage the woman to talk about her baby and to ask questions; the midwife
giving comforting answers and explanations. It may console the mother to be told
that the cause of death (e.g. anoxia) could have had a detrimental effect on the
child's development had he lived. Unless the mother proposes the subject it might
be advisable not to suggest naming the baby or starting another pregnancy. If the
parents express guilt feelings they should be given assurance.

**The doctor will also discuss with them the cause of death** and other matters. Some
paediatricians advise that the parents should see and handle the baby, but their
wishes should be ascertained and complied with. Whether the mother should see a
seriously malformed infant is controversial and should be left to the discretion of
the father.

**Counsel regarding registration of stillbirth** or birth and death is given as
appropriate. Arrangements concerning funeral and burial may be discussed with
the hospital chaplain. The Area Health Authority (Eng.); Health Board (Scot.),
will arrange for and meet the cost of the burial of a baby stillborn in hospital if the
parents desire this; should they prefer to make private arrangements they are
required to meet the cost themselves.

**Early transfer home is a wise policy** to avoid (*a*) the anguish of seeing other
mothers handling their babies; (*b*) being within sound of the nurseries; (*c*) to enable

the mother to find solace in her familiar home surroundings with the sustenance of relatives and friends who should be advised to encourage her to talk about the baby.

**Crying has therapeutic value** and should not be suppressed. One of the joys of womanhood has been snatched from her grasp: all her plans, preparations and the travail of labour have been in vain, she is submerged in despondency and needs compassionate understanding.

**Sedatives are not prescribed so freely** for the grieving mother as was done formerly. It is now considered that sedatives postpone the phase of depression and that it is better for the woman to cope with the grieving process by crying and expressing her feelings about the loss of her baby.

**Time spent by the midwife in comforting the bereaved parents** will give them consolation on a day that should have been one of gratitude and gladness.

## Immunisation of Infants

Midwives should be aware of the protective measures available whereby babies can be inoculated against diseases such as whooping cough, diphtheria, poliomyelitis and measles. They can inform mothers regarding the need for this as well as assuring and persuading those who are apprehensive or reluctant regarding inoculation which is provided free by the family doctor and at child health clinics.

### SMALLPOX

The routine vaccination of babies is no longer recommended by the Department of Health and Social Security— (July 1971) except when an epidemic occurs. Smallpox vaccination is a prerequisite for travellers to countries where the disease remains prevalent. Failure to thrive and eczema are contraindications.

### POLIOMYELITIS

This disease rarely occurs during the first six months of life. The Sabin type vaccine is the method of choice; three oral doses are given, and a booster dose at school entrance.

### WHOOPING COUGH (Pertussis)

The risks associated with whooping cough, and the mortality rate, are greatest during the first year of life. Three injections for a primary course are required, given at intervals of 6 to 8 weeks between first and second doses and 4 to 6 months between second and third (see Schedule).

### DIPHTHERIA

About 50 per cent of mothers have no immunity to diphtheria so their babies are susceptible from birth.

Triple antigens are given to avoid giving multiple injections; combined pertussis, diphtheria and tetanus antigens are given. (Quadruple vaccines for diphtheria, pertussis, poliomyelitis and tetanus are sometimes used.)

### MEASLES

A live modified measles virus vaccine is now available for protection against this disease. One injection only is given, not before 9 months of age and preferably soon after the first birthday. Immunity seems to be fairly prolonged.

## SCHEDULE OF VACCINATION AND IMMUNISATION PROCEDURES

*Department of Health and Social Security*

| Age | Vaccine | Interval | Notes |
|---|---|---|---|
| During the first 10 months of life<br><br>First dose at 3 months | Diph./Tet./Pert. and oral polio vaccine. (First dose)<br>Diph./Tet./Pert. and oral polio vaccine. (Second dose)<br>Diph./Tet./Pert. and oral polio vaccine. (Third dose) | Preferably after an interval of 6–8 weeks.<br>Preferably after an interval of 4–6 months. | The earliest age at which the first dose should be given is 3 months. |
| During the second year of life | Measles vaccine | After an interval of not less than 3 weeks | |

### Additional Notes

1. The basic course of immunisation against diphtheria, pertussis, tetanus and poliomyelitis should be completed at as early an age as possible consistent with the likelihood of a good immunological response. Live measles vaccine should not be given to children below the age of nine months, since it usually fails to immunise such children owing to the presence of maternally transmitted antibodies.

2. Examples of timing of basic course of immunisation:

|  | 1st dose | 2nd dose | 3rd dose |
|---|---|---|---|
| Age | 3 months | 5 months | 9–12 months |
| | 4 months | 6 months | 10–12 months |
| | 5 months | 7 months | about 12 months |
| | 6 months | 8 months | about 12–14 months |
| | | Interval<br>6–8 weeks | Interval<br>4–6 months |

3. The desirable commencing age for immunisation is six months of age because: (a) before this age the antibody response may be reduced by the presence of maternal antibody; (b) the child's antibody-forming mechanism is immature in the early months of life; and (c) severe reactions to pertussis vaccine are less common in children over six months old than at three months of age.

## QUESTIONS FOR REVISION
### VITAL STATISTICS. IMMUNISATION

**What advice would you give** to the parents regarding registration of births? Define the following mortality rates: infant, neonatal, perinatal, stillbirth, maternal. State the obstetrical causes of stillbirths and neonatal deaths. Name the factors which have helped to reduce these death rates.

**C.M.B.(Scot.).** Define maternal mortality rate. What are the main causes of maternal mortality? What steps should be taken to reduce the rate still further?

**(N. Ireland) 30-min. question.** How can good antenatal care prevent stillbirths? Describe in what way the midwife can help to reduce stillbirths during labour.

**C.M.B.(Eng.) 30-min. question.** What is meant by the term 'neonatal death'? What are the chief causes? Indicate what preventative measures may be taken to avoid neonatal deaths.

**C.M.B.(Eng.) 30-min. question.** Explain how antenatal care helps to reduce the perinatal mortality rate.

**C.M.B.(Eng.) 30-min. question.** What factors have contributed to the reduction in maternal and infant mortality?

**C.M.B.(Scot.) 30-min. question.** Define perinatal mortality. What steps can be taken to reduce the current incidence?

**C.M.B.(Scot.) 30-min. question.** Give an account of the factors contributing to the reduction in maternal mortality.

**C.M.B.(Eng.) 30-min. question.** Outline a talk to expectant mothers on the immunisation facilities for their babies and give a suggested programme.

**C.M.B.(Eng.) 30-min. question.** Outline the immunisation procedures in infancy which are at present in common use.

**C.M.B.(Scot.) 30-min. question.** What information and supportive measures can be given to the parents following a stillbirth or a neonatal death?

**C.M.B.(Scot.).** What advice would you give a mother about registration of births.

**What are the three classes** under which live and stillborn babies are registered? In which district is a baby registered, and by whom? **To whom are births notified?** Why? What is the duty of the midwife *re* notification of births?

**An unwed mother asks you:** (*a*) regarding registration of the birth of her baby to the man she is co-habiting with; (*b*) if the fact that the baby is illegitimate will be recorded on the birth certificate; (*c*) if the father can register the birth?

A birth is registered in England within ........................ days: in Scotland within ........................ days: a birth must be notified within ............................

Differentiate between: (*a*) notification and registration of births; (*b*) neonatal and infant deaths; (*c*) stillbirth and perinatal death.

Discuss the midwife's role in the prevention of: stillbirths; maternal deaths; perinatal deaths. Preventive medicine has reduced the perinatal mortality rate. Write 10 lines elaborating this statement.

**C.M.B.(Eng.) 30-min. question.** Describe the midwife's role following a stillbirth; the legal requirements, record keeping, advice and support for the parents.

**N.Ire.** Management of a mother whose child is stillborn.


## England C.M.B. Short Questions

What is meant by the term vital statistics? Maternal mortality? Perinatal mortality? Discuss the value of vital statistics in obstetrics. Define the maternal mortality rate. Give the main causes of perinatal death. What is meant by notification of birth? What is meant by registration of births? The duties of a midwife when a stillbirth occurs in her practice. Notification procedure following a stillbirth in the home. Why do we have vital statistics? What factors have contributed to the decline in perinatal mortality? Describe the notification, registration and disposal of a stillborn child.

Whooping cough vaccination. Sudden infant death (cot death). Neonatal mortality. Recording of vital statistics. Notifications following a stillbirth. **Eng.** The notification, registration and disposal of a stillborn child.


## Scotland C.M.B. Short Questions

Neonatal mortality: give the definition of a stillbirth: causes of maternal mortality. What do you understand by notification of births? What certificates of registration of births are available? To what period of time is the term 'perinatal' applied? What is the latest figure for maternal mortality? Within what time must a birth be notified? What is the most common cause of perinatal death? Stillbirth rate. Define infant mortality. Within what time must a birth be registered?

**Scot.** Differentiate between Registration and Notification of Births.

Infant mortality rate and perinatal mortality rate.

Infant immunisation. **Scot.:** Name one disease prevented by triple vaccine.

# 41
# The Social Aspect of Obstetrics

*Socio-economic factors. Social trends, pressures, problems, behaviour. Socio-obstetric aspects. Immigrant groups. The midwives role. Provisions by the State. Unmarried mother and her child. Adoption. Children in care; foster child, deprived child, delinquent child. The battered baby. Sex education. Counselling by midwives. Ethical problems.*

---

**Social factors have a profound influence** on the processes of child bearing and rearing. The pregnant woman's health and skeletal structure may have been adversely affected, her reproductive ability impaired by substandard social conditions during her fetal life, infancy, childhood and adolescence.

The fetus *in utero* is a potential parent and good social conditions can have a beneficial effect on fetal growth and well-being. Midwives should stress fetal welfare when advising mothers-to-be.

**Socio-economic factors** determine the conditions under which the pregnant woman spent her formative years: poverty, poor housing, overcrowding, and malnutrition do not favour a healthful standard of living. Preterm labour is more common; the infant death rate higher in the lower socio-economic group.

**Social effects on perinatal mortality** are causing concern. The perinatal death rate is high in social groups where the parents are financially unable or intellectually incapable of providing a healthy way of life: the mortality rate being twice as high in the unskilled workers than in the professional class.

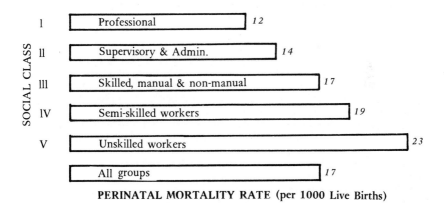

PERINATAL MORTALITY RATE (per 1000 Live Births)

Fig. 41-1

**Social disadvantages are difficult to overcome.** Living in impoverished conditions with dirty, drab surroundings saps the physical and mental vitality. It takes willpower, energy, pride, ambition and some degree of intelligence to budget effectively, manage a family and home successfully and to rise above squalid circumstances. Parents in such a situation need sympathetic understanding and much helpful advice.

**Social awareness is now more obvious throughout Britain.** The recent improved standard of living has enhanced the way of life, including education and nutrition, of childbearing women who have become increasingly interested in achieving maternal, fetal and child wellbeing. The media and women's magazines are helping to meet the need for education on physical and mental health and on the reproductive process. The midwife should motivate expectant mothers to take advantage of the health education talks, demonstrations and discussions.

## Social trends

These have, in various ways, influenced maternity care, e.g. at the beginning of this century 90 per cent of babies were born at home; now, over 98 per cent are born in hospital. The acceptance of prenatal care, and family planning, are social rather than medical decisions. Large families, with worn out overworked mothers, are now outmoded. Women at work outside the home have changed the domestic and nutritional way of life. The pregnant woman in employment may be deprived of sufficient rest which can have a detrimental effect on fetal and maternal welfare. The wise counsel of midwives is needed. Transfer home 24–48 hours after delivery originated as an expedient for the shortage of maternity beds; the mothers approved and now it has become a social preference.

### SOCIAL PRESSURES

These can have a powerful influence in directing social trends. Such pressures have been responsible for the decline in breast feeding.

**Smoking is a social habit** which, during pregnancy, has an adverse effect on fetal growth. Alcohol can damage fetal brain cells.

**The use of contraceptives** has promoted a more permissive attitude to sex: premarital sexual relations being condoned by many. Social acceptance of the unwed mother, and of cohabitation prior to marriage, denotes the changed social attitude to sexuality.

That abortion is needed for so many schoolgirls is a disturbing outcome of social pressures regarding sex in that immature group.

### SOCIAL BEHAVIOUR

Social behaviour is one of the skills that babies have to be taught; they must learn to conform to socially acceptable standards of behaviour, as in feeding, sleeping and elimination. The natural urge to demand immediate gratification of his needs and desires has to be brought under control; this being accomplished by discipline applied as kindly consistent guidance. Much patience is required.

To achieve a harmonious marital relationship both parents must exercise self-discipline: well controlled social behaviour being a good example to their offspring. Any unsocial, irresponsible behaviour as may be evident in some teenagers should be frowned on: truancy, vandalism and violence are the sequelae to lack of self-discipline.

**Midwives can advise mothers** regarding how to motivate their children to acquire acceptable standards of social behaviour.

## Social Problems

These may arise when the young husband and wife are irresponsible, undomesticated and financially insecure; pregnancy puts an additional strain on the marital situation. The mother-to-be should be made aware of the social benefits to which she is entitled and given advice re suitable infant clothes and equipment, as well as in organising baby's daily routine.

**Alcoholism,** marital infidelity, desertion and husbands in prison are serious social problems that hospital midwives meet and will refer to the social worker.

**Immigrant groups** present a social problem that midwives have to deal with: diseases with social connotations, such as rickets and tuberculosis, are not uncommon in immigrant families: unusual forms of anaemia need expert care. Language difficulties can be helped by the use of videotapes. Cultural traditions re health, food and childrearing that may be deleterious, are not easily remedied so much patience and perseverence are necessary.

### SOCIO-OBSTETRIC ASPECTS

These are concerned with improving the quality of fetal life, preventing complications and lowering the perinatal death rate. This can only be accomplished when pregnant women can be persuaded to collaborate by carrying out the measures advocated in a programme of health education which includes good nutrition, adequate rest, and the avoidance of teratogenic agents.

**Early booking,** regular attendance at the prenatal clinic, aiming at about 12 visits, should be advocated by midwives and the mothers persuaded and encouraged to co-operate.

**Care of the unsupported child,** family planning, subfertility, prevention of cervical and breast cancer, and sexually transmitted disease are social aspects of obstetric care. The midwife should be aware of the facilities available for such conditions.

## THE ROLE OF THE MIDWIFE

**Social aspects of obstetrics have widened the midwife's function,** and broadened her outlook. She should, therefore apply her socio-obstetric knowledge in the practice of midwifery. Knowledge of the expectant mother's social circumstances will enable the midwife to give personal advice more effectively. Family centred maternity care must be orientated to meet the woman's social and educational needs.

**As an educator, the midwife plays an integral part** in motivating the expectant mother to observe the rules of health and to utilise the various resources provided by the state.

**Social influence on the adolescent** can be compelling although insidious. The midwife can suggest ways in which parents can take an interest in and try to influence their children's choice of leisure pursuits.

This is needed especially to counteract retrograde social pressures in an era when moral values are being demoted and respect for authority disparaged or ridiculed.

**Education of childbearing parents is one of the cardinal functions of the modern midwife** and a socio-obstetric duty she has an obligation to fulfil.

# SOCIAL AND HEALTH BENEFITS PROVIDED BY THE STATE

**Clinics.** Prenatal; postnatal; child health; special clinics, e.g. dental, chest, cardiac, diabetic, haematological, urological, sexually transmitted diseases, family planning, infertility.

**For hospital confinement.** General, specialist and intensive care for mother and child; obstetricians; physicians; paediatricians; anaesthetists; radiologists; bacteriologists; midwives; family planning facilities. Ambulances are provided when necessary.

**For home confinement.** Doctor; consultation by obstetrician; paediatrician; care by midwife; mobile obstetric and paediatric resuscitation units. Maternity packs with sterile supplies (issued free).

**Home help services.** Each local government district council is required to make provision for a home help service. Social workers usually make the necessary arrangements and a charge can be made for the service which is available for illness, the ailing elderly, maternity cases and the welfare of young children. The home help attends for a number of hours during week days or as directed.

**Milk and vitamins.** These are available for expectant mothers and all children under school age in families who are receiving supplementary benefits, family income supplement or are in special need because of low income. Liquid milk 600 ml daily or modified dried milk 2 packs per week. Vitamins A, D, C children's vitamin drops 2 bottles every 13 weeks, expectant mothers vitamin tablets, 2 containers every 13 weeks. If not entitled to free milk and vitamins, dried milk and vitamins can be bought without tokens at low prices at places where these products are distributed, usually at health centres. The midwife may issue a certificate of expected confinement to enable the eligible woman to obtain milk and vitamins.

## FINANCIAL

As maternity benefits are increased from time to time the midwife should consult the most recent issue of Leaflet N.I. 17A. The midwife may issue a certificate of expected confinement not earlier than the 14th week prior to the EDD in order that the woman may claim the maternity allowance and grant (at the local office of the Department of Health and Social Security).

**Maternity Allowance** is paid weekly for 18 weeks, beginning 11 weeks before the expected week of confinement, and is claimed by the employed woman who has paid the required number of contributions. She must cease paid work during this period.

**Maternity Grant** is paid to all mothers giving birth to a live or stillborn child after 28 weeks' gestation. It is claimed on their own or their husband's insurance, but not both; application for the grant being made between 9 weeks before the baby is expected and 3 months after the baby is born. In case of multiple births an extra grant may be paid for each additional baby who is alive 12 hours after birth. Pregnant women should obtain leaflet N.I. 17A and the claim form from the local Department of Health and Social Security office not later than 14 weeks before the expected date of confinement. In 1982 the maternity grant will be non-contributory. There will be a residence test of six months.

The pregnant girl under 16 years does not receive maternity grant or allowance. Her parents can claim supplementary benefit for her as a dependent child.

**Child benefit** is paid weekly for every child during the period until the child reaches the 16th birthday. Supplementary Allowances are granted in necessitous cases, on application to the local Department of Health and Social Security office.

### Employment of pregnant women

The opinion of the midwife may be asked as to whether a pregnant married woman should continue to work beyond mid-term. The need for extra money is sometimes urgent, but it is an unwise measure in the long run for only the strongest type of woman can keep house successfully and carry on a full-time job as well. An industrial nurse may have to approach the factory personnel officer on behalf of a pregnant woman, regarding the suitability of a job which involves heavy work. Occupations necessitating exposure to certain chemical or radio-active substances may be safe for the non-pregnant woman but hazardous during pregnancy. A doctor should be consulted. Although the Factory Act does not forbid a woman to work during the latter weeks of pregnancy, she should be dissuaded from doing so. The maternity allowance paid to employed persons after the 28th week is intended to enable them to cease work then.

A number of professional women tend to devote about 10 years to child bearing and rearing and then return to their careers on a part or whole time basis.

## MATERNITY LEAVE AND PAY

Under the Employment Protection Act 1975 a woman, married or unmarried, who has worked for her employer for 6 months cannot be dismissed because she is pregnant. Suitable alternative work may be offered. If she has worked for her employer for 2 years up to the eleventh week before her baby is due she has the right to receive from him maternity pay amounting to nine tenths of her normal weekly pay, for the first six weeks she is away from work. The amount of the standard social security maternity allowance is deducted from maternity pay. She is entitled to maternity pay whether or not she intends to return to work after the baby is born.

If she has worked for her employer for 2 years she has a right to return to her job or another of the same kind, any time up to 29 weeks after the birth of the baby. Full details are available in Leaflet 4, 'New Rights for the Expectant Mother,' from the Department of Employment.


# THE UNMARRIED MOTHER AND HER CHILD

The term 'unsupported mother' is sometimes used to include pregnant women who are single, divorced, separated or widows.

Some 9 per cent of births in Great Britain are illegitimate, and this amounts to about 55,000 annually with a marked increase in young teenage unwed mothers. The unmarried mother is emotionally distressed and in dire need of guidance and help; but there are so many aspects of her problem, social and psychological as well as obstetrical, that expert handling is essential for their solution. The midwife should put the girl in touch with the social worker employed by the Local Government Regional Council or maternity hospital. The workers will make the necessary contacts with the most suitable organisation to help the unwed mother, and will follow up the case until the social problem has been solved, e.g. the National Council for One Parent Families. Religious and other voluntary bodies provide homes for the unmarried mother and her child and are given financial support by Local Government. Almost 10 per cent of families in Britain are 'one parent'.

**Affiliation Order**

This is a court order to establish the paternity of an illegitimate child on a putative father, for the purpose of paying for maintenance of the child until he is 16 years of age. The court decides how much the father will pay but if the child is adopted the father does not pay for maintenance of the child. The father of an illegitimate child cannot be made to provide financial aid unless an affiliation order is enforced against him. Even when the father admits paternity and is willing to make payment towards the upkeep of the child such arrangements should always be made through the court. Legal aid may be provided.

**Baby of the unwed mother.** Fortunately many are now accepted into the grandparents' home: some of the younger girls have their babies adopted. A number of older or more intelligent mothers wish to care for their babies themselves and it is humane to encourage them to do this: an undertaking that involves hard work, restricted leisure and social life. Hostels and blocks of flats with nurseries are provided in some areas, a more convenient arrangement than having to take the infant to a day nursery or child minder: the mothers sharing baby sitting.

# ADOPTION

Adoption should always be arranged through a registered adoption society or the Local Government Social Service Department to whom the midwife will refer her patient. The midwife would be well advised to refrain from using her influence either for or against adoption and to leave the solution of the problem in the hands of those who have greater knowledge and experience of all its aspects.

No action will be taken until the child is born. The infant must be at least six weeks old before the mother can give her consent to adoption, although the infant may be placed with prospective adopters before this age. Sometimes the mother remains with her baby in a mother and baby home until she decides about adoption. In other instances, if the mother is unable to look after her infant but has not made up her mind about adoption, the infant may be taken into care by the Local Government Social Service Department.

**The adopters must notify the Local Government Social Service Department** when they intend to apply for an Adoption Order. This is granted by the High Court, County Court or Magistrates Court (Eng.). By the Court of Session or Sheriff Court (Scot.). The adopters must also have had the child in their care for thirteen consecutive weeks immediately preceding the date of the adoption order being granted: this being over and above the period of six weeks before the mother consents to adoption. The granting of an Adoption Order by the court is legal and binding; the parent or parents of the child give their written consent and relinquish all further claim on the child.

The character, health, race and financial status of the adopters are investigated; the home must also be satisfactory. The baby's mental and physical health, as well as the parental background are investigated.

Classes in preparation for parenthood for adoptive parents are held at some maternity hospitals.

**A protected child.** When notice of intention to apply for adoption is made the court appoints a person to act as guardian *ad litem* (in law) Eng., curator *ad litem* (Scot.) with the duty of safeguarding the interest of the infant before the court. An officer of the Local Government Social Service Department may be appointed: the infant becomes a protected child.

## *Adopted persons*

**Adopted persons who have reached the age of 18 years** (17 years in Scotland) may, under the Children Act 1976, apply for their birth certificate from the Registrar General who also provides a counselling service. The mother should be told that her relinquished child, being entitled at 18 years to trace his parents, may seek to do so.

**The adoptive parents get a new birth certificate** for the child.

## MARITAL DIFFICULTIES

A pregnant married woman may have an urgent social problem and the midwife should refer her to a social worker. When financial help is required, they will recommend the appropriate association or advise application for a supplementary allowance. If the marriage is in danger of breaking up, the Marriage Guidance Council may be consulted. Legal advice will be arranged for in such instances as neglect, cruelty or desertion.

**Alimony.** Financial allowance for support made by a man to a woman pending or after her legal separation or divorce from him.

**Children in care.** It is the responsibility of the Local Government Regional Council to receive into care any child in the area who is deprived of a normal home life. Every effort is made to avoid having the child removed from his home if he can be looked after by relatives or at a day nursery or by a child minder.

**Day nurseries** are provided by the Local Government Social Service Department to care for children from a few weeks of age until they are 5 years old. Unwed, unsupported mothers, and those with ailing husbands would get priority: the charge made depends on what they can afford to pay. Day nurseries must be registered under the Nurseries and Childminders Act and are subject to supervision by the Local Government Social Service Department.

**Child minder.** If a person looks after children under 5 years of age or takes children into his or her home for gain for more than 2 hours per day, he/she must be registered with the Social Service Department as a child minder. If the children are relatives, no registration is necessary. The Local Government Authority may limit the number of children to be looked after, and require that precautions against infectious disease are taken. They may also determine the qualifications and experience of those who are to look after the children: the equipment, safety and maintenance of the premises or house, the feeding of the children, and the records to be kept. Some local authorities have training programmes for child minders to improve the standard of care.

**A foster child** means a child under school-leaving age who is cared for by someone other than a guardian or relative for a period of more than six days. Any person proposing to care for such a child is required to notify his intention to the Local Government Social Service Department in writing, two weeks in advance, unless the child is received in an emergency in which case the Local Government Authority must be informed within seven days of the child being received. This Authority may 'board out' children 'in care' with foster parents who are paid a small fee that does not allow for profit making. Although relatives are not regarded as foster parents they may also be paid if they cannot afford to support the child. Fostering may be arranged and paid for privately, but in all cases the Social Service Department must be notified so that the appropriate investigations can be made. Visits will be paid by the social worker to ensure that the child is happy and well cared for and to give such advice as may appear to be needed.

**The deprived child.** Any child up to the age of leaving school, who does not have a normal home life with the necessary food, care and shelter, is deprived. Many of the long-term cases are mentally retarded or physically handicapped and sometimes illegitimate. Those who have been abandoned, neglected or treated cruelly are referred by the Juvenile Court (Eng.), Children's Panel (Scot.) to be taken into care by the Local Government Social Service Department. The majority are boarded out with parents to give them a stable home life.

**The delinquent child** may have committed a criminal offence or be beyond control and the court may refer him for compulsory care. They will decide whether the child ought to be placed in a residential home or under the supervision of the Social Service Department or a voluntary agency.

## THE BATTERED BABY

*The Abused Baby—Non-accidental Injury*

In Britain every year over 4500 babies suffer non-accidental injuries 3000 being severely damaged, about 700 being fatal. (The figures are even higher in other sophisticated countries.) One survey showed that 60 per cent of the infants were less than 9 months old and 30 per cent under 6 months. Injuries include deliberate burning by a cigarette, electric fire or hot poker: fracture of long bones, ribs and skull: brain damage due to whiplash and jerking caused by gross shaking and banging the head on the wall. Battering by striking the mouth is so common as to arouse strong suspicion: diagnosis of multiple old fractures on radiological examination is very suggestive. Extensive bruising may be present. The children are mostly under 3 years of age and therefore cannot give an account of what happened. Suspicion is aroused when there is delay in seeking medical assistance and when the explanation given does not coincide with or justify the extent of the damage done.

### Type of parents

Only 10 per cent of the parents are psychopaths, although the sadistic violence inflicted suggests otherwise. Many are young, immature and unstable: a number of parents have low intelligence and over 50 per cent come from poor homes. The situation arises most commonly when the home conditions are squalid or over-crowded. The poor-quality father, improvident, bad tempered and addicted to alcohol is more likely to injure his child.

## THE PREVENTIVE ROLE OF THE MIDWIFE

Midwives and health visitors who are responsible for instructing pregnant women will be deeply disturbed at the immensity of this social problem and must wonder whether they have effectively prepared parents to understand and meet the needs of their infants. A series of talks at prenatal clinics, and discussions in the postnatal wards could be arranged. It would not be prudent to talk to the parents as though they were potential child abusers so the subject could be introduced indirectly via (1) the crying baby and what to do, (2) babies need tender loving care, (3) how normal babies grow and behave.

### THE PERSISTENTLY CRYING BABY A CAUSE OF BATTERING

Much non-accidental injury inflicted during the first six months of life is due to the mother's or father's exasperation from the incessant crying of the infant: anger mounts and the parent is unable to control the aggressive impulse that overwhelms him/her. The mature well-adjusted person can subdue any urge to inflict corporal punishment on a baby but all parents are not mature or well adjusted: they need counsel and it is this preventive aspect of baby battering that concerns midwives.

**Many babies cry because of thirst** rather than hunger. One such condition with serious consequences (hypernatraemia) is due to giving babies too much sodium by heaping or pressing the dried milk in the measuring scoop. (Cows milk contains 4 times as much sodium as human milk.) The baby becomes thirsty and cries, the mother thinking he is hungry gives more dried milk so thirst is intensified and crying continues. Dehydration and brain cell damage may ensue. Crying is the baby's language: his only means of 'asking' or 'complaining' and mothers should be advised to find the reason why and to consider whether they may be at fault in not meeting his needs. They should be told to go to the Child Health Clinic or their general practitioner if deprived of more than one night's sleep. A 24-hour telephone service where mothers could contact a midwife or health visitor for advice re crying or any urgent baby problem would be invaluable.

Undue crying in babies over 6 months of age may be caused by repeated thwarting of the child's natural impulses. He is emerging as an independent human being with a will of his own, deeply resentful of physical or emotional restraint, yet he has to learn to conform to acceptable social behaviour patterns. The baby has a tremendous amount to learn regarding movement, locomotion, speech, spoon feeding, bladder and bowel control. Some mothers do not understand how difficult this is and expect too much of a baby: life can be very frustrating when everything he does evokes a reprimand. He should feel loved even although his behaviour is not approved of: shouting angrily at a child only teaches him to do likewise. Babies respond to a soothing tone of voice and gentle handling: cuddling and caressing are essential as a means of expressing love and babies thrive emotionally when they get adequate affection. Smacking is rarely necessary until the second year and should be no more than a tap on the hand to stop him from touching a hot or otherwise dangerous object: the tone of voice is usually a sufficient deterrent.

During the second year the child objects strongly to being thwarted and is unable to control his feelings of rage (temper tantrums are evidence of this). The child of 2 years can be very difficult: he cannot be reasoned with: he has learned to use the powerful word 'no' and this may be interpreted as defiance when it is only his way of saying 'I don't want to' with his limited vocabulary. A clash of wills should be avoided; changing the subject or diverting his attention to another object usually succeeds if done good naturedly. He must be given scope to experiment with things in order to learn to use his hands. Toleration is needed in handling the turbulent toddler.

### PARENTS AT FAULT THROUGH IGNORANCE

Many teenage parents reared in this age of violence, where the tender emotions seem to be subordinated, are unaware of the gentle loving care that babies need. Some come from broken homes, others have been exposed in childhood to verbal or physical abuse. The disgruntled adolescent mother is a product of the modern attitude to life which inculcates expectation of extensive social pleasures. A more serious state of affairs exists when the mother states active dislike for her child who may be unresponsive, unattractive or unwanted. This problem needs expert psychological advice, the fault usually being parental, for most babies respond happily to affection.

## Tender loving care is needed

Parents usually respond positively to the helpless dependence of their babies: tender protective emotions are aroused and loving care is provided: the most ferocious wild animals treat their young with toleration and affection. The mother is imprinting her children to be gentle with babies when she herself shows gentleness: children should be encouraged to be kind to pets and to give loving care to dolls and toy animals. But even well-balanced mothers find themselves being exasperated almost beyond endurance, by the whining, crying infant so husbands should be made aware of the emotional strain in caring for two, or even one child all day. The mother becomes overwrought when her tolerance and patience are exhausted: usually one parent intervenes to relieve the emotional tension before it gets out of hand. Mothers should be encouraged to have a daily outing (a pram is essential): a weekly evening out is a wise indulgence (a baby sitter being arranged for).

## Therapeutic Measures

Medical, social and psychological workers are all concerned with diagnosing parents who are potential batterers as well as in protecting the abused child. Such parents are in dire need of help, understanding and guidance but their violent actions are criminal offences that cannot be condoned.

**Social measures** such as improving squalid home conditions and increasing child allowances would help. Teaching mothers how to budget economically, create a happy home and to nurture their children with compassion could have social repercussions. Providing day nurseries or play groups where a mother could place her child for a few hours' respite would improve the situation and ease the intolerable strain. The desperate mother who seeks help because she fears she will lose control and harm her child is in dire need: her cry for help must not be ignored.

### Inculcating wholesome parental attitudes

The great need is to create in parents a loving protective, nurturing attitude to their children. The church, school, broadcasting media, grandparents can all contribute: midwives have an unrivalled opportunity to influence the attitude of young mothers. Babies can be a source of great joy and young parents should be made aware of this. It might be possible for the midwife to inaugurate 'Mothering Groups' where young mothers separated by distance from their parents could meet kindly grandmotherly women in a social situation. Their example in handling babies in a loving manner, discussing from experience problems *re* the emotional development of babies could be helpful. By invitation some might visit the homes as baby sitters. This social need is urgent and as in other situations prevention is better than cure.

# SEX EDUCATION

It is desirable that children should be given reliable education about sex, as an integral part of growing up: but such knowledge when given formally ought to be presented in a responsible manner and suited to their age and maturity. The eight-year-old child is not aware of the emotions associated with sexuality: at that age it would be advantageous to avoid the word 'sex' and to teach the subject as human reproduction in the context of biology. Menstruation, fertilisation and growth of the fetus could be shown on films.

Arousing undue curiosity in the generative organs and concentrating attention on sex as it is commonly depicted today, is not advisable at an age when the child would be better occupied in outdoor pursuits and group activities.

**Nearer puberty** sex education could be more specific but should not be delineated as an isolated experience. It should be related fundamentally to increased interest in and response to the opposite sex, choosing a life partner, marriage, home building, child bearing and rearing.

**Parents play a large part in conditioning their children's conception of sexuality** and in fostering emotional and psychosexual maturity. When the bond of affection between parents, as well as between parents and children, is strong the subjects related to sex can be presented in daily life and discussed under ideal conditions. In a stable home atmosphere children are exposed to influences that give them an awareness of responsible attitudes and behaviour to the opposite sex.

**Girls of eleven years in Britain have in recent years become mothers; boys of fourteen years, fathers,** so it would be expedient to discuss with them, prior to that age, the subject in greater detail. In an ideal situation the parents should give sex education but some parents and many teachers, find this too embarrassing. Nor are young teenagers easy to teach: they have been exposed to the permissive ideas of individuals in the media: jokes on sex give rise to hilarity in adults, sex is debased in pornographic literature and denigrated in obscene publications. In a society which is blatantly sex conscious it takes courage and conviction to advocate self discipline and moral restraint. The teacher should be mature, well adjusted, happily married and competent to cope with the 13 year old, who may be blasé, asks the teacher personal questions on sex, makes rude remarks and 'shows off' generally; a testing experience for any teacher.

Although modern methods of contraception have changed the whole sexual scene, sex should be presented as emotional fulfilment within marriage based on love and affection. Children are idealistic and this should be fostered; many will live up to a high standard of behaviour when expected to, and a good example is set. Most girls have sufficient control to repel unwanted sexual advances but they ought not to tempt or encourage boys sexually: teenagers should be made aware of the overwhelming power of the sex drive in some people.

Giving contraceptive advice is not necessarily an essential part of sex education. Prescribing the pill for girls at puberty has dangers not yet fully understood or realised: this may be the easy way out but not the honourable one: it anticipates sexual relations and provides a passport to promiscuity.

**It is illegal** for a man or boy to have sexual intercourse with a girl under the age of 16 under the Sexual Offences Act 1956. This is a logical reason for refraining from prescribing the contraceptive pill to girls at puberty.

**Boys ought to be told that they have no right to expect girls to be permissive:** if pregnancy occurs both are embarrassed and disturbed; they also have to suffer the distress of their parents. The girl bears the brunt of abortion or childbirth, her career and future marriage prospects may be jeopardised.

Adolescents who indulge in sex should receive explicit warning regarding the possibility of pregnancy and the risk of contracting venereal disease.

Most school children respond to the principle of sex within the marriage relationship, one of love and trust. Why should young girls be reared under circumstances in which they are expected to be sexually permissive? The result for individuals, family and society cannot be meritorious. Parents, teachers and preachers should urgently endeavour to create a society that is morally safe for young people to grow up in. Midwives ought to give serious consideration to this problem.

## COUNSELLING BY MIDWIVES

Part of the caring role of the midwife is concerned with counselling expectant mothers. During childbearing stressful marital situations may arise for which the woman needs information and advice.

True counselling is concerned more with alleviating emotional distress and assisting the woman who is unable to make decisions that will solve her problem. The midwife must learn the art of counselling, which is a delicate and sensitive process.

### Examples of likely problems

**Marital incompatibility, infidelity and battering** can produce distress and despair. Such cases the midwife would refer to the social worker or Marriage Guidance Counsellor for expert handling of the situation. In the meantime, the midwife could talk over the problem with the woman and help her to clarify her thoughts.

**The unwed mother-to-be** needs financial support and probably shelter but she may need counsel re the questions of informing her parents, marriage, adoption, fostering or keeping the baby.

**The mother of a subnormal baby** will need information regarding how she can best give her infant the care he will require. She will be upset that she has given birth to a subnormal child: dealing with any guilt feelings and her emotional turmoil need counselling. (Bereavement has been discussed on p. 687.)

### THE COUNSELLING PROCESS

Counselling involves the personal interaction between a client with an individual problem she cannot solve, and a counsellor who will help to elucidate the situation and enable the woman herself to decide what is right for her in the existing circumstances. The counsellor does not dictate, use pressure, or suggest a specific course of action: the client personally makes the decision. By inducing the woman to talk and express her feelings, fears, and anxieties and by encouraging her to analyse her motives, she gains insight into the behaviour which led up to the stress situation. The client may, by the effort of discussing the situation, see a solution to the problem.

### THE QUALIFIED MIDWIFE AS COUNSELLOR

**The counsellor should be a stable, mature person,** friendly and approachable: tact is needed and the ability to see the other person's point of view. She should be tolerant regarding the frailties of human nature: being neither critical nor judgmental: humility regarding her own ability being an admirable quality, enabling her to maintain a good relationship with the client. It is essential that she is interested in people: meaningful conversation and above all willingness to listen are essential. The midwife counsellor should refer all cases that are specialised to a social worker who, by her professional qualification, can recommend the agency best equipped to help. If the midwife has religious views that forbid abortion, family planning or divorce, and strong moral objections to the current behaviour patterns, she should not be a counsellor.

### THE STUDENT MIDWIFE

During her training the student midwife will learn about counselling but she is a novice and should not aspire to giving counsel until she is qualified to do so. Counselling is a very delicate undertaking that encroaches on personal feelings and private behaviour so it would be wise for her to read about counselling and ancillary subjects such as psychology, marriage guidance, sexuality, human behaviour and to watch an experienced counsellor at work. She ought to endeavour to prepare herself prior to assuming the role of a counsellor.

## ETHICAL PROBLEMS

Although midwives may be extremely interested in many ethical problems they should be very guarded in expressing their opinions or in giving advice to parents regarding problems with an ethical background. The midwife may feel justified in objecting to termination of pregnancy; her religious belief may dictate that an abortion must not be performed even when the mother's life is at stake, but her convictions should be applied to her own behaviour, i.e. she may legally refuse to assist in the performance of an abortion. The patient, doctor and 'the law', decide whether an abortion shall be carried out or not.

### SPINA BIFIDA

There is much controversy on the subject of non-interference: if left to nature, the baby is likely to die within 6 weeks. A number of paediatric surgeons who previously operated on the spina bifida baby at birth, are now reluctant to do so. Some of these children spend much of their lives in hospital having repeated operations; they suffer physical pain, mental and emotional deprivation so the quality of life they lead is very poor. Wide knowledge of the subject is needed.

### DOWN'S SYNDROME

Whether the mongoloid child stays at home, and this has been proved best for the child, or in an institution, ought to be decided by the parents. Midwives should refer such cases to experts who have wide knowledge of all aspects of the situation and experience of what caring for handicapped children involves and has done to parents and their families (see p. 595).

The parent's point of view must be given serious consideration and using phrases such as 'human life is sacred', 'reverence for life', adds to their anguish. The parents must make the decision and this is not easy: what they would like to do and what they are capable of doing may be poles apart. A child with severe brain damage needs constant devoted care and can be a life-long responsibility: the burden imposed may be more than the parents can cope with or bear. The non-expert may not comprehend the complexities of the situation.

## MEDICAL AND OTHER PROBLEMS

There are many ethical problems regarding which midwives are concerned.

(1) **Whether married mothers of young children should go out to work:** financial reasons are compelling but not necessarily wise; sympathetic understanding is needed when necessities as well as luxuries are needed in the home.

(2) **Induction and acceleration of labour** has ethical and psychological overtones for some expectant mothers. If induction is safe for abnormal cases it ought to be safe in normal labour too. Childbearing women should be given the benefit of modern technical advances and midwives with limited experience of induction should not condemn the procedure. Midwives should have a flexible mind, receptive to new ideas that are beneficial to mother and child.

(3) **Whether certain vaccines should be administered.** The benefits may outweigh the disadvantages and the medical profession is likely to be aware of research that has been done on the subject.

(4) **Should girls at puberty be given the pill?** The long term endocrinological and medical effects are not yet known. Does this not anticipate sexual relations under sixteen when it is illegal? Midwives should uphold a high code of moral behaviour: their work brings them in contact with the disastrous effects, on personal and family stability, of the permissive society; broken homes as well as unwanted babies and children in care.

(5) **Clinical research on well babies.** This may disturb some midwives. Expert committees are appointed (midwives are members of such committees) to permit or forbid such research projects in most hospitals or areas. Their medical knowledge and reasoned judgment should be respected: the Helsinki Declaration (1964) contains basic principles for a code of ethics in medical experimentation (clinical research). These are observed by the medical profession in the United Kingdom.

**Most ethical problems have reasons for and against them,** based on humanitarian, medical, religious or cultural grounds. The short- and long-term effect on the welfare of the child, parents, and family are considered: as well as the benefit to future generations.

### THE MIDWIVES' ATTITUDE

**The student midwife should refrain from adopting a censorious attitude** regarding parental or medical decisions on ethical problems. It is sometimes too easy to voice destructive criticism: her knowledge of all the features of the situation may be slight; her experience of life rather limited; her ethical judgments somewhat immature. Emotion and prejudice are not a sound foundation on which to base important decisions.

**Midwives can and should demonstrate their interest in research,** remembering that most of the meritorious therapeutic advances have resulted from research.

---

## QUESTIONS FOR REVISION

Differentiate between: adoption and fostering, deprived and delinquent child, unsupported and protected child, affiliation order and alimony, day nursery and nursery school.

How do counselling and advising differ? Name 3 examples for which (*a*) a married (*b*) an unwed expectant mother might seek counsel. Why should the student midwife refrain from giving counsel?

Ethical problems are based on various grounds; name three. What is the Helsinki Declaration? State briefly your views on (*a*) Giving the pill to girls at puberty (*b*) giving whooping cough vaccine to babies.

## *C.M.B. Short Questions*

**C.M.B.(Eng.).** A mother in your care has given birth to a baby with Downs syndrome (mongolism). Discuss the likely progress of the child's development and the educational and social service provisions which may be needed.

**C.M.B.(Eng.).** Discuss the problems of one parent families. What help is available to them?

**C.M.B.(Scot.).** What is child abuse (non accidental injury)? What are the predisposing factors? Indicate the preventive measures which may be adopted.

**C.M.B.(Scot.)** What are the legal requirements for (*a*) fostering and (*b*) adoption of children?

**C.M.B.(Eng.)** What do you understand by a deprived child? How may this child be recognised by members of the Primary Health Care Team? Outline the help that could be offered.

**C.M.B.(Eng.).** Describe the help which may be needed for an unmarried primigravida, fifteen years of age.

**C.M.B.(Scot.).** What facilities are available for the unsupported woman during pregnancy and the postnatal period?

**C.M.B.(Eng.).** What services are available to give help and support to the parents of a physically handicapped child?

**C.M.B.(Eng.).** What facilities are available for the care of children in single parent families?

**C.M.B.(Eng.).** One parent families. Child benefit. Home help service. Foster parents. Attendance allowance. Child Health Clinics. Maternity allowance. Discuss the functions of a child health clinic. Affiliation Order. Nursery schools. Battered baby syndrome.

**C.M.B.(Scot.).** Maternity allowance and maternity grant. Family income supplement and family allowance. Registered child minder and foster parent. Affiliation Order and Adoption Order. Maternity Leave. Adoption and fostering. The law regarding fostering. Registered child minder.

# 42
# The National Health Service
### ENGLAND SCOTLAND WALES
# Local Government
### ENGLAND, SCOTLAND

*Reorganised unified system. Central administration. Regional Health Authorities Area Health Authorities (Eng.). Health Boards (Scot.). Districts. Nursing Officers in top management. Advisory bodies. Public participation. Comparative structure and nomenclature between England and Scotland Health Service. Health Service in Wales.* **Local Government Reorganisation** *(England and Scotland). Reallocation of some health and social functions.*

---

## THE NATIONAL HEALTH SERVICE 1948

Under the National Health Service Reorganisation (England) Act 1973 and the National Health Service (Scotland) Act 1972, the administration of the National Health Service was restructured to function on a unified basis, commencing on 1st April 1974: one authority instead of three providing all personal health care and taking responsibility for health services in hospital and in the community.

## CENTRAL ADMINISTRATION

**In England** the central department at national level is the Department of Health and Social Security (DHSS), the Secretary of State being in charge.

**In Scotland** the Scottish Home and Health Department, Edinburgh, is the central governing body, the Secretary of State for Scotland being responsible for the Health Service.

These Central Departments have a strategic planning role and are responsible for monitoring the works of the health service as a whole. They are concerned with delineating long-term national objectives, determining priorities in financial expenditure and allocating financial resources to the Regional Health Authorities (Eng.), the Health Boards (Scot.).

### REGIONAL HEALTH AUTHORITIES, ENGLAND

*There are no Regional Authorities in Wales and Scotland*

**In England** there are 14 Regional Health Authorities (RHA) each administered by a regional team of officers which includes a Regional Nursing Officer. Each Regional Health Authority is supported by a team of officers through which work delegated by the Authority to its officers will be co-ordinated. The RHA is directly accountable to the Department of Health and Social Security (DHSS), and responsible for capital projects, planning, regional services (e.g. blood transfusion), and the allocation of resources to the Area Health Authorities (AHA), together with the monitoring of their activities.

**In Scotland** the blood transfusion service and the ambulance service are co-ordinated at Central level under the Common Services Agency.

**Local Supervising Authority**

On 1st April 1974 the statutory responsibilities of the local supervising authority under the Midwives Act 1951 were transferred in England to the Regional Health Authority; the Health Boards in Scotland. Certain statutory supervisory duties may be allocated by the RHA through the Area Health Authority to Supervisors of Midwives in Health Districts, e.g. notifications required under the Central Midwives Board Rules, e.g. intention to practise and change of name or address. The AHA provides or arranges for refresher courses for practising midwives.

**Statutory supervision of midwives (Scot.).** This rests with the Health Boards. Each Board decides how best to carry out its duty to exercise general supervision over all certified midwives practising within its area.


# AREA HEALTH AUTHORITIES (ENGLAND)
# HEALTH BOARDS (SCOTLAND)

**In England** there are 90 Area Health Authorities whose boundaries match those of the non-metropolitan counties and metropolitan districts of local government. In London, AHA boundaries are conterminous with London boroughs or combinations of London boroughs.

**Area Health Authorities (Eng.) and Health Boards (Scot.)** are the statutory administrative tier responsible for planning, organising and administering a comprehensive health service to the population within their geographical area.

The AHA has an area team of officers which includes an Area Nursing Officer.

Birth Notifications are received by the Area Medical Officer.

**In Scotland** there are 15 Health Boards whose areas are largely conterminous with the new local government boundaries. The Health Boards are directly responsible to the Secretary of State for Scotland.

**Notification of births (Scotland).** Births are notified to the Chief Administrative Medical Officer of the Health Board.


# HEALTH DISTRICTS

Geographically large, or heavily populated areas may be sub-divided into Health Districts, which are each administered by a District Management Team (Eng.): District Executive Group (Scot.) responsible for providing a full range of health services within the district, and directly accountable to the Area Health Authority Health Board (Scot.). **The district is the basic unit** responsible for the actual integration and management of hospital, community and other health services at patient care level. It is the key operational unit with a planning function and concerned with the provision and maintenance of high standards of day-to-day health care; facilitating decentralisation of authority and a more personalised service.

## NURSING OFFICERS IN TOP MANAGEMENT

At Region, Area and District levels, the Nursing Officer is a full and equal member of the administrative team. This ensures that the nursing and midwifery services are fully represented, and their interests supported at all levels of policy making and implementation within the National Health Service.

## ADVISORY BODIES
### STANDING ADVISORY COMMITTEES

These committees present the view of their various professional organisations—doctors, dentists, nurses and midwives, pharmacists—to the Secretary of State (DHSS), on their specific interests within the health service, e.g. Standing Nursing and Midwifery Advisory Committee (Eng.). Health Services Planning Council (Scot.).

### PROFESSIONAL ADVISORY MACHINERY

These Regional and Area Committees are set up by the professions themselves, and in the case of the Nursing and Midwifery Committees, are composed entirely of nurses and midwives who represent all aspects of administration, clinical practice and teaching.

They advise the RHA and AHA on matters relating to professional practice and care, and are required to respond to remits from these authorities.

### HEALTH SERVICE COMMISSIONER *(OMBUDSMAN)*

An ombudsman has been appointed by central government to investigate complaints from members of the community, when these complaints have failed to be satisfactorily resolved at Area level.

## PUBLIC PARTICIPATION

### Community Health Councils (Eng.)
### Local Health Councils (Scot.)

These Councils are set up by the Area Health Authorities (Eng.), Health Boards (Scot.) for each District, and approved by the Secretaries of State DHSS (Eng.) and SHHD (Scot.). They consist of 20 to 30 members of the public who will provide consumer participation and have an effective voice in the local operation of the Health Service. The council will represent the interests of those who are at the receiving end of medical care and enable the Area Health Authority (Health Board, Scot.) to be aware of what the people's views are on the Health Service provided.

### COMPARATIVE STRUCTURE AND NOMENCLATURE BETWEEN ENGLAND AND SCOTLAND N.H.S.

**England:** A two-tier structure: Regional and Area Health Authorities.
**Scotland:** A one-tier structure: Health Boards.

**England:** An Area Medical Officer.
**Scotland:** A Chief Administrative Medical Officer.

**England:** An Area Nursing Officer.
**Scotland:** A Chief Area Nursing Officer.

**England:** A District Community Physician.
**Scotland:** A District Community Medicine Specialist.

**England:** Regional, Area and District Management Teams.
**Scotland:** Area and District—Executive Groups.

**England:** Family Practitioner Committee.
**Scotland:** Family Practitioner Council.

**England:** Consumer participation by Community Health Councils.
**Scotland:** Consumer participation by Local Health Councils.

**England:** Regional Health Authorities have statutory responsibility of local supervising authority (Midwives Act 1951).
**Scotland:** Health Boards have statutory responsibility of local supervising authority (Midwives Scotland Act 1951).

**England:** Births are notified to the medical officer of the Area Health Authority.
**Scotland:** Births are notified to the Chief Administrative Medical Officer of the Health Board.

**England:** Regional, Area and District Nursing Officers are not in line management.
**Scotland:** Area and District Nursing Officers are in line management.

**England:** Blood Transfusion and ambulance Service is co-ordinated at Regional level.
**Scotland:** Blood Transfusion and ambulance Service is co-ordinated at Central level (Common Services Agency).

# WALES

### NATIONAL HEALTH SERVICE

The Welsh National Health Service was restructured administratively on 1st April 1974: overall responsibility resting with the Secretary of State for Wales acting through the Welsh Office. There is no Regional tier.

### AREA HEALTH AUTHORITIES

Eight Area Health Authorities carry delegated responsibility for planning and managing the Health Services in their areas, subject to the strategic guidance and control of the Welsh Secretary of State.

### THE WELSH OFFICE

The Welsh Office has various responsibilities, i.e. a Health and Social Work Department and within this the Nursing Division set up in 1972, has a number of senior professional nurses and midwives who advise the Secretary of State on policy matters affecting nursing and midwifery, and interpret Welsh Office policies to authorities and professional organisations.

**Supervision of Midwives** is delegated to the Areas: the Welsh Office carrying out a co-ordinating as well as a departmental role.

# LOCAL GOVERNMENT

Reorganised Local Government in England was introduced on 1st April 1974, simultaneously with reorganisation of the National Health Service. In Scotland reorganisation of Local Government was established in May 1975.

The Social Service Department of the County Councils and Metropolitan District Councils (Eng.) and the Social Work Department of the Regional Councils (Scot.) are now responsible for care of the unsupported mother and her child; adoption; fostering; children in care; day nurseries; residential nurseries; child minders; the home help service; the social aspects of physically and mentally handicapped children; day care of pre-school children.

## SOME LOCAL GOVERNMENT FUNCTIONS

| County Council (Eng.)<br>Regional Council (Scot.) | District Council (Eng.)<br>District Council (Scot.) |
|---|---|
| Registration of births, marriages and deaths. Social Service (England). Social Work (Scotland). Education. Roads. Police. Fire. Water supply. Food standards. Weights and measures. | Housing. Environmental health, including food hygiene, milk sampling, cleansing, clean air. |

## REALLOCATION OF HEALTH AND SOCIAL FUNCTIONS

| Area Health Authorities (Eng.)<br>Health Boards (Scot.) | Local Government | |
|---|---|---|
| | County Councils (Eng.)<br>Regional Councils (Scot.) | District Councils (Eng.)<br>District Councils (Scot.) |
| **HEALTH CARE** | **SOCIAL SERVICES** | **ENVIRONMENTAL HEALTH** |
| Hospital service, including doctors, nurses, midwives and para-medical staff. Specialist services, family practitioners, community nurses, midwives and health visitors. Dental care. General surveillance of the health of the population, epidemiology of disease. School health service. Maternal and child health. Family planning. Health education. Prevention, care and after care of illness. Immunisation and vaccination. Registration and supervision of nursing homes. | The unsupported mother and her child, mother and baby homes. Adoption. Foster children. Children in care. Day and residential nurseries. Day care of pre-school children. Child minders. Social aspects of physically and mentally handicapped persons. The home help service. Social work with the mentally ill and the elderly. | Pure food, milk and water. Efficient sanitation, disposal of waste. Nuisances. Pest control. Clean air. Disinfestation. Communicable diseases. |

**All aspects of environmental health** are the prime responsibility of local government, although there is close liaison with the area medical specialist in environmental health and district community physicians.

## QUESTIONS FOR REVISION

**C.M.B.(Scot.) 30-min. question.** What are the Central Midwives Board for Scotland rules regarding (a) antenatal visits, (b) postnatal visits by the domiciliary midwife, (c) examination of the placenta?

### C.M.B. Short Questions

**Eng.:** What is a 'Local Supervising Authority'? **Eng.:** The Central Midwives Board? **Eng.:** What is a medical aid form and when is it used? **Scot.:** How frequently is a practising midwife required to attend a refresher course? **Scot.:** What is the Central Midwives Board? **Scot.:** The Central Midwives Board for Scotland rule regarding attendance at refresher courses?

**Eng.:** District Management Team. **Scot.:** Health Board and Local Health Council. **Scot.:** Local Supervising Authority.

# 43
# History of Midwifery
### With emphasis on the part played by midwives
*Pre-historic times. Biblical times. First to eighteenth century. William Smellie. The British midwife. The Royal College of Midwives. The Central Midwives Boards. Progress in obstetrics*

### Pre-historic times
Although one might surmise that in the remote ages the first woman who helped another in childbirth was a midwife, this is probably not quite correct, for only a husband or a female relative was permitted to attend the woman in labour. Later, women outside the family circle earned their livelihood in this way and became known as midwives.

Tribal customs during labour were based on belief in magic; charms and incantations being used to ward off demons. Practices during prolonged labour were crude, even cruel, for the midwives had no understanding of the process of birth.

Models are in existence (5000 B.C.) of the woman squatting during childbirth, supported behind by another woman in a similar attitude. Birth stools were a later development and are mentioned in the Old Testament.

The healing of the sick was in the hands of witch doctors and medicine men, and although priests and other men of learning took over the practice of medicine, midwifery remained in the hands of uneducated midwives, so progress did not take place.

### Biblical times
Midwives are mentioned in the Old Testament, Genesis chap. 35, verse 17, and chap. 38, verse 28, also in Exodus chap. 1, verses 15–21, when Pharaoh, King of Egypt, commands the midwives to slay all the Jewish infants of the male sex. The midwives feared God so they disobeyed this order, saying unto Pharaoh, 'Because the Hebrew women are not as the Egyptian women; for they are lively, and are delivered ere the midwives come in unto them'. And so the story of Moses, hidden in the cradle of bulrushes came to be told.

### The Hippocratic era (470 to 370 B.C.)
In ancient Greece, Hippocrates, the Father of Medicine, inaugurated the scientific approach to the healing of the sick. He believed that disease was due to natural causes, so he discarded practices based on superstition or magic, as well as on religious rites and priestcraft. Midwifery still remained in the hands of midwives who sought the advice, but not the help, of physicians in difficult cases only. Hippocrates took some part in the management of childbirth, and the midwives contemptuously called him a 'he-grandmother'.

### The first to the fourth century A.D.
Soranus of Ephesus, who lived during the second century, studied and taught midwifery and the treatise he wrote became the basis of various books on the subject. During the third and fourth centuries midwifery was ignored by physicians, and by custom and law they were prohibited from attending women in labour.

### The fifth to the fifteenth century

With the decline of the Roman Empire the teaching of Hippocrates and Soranus fell into disuse. During this period of intellectual stagnation, herbs, potions and incantations were again used in healing the sick, and superstitious untrained midwives had complete control of midwifery. The assistance they gave during labour was in dilating the cervix manually, massaging the abdomen, and supporting the perineum with a linen cloth. Pulling on the cord and manual removal of the placenta were also practised.

In the fifteenth century it was the established continental practice for midwives to be examined by members of the medical profession regarding their methods of procedure.

### The sixteenth century

The invention of printing gave great impetus to learning, and in Germany, in 1513, the first book on midwifery was printed. This book, based on Soranus's teaching, was, in 1540, translated into English as *Ye Byrth of Mankynde,* and for a century and a half was the only book on midwifery printed in English. Few midwives could read, so their abysmal ignorance persisted.

Doctors were rigidly excluded from the birth chamber, and a physician in Hamburg in 1522, who dressed as a woman in order to witness the birth of a baby, was punished by being burned to death. In 1580 a law was passed in Germany preventing swineherds and shepherds from attending women in labour.

Although some progress was being made in medicine and surgery, knowledge of obstetrics lagged far behind. Childbearing women were therefore deprived of the benefits which could only accrue if the physicians, with their education and access to further learning, were permitted to enter the field.

### *The Dawn of Progress—Ambroise Paré (1510 to 1590)*

This celebrated French surgeon laid the foundation of the modern art of obstetrics. He advocated the operation of podalic version (mainly for shoulder presentation), and his skill in delivering the child alive enhanced his prestige with the midwives. He was the first to deliver women in bed instead of on the birth stool; he also sutured the perineum. Paré founded a school for midwives at the Hotel Dieu in Paris, and those trained there were able to recognise abnormalities and were willing to seek the help of the surgeons who had taught them. Louise Bourgeois, a midwife of outstanding character and ability, was trained under Paré and attended the ladies of the French court. Her writings on obstetrics were quoted in many subsequent publications.

### The seventeenth century

William Harvey (1587 to 1657), who discovered the circulation of the blood, drew attention to the deplorable ignorance of midwives and to the multitudes of women who had perished because of this.

The reluctance of women to be delivered by men continued. In 1658 a practising midwife, the daugher of Dr Willughby, a Middlesex physician, was perturbed because of a breech presentation. She requested her father to creep into the birth chamber on his hands and knees, unknown to her patient, and persuaded him to remain and assist her with the delivery.

Gross pelvic deformity caused by rickets necessitated the assistance of a physician or surgeon to deliver the woman. Midwives did not usually seek medical aid until labour was hopelessly obstructed, and the ensuing death of mother or child gave physicians unwarrantably bad reputations.

During 1663 Louis XIV employed a surgeon from Paris to attend one of his mistresses, in preference to the gossiping midwives. He was pleased with the decorous conduct of the man-midwife and honoured him with the more dignified title of accoucheur. The fashion spread amongst the ladies of the court and was followed by the women of France. The French accoucheurs, therefore, gained vast experience and built up a school of midwifery which attracted doctors from all over Europe to study there. Mauriceau published in 1668 a treatise on midwifery, far ahead of any other book on the subject, which was translated into English in 1672 by Hugh Chamberlen, of forceps family fame, and greatly assisted the progress of midwifery in Britain.

## The eighteenth century

Midwifery forceps to deliver a live child were invented by one of the Chamberlens, a Huguenot family of whom four generations practised medicine in England from 1569 to 1683. They went to great lengths to keep their instrument a secret, but knowledge of it leaked out and in 1733 Edmund Chapman, an English obstetrician, gave the first description of the Chamberlen forceps. In 1813 the Chamberlen forceps were found under the floor of an attic in a house near Malden, Essex, where they were hidden in 1683 on the death of Dr Peter Chamberlen because he had no son to succeed him.

### The First School of Midwifery in Britain

Queen Charlotte's was the first maternity hospital in Britain. It was founded in 1739 and in 1752 it became the General Lying-in Hospital, and later (1791) the name was changed when Queen Charlotte became its patron. Three other London maternity hospitals were opened in 1747 to 1750.

The Edinburgh Royal Infirmary allocated four beds for midwifery in 1752 and medical students were permitted to attend, but not until 1833 in Scotland and 1886 in England did the subject of midwifery become compulsory for medical students.

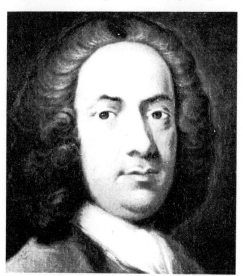

Fig. 43-1   William Smellie, 1697–1763
*(From a painting by himself at 22 years of age)*

#### WILLIAM SMELLIE, 1697 to 1763

William Smellie, the Master of British Obstetrics, gained his knowledge of medicine as an apprentice and began his career as a doctor in Lanark, Scotland, in

1720. At this time midwives sought the help of doctors only for preternatural labours (not head first), and Smellie was perturbed over the loss of so many babies. Wishing to study normal labour and to learn more about the application of forceps, he travelled to London, a journey which took 13 days, and to Paris. In 1739 he set up in practice in London, where he taught midwifery in the homes of the poor to classes of 4 to 12 doctors. During a period of 10 years over 1000 doctors attended his courses of lectures and clinical demonstrations, some coming from the Continent and America, such was his fame. With no university education and no research facilities, his achievements were remarkable. He discarded the superstitious notions regarding childbirth and laid the foundation of the art and science of obstetrics as we know it today.

Smellie described the pelvis and fetal skull and their measurements, and demonstrated how to diagnose the positions of the vertex vaginally by the sutures and fontanelles. It was he who explained the mechanism of labour. He also devised a lock for midwifery forceps, which permitted each blade to be inserted separately.

Smellie's influence on obstetrics was profound, and it has been said that he accomplished for midwifery in his lifetime more than any individual before or since. His volumes on midwifery are full of obstetrical wisdom which is still valid.

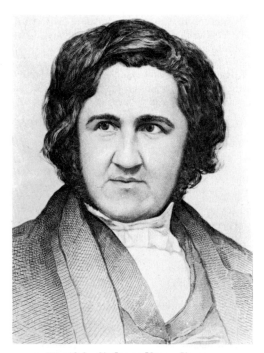

Fig. 43-2   Sir James Young Simpson

### SIR JAMES YOUNG SIMPSON

Sir James Young Simpson will be remembered as one of the pioneers who attempted to alleviate the pains of childbirth. In the year 1847, while Professor of Midwifery in Edinburgh, he first used chloroform for this purpose; but strenuous objection from the clergy, the medical profession and the laity was encountered. Six years later, chloroform was administered to Queen Victoria during the birth of her seventh child, and her enthusiastic appreciation of the drug did much to break down the opposition to its use. Chloroform has been superseded by substances which do not have its disadvantages and dangers.

### J. W. BALLANTYNE

Dr. J. W. Ballantyne, who has been called 'the father of antenatal care', was lecturer in antenatal pathology at the University of Edinburgh. He wrote a paper deploring how little progress had been made in antenatal pathology and urged that a 'pro-maternity' hospital was necessary. The anonymous gift of £1,000 to endow a bed in the Royal Maternity and Simpson Memorial Hospital enabled him, in the year 1901, to set apart the *first bed ever to be used* for the study of the pregnant woman.

During the same year, in Boston, U.S.A., visits were paid to some patients in their homes, and the first antenatal clinic was opened there in 1911, others in Sydney during 1912 and in Edinburgh during 1915.

### HISTORY OF PUERPERAL SEPSIS

Puerperal sepsis was known at the time of Hippocrates, but epidemics of the disease coincided with the establishment of lying-in hospitals. Charles White of Manchester (1773) and Alexander Gordon of Aberdeen (1795) were the first to state that puerperal fever was infectious and could be carried from patient to patient. Oliver Wendell Holmes in the United States of America (1843) maintained that epidemic fever in the puerperium was due to lack of cleanliness. Semmelweis of Vienna (1844) noticed that the death rate in the wards where medical students and doctors delivered the woman was three times greater than in the midwives' wards, because doctors carried infection from the post-mortem examinations they made.

The invention of the microscope and the work of Pasteur and Lister led to the recognition of the causative organisms and the employment of methods of combating them. Improved techniques, the avoidance of unnecessary interference and the introduction of chemotherapeutic agents and antibiotics have reduced still further the incidence of puerperal sepsis.

## THE BRITISH MIDWIFE

### *Sixteenth to Twentieth Century*

Few records are available regarding the practice of midwifery in Britain until the 16th century. Following the Reformation, the Church of England accepted responsibility for issuing, by the Bishops, of licences for midwives to practise. Midwifery was practised entirely by midwives, who were completely ignorant of the most elementary facts of anatomy and obstetrics, and in 1616 a petition was made unsuccessfully to James I by Peter Chamberlen, 'That some order may be settled by the State for the instruction and civil government of midwives'. A second petition, submitted in 1687 by a midwife, suggested the establishment of a corporation of midwives, but the College of Physicians of London opposed it.

The first chair of midwifery, anywhere, was created in Edinburgh during 1726 for the purpose of giving instruction to midwives. (Later, medical students were permitted to attend the lectures given by the Professor.) The magistrates of Edinburgh insisted upon the production of certificates from a physician or surgeon testifying that the midwives had received instruction prior to practising their profession. Courses of instruction were given to midwives in various centres throughout Britain during the 18th century, and a few hospitals issued certificates.

In 1756 Dr John Douglas wrote a pamphlet, deploring the lamentable state of midwifery practice in London and suggesting (1) proper courses of instruction for midwives; (2) the establishment of training schools in maternity hospitals, and (3) an examination before a certificate to practise was granted. The pamphlet was a fertile seed which eventually bore fruit.

In 1813 the Society of Apothecaries tried to persuade Parliament to pass a law forbidding women to practise as midwives for gain without having undergone an examination and obtaining a certificate of their ability to practise as midwives. The Committee of the House of Commons would not permit any mention of midwives, who at that time were of the lowest strata of society, unable to read or write, the gin-drinking type, later immortalised by Dickens as Sairey Gamp.

The Ladies' Obstetrical College, London, was found in 1864, and the daughters of professional men attended lectures and became midwives. In 1872 the Obstetrical Society of London proceeded to constitute an examining Board, which awarded certificates to successful candidates, testifying to their competence to attend normal confinements.

## THE ROYAL COLLEGE OF MIDWIVES

This body was set up in 1881 as The Midwives Institute, and was responsible for the promotion of the first Midwives' Bill, which was introduced into the House of Commons in 1890, but the Bill was bitterly opposed by untrained midwives as well as the medical profession and failed to pass into legislation. A further seven Bills were introduced between 1891 and 1900, but were unsuccessful. At last, in 1902, the first English Midwives Act was passed, and State registration of midwives became compulsory by law. Scotland followed in 1915 with a similar Act. The Midwives Institute celebrated its 60th anniversary in 1941, and the title was changed to the College of Midwives. In 1947 the Royal prefix was granted. 1981 is the Centenary year. The aim of The Royal College of Midwives is to advance the art and science of midwifery and to maintain high professional standards. To provide information on midwifery in the United Kingdom. An exchange of ideas and information on midwifery throughout the world is encouraged. Research by midwives is promoted.

The College is an advisory body, negotiating with Government departments and other groups concerned with the maternity services in the United Kingdom.

It represents the midwives' interests, and has been the chief instrument in promoting progress in the practice of midwifery by midwives and the means of improving their education, conditions of service, salary and status.

## THE CENTRAL MIDWIVES BOARDS

The Midwives Act of 1902 (Eng.) sanctioned the setting up of a statutory body, the Central Midwives Board, prescribed its constitution and laid down its duties and powers. The Board was authorised to frame rules regulating the training and practice of midwives, to conduct examinations and maintain a roll of persons who had been awarded its certificate. The Board also organises examinations for the Midwife Teacher's Diploma.

The primary function of the Central Midwives Board is to protect the public by providing well-trained midwives who must carry out a code of practice as laid down by the Board. The actual duty of supervising the midwife in practice is the responsibility of the Regional Health Authority in England, the Health Board in Scotland.

The training period for midwives has gradually been lengthened to meet advances in knowledge and improved methods of practice. From the year 1902 to 1916 the training period lasted three months. Since 1938 it has been one year for trained and two years for untrained nurses. It is anticipated that in 1981 the training period will be 18 months for Registered nurses and 3 years for untrained nurses. In Scotland only nurses who are State Registered are eligible for training.

The Midwives Act of 1902: (Scotland, 1915), gave protection to the title 'Midwife' and made it a legal offence for any woman to use the title when not certified as such. The Act required all practising midwives to notify the Local Supervising Authority in January every year of their intention to practise and to notify the Central Midwives Board of any change of name or address, whether practising or not.

### ADDRESSES OF CENTRAL MIDWIVES BOARDS

**England**—39 Harrington Gardens, South Kensington, London SW7 4JY.
**Scotland**—24 Dublin Street, Edinburgh, EH1 3PU.
**N. Ireland**—Council for Nurses and Midwives, 216 Belmont Road, Belfast, BT4 2AT.

### NOTIFICATION TO THE CENTRAL MIDWIVES BOARDS

*(1980 certain modifications of existing notification are being made)*

**England** The midwife sends an official notification (special form) of **intention to practise** to the Central Midwives Board: it is also sent in January of each subsequent year.
*(The midwife informs the C.M.B. by letter of any change of name or address whether practising or not)*

**Scotland** The midwife sends an official notification (special form) to the Central Midwives Board for Scotland on the following occasions. (1) **Intention to practice:** (this is repeated in January of each subsequent year). (2) **Death of mother or child.** (3) **When patient refuses to seek medical advice.** (4) **When for home confinement the patient's accommodation is not suitable.**
*(The midwife informs the C.M.B. by letter of any change of name or address whether practising or not)*

### REFRESHER COURSES

These must, according to the Central Midwives Boards Rules, be provided or arranged for by the Regional Health Authority (Eng.) who may delegate this function to the Area Health Authority, The Health Board (Scot.). Practising midwives are required to attend such a course in England and Scotland within five years of having passed the C.M.B. examination or having attended such a course.

## THE NURSES, MIDWIVES AND HEALTH VISITORS ACT, 1979
*(some excerpts that concern midwives)*

When this Act comes into force, The General Nursing Councils and the Central Midwives Boards will be dissolved.

**A United Kingdom Central Council** for Nursing, Midwifery and Health Visiting will be set up.

**National Boards for Nursing, Midwifery and Health Visiting** will be set up in England, Wales, Scotland and Northern Ireland.

**A Midwifery committee** will be constituted as a standing committee of each National Board; the majority of the committee members shall be practising midwives. Each National Board will consult its midwifery committee on all matters relating to midwifery. The Act will make new provision with respect to the education, training, regulation and discipline of nurses, midwives and health visitors. There are provisions in the Act for making the rules for midwifery practice, supervision of midwifery practice and limiting attendance on a woman in childbirth.

**Registration**

**The Central Council shall prepare and maintain a register** of qualified nurses, midwives, and health visitors. Midwives will be **'registered' not 'certified'**. 'Pupil midwives' will be 'student midwives'.

**Local Supervising Authorities**

**In England and Wales**—Regional Health Authorities.

**In Scotland**—Health Boards.

**In Northern Ireland**—Health and Social Services Boards.

## PROGRESS IN OBSTETRICS

Not until the medical profession entered the field of obstetrics was any real progress made. Only then did childbearing women derive any benefit from the advances made in medicine and surgery which could be applied to obstetrics. The invention of midwifery forceps gave men practitioners a great advantage. The introduction of anaesthetics, as well as the knowledge of antisepsis and asepsis, made obstetrical operations possible. Advances in physiology, biochemistry, bacteriology, anaesthesiology, haematology, radiology, ultrasonography, endocrinology, immunology, genetics and pharmacology have brought obstetrics and neonatology to a level which could never have been attained by midwives alone.

Both doctor and midwife are essential, even for normal cases, if the woman is to receive the maximal benefit of all modern investigations and treatment during pregnancy and labour. The proficient midwife of today is an expert in the care of women in normal pregnancy, labour, the puerperium and in neonatal paediatrics, as well as a helpful collaborator with the obstetrician when dealing with abnormal or operative obstetrics. She is also a teacher of health, preparation for childbirth and early parenthood and a counsellor on family planning and other relevant subjects.

### TEAM WORK

The midwife co-operates as one of a team, which includes:

**OBSTETRICIANS, PHYSICIANS, PAEDIATRICIANS, ANAESTHETISTS, ENDOCRINOLOGISTS, GENERAL PRACTITIONERS, BACTERIOLOGISTS, RADIOLOGISTS, ULTRASONOLOGISTS, HAEMATOLOGISTS, GENETECISTS**

aided by:

**HEALTH VISTORS; DIETITIANS; SOCIAL WORKERS and PHYSIOTHERAPISTS**

all of whom are concerned with the welfare of mothers and babies.

---

## QUESTIONS FOR REVISION

**C.M.B.(Scot.) 30-min. question.** What are the Central Midwives Board for Scotland rules regarding (*a*) antenatal visits, (*b*) postnatal visits by the domiciliary midwife, (*c*) examination of the placenta?

### C.M.B. Short Questions

**Eng.:** Who is the 'Local Supervising Authority'? **Eng.:** The Central Midwives Board? **Eng.:** What is a medical aid form and when is it used? **Scot.:** How frequently is a practising midwife required to attend a refresher course? **Scot.:** What is the Central Midwives Board? **Scot.:** The Central Midwives Board for Scotland rule regarding attendance at refresher courses?

What are the provisions of the Nurses, Midwives and Health Visitors Act 1979 that are of concern to midwives.

# 44
# The use of Medicines by Midwives

*Legislation re drugs: Acts; Regulations. Central Midwives Board Directives: The use of pethidine by midwives: Addition of drugs to i.v. fluids. Giving drugs i.v. and i.m. to the neonate: 'Topping up' epidural analgesics: Drug interaction: Expiry date, teratogenic drugs: Ensuring safety of drugs: SI Units: Fahrenheit to Celsius.*

Midwives administer a large number of drugs in the practice of their profession; many of these having been described throughout the text. Drugs for the relief of pain in labour are discussed on p. 259; basic information re epidural analgesia is given on p. 623 topping up on p. 629.

*The need for drugs in the practice of midwifery is concerned mainly with:*

(1) **Relief of pain in labour;**
(2) **Resuscitation of the newborn;**
(3) **Prevention and treatment of haemorrhage;**
(4) **Treatment of medical complications.**

### LEGISLATION GOVERNING THE USE OF MEDICINES AND DRUGS (BY MIDWIVES IN BRITAIN)

**Midwives must be familiar with the laws that govern the administration of 'Controlled Drugs' and 'Prescription Only Medicines'** that midwives are permitted to use. They should also be aware that if a drug mistake leads to litigation, ignorance of the law is no excuse.

*The main legislation controlling the use of drugs by midwives in Britain is as follows:*

(1) **Medicines Act 1968;** (2) **Misuse of Drugs Act 1971;** (3) **Misuse of Drugs Regulations 1973;** (4) **Misuse of Drugs (Amendment) Regulations 1974;** (5) **Medicines Prescription Only Order 1977.**

### (1) The Medicines Act 1968

**This Act is concerned with regulating the legitimate use of medicinal products.** Certain medicines normally issued on a doctor's prescription may be supplied to midwives for use in their practice. These medicines are now listed in schedule IV of the 'Prescription Only Medicines' Order 1977 (see No. 4, p. 720).

### (2) The Misuse of Drugs Act 1971

**This Act is concerned with the abuse of Controlled drugs.** The supply, possession, and use of drugs of dependence (addiction) such as pethidine, morphine, diamorphine and other synthetic morphine-like compounds, is prohibited except as provided by Regulations issued by the Home Secretary.

### (3) The Misuse of Drugs Regulations 1973

**These Regulations stipulate the conditions under which Controlled Drugs can be used by medical practitioners and certain others.** A registered midwife who has, in accordance with the provisions of the Midwives Act 1951 or the Midwives (Scotland)

Act 1951, notified to the local supervising authority her intention to practise, is hereby authorised, as far as is necessary in the practice of her profession or employment as a midwife, to be in possession of pethidine which she has procured upon furnishing to the supplier thereof, a midwife's supply order duly signed (see below only applicable to community midwives).

### (4) The Misuse of Drugs (Amendment) Regulations 1974

**These Regulations outline (A) the safe custody of controlled drugs; (B) the procedure by which midwives may surrender stocks of unwanted pethidine** to an appropriate medical officer but not to a supervisor of midwives. The midwife may destroy pethidine which is no longer required only in the presence of an authorised person, who may be: (1) a police officer; (2) an Inspector of the Home Office Drugs Branch; (3) an Inspector of the Pharmaceutical Society of Gt. Britain.

### (5) Medicines Prescription Only Order 1977

Prescription Only Medicines are prescribed by a doctor but practising midwives are permitted to obtain certain prescription only medicines under:

**Statutory Instrument No. 2127, The Medicines Prescription Only Order 1977** for use in their professional practice, viz. Ergometrine maleate, oxytocins (natural and synthetic), naloxone (Narcan), pentazocine lactate (Fortral), promazine hydrochloride (Sparine), chloral hydrate, dichloralphenazone (Welldorm), (lignocaine has been added to this list). In Scotland only ergometrine, Syntometrine and lignocaine may be administered without a medical prescription.

#### EXCERPTS FROM THE CENTRAL MIDWIVES BOARD (RULES AND CODE OF PRACTICE)

Midwives are required by the CMB to observe the Statutory Acts and Regulations governing the administration of drugs and the Memoranda issued by the DHSS (Eng.), The Scottish Home and Health Department, e.g. The Aitken Report (Eng.) and the Roxburgh Report (Scot.) (see p. 721).

**The CMB rules state:** 'A practising midwife must not on her own responsibility use any drug, including an analgesic unless in the course of her training, whether before or after enrolment, she has been thoroughly instructed in its use and is familiar with its dosage and methods of administration or application.' Also 'When a midwife administers or applies in any way any drug other than an aperient, she must forthwith make a proper record of the name and dose of the drug and the date and time of its administration or application'.

**According to the CMB the following preparations would ordinarily be carried by community midwives:** aperients, sedatives and analgesics, a preparation of ergot for intramuscular injection, approved agents for maternal and neonatal resuscitation.


## ADMINISTRATION OF PETHIDINE BY MIDWIVES

**The Misuse of Drugs Regulations 1973 and the Misuse of Drugs (Amendment) Regulations 1974** permit registered midwives who have notified their intention to practise in accordance with the requirements of the Midwives Act 1951, to possess and administer pethidine so far as is necessary in the practice of their profession. Pethidine can only be obtained by midwives on the authority of a midwife's supply order signed by (a) an appropriate medical officer who is authorised in writing by the Local Supervising Authority or (b) a person appointed by the Local Supervising Authority to exercise supervision over midwives within their area.

**These Regulations are applicable only to midwives who are practising in the community.** The supply order must specify the name of the midwife, the purpose for which the pethidine is required and the quantity to be obtained. The midwife is required to record in her Drugs Book the name and quantity of the controlled drug (pethidine): the name and address of the firm or person from whom it was obtained, including the amount: the date, name and address of the person to whom the drug was administered including the amount of the drug given.

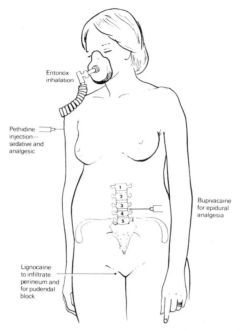

Entonox inhalation

Pethidine injection— sedative and analgesic

Bupivacaine for epidural analgesia

Lignocaine to infiltrate perineum and for pudendal block

Fig. 44-1 Drugs administered by inhalation—injection-epidural

### Administration of pethidine by midwives in hospital

Midwives supply orders are not issued to midwives practising in hospital. The Aitken Report (Eng.) and the Roxburgh Report (Scot.) state that midwives practising in a maternity hospital have no 'rights' in regard to giving pethidine on their own authority.

**The DHSS Circular G/M 152–(1972)** advises that a procedure should be followed to eliminate the possibility of a woman in hospital failing to receive a drug such as pethidine to relieve pain in labour because no doctor is available to prescribe it. In such circumstances, the procedure to be followed should be agreed on by doctors and senior midwives and a statement of the agreed procedure signed by the obstetrician or doctor should be displayed in each labour unit. Otherwise midwives in hospital are not authorised to give drugs such as pethidine on their own initiative.

#### STORAGE AND SAFE CUSTODY OF CONTROLLED DRUGS

**The community midwife** must keep controlled drugs such as pethidine in a locked receptacle that can be opened only by her.

**In NHS hospitals** the pharmacist (or in hospitals that have no pharmacist the officer in charge of nursing services) is responsible for obtaining and issuing supplies of controlled drugs and maintaining a controlled drugs register. The sister or acting sister is responsible for the safe custody and for checking and recording the stock of controlled drugs as directed by her employing authority.

**Controlled drugs must be kept in a locked compartment** within a locked cupboard; the keys being carried by the sister in charge.

## ADMINISTRATION OF MEDICINES INTRAVENOUSLY

This is an extension of nursing and midwifery practice, and each employing Authority lays down detailed polices which should be studied and adhered to.

**Midwives are permitted by the CMB** to administer ergometrine intravenously in the emergency treatment of post partum haemorrhage.

Many medicines administered intravenously are given through an indwelling cannula which should have been inserted by a doctor, and the prescription including full instructions should be written up beforehand. The midwife should ensure that the dose of the medicine and its administration is witnessed by a second trained member of staff. Drugs given intravenously are more commonly added to infusion fluid e.g. oxytocin, but not to blood or plasma.

**The doctor, delegating responsibility to a registered nurse or registered midwife** for i.v. therapy, must satisfy himself that she is competent to undertake the procedure. Medicines should not be added to i.v. fluids by a nurse in training.

### Statement by the Central Midwives Board, 1978

'In the Board's view, the giving of intravenous injections is a procedure within the province of a midwife provided she has been properly instructed, and her employing authority is satisfied as to her competence'.

'Similarly the setting up of an intravenous infusion on medical authority would be regarded as being within the proper sphere of the midwife, although the Board would not expect her to initiate such a procedure on her own behalf'.

### THE MIDWIFE'S RESPONSIBILITIES INCLUDE

**Obtaining theoretical and practical instruction** on the pharmacology, storage, inspection and administration of drugs and the infusion fluids to which they are added; including hazards of the procedure.

**Achieving competence** prior to adding medicines.

**Limiting the drugs used to those within the scope of locally agreed policy.**

**Reading instructions carefully.**

**Carrying out the necessary aseptic technique** and other instructions laid down by her employing authority.

**Confirming** (a) **that the pharmacological name of the medicine to be administered is written clearly in capital letters;** (b) prescribed dose, amount of fluid and other instructions signed by the doctor.

**Checking** (a) **of the dose of medicine and amount of fluid by another nurse or midwife;** (b) that medicine and fluid are properly mixed by inverting the container 2 or 3 times.

**Reporting** (a) **cracks in the glass container,** presence of cloudiness, particulate matter (b) turbidity, change of colour, precipitation of fluid on addition of the medicine.

**Ensuring that** (a) **air is expelled from the syringe;** (b) the intravenous line is patent; (c) flow is at the prescribed rate; (d) site of injection shows no evidence of infection or needle displacement.

**Observing the condition of the patient** and (as with oxytocin) the effect on the fetal heart rate, uterine contractions, blood pressure and pulse rate.

**Keeping the required records;** applying additive labels to confirm content, dosage, date and time of administration.

#### RESUME OF SOME HAZARDS

**Medicines should not be injected into infusions of blood,** plasma, parenteral amino-acids, lipids and infusions of mannitol or sodium bicarbonate. No more than one medicine should be added to i.v. infusion fluid.

**Overdosage;** illegible writing of prescriptions; wrong interpretation of SI doses. Giving the medicine into the tubing when it should have been mixed with the infusion fluid increases the dose and may cause an adverse effect on the patient.

**Medicines may be incompatible** with the fluid.

**Injecting too much fluid** or giving it too quickly can upset the fluid and electrolyte balance.

## *Discontinuation of IV fluids*

Midwives who are permitted to remove i.v. apparatus on the completion of the regime must ensure that the cannula is complete.

## INTRAVENOUS MEDICINE THERAPY IN NEONATAL INTENSIVE CARE UNITS

The umbilical blood vessels are rarely available after the first week; one of the scalp veins is more commonly used and a small plaster of Paris support prevents dislodgement of the needle. Swelling of the scalp should be reported as this indicates displacement of the needle.

**Disposable scalp vein sets are available;** a wing fixes the needle to the scalp. To prevent the flow being too rapid and the volume excessive, a subsidiary chamber containing 30 ml or more of infusion fluid is connected to the main infusion bottle by a 'shut off' valve. Servo controlled electronic drop counters and high precision roller pumps are used to control the flow and avoid over burdening the baby's circulation and upsetting the fluid balance.

**Midwives must find out** whether the medicine is to be added to the infusion bottle or to the drip chamber from which the drug will be administered in a more concentrated form.

**Close observation of the baby is essential.**

## 'TOPPING UP' AN EPIDURAL ANALGESIC

*(See also p. 623)*

### *Statement by the Central Midwives Board*

'Midwives are permitted by the Central Midwives Board (Scot.) to give "topping up" doses, provided the following safeguards are observed.

1. That the ultimate responsibility for such a technique should clearly rest with the doctor.

2. **That written instruction as to the dose should be given by the doctor concerned.**

3. **That the dose given by the midwife should be checked by one other person.**

4. **That instructions should be given by the doctor** as to the posture of the patient at the time of injection, observations on the blood pressure and measures to be taken in the event of any adverse side effects.

5. **That the midwife should have been thoroughly instructed** in the technique so that the doctor concerned is satisfied as to her ability.'

#### MIDWIVES DUTIES

1. The midwife should ascertain that the initial dose with the recommended local analgesic agent has been given by an anaesthetist through the catheter system and that it worked successfully.

2. A 10 or 20 ml syringe should be used; the concentration and dose checked according to regulations.

3. The rubber bung is removed, syringe nozzle attached to the millipore filter; solution injected slowly 5 ml/30 seconds. The bung is replaced when the 'top up' is completed.

THE ANAESTHETIST IS INFORMED IF

**THE ANAESTHETIST IS INFORMED IF**

1. **A fall in blood pressure** or deceleration of the FH rate occurs which is not rectified within 5 minutes by turning the patient on her other side.

2. **Ringing in her ears, drowsiness** or **slurred speech** is present.

3. **Blood appears in the epidural catheter.**

## Points to Note

(a) **Always use a syringe of 10 ml capacity or larger.**

(b) **Never aspirate: never remove the filter.**

(c) **Never inject into an epidural catheter without a filter.**

(d) **Do not administer a stronger concentration, a larger volume or a different local analgesic from that which is ordered.**

## PROVISION FOR THE SAFETY OF MEDICINES

**New medicines are subjected to rigorous tests** before being released for clinical use. Following the thalidomide tragedy in 1962, when hundreds of babies were born without one or more limbs, the Government set up a Committee on the Safety of Drugs. Every new drug is tested for activity, potency and toxicity: it is also tested on pregnant laboratory animals. The Committee reviews evidence regarding toxicity tests, as well as animal and human pharmacology.

### TERATOGENIC EFFECTS

**The fetus in utero is particularly vulnerable to the effect of medicines.** Some medicines that are harmless to the pregnant woman have an adverse effect on the fetus. A number of medicines cause fetal abnormalities (teratogenic drugs) and this occurs during the first 12 weeks of pregnancy (particularly the first 8 weeks) when the limbs, eyes, ears and other organs are forming: the child may be born with one or more limbs absent. Medicines found in the home, and considered innocuous, such as aspirin, mild sedatives, and anti-emetic medicines should be treated as suspect. It is prudent to assume that all medicines given to the pregnant woman are also given to the fetus: the placenta is not an effective barrier. **Only medicines prescribed by the doctor should be administered during pregnancy.**

### Potential mothers should be given instruction

Because the majority of pregnant women do not come under the care of doctor or midwife until after the 12th week of pregnancy, it would be a commendable prophylactic measure to give senior schoolgirls teaching in preparation for motherhood. They should be told about the thalidomide disaster so that they are aware of the danger of taking medicines in the early weeks of pregnancy.

### EFFECT OF DRUGS ON THE FETUS DURING LABOUR

It is well known that narcotic drugs such as morphine and diamorphine have a depressant effect on the fetal respiratory centre, so they are not administered to the woman in labour within 4 hours of the anticipated time of birth. Tranquillisers such as diazepam (Valium) and promazine (Sparine) have a hypotonic action on the fetus, the neonate is born limp, as well as being hypothermic and drowsy, so the dose given should be minimal. Lorfan may have a depressant effect on the fetus so the use of pethilorfan is not now advocated: pethidine is safer. Most hypnotic, analgesic and general anaesthetic drugs administered during labour have a restrictive effect on the initiation of respiration.

**Medicines given to the neonate** should be dispensed in paediatric doses by the manufacturer or pharmacist to avoid the errors that occur when calculations are made from adult doses.

**Midwives should be aware of the inadvisability of using some of the older stimulant medicines to initiate respiration,** e.g. nikethamide, Vandid and levallorphan. Naloxone (Narcan neonatal), an effective and much safer drug, is now preferred.

**Streptomycin and gentamicin in repeated or large doses may damage the auditory nerve** and cause deafness. The tetracyclines will stain the teeth yellow and may be toxic to the liver. Chloramphenicol is toxic to the preterm baby.

**When giving medicines to babies intramuscularly** the needle must be inserted on the slant and not at right angles; the tissues are shallow: periosteum and bone may be penetrated. To avoid injury to the sciatic nerve or hip joint, the upper outer quadrant of the buttock is preferred. The anterior area of the thigh may be used but the needle must point towards the knee to avoid penetration of blood vessels in the groin. Intramuscular injections should not be given into the arm of a baby.

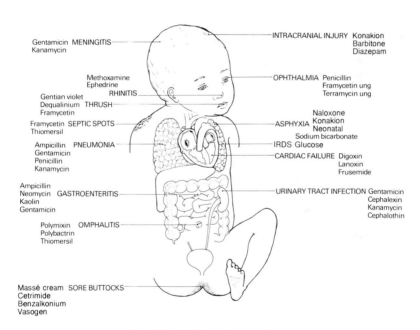

Fig. 44-2   Medicines for the Neonate

### DRUG INTERACTION

When two potent medicines are administered together, the action of one medicine may lead to an increase, reduction, or modification of the effect of the other medicine, e.g. monoamine oxidase inhibitors such as phenelzine (Nardil), will potentiate the action of drugs such as pethidine or morphine and may produce coma. Alcohol will increase the sedative effects of most central depressant drugs and in high doses may cause severe respiratory depression. It may damage the fetal brain cells during pregnancy.

## EXPIRY DATE OF DRUGS

Midwives should be vigilant in noting whether a liquid medicine, such as would be used for ophthalmia neonatorum, has evaporated: if so, the concentration of the medicine could have trebled. Serious and fatal accidents have happened when old solutions of nepenthe and of paraldehyde were administered.

Syntometrine must not be used after the expiry date stated on the label = 9 months after manufacture. It should be kept in a cool place. Light is harmful so the ampoules should be kept in the box and not exposed on a tray in the delivery room.

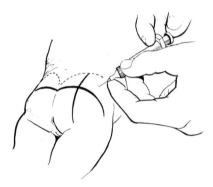

Fig. 44-3    Injecting upper outer quadrant

### PHARMACOLOGICAL AND PHARMACEUTICAL DRUGS

Pharmacological (approved) drugs have no capital letter, e.g. promazine, naloxone, methyldopa.

Pharmaceutical drugs, proprietory or trade names are written with a capital letter; sometimes italics are used, e.g. Sparine, Narcan, Aldomet.

# SYSTEME INTERNATIONAL d'UNITES (SI)

*(International System of Units)*

**A selection of facts re SI units that are of interest to midwives**

SI, an internationally agreed version of the metric system, has been used in scientific work and in industry since 1960. The British medical profession accepted the SI system of measurement in 1977 in order to unify and simplify practice in medical measurement and conform to the international system of measurement.

**Great care must be exercised during the period of change over to SI units in the administration of medicines** and in reading laboratory reports. In pharmaecutical work, changes involving SI units are minimal; metric measurements have been used by midwives in Britain for a number of years, and this has simplified the introduction of SI units:

**Medicines are administered** in milligrams, grams, and millilitres: intravenous solutions in litres.

**Babies are measured in centimetres,** weighed in grams. Adults are measured in metres and centimetres, weighed in kilograms.

**Temperature is recorded on the Celsius scale,** °C.

**In laboratory reports,** millimoles may replace milligrams, e.g. blood glucose is now recorded in millimoles per litre (mmol/l) instead of mg/100 ml. Bilirubin is recorded in micromoles per litre—micromole/l instead of mg/100 ml.

## SI BASIC UNITS

*There are 7 units that form the basis of the SI system*

| PHYSICAL QUANTITY | SI UNIT | SYMBOL |
|---|---|---|
| **length** | **metre** | m |
| **mass** | **kilogram** | kg |
| **time** | **second** | s |
| **electric current** | **ampere** | A |
| **thermodynamic temperature** | **kelvin** | K |
| **amount of substance** | **mole** | mol |
| **luminous intensity** | **candela** | cd |

### THE KILOGRAM

*The kilogram is the basic unit of mass (2·2 lbs)*

**One kilogram** (kg) = 1000 grams (g). **One gram** (g) = 1000 milligrams (mg). **One milligram** (mg) = 1000 micrograms ($\mu$g). **The word microgram should be written out in full** to avoid misinterpretation of the $\mu$g symbol.

### THE METRE

*The metre is the basic unit of length = (39·3 inches)*

**One kilometre** (km) = 1000 metres.
**One decimetre** (dm)  = 0·1 metres (one tenth metre).
**One centimetre** (cm)  = 0·01 metres (one hundredth metre).
**One millimetre** (mm)  = 0·001 metres (one thousandth metre).
**One micrometre** ($\mu$m) = 0·000 001 metres (one millionth metre).

*There are 10 millimetres in one centimetre (as on a ruler).*

*There are 2·5 centimetres in one inch.*

### THE MOLE

**The mole is an additional SI Unit** and is the unit of 'amount of substance' (weight).

The reporting of analyses in clinical chemistry laboratories is now made in millimoles per litre mmol/l instead of milligrams per 100 millilitres (mg/100 ml).

**Conversion.** Serum glucose mmol/l × 18 = mg/100 ml.

**In laboratory work** the mole will replace mass units such as the gram and milligram. The mole will also replace the milliequivalent for certain constituents of intravenous fluids.

### Prefixes

**decimole** is one tenth of a mole (dmol/l).
**millimole** is one thousandth of a mole (mmol/l).
**micromole** is one millionth of a mole ($\mu$mol/l) (micromole should be written out in full).

### THE LITRE

**The litre,** which is a non-SI unit, is accepted as the reference unit of volume for all concentrations and cell counts.

**One litre** equals 1000 millilitres (ml).
**One litre** equals  100 centilitres (cl).
**One litre** equals   10 decilitres (dl).

**One decilitre** (dl) equals 100 millilitres (ml): haemoglobin is recorded in grams per decilitre (g/dl) instead of grams per 100 millilitres (g/100 ml): (g/dl and g/100 ml are similar in amount).

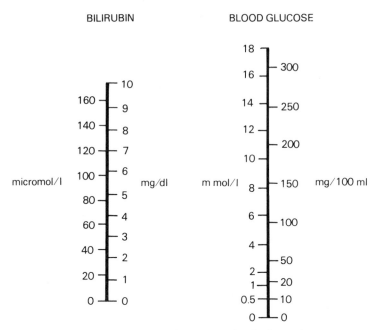

Fig. 44-4   Conversion of mg to mmol and micromols

*There are 18 derived units, three of which are of interest to midwives*

### (1) Celsius temperature scale (°C)

The centigrade temperature scale is now known as Celsius (°C) after the scientist who introduced it. Freezing point is 0°C and boiling point is 100°C.

### (2) Pressure

The action of force on an area has been given the name pascal (Pa). The partial pressure of blood gases $pO_2$ and $pCO_2$ are expressed as kilopascals (kPa) instead of millimetres of mercury (mmHg). 1000 pascals (Pa) = 1 kilopascal (kPa).

*Blood pressure continues to be measured in mm Hg; the change over to kilopascals will take place in a few years time*

### (3) The Joule (J)

This term, named after a famous scientist, is used in nutritional science for the calorie, and denotes the quantity of heat and energy released when food is utilised (burnt) by the body; or the heat and energy produced by fuel. The large or kilocalorie equals 4·184 kilojoules (approximately 4). 1000 joules (J) equals one kilojoule: 1000 kilojoules (kJ) equal one mega joule (MJ), which is one million joules.

## SUBMULTIPLES AND MULTIPLES

*These are denoted by the addition of prefixes*

| PREFIX | SYMBOL | SUBMULTIPLE | |
|---|---|---|---|
| deci | d | one tenth | $10^{-1}$ or $0 \cdot 1$ |
| centi | c | one hundredth | $10^{-2}$ or $0 \cdot 01$ |
| milli | m | one thousandth | $10^{-3}$ or $0 \cdot 001$ |
| micro | $\mu$g | one millionth | $10^{-6}$ or $0 \cdot 000\ 001$ |
| | | MULTIPLE | |
| deca | da | ten times | $10^1$ |
| hecto | h | one hundred times | $10^2$ |
| kilo | k | one thousand times | $10^3$ |
| mega | M | one million times | $10^6$ |

When dealing with large numbers, the zero figures are indicated as a raised number, $10^2$ (has 2 zeros) = 100; $10^3$ (has 3 zeros) = 1000; $10^6$ (has 6 zeros) = 1 000 000.

When the amount is less than one (a fraction) a minus sign is placed before the raised number, $10^{-2}$ = one hundredth $0 \cdot 01$; $10^{-3}$ = one thousandth $0 \cdot 001$; $10^{-6}$ = one millionth $0 \cdot 000\ 001$.

### SUBMULTIPLES

**Micro** is one millionth part, $0 \cdot 000\ 001$, e.g. microgram ($\mu$g); micromole ($\mu$mol); micro metre ($\mu$m).

**Milli** is one thousandth part, $0 \cdot 001$, e.g. milligram (mg); millimetre (mm); millilitre (ml).

**Centi** is one hundredth part, $0 \cdot 01$, e.g. centigram (cg); centimetre (cm).

**Deci** is one tenth part, $0 \cdot 1$, e.g. decigram (dg); decimetre (dm); decilitre (dl).

### MULTIPLES

**Kilo** is one thousand times. Kilogram (kg) = 1000 grams; kilometre (km) = 1000 metres; kilolitre (kl) = 1000 litres.

Midwives should be aware of the danger in confusing the symbols for microgram ($\mu$g) and milligram (mg). One mg (milligram) is the equivalent of 1000 micrograms: the symbol for micro being the Greek abbreviation $\mu$.

**The prefix micro should always be written out in full,** e.g. microgram, micromole, when prescribing or labelling drugs.

### POINTS TO BE NOTED

#### Plural units

The symbol for a unit does not have an 'S' added when plural. Kilograms = kg (not kgs). Decilitres = dl (not dls).

#### The use of small and capital letters

There is a vast difference between small and capital letters used as symbols. Capital 'M' is the symbol for Mega which is one million times. The small letter 'm' signifies milli which is one thousandth part: a millimole (mmol) is 1/1000th of a mole: a millilitre (ml) is one thousandth part of a litre. The small letters, kg, are the symbol for kilogram. The use of Kg, KG, or kG is wrong.

### The sign for 'per'

A sloping dash, /, is the sign for 'per', i.e. grams per decilitre = g/dl: millimoles per litre = mmol/l. The dash should be used once only in each unit: the small letter 'l' is used for litre.

### Decimal points

When denoting figures less than 'one', the decimal point should always be preceded by a zero; 0·5 (not ·5). Otherwise the dot may be ignored and 10 times the dose given. A period is not used following symbols for units, eg 0·5 (not 0·5.); 10g (not 10g.); unless to end a sentence.

### FAHRENHEIT TO CELSIUS CONVERSION TABLE

Celsius introduced the centigrade scale Freezing = 0 °C: Boiling 100 °C.
Fahrenheit: freezing 32 °F: boiling 212 °F.
To convert Celsius to Fahrenheit, multiply by 9, divide by 5, add 32.
To convert Fahrenheit to Celsius, subtract 32, multiply by 5 and divide by 9.

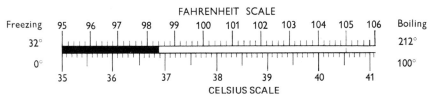

Fig. 44-5    Fahrenheit to Celsius scale

---

## QUESTIONS FOR REVISION

### *Drugs and SI Units*

**C.M.B.(Eng.) 30-min. question.** Name the drugs you may have to use in your midwifery practice, and give the indications for the use of each. What rule relating to the use of drugs does the Central Midwives Board lay down?

**C.M.B.(Eng.) 30-min. question.** What drugs may a midwife use during the course of labour? Give the (a) indications, (b) dosage, (c) method of administration in respect of each drug.

**How does a community midwife ensure safe custody of controlled drugs?** What is meant by the thalidomide tragedy? What is a teratogenic drug? At what period in pregnancy are drugs most likely to damage the fetus?

How are community midwives authorised to obtain pethidine? What is the procedure when a midwife wishes to surrender surplus pethidine? How do hospital midwives proceed when no doctor is available to prescribe pethidine?

**What are prescription only medicines (POM)?** and which are midwives permitted to administer?

**What is the Central Midwives Boards policy** regarding the administration of drugs by midwives? What does the midwife record in the Midwives' Drugs Book? What is a Midwives Supply Order?

**What is the responsibility of the ward sister regarding** (a) the custody of controlled drugs; (b) fluid medicines that have been in stock for a prolonged period?

**What precautions do you take** when injecting a drug i.m. to the neonate to avoid (a) the sciatic nerve; (b) groin blood vessels; (c) injuring periosteum?

**What are the hazards of adding drugs to intravenous infusion fluids?**

**Differentiate between:** (a) pharmacological and pharmaceutical drugs, which group requires a capital letter? (b) Natural and synthetic oxytocins: (c) Syntometrine and ergometrine: (d) Kilo, centi, micro, milli, deci.

### Give the symbol for

Kilogram (     ); litre (     ); milligram (     ); microgram (     ); millimole (     ); kilometre (     ); decilitre (     ); grams per decilitre (     ); millimoles per litre (     ); milligrams per decilitre (     ).

## How many

Milligrams in one gram (    ); micromoles in one mole (    ); grams in one kilogram (    ); millimetres in one centimetre (    ); centimetres in one metre (    ); decilitres in one litre (    ); metres in one kilometre (    ); millimoles in one mole (    ).

### SHORT C.M.B. QUESTIONS

**C.M.B.(Eng.).** Outline the procedure whereby the domiciliary midwife is authorised to possess and administer controlled drugs. How does the domiciliary midwife obtain a supply of drugs for use in her practice? Central Midwives Board rules regarding drugs. What is a midwife's drugs supply order? The drugs which a midwife may use in her routine work.

**Write notes on:** (Eng.) laws relating to drugs and the midwife. (Scot.) Syntometrine, Prostaglandins, Syntocinon. (Eng.) Controlled drugs. (Scot.) Midwife's Supply order form. (Scot.) Regulations regarding the storage of Controlled drugs. (Eng.) Regulations governing the use of Controlled drugs by midwives. (Eng.) The midwives responsibility for the safe keeping of Controlled drugs.

# 45
# Preparation for Childbirth
## by EXPERIENCED MIDWIVES

*The midwife a health educator. Preparation for labour. Planned course of instruction. Programme of 10 classes. Relaxation. Hypnosis. Rehearsal for labour. Keeping fit. Nutrition. Protect your unborn baby. Beauty hints. Breast feeding. Stork on the way. Rehearsal for analgesic gas. A word to the expectant father*

Expectant mothers today, having been subjected to mass media of communication on the subject of health education, including human reproduction, expect to receive information and advice that will equip them to approach and participate in the childbearing and rearing process happily and successfully. Their need is urgent. Many are aware of their inadequacy as future parents and are eager to attend courses of instruction: emotional problems and fears disturb their peace of mind; these should be clarified or dispersed.

Prospective parents are entitled to receive the necessary education from the professional group best qualified to provide this i.e. midwives.

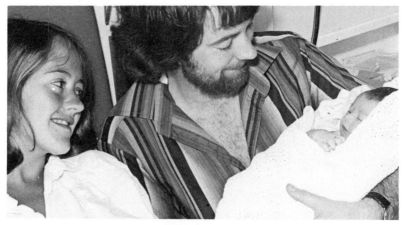

Fig. 45-1   Parents admiring their baby one hour after birth.
*Maternity Unit, Southern General Hospital, Glasgow.*

### CHILDBEARING TODAY

The birth process is easier and more successful than it has ever been. Improvement in the quality of infant life in Britain, is now apparent, due in some measure to monitoring by ultrasonic and electronic screening equipment, as well as diagnostic techniques and modern methods of treatment by obstetricians, paediatricians and midwives. Expectant mothers should be told this.

**Second and third pregnancies are the safest;** the first being the least predictable. The outlook is more favourable for the well educated woman who is more likely to obtain relevant information by reading as well as seeking and following professional advice. Midwives should make an effort to motivate and instruct the less intelligent mothers-to-be.

## THE MIDWIFE A HEALTH EDUCATOR

Midwives are licensed to give obstetric care to women during normal pregnancy, labour and the puerperium: teaching is an integral part of that care. Their expert knowledge of midwifery and vast experience in dealing with women during pregnancy and labour qualify them as unrivalled teachers of expectant mothers. Midwives must therefore be given, and accept, responsibility for this duty.

**The midwife understands the mothers' needs,** obstetrical, educational, social and psychological. To meet these needs she will arrange a balanced programme, no more time than is justified being devoted to any particular aspect. Although the subject of labour looms large on the woman's horizon and she has an insatiable desire to hear or talk about it, the wellbeing of the unborn and the newly born child is equally important.

**Family centred health education is provided by midwives** as a preventive, promotive and therapeutic service: the family being considered as a unit. Resources available through the health service for their physical and emotional wellbeing should be recommended when deviation from normal behaviour is apparent, such as marital maladjustment, alcoholism, incipient signs of baby abuse. The woman is referred to the agency equipped to render the appropriate therapy.

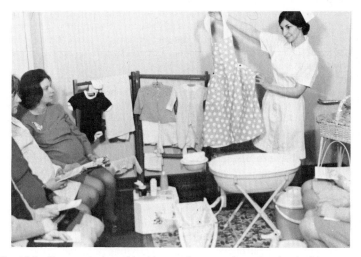

Fig. 45-2  Demonstration of bathing equipment—sister showing bathing apron.
*Mothercraft Department, Royal Maternity Hospital, Rottenrow, Glasgow.*

Midwives have always given individual instruction to their patients at prenatal clinics, in hospital and in the home; they should continue to do so. But individual teaching, although useful, is limited in scope and often confined to prescribing the remedy for some minor ailment. Organised group teaching is modern and preventive in outlook; it covers a more comprehensive field and is economical in teaching time. Certain aspects in preparation for childbirth and early parenthood the midwife may delegate to other members of a team who are qualified to contribute to the welfare of mother and child but she must assume team leadership: hers is the key role: arranging and organising the programme, teaching the obstetric subjects and applying the subsidiary information given by other groups to the obstetric situation.

## PSYCHOPHYSICAL PREPARATION FOR LABOUR

Midwives have in the past, by their kindly manner and understanding care, unknowingly employed psychophysical techniques, giving the woman sympathetic support and enabling her to achieve satisfaction in coping with the stresses of labour in a serene and dignified manner. They have, however, tended to rely to a greater extent on the pharmacological method for relief of pain but the midwife with vision will realise that she must actively participate in the prenatal teaching of psychophysical techniques if women in labour are to achieve emotional satisfaction and adequate pain-relief.

**There is no mystique or miraculous element in any of the methods** of preparation including psychoprophylaxis, nor is there any justification for adopting a fanatical degree of fervour which demands absolute adherence to the minute details of the procedures taught.

*The psychological principles are:*
### SUGGESTION    DISTRACTION    CONFIDENCE AND ASSURANCE

**Suggestion** is extensively used in hypnosis, which is a trance-like state: but suggestion could be used by midwives without carrying it to the stage of hypnosis. The hypnotised woman feels no pain when her hand is pricked with a needle, because it has been suggested to her that her hand is numb. This proves the influence of the mind over the body. If the midwife uses a persuasive manner and a pleasant tone of voice the expectant mother becomes more receptive to the teacher and to what she is being taught.

During pregnancy the midwife's attitude influences the expectant mother's approach to childbirth and when labour-ward midwives have the opportunity to meet the women whom they will eventually be looking after, their competent bearing and proficiency in describing the management of labour gives assurance. During labour, the friendly welcome, the calm unhurried manner suggest kindliness and competence; encouraging remarks *re* progress suggest a successful labour. Midwives are well aware of the power of suggestion; hypnotic drugs having no analgesic effect are alleged by patients to relieve pain.

**Distraction** is probably the most powerful and the most widely used factor. Awareness of pain is reduced when attention is diverted by listening to an engrossing radio programme, by looking at some interesting performance or by doing something, i.e. house-work, knitting.

Midwives will utilise harmless distracting activities, e.g. the radio, television, companionship. Controlled breathing with a sighing expiration is one of the most helpful distracting activities used in labour today (see p. 743).

**Confidence** is a psychological state stemming from knowledge and experience and is an excellent antidote to fear. Every method of preparation for childbirth makes use of giving instruction that will enable the woman to comprehend the processes of pregnancy and labour in so far as they will affect her. Talks, demonstrations, films, visual aids and discussion should all be used to instruct the expectant mother. Giving assurance to the woman is a means of instilling confidence in her ability to cope with the childbearing and rearing situation.

#### THE WOMAN'S EMOTIONAL REACTION TO LABOUR

Every woman is entitled to approach the emotional aspect of childbirth in her own way: no person has the right to pontificate to another individual as to how she ought to feel or behave during labour. How a woman reacts to the pain of labour or feels towards her newborn baby depends on the type of person she is, her attitude to love, marriage, motherhood and to life in general. Not all have the emotional endowment to glorify the pain of labour and to interpret it as being pleasurable, nor to find enrichment in the process. The majority of women describe what they feel during a uterine contraction as pain. The use of the word 'contraction' for 'pain' does not lessen the sensation the woman experiences as pain. If she is led to expect a painless labour she reacts very badly when she feels pain whether it has been described as tightening, hardening or discomfort. The modern idea is to use the word 'pain'. Everything possible should be done to enable women to have as comfortable a labour as is possible, and to achieve emotional satisfaction.

None of the exponents of psychological methods today promise a painless labour but women can be helped to cope with pain. Many of the techniques employed are designed to lower the receptivity of the cortex of the brain to painful stimuli: they raise the pain threshold. Persons with a low pain threshold would feel acute pain from a pin prick; those with a high pain threshold would scarcely notice it.

## PLANNING A COURSE OF INSTRUCTION

### Aims of the Course

A. *Physical and Mental Health Education*

**To give instruction** on how to achieve the physical fitness, by healthy living and good nutrition, to produce a well-formed, mature vigorous child without depleting the mother of vital body-substances.

**To provide sympathetic assurance** and understanding, aiding the woman in the enjoyment of a serene outlook during pregnancy, in labour and in caring for her child.

**To give suitable advice** regarding the fears and anxieties that disturb prospective parents, often due to lack of knowledge.

B. *Preparation for Childbirth*

**To employ modern means of communication** in presenting the appropriate methods of coping with the stress of labour: providing practice class demonstrations of exercise, relaxation, rhythmic breathing and labour positions.

**To inform** regarding the elementary processes of childbearing, giving also a brief explanation of some common deviations from normal to enable the woman to approach labour in an enlightened, confident manner.

**To assure** regarding the provision of emotional support, kindly professional companionship and supervision and the use of modern means of pain relief during labour including epidural analgesia.

**To integrate the instruction** given during pregnancy with the realities of labour by permitting labour ward midwives to participate actively in the teaching programme.

Induction and acceleration of labour are now commonplace, so to avoid apprehension when an intravenous drip is set up or the cardiotocograph used, it would be expedient to show these. Parents recently questioned stated that they would prefer to see obstetric forceps. (Wrigleys would be suitable, see Fig. 45–3.)

Admitting the woman in labour into a room with electronic equipment without having given her previously some information and explanation of their function and benefits is unwise. Visiting the labour ward and intensive care nurseries during pregnancy has an assuring influence.

C. *To arrange for and give instruction in Baby Care.*

D. *To discuss subjects that concern inexperienced parents,* e.g.

State benefits, budgeting for baby, family planning, family relationships and responsibilities.

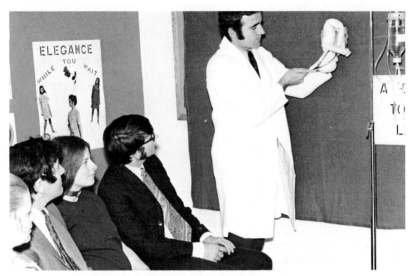

Fig. 45-3　Obstetrician showing low forceps, also intravenous drip to induce labour.
*(Parents were consulted and expressed great interest.)*
*Maternity Hospital, Stirling.*

**The midwife who is alert to current tendencies** is aware that some mothers-to-be wish to be consulted regarding certain aspects of childbearing. If expectant mothers knew of the high maternal, fetal, and neonatal death rates that occurred when the majority of babies were born at home, they would appreciate the safety of modern maternity hospitals. There, doctors and midwives are experienced experts; using electronic monitors that safeguard the quality of maternal and fetal life, mental as well as physical.

**Midwives should be eager to explain the benefits of the procedures women object to,** such as hospital delivery, drip induction, episiotomy, fetal monitoring. Discussion groups would provide an excellent medium for spreading greater optimism among pregnant women.

## TEAMWORK AND CONTINUITY

**To ensure integration and continuity** between what is taught during pregnancy and practised during labour it is imperative that instruction regarding childbirth should be given by midwives. Labour ward midwives only, should apply relaxation techniques concerning labour because they understand the physiology and management of labour and can speak with the authority of sound knowledge and practical experience.

Without continuity in teaching, the woman in labour cannot effectively carry out the instruction she has been given at prenatal classes. The labour ward midwives are deprived of the opportunity to give the necessary emotional support and physical relief.

**10 CLASSES OF 2 HOURS**

| Member of Team | No. of Classes | Length of class |
|---|---|---|
| Obstetrician | 2 | 30–40 minutes |
| Organising Sister | 10 | 30–40 ,, |
| Labour Ward Sister | 4 | 30 ,, |
| Nursery Sister | 4 | 30 ,, |
| Postnatal Sister | 2 | 30 ,, |
| Health Visitor | 2 | 30 ,, |
| Physiotherapist | 4 | 30 ,, |
| Dietitian | 1 | 30 ,, |
| Social Worker | 1 | 30 ,, |
| (Discussion and Tea) | 10 | 20 ,, |
| | | **20 hours** |

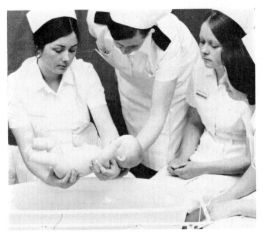

Fig. 45-4   Mothercraft sister teaching student midwives how to demonstrate baby-bathing to expectant mothers.

*Aberdeen Maternity Hospital.*

**An obstetrician would be present at the first class to explain** (1) the physical and emotional changes during pregnancy, (2) what is done at the prenatal clinic, (3) avoiding drugs and infections. Following the tea break he could talk to husbands while Sister demonstrated a model layette to the expectant mothers.

Ten classes, each lasting 2 hours with a 20 minute discussion and tea break, would be ideal. Four subjects could be taught at one session by different people. Demonstrations of baby care, exercises, relaxation, require little mental effort; if the talks are short and given in a bright, chatty style, interspersed with opportunities for comments and questions, the mothers-to-be should not suffer mental fatigue. If a film depicting baby's birth is shown it should be the culmination of visual teaching during which parents are gradually introduced to and prepared for viewing a photographic presentation of the birth process. To some women this may be an emotionally traumatising experience when they personally are approaching a similar event. Married couples are sometimes so distressed that they leave the room. A permissive attitude regarding attendance should be adopted. A tour of the labour wards and normal baby nurseries is usually enjoyed and the staff on duty should be prepared to talk to the mothers-to-be and show the facilities available, e.g. admission room, analgesic gas machines, electronic monitoring equipment, intravenous drip for induction of labour. Fathers should be encouraged to attend.

### TIMING THE CLASSES

The need for one class, not later than the 8th week of pregnancy, is urgent in order to warn expectant mothers of the dangers in taking drugs not prescribed by the doctor. They must also be told to avoid contact with certain infectious diseases such as rubella and could be advised regarding good food and the prevention of anaemia, minor disorders, and baby's layette. This early class could be held in the evening once every month and husbands invited to attend. The other nine classes could start at the 20th week, and in order that they are not completed too soon, they can be given every two weeks until the 36th week. Special evening classes should be arranged between the 20th and 28th weeks for those who go out to work. Duplication of classes will be necessary. A number of maternity hospitals in Great Britain give classes, 12 times per week. Expectant mothers will undoubtedly attend if the talks are enjoyable and instructive.

### PROGRAMME OF 10 TWO-HOUR CLASSES

#### *(With Discussion during 20-minute Tea Break)*

| Subjects | Minutes | Lecturer |
|---|---|---|
| **1. At 6 Weeks** | | |
| What happens at the clinic and during labour. Avoiding drugs and infections. | 40 | Obstetrician |
| Keep fit—walk tall. Minor ailments. The expectant father. | 40 | Sister in Charge |
| Baby's layette. | 20 | Nursery Sister |
| **2. At 20 Weeks** | | |
| Childbirth never so good. The womb and baby growing inside it: fashionable maternity wear. | 40 | Sister in Charge |
| Waiting for the stork. How we will help you. Controlled breathing. | 20 | Labour W. Sister |
| Limbering up: posture, relaxation. | 30 | Physiotherapist |
| **3. At 22 Weeks** | | |
| Baby's outward journey. False and true labour. | 30 | Sister in Charge |
| Dress baby for comfort. Nappies new and old. Handling and dressing baby. | 30 | Nursery Sister |
| Good food: food supplements. | 20 | Dietitian |
| Exercises: posture: relaxation. | 20 | Physiotherapist |
| **4. At 24 Weeks** | | |
| Budgeting for baby. Equipment needed. Words heard at the clinic. | 30 | Sister in Charge |
| What to expect during and after labour. | 30 | Obstetrician |
| Stork on the way: coping with pain: relaxation and controlled breathing, monitoring equipment. | 20 | Labour W. Sister |
| Exercises: posture: relaxation. | 20 | Physiotherapist |
| **5. At 26 Weeks** | | |
| The first and second stages. Positions for relief of backache. Epidural. | 20 | Sister in Charge |

| Subjects | Mintues | Lecturer |
|---|---|---|
| Equipment for baby. Positions for bathing. Why baby cries. | 30 | Nursery Sister |
| Family relationships and responsibilities: safety in the home. The Child Health Clinic. | 30 | Health Visitor |
| Posture: lifting: relaxation. | 20 | Physiotherapist |

**6. At 28 Weeks**

| | | |
|---|---|---|
| Induction of labour: labour positions: baby's birth, analgesic gas. Bonding | 40 | Labour W. Sister |
| Breast feeding. | 30 | Nursery Sister |
| Maternity benefits: State help. | 20 | Social Worker |

**7. At 30 Weeks**

| | | |
|---|---|---|
| Twins. Breech. Caesarean birth. Relaxation. Controlled breathing. The new father. | 40 | Sister in Charge |
| Demonstration of bathing baby: baby care. | 40 | Nursery Sister |
| Baby and you in hospital: reasons for routine. | 20 | Postnatal Sister |

**8. At 32 Weeks**

| | | |
|---|---|---|
| Planning baby's day. Registering the birth. | 30 | Sister in Charge |
| Rehearsal for labour. Why be afraid? | 30 | Labour W. Sister |
| Health visitor will call. Attending baby clinic. Immunisation. | 30 | Health Visitor |

**9. At 34 Weeks**

| | | |
|---|---|---|
| Family planning. | 10 | Sister in Charge |
| Tour of hospital. | 40 | Sister in Charge |
| Bottle feeding. | 40 | Nursery Sister |
| Taking things easy at home. Attending for post-natal examination. Postnatal blues | 20 | Postnatal Sister |

**10. At 36 Weeks**

| | | |
|---|---|---|
| Film of labour. | 30 | Sister in Charge |
| Your views aired: your questions answered. | 30 | Two of the Lecturers |

Fathers are invited to attend: evening classes will be held.

## SCHEME FOR TEACHING EXPECTANT MOTHERS

In the following scheme, drawn up for practising midwives, a number of procedures are incorporated which have been used in psychophysical preparation for childbirth. Only techniques that are obstetrically safe and physiologically beneficial have been selected. Experienced midwives are perfectly capable of instructing expectant mothers in all the simple procedures necessary in preparation for childbirth.

*The procedures are:*
### EXERCISES, ACTIVE RELAXATION, CONTROLLED BREATHING, POSITIONS FOR LABOUR

In the past a great deal of time and energy has been expended carrying out exercises in preparation for labour. They may have some psychological value in that the woman is doing something that she expects will help her. As a means for limbering up and keeping fit during pregnancy they are admirable but there is no proof that they have any beneficial effect on the course or the outcome of labour.

Midwives are aware that the pelvic joints are in a relaxed state due to endocrine action during pregnancy; strenuous pelvic rocking could therefore overstretch relaxed ligaments: hyperextension of the spine is not advocated. Pelvic floor exercises will not prevent lacerations nor improve the performance of the pelvic floor during labour; they are beneficial in the postnatal period to tone up a relaxed pelvic floor.

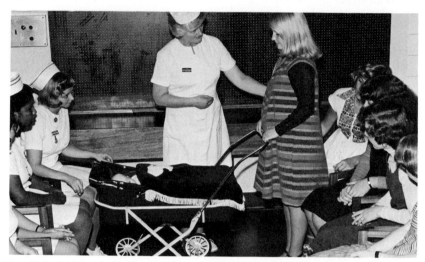

Fig. 45-5  Pushing the pram; The back ought to be straight and the tendency to bend forwards resisted. Elbows are held close to the body. Arms and hands should be relaxed and the handle grasped lightly, not clutched in a tense manner. The pram handle is kept close to the mother's body. The shoulders are relaxed and held back and down, chest raised and ribs expanded sideways to facilitate deep breathing.

*Maternity Hospital, Bellshill, Lanarkshire.*

### The Talk as given to Expectant Mothers

**'You will want to look and feel fit for baby's birthday** so we will show you a few simple exercises to limber up your joints and muscles, improve your circulation, and give you a feeling of wellbeing. Good posture enables you to cope with the discomforts that occur in pregnancy due to alterations in your balance: as your abdomen grows larger and heavier you will tend to lean back too far and to walk in a slouching fashion, even to waddle, instead of carrying your baby with poise and grace. Bad posture gives rise to low backache, aching limbs and feet as well as general fatigue. You must first of all walk tall, feel tall, hold your head high and show you are proud to be pregnant . . .. Relax your shoulders, hold them back and downwards, not stiffly. You will of course, have to hold your shoulders back to maintain your balance but don't overdo this. Gently straighten your knees . . .. Stand with your feet 22 cm apart, toes pointing straight forwards; don't lean back on your heels . . .. Take in a few deep breaths now, expanding your ribs sideways without raising your shoulders . . .. Will you now take a dozen steps? Swing your legs from the hips, lean slightly forwards and propel your weight from your heels on to the balls of the feet and tips of the toes. Don't clamp each foot down as a solid mass: walk with a lilt in your step.'

### LIMBERING UP STIFF JOINTS

**Feet.** 'Sit down and take off your shoes. Let the outer edges of the feet rest on the floor, curl your feet and toes; relax—repeat 6 times.'

**Ankles.** 'Stretch your leg forwards and rotate the foot in an inward direction six times, then with the other foot in an outward direction—6 times. Stand tall, rise on tiptoes and lower six times: then raise and lower alternate heels. This exercise will strengthen your arches for the extra load you are carrying.'

**Arm swinging.** 'Stand tall, stretch your arms forwards and upwards while raising yourself on tiptoe: lower arms in a backward direction, lower heels—repeat 6 times.'

**Shoulder rolling.** 'Stand upright, finger tips on shoulders. Raise and swing shoulders backwards with a circular movement slowly; reverse movement in forward direction—repeat 6 times.'

**Spine rotation.** 'Stand with head high: arms outstretched at shoulder level: turn head and body to left, keeping the knees pointing forwards: then turn to right.

# RELAXATION

Less time is spent teaching relaxation today, since accelerated labour lasts 8 to 12 hours in many cases and epidural and other forms of pain relief are utilised.

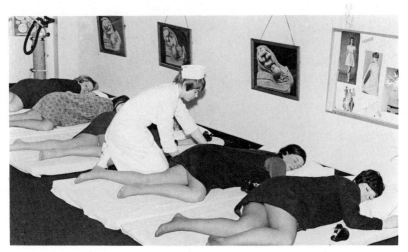

Fig. 45-6   Labour Ward Sister with relaxation class.
*Simpson Memorial Maternity Pavilion, Edinburgh.*

### *The Talk as given to Expectant Mothers*

*The midwife speaks quietly using a low pitch and soothing tone:*
'Today we will consider how to relax your body and your mind in preparation for a tranquil labour. Later you will learn about, and practise active relaxation.'

#### PASSIVE RELAXATION

'Will you lie down on your left side, the position you may use during the first stage of labour . . .. Place one pillow for your right knee and ankle to rest on: pull the end of the head pillow down and forwards . . .. Bring your under arm in front with forearm across the chest. Bend your right leg at the knee and place knee and ankle on the pillow.

'Get yourself into a really comfortable position: we will begin relaxing at the head and work downwards. Close your eyes gently, smooth all the wrinkles from your brow, relax your scalp ... allow your lower jaw to sag but keep your lips closed lightly, let your tongue be limp . . .. Loosen the muscles of your neck and let your shoulders droop, at ease . . .. Allow your back to sink into the mattress, . . . relax your rib cage and the muscles of your abdomen. This is important as it will play some part in lessening labour pain. Slacken the muscles of your buttocks and thighs . . .. Let your knees and ankles go limp as they sink into the mattress, wriggle your toes then think of them as being lax and floppy: feet 25 cm apart.

'Breathe quietly and you will soon feel drowsy.' (The midwife should silently pass from one to the other testing for tension by gently lifting elbow or fingers. . . .) 'Sit up slowly because when you are so completely relaxed you might feel faint if you jumped up quickly . . .. Will you practise relaxing like this at home? And do concentrate on relaxing the abdominal muscles. At the next class we will practise active relaxation and the positions for the late first and the second stage of labour.'

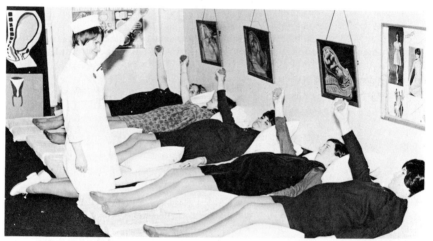

Fig. 45-7 Labour Ward Sister demonstrates squeezing a tennis ball to simulate the contracting uterus (in pregnancy) while relaxing voluntary muscles.

*Simpson Memorial Maternity Pavilion, Edinburgh.*

### ACTIVE RELAXATION

The method of active relaxation requires that the woman shall be mentally alert during labour, usually concentrating on some distracting activity such as controlled breathing. Active relaxation must never be carried to excess or the woman in labour becomes exhausted, as has occurred when women under psychoprophylaxis have used forced breathing for 12 hours, refusing sedation and remaining awake during that time. Sedative and analgesic drugs should be administered as required. It is quite unnecessary to insist on the woman remaining alert between contractions: there is no reason why she may not close her eyes and relax. The midwife will rouse the woman when she feels the uterus contracting, in time for her to relax actively before she experiences pain.

**To simulate a uterine contraction** the expectant mother grasps and squeezes a tennis ball (or a ball of newspaper) with her arm extended, for 60 seconds; while maintaining all her voluntary muscles in a state of relaxation.

When a woman in labour concentrates on the rhythm of her breathing, which should be at her own normal rate, it becomes a distracting activity that helps to take her mind off the pain she experiences. Many women have stated that 'The Breathing' was the most helpful agent in relieving pain. To make rhythmic breathing more purposeful to the woman it is described to her in detail. She is asked to breathe in through her mouth and to accentuate the expiration which should be audible like a sigh with a 'pooh' sound, made by the lips. This soothing sound seems to have a calming effect and is a psychological, harmless, distracting activity. Natural rhythmic breathing must not be confused with the type of breathing at abnormal levels and rates advocated by certain groups: research has proved these to be harmful to both mother and fetus. Women in labour frequently breathe more rapidly at the acme of a contraction but should be advised not to do so. Persistent rapid breathing or breath-holding is usually a sign of panic.

Slow deep breathing can, by hyperventilation, induce alkalosis with an increase in the pH of maternal blood and a lowered serum calcium which produces fetal acidosis. Tingling of fingers occurs which may proceed to carpopedal spasm and even tetany. Rapid shallow breathing or panting is only tracheal and, as very little air reaches the lungs, hypoventilation occurs and the fetus may be deprived of oxygen. In cases of placental dysfunction or incipient fetal distress the effect of panting could be harmful. Panting is not now practised. To counteract any contra-indicated expulsive effort, the woman can be taught to open her mouth and throat (*to avoid closing the glottis*) and to accentuate inspiration rather than expiration. This type of breathing can also be used during the actual expulsion of the baby's head.

### ACTIVE RELAXATION–WITH RHYTHMIC BREATHING

#### *Talk as given to Mothers*

'First we will repeat the method of physical and mental relaxation you learned at the previous class, using a tennis ball for an imaginary contraction of the uterus . . .. Now we will practise active relaxation during which you will remain mentally alert, concentrating on rhythmic breathing. This type of relaxation is very good when the labour contractions are strong. . . .

'Will you all lie on your backs now with a wedge, or two pillows, to prop up your head and shoulders, and one pillow under your knees. Have your feet about 30 cm apart, toes pointing outwards, all muscles relaxed . . . . Let us now practise the special type of controlled or rhythmic breathing.—"Breathe in" naturally through your nose and mouth . . . you will relax better by breathing with an open mouth. Concentrate on the rising of your relaxed abdominal muscles as you "breathe in" and the falling of them as you sigh your breath out with a soft soothing "pooh" sound made with your lips like this . . .. I will time your breathing at an average rate of about 18 per minute—in—out, in—out. . . .

'We will now practise breathing during a labour contraction while holding the tennis ball . . . squeezing the ball gently at first then harder and harder. A contraction is starting now! Breathe steadily in and out; let me hear the "pooh" sound. Relax all your muscles except the arm that is holding the ball. Gradually reduce your grip . . .. We will repeat that.'

## POSITIONS IN LABOUR

**'Let us now rehearse the positions you will adopt during the first stage.**

'In the second stage you may be lying on your back using rhythmic breathing during contractions; resting and relaxing between them. The midwife will tell you when a contraction is starting so that you can be alert and ready to cope with it.

When the time for pushing arrives you will be lying propped up on two foam wedges and a pillow; you will then adopt a special position at the beginning of each contraction; flex your legs at the hips and knees, widely separate them and with your hands grasping the thighs under the knees, raise your legs; at the same time bend your spine forwards, chin on chest. Take one or two deep breaths, close your mouth firmly, tighten the throat muscles (close the glottis) hold your breath and push (bear down). You will be inhaling gas and oxygen and you may take another quick breath of gas and push again so long as the uterus is still contracted . . . . One sustained push is more effective than a series of short ones.

'**Towards the end of the second stage you will have a very strong urge to "push"** when baby's head descends on to the pelvic floor: but you must not bear down until the midwife tells you to do so. To counteract this desire to "push", open your mouth and your throat, relax the muscles of your neck: concentrate on "breathing in" deliberately, rather than on "breathing out", do not use the "pooh" sound. The second stage of labour is not as painful as you might expect: with every contraction baby descends a little farther until he is ready to be born.

'We will practise the second stage position now using the tennis ball and the analgesic gas mask. . . .'

### Birth of baby's head

'To enable baby's head to be born easily you must relax your pelvic floor at the time the head is actually being born. The perineum will be fully stretched, but don't worry, it will have a numb feeling. You will have a tremendous urge to push but this is where your training in relaxation enables you to be in control and to refrain from pushing. Keep your mouth and throat open and breathe as described previously. If you pushed baby's head out quickly your perineum might tear.'

#### HYPNOSIS

**This is a trance-like state** produced in the person who is willing to co-operate with the hypnotist. Through the power of suggestion the threshold for the perception of pain is raised; the degree of hypnosis used in obstetrics does not place the woman under the complete dominance of the hypnotist; she is rendered more responsive to suggestion and co-operates more willingly. Midwives could use suggestion without carrying it to the hypnotic state. During pregnancy the woman can be told: (a) that the instruction she is given will enable her to control her reaction to pain; (b) that uterine contractions have a beneficial function, each one bringing the baby nearer to being born.

**A soothing and pleasantly monotonous tone of voice** and a persuasive manner are necessary to induce a tranquil frame of mind and engender a receptive attitude. The midwife's attitude during pregnancy should be optimistic, suggesting that all is well, instilling confidence without being assertive. During labour the midwife's calm, competent bearing radiates confidence, encouraging remarks *re* progress suggest a successful outcome. Midwives are well aware of the power of suggestion, e.g. that a placebo relieves pain as do hypnotic drugs that have no analgesic properties.

---

## KEEPING FIT DURING PREGNANCY

A woman ought to look after her health during pregnancy for her own sake, but she is much more likely to do so for the sake of her baby. In order to appeal to expectant mothers the subject should be presented in such a way that the welfare of the baby predominates.

In a very elementary manner a few facts regarding the embedding and development of the ovum could be taught. Simple illustrations showing how the baby is sheltered and nourished for nine months will interest the woman of average intelligence; such information being given only to stress the fact that the growing baby is dependent on the mother's food, on the fresh air she breathes and on her good general health.

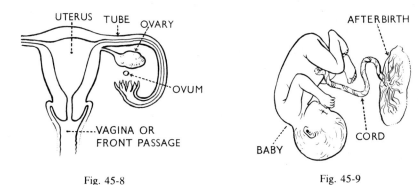

Fig. 45-8                                         Fig. 45-9

### The Talk as given

'Everyone knows that babies need good food and fresh air after they are born, but do you realise that babies need these before they are born as well? Babies get milk and vitamin drops to make them healthy and strong, so if you take these foods now, the baby growing inside your body will also get the benefit of them.

'We see babies out in their prams, getting fresh air, but baby needs oxygen before he is born, too, so take him out for an airing every day, rain or shine. On sunny days sit in the garden or go to the park. The baby inside the uterus gets all the substances he needs for growth and good health from his mother's blood, and these substances in her blood come from the food she eats. If your meals contain the necessary body-builders, calcium, iron and vitamins, baby will get them too and he will be strong and vigorous. Just think of the gardener for a moment. To ensure hardy plants he sows the seeds in well-prepared soil in a sunny garden. He tends the growing plants by watering them and keeping the weeds in check. He knows he won't get a good harvest otherwise.'

#### HOW YOUR UNBORN BABY GROWS

'**Your baby grows from two tiny cells,** no larger than the point of a fine needle, until he weighs about 3·2 kg (7 lb) on the day he is born. He obtains his food during this time without having to swallow or digest it, and gets oxygen without having to breathe. Both food and oxygen pass from mother to baby along the umbilical cord, which you see in the diagram is attached to baby's navel at one end and to the afterbirth at the other.

'The afterbirth or placenta, is a mass of tissue which can be likened to the roots of a plant. These roots are embedded in the wall of the uterus, and by penetrating the small blood-vessels of that organ they absorb from the mother's blood the necessary food and oxygen.

'**Body-building foods are needed for baby's growth and vigour:** they include meat, fish, eggs, cheese and milk. You should have one of these at each of the three main meals. To give baby strong white teeth and straight limbs drink 1200 ml (2 pints) of milk every day. If you want your infant to have rosy cheeks when he is three months old, give him iron now; take the iron tablets we have given you and eat foods such as liver, wholewheat bread and green vegetables. But we must think of you as well as baby. If you don't replace what baby is taking from your blood, you will become weak, easily tired and breathless, with no energy for housework, shopping and recreation.

'An expectant mother should feel better than usual, except for the little ailments such as morning sickness and heartburn; pregnancy isn't an illness, and life shouldn't become drab and the carrying of a baby a burden. Plan your work so that you have time to rest and to go out. Get yourself maternity clothes, so that you will enjoy walking out of doors, even during the last month. Wear sensible shoes to prevent backache, and I would recommend a maternity belt or corset during the last three months to give extra support.

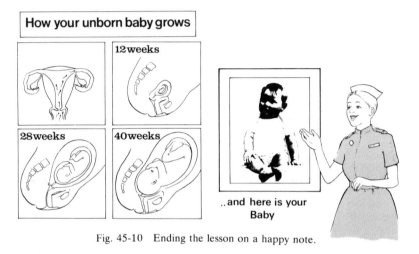

Fig. 45-10   Ending the lesson on a happy note.

'Go to bed early, so that you will have nine hours' sleep. During the last three months you will get tired towards the end of the day, so lie down for an hour after the midday meal.

'Be sure that you bowels move every day. Drink plenty of water and eat fruit and vegetables. If you are constipated, take a mild laxative, such as Senokot.'

### SEE THE DOCTOR REGULARLY

'There are early signs by which the doctor can tell that things are not as they should be although you may feel perfectly well. Notify the doctor or clinic if you are ill and cannot attend. Do what the doctor advises. If he suggests more rest there is a reason why you should have it. If you are told to come into hospital but you feel you are needed at home, remember that this advice is in the interests of your baby and your family as well as yourself. We want you to bloom with good health in readiness for your baby's birthday. If you do, you won't get so tired during labour; you will have a better supply of breast milk; on getting up, you will feel stronger, ready to enjoy looking after your baby, family and home.'

## FAMILY CENTRED NUTRITION

The teaching of nutrition to expectant mothers is an essential part of prenatal care. Many pregnant women are malnourished although few are underfed; they are anaemic and flabby, some overfed with the wrong kinds of food. Many women have no knowledge of the foods that are beneficial or even necessary for the pregnant woman. Although the midwife may be aware of what constitutes a well-balanced diet and has scientific reasons for advocating certain foods, the factors that influence people in their choice of food and methods of cooking must be kept in mind, otherwise she is less likely to persuade expectant mothers to improve their dietary habits. The primigravida may have acquired poor dietetic habits during adolescence so she must be given advice to safeguard the nutritional wellbeing of the fetus in utero.

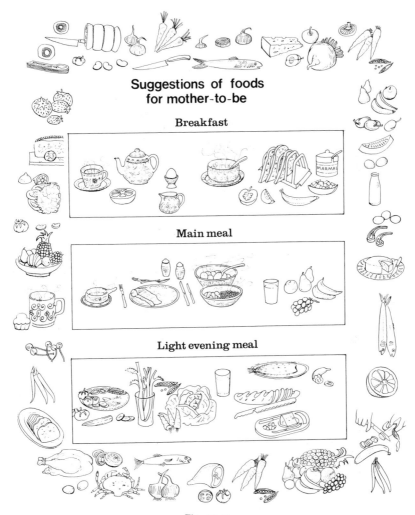

### Suggestions of foods for mother-to-be

**Breakfast**

**Main meal**

**Light evening meal**

Fig. 45-11

The food eaten in different countries varies according to climate, foods available, and custom. But even in a land such as Great Britain where a variety of foods is available, factors such as tradition, geographical location, religion, race, intelligence, education, social and economic status may influence the choice of food.

Married women in industry have increased the demand for processed, tinned and quickly prepared articles of food. All women should be taught more about what constitutes an adequate wholesome diet and how to plan and cook nutritious appetising meals for their families.

The midwife is well aware of the functions of food and a few facts could be passed on to mothers, e.g. body-builders such as meat, fish, eggs, milk, cheese are needed for the health and growth of all the tissues of the body including the ovum and sperm from which the baby develops. During pregnancy body-builders are needed for the growth of baby, the mother's uterus, blood and breasts.

Carbohydrates such as bread and potatoes are reasonably cheap, readily available and satisfying, but they contain little of the vital body-building food factors. Savoury foods are mostly proteins and although they are preferred because they appeal to the palate, unfortunately, they are expensive and that fact cannot be ignored. Midwives should recommend beans, lentils, peas, wholemeal bread: cheese, eggs and the cheaper fish should be utilised to replace meat which is too costly for many families. Vegetables contain the essential minerals but are not so appetising but women must be persuaded to eat them because of the minerals and vitamins they contain. Fortunately, many body-building foods are also rich in minerals and vitamins, e.g. liver, eggs, milk, cheese. Proteins, iron, calcium and vitamins are the important constituents of food for the pregnant woman and she must be convinced of the need for these for her husband and family.

## HINTS ON TEACHING NUTRITION

Telling a woman to take a nourishing diet has little educational value, for each woman will have a different conception of what constitutes a nourising diet. She may consider macaroni, ice-cream, cakes with cream filling to be highly nutritious, yet they contain no protein. Ambiguous terms such as 'good', or 'plenty', ought to be avoided.

**Food should be discussed in terms of meals** rather than proteins, carbohydrates, fat and calories. The women can visualise and understand food values better when the food under discussion is what is served at meal times. The statement 'three cooked meals a day' conveys immediately the idea of the body-building foods we advocate. Breakfast should be discussed, and kidney, eggs, bacon (not salty), fish, high quality sausages can be recommended. (*Many packaged cereals have little food value other than the sugar and milk added to them.*) The need for a daily helping of meat, liver, chicken or fish at least 113g at the main meal should be stressed. Vitamins and minerals will be contained in the potatoes and green vegetables served with the meat. Raw or stewed fruit should be advocated in preference to greasy suet puddings or very sweet desserts. Suitable supper dishes can be suggested which incorporate eggs, cheese or fish and salad.

**The need for iron should be introduced on every possible occasion** and by giving talks on subjects such as:

| | |
|---|---|
| **Feed baby before birth.** | **Beauty hints for mothers-to-be.** |
| **Why mothers are anaemic.** | **Eat wisely for baby's sake.** |
| **Meals for ladies-in-waiting.** | **Keep fit during pregnancy.** |

The harmful effect of excessive salt in the diet should be explained: foods high in salt mentioned and condemned. Merely giving a list of foods to be taken or avoided does not constitute a well-rounded lesson.

### TEACHING AIDS

A cooking demonstration would be appreciated by the primigravid women who have limited experience in housewifery. Fresh foods should be displayed in preference to models which tend to look drab. Salads are always colourful, attractive, and give vitality to the demonstration; new salad recipes should be introduced. A bottle of milk should be on display as a constant reminder of the baby's need for calcium.

Posters are valuable visual aids. Cut-outs from the glossy magazines can be used to lend a gay tint of colour to the talk-demonstration. Trays can be set with an ideal breakfast, lunch, dinner or supper. (*It is better to depict what is good rather than what is bad.*) Body-building foods for one day. Foods rich in iron. Foods that keep weight under control.

## EAT THE FOODS THAT KEEP BABY AND YOU FIT

### *The Talk as given to Multiparous Women*

'It is always mother who "does without", whether it is food, clothes or leisure. She is so busy providing father with good meals because he works hard; giving the children her share because they are growing fast and always hungry. But the expectant mother is the most important member of the family. Baby depends on you for the food he gets before birth. He grows from a speck the size of the point of a needle until he is a sturdy infant weighing 3·2 kg (7 lb). If you don't take in your diet the foods baby requires, he will rob your body of the substances he needs, and you will become anaemic and tired. Baby gets his rosy cheeks at your expense so try to provide the food needed to keep baby and you strong and healthy.

'Baby requires, body-building foods, iron and calcium (*lime*). Body-builders are foods such as meat, chicken, liver, eggs, milk and cheese: any one of which you should have at the three main meals. They are the only foods that build tissue (*or flesh*). Starchy foods and fats produce heat and energy and when taken in excess make you fat.

'600 ml of milk contains one fifth of your needs in body-builders. If you are overweight skim off the cream which is only fat and is not a body-builder.'

### HAVE THREE COOKED MEALS EVERY DAY

#### 'For breakfast

'Bacon (not salty), egg, fish, or high grade sausages. If you can take porridge and milk also, so much the better; the crisp cereals contain less body-building substance.

#### 'For the main meal

'Have 113 g of meat, liver, chicken or fish every day without fail. You won't take too much: few people could afford to eat more than they need of body-builders, as these valuable foods are expensive.

#### 'At supper time

'Take another egg, fish, cheese or blood sausage.'

### *The Need for Iron*

'Iron is the next most important substance needed by the mother-to-be. So many women are anaemic (bloodless) and this makes them feel tired and breathless. You need extra iron during pregnancy to supply iron for baby and for the additional blood you have to make for yourself at this time. During the years that you are having your babies you are very liable to become anaemic. That is why the doctor gives you iron tablets, but foods rich in iron are needed too.

'Women lose blood during menstruation and there is always the unavoidable loss of blood at childbirth. Baby takes iron from you for his own blood and he also stores up a supply for the first three months of life for the milk he will get has no iron in it. Having three or four babies quickly, especially twins, is a terrific drain on the mother's supply of iron. Six slices of wholewheat bread gives you half of your day's supply of iron. Liver is best of all, but red meat, blood sausage, green vegetables, prunes and raisins are very good.'

## PROTECT YOUR UNBORN BABY

**As soon as your baby is born** the first thing you will probably ask, after being told 'boy or girl', is likely to be 'Is he/she all right?' Of course we hope your baby will be beautifully healthy and perfectly formed, but occasionally a few, (about two in every 100) are born with a physical defect; some minor, others more serious.

**We want to advise you** how you can help to avoid such disappointing happenings. Remember that your unborn baby gets his needs for growth and health from you. The food you eat is digested and then absorbed into your bloodstream. It passes through the placenta and goes to baby by the umbilical cord.

**Make up your mind to eat fresh wholesome food.** Baby needs the protein that is present in meat, poultry, fish, eggs and cheese to build a sturdy body. You should have protein in two meals every day. The calcium in milk helps to form strong bones and good teeth, so drink at least one pint daily. Fruit and vegetables will supply the minerals and vitamins needed and iron is very special for rosy cheeks. The vitamins found in most of the foods I have mentioned will help your baby (and you also) to bloom with health.

### FRESH AIR

No doubt you are planning to buy a pram later on so that baby can be outside every day in the fresh air. Think of baby now; he needs fresh air and will benefit from the sun that shines on you. You will both benefit from a daily outing so take him to the park or for a walk in the suburbs every day, rain or shine.

### REST

**Be sure to take sufficient rest** especially during the last three months. Lie down for an hour or more after the mid-day meal for a 'shut eye': avoid late nights and try to have 9 hours in bed at night. Rest helps to keep down your blood pressure and ensures a good flow to the uterus of blood from which baby gets nourishment and oxygen.

If you lead a healthy life you are more likely to have a vigorous baby: it is well worth making the effort.

### *The Cause of Defects*

**During the first 12 weeks of pregnancy** and particularly before the 8th week, baby's organs are forming. As you would expect, they are tiny, delicate structures especially the eyes and the heart. Their normal growth can very easily be disturbed by drugs and infections: expectant mothers should know about these and try to avoid them.

### AVOID MEDICINES

**When taken by the pregnant woman during the early weeks,** certain drugs can slightly or seriously affect the unborn child. You may have heard of the thalidomide tragedy that occurred in 1960–1962 when hundreds of babies in Germany and in Britain were born without one or both arms or legs because their mothers took the drug thalidomide as a sedative or for sleeplessness or to treat morning sickness. All drugs must now be tested rigorously to ensure that if given to pregnant women they will not harm the fetus. You need not worry about this; doctors are very reluctant to prescribe drugs at all in early pregnancy and only when they are absolutely necessary and safe for mother and fetus. Even simple drugs, commonly found in the home (aspirin, or drugs for morning sickness) are suspected of harming the fetus. **Do not take any drug whatsoever unless your own, or the clinic doctor prescribes it.**

### AVOID INFECTIONS

It has been proved that infections such as rubella and influenza affecting the pregnant woman, can seriously harm (*a*) the eyes of the fetus and cause cataract, even blindness; (*b*) when the ears are damaged the baby is born deaf; (*c*) if the fetal heart is damaged the baby will have heart disease and (*d*) if the brain is affected the baby may be mentally handicapped. Over 200 babies in Britain are born damaged by rubella every year.

Of course, you will try to prevent these disasters. Ideally every schoolgirl should have her blood tested for rubella antibodies and if they are absent she should be vaccinated against rubella. At the prenatal clinic the expectant mother's blood is tested but if rubella antibodies are not present she will not be vaccinated until after the baby is born.

**Pregnant women should avoid persons who are suffering from rubella.** Tell your doctor should you come in contact with someone who has the disease. Termination of the pregnancy is usually considered advisable by obstetricians when rubella occurs during the first three months, if the parents agree that this should be done. This is legal to avoid the risk of a malformed baby.

### SMOKING

**Nicotine retards fetal growth;** even 5 cigarettes per day will harm the fetus. It causes premature labour and small babies do not tolerate labour well and are more difficult to rear. Smoking also causes an increased risk of abortion and stillbirth, when the woman is a heavy smoker: baby's mental capacity may be reduced. You are strongly advised to give up the smoking habit—which is really drug addiction or nicotine dependence, but if you find this is impossible, then severely reduce the number of cigarettes you smoke. When you go home with baby, and if you and your husband are both smokers, baby will have to breathe your exhaled cigarette smoke. This is not good for his lungs or health nor is it fair to subject an infant to a polluted atmosphere. For the sake of baby's health as well as your own, give up smoking.

### ALCOHOL

Take very little alcohol: it has a harmful effect on fetal brain cells and may retard baby's intelligence.

## BEAUTY HINTS FOR LADIES-IN-WAITING

The title of this talk will no doubt appeal to the younger group of expectant mothers, but its real purpose is to stress health rather than beauty, with emphasis on nutrition. The midwife will find it well worth while going to some trouble in order to demonstrate the foods that are of value to pregnant women. Young inexperienced housewives will appreciate being shown new ways of preparing meals, and the aid of a dietitian would be invaluable: cookery classes could be arranged. The parentcraft teacher should stress that green vegetables and citrus fruits aid the absorption of iron.

### Teaching aids

Posters of sturdy babies should be on view, and will enable the midwife to correlate the mother's health and the baby's welfare. The colourful salad mentioned in the talk should be freshly prepared and exhibited, as well as a tray of foods rich in iron and a bottle of milk, vitamin and iron tablets. These are shown to the class as they are mentioned.

### *The Talk as given*

'Of course you are thrilled to be one of the fortunate "ladies-in-waiting." Let me assure you that the expectant mother can be more beautiful than ever, so banish the thought that you will be less attractive just because you are going to have a baby. There is something radiant in the glowing cheeks, sparkling eyes, and natural red lips of the healthy, happy mother-to-be. Remember too that if you are blooming with good health, you will feel fit and enjoy your pregnancy. Don't forget that the baby you are carrying also gets the advantages of your aids to beauty; the nourishing food, the vitamin tablets, the fresh air and sunshine. Motherhood is the crowning glory of a woman's life, and your body at this time does its utmost to help you to produce a sturdy infant, so if you do your part you will be amply repaid in every way.

'I'd like to recommend nature's lipstick. You get it in foods that are rich in iron, such as liver, meat, eggs, wholewheat bread and green vegetables; the tablets the doctor orders for you are a great help, but the iron in food is better still. Fresh air and sunshine are also needed to make the red blood which gives that rosy glow to your cheeks. Iron is a substance you must take a great deal of when you are pregnant, because your baby removes a tremendous amount of it from your blood during the last three months. The reason for this is that baby's food after he is born, whether it is your milk or cow's milk, contains very little iron; baby therefore stores the iron that he takes from you and uses it during the first four months of life, until he is given foods rich in iron, such as egg yolk. Your supply must therefore be sufficient for baby's needs as well as your own.'

#### CLEAR SKIN AND BRIGHT EYES

'If you would have a clear skin drink at least two glasses of water daily; flavour it with fruit juice for a change. Your complexion will be dull and pasty if you become constipated, but if you take plenty of fresh vegetables and fruit, as well as the water I have already mentioned, your bowels should move every day. For bright eyes we recommend fresh fruit and vegetables with their health-giving vitamins and minerals. Have you ever tried vegetable salad during the winter months? Raw carrot, turnip and beetroot are delicious when grated; add raisins to the carrot if you like, and arrange each vegetable separately in the salad bowl. Finely shredded raw cabbage is excellent if you add sufficient salad dressing to it. Chopped apple, with a sprinkling of crushed walnuts, well mixed with mayonnaise makes a very special salad, and if you add a little celery the flavour is quite delightful. Try it sometime. These foods are excellent for baby and you.

'**Do drink 1000 ml (2 pints) of milk every day;** use it for puddings; add cocoa, Ovaltine or any flavour you choose if raw milk doesn't appeal to you. Cheese is also a rich source of calcium. Your nails may tend to break off at the tips; this may well be because baby is taking a big share of the calcium (or lime) from your body to build for himself strong, straight limbs and a fine set of teeth. Milk is a rich source of calcium.

'Tone up your hair by five minutes of scalp massage and 100 brush-strokes at night. Many expectant mothers complain that their hair is dull and lifeless, but this occurs when they are not replacing, by taking nourishing food, the substances baby is taking from their bodies. A permanent wave doesn't always "take" well during pregnancy, so it might be better to wait until three months after baby is born.'

#### GOOD POSTURE

'**The biggest change is, of course, in your figure,** but there is no reason why you cannot carry your precious burden with grace and dignity. Good posture is the first essential; head erect, chest raised, shoulders well back without lifting them, and the lower abdomen drawn in. An uplift brassière will support the breasts which become so much heavier and have a tendency to sag.

'A maternity "roll on" makes the pregnancy less noticeable, and the support it gives during the later months prevents backache and the tired feeling some women complain of. Do wear sensible shoes with a moderately low heel; extra support is required because the arches of your feet are carrying an additional load. Looking lovely and at your elegant best depends greatly on the clothes you choose, but good posture enables you to wear them with poise and style.

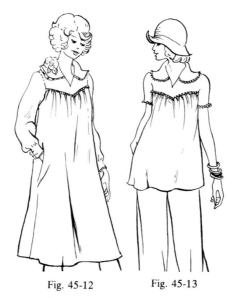

Fig. 45-12      Fig. 45-13

*Courtesy of Vogue Pattern Service.*

### ATTRACTIVE CLOTHES

**Modern maternity wear is wonderfully flattering** to those with great expectations. There is no reason why the mother-to-be should not be graceful and attractive while pregnant. Simple uncluttered lines are best.'

'**Suitable maternity garments are a necessity, not a luxury,** and should be comfortable as well as becoming. You can then enjoy the same outdoor recreation as any other woman, so long as the games are not too exciting or strenuous. Crease-resistant nylon tricot print dresses are flattering to the figure. Dicel dresses are practical for housework, gay coloured floral ones you can wear at parties.

'For wear in the mornings flared slacks with an expanding waistband or velcro fastening overlap in ribbed polyester or acrylic jersey with a shirt top in knitted polyester are popular with the trim, young mothers-to-be. The simple flared pinafore dress, coordinated with a gay contrasting jumper or check blouse is excellent from the fourth to the seventh month. Straight coat dresses are splendid for the tall girl but they are very revealing after the sixth month. Avoid front button-up dresses'; they tend to gape later on. A Crimplene machine-washable non-iron dress with mandarin collar is a useful standby. Long-sleeved blouses team-up well with polyester and cotton pinafore dresses. Woven twill or stretch slacks with flared leg line are ideal for the expanding waist-line. Kayser maternity tights with adjustable waistband can be worn with short dresses of printed Crimplene. A gay scarf with a jaunty bow takes the eyes of passers-by away from coming events. For good camouflage you can't improve on the box-jacket and the flared coat.

'You need not wear maternity clothes until the fifth month. If you put them on too soon, you will be tired of them before the end of the ninth month, when you can't wear anything else. Pregnancy itself is an aid to beauty, for this new experience enriches your personality and gives to your face an expression of tranquillity and happiness. The understanding and tenderness shown by your husband helps to produce the serenity of mind which is so essential at this time, and which enhances the natural beauty of the lady-in-waiting.'

# BREAST FEEDING

### *The Talk as given*

'**Everyone agrees that breast milk is the best food for babies** and more mothers are now breast-feeding their babies. There is no danger of the baby getting too much salt as can happen when giving dried milk. The babies have fewer illnesses during the first year and recover better from the ones that do occur.

'The baby snuggled at the breast enjoys the warmth, the cuddling, the physical nearness of his mother. This induces a contented frame of mind, which, if it becomes a habit, may lay the foundation of a happy disposition. And what satisfaction it gives a mother to be aware that she is so necessary to her infant, for one of the joys of motherhood is to be needed. She sees her baby thriving on food she has produced, and knows she is giving her child a good start in life.

'From your point of view it is more convenient, for there are no bottles and pans to wash and no feeds to be heated at 06.00 hours in the morning. Breast feeding completes the process of childbirth and helps to restore your figure to what it was before you became pregnant.'

#### GOOD FOOD IS ESSENTIAL

'To ensure that you will have plenty of milk for your baby, start now. During these waiting months you should be having body-building foods, such as milk, eggs, fish, poultry and meat. They are the foods that help to produce milk.

'After baby is born you need the same good diet, but two other things are then important in helping to keep up a good supply of milk. These are calmness and sufficient rest. Make up your mind to take life easily for a week or two until baby and you have got the food question nicely settled. Shut your eyes to all the things that need polishing, and enjoy being lazy for a week or two. If he is your first baby, you may feel a little flustered with the responsibility of looking after your precious infant. Learn all you can about babies, but don't worry whatever you do. The health visitor will advise you and you can also attend the child health clinic.'

#### DIFFICULTIES CAN BE OVERCOME

'There may be a few difficulties to overcome during the first few days, but you will be helped with these when the need arises. Rarely does the breast-milk upset baby, any difficulty that occurs is due to the method of feeding: it is possible that baby may take the milk too quickly or take too much. On the other hand, you may not have enough at first, but all of theses things can be put right. To prevent your nipples from getting sore, we will show you how to look after them before baby is born.

'You may imagine that you will have to curtail your interests and pleasures outside the home if you breast-feed your baby, but that really isn't so. During the first six weeks you will be resting more anyhow, and by that time baby will be on four-hourly feeding, and you can enjoy a visit to friends or the theatre within that time. Persevere and you will succeed in giving your baby the food nature intended for him, as well as the contentment he enjoys when cuddled at his mother's breast.'

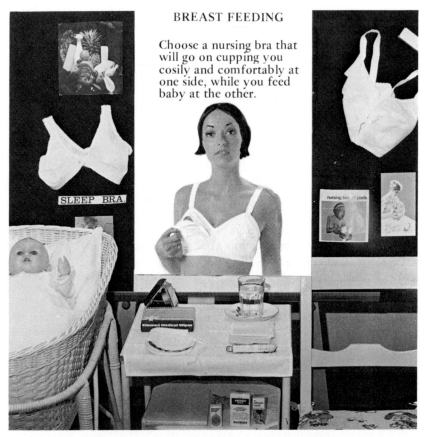

**BREAST FEEDING**

Choose a nursing bra that will go on cupping you cosily and comfortably at one side, while you feed baby at the other.

Fig. 45-14   Display for discussion on breast feeding.
Doll in cot to demonstrate breast-feeding position and bringing up wind. Comfortable nursing chair. Various nursing bras, including one by Mothercare. Clock, glass of water, feeding bib, tissue wipes, tube of Masse cream, pads to cover nipples. *Lower shelf:* children's vitamin drops; Abidec.

*Royal Maternity Hospital, Rottenrow, Glasgow.*

## STORK ON THE WAY

### *The Talk as given*

'You are looking forward to the important day that lies ahead, your baby's birthday. This is not the day of hard work that was common 20 years ago. So much can be done to make things easier for you during labour.

'Here is a drawing of the uterus; this is the baby, lying head downwards in the bag of water which has protected him during pregnancy. You can see baby's cord attached to the afterbirth. The neck of the uterus protrudes down for about 2·5 cm into the vagina or front passage. Note that the opening into the uterus is closed and sealed with a plug of mucus. When labour starts, the neck of the uterus opens up and the plug of mucus escapes, with a slight staining of blood. That bloodstained mucus we call the "show", and you will see it a few hours before or after labour begins; it is one of the signs of labour.'

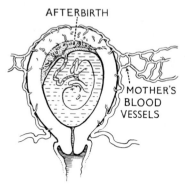

AFTERBIRTH

MOTHER'S BLOOD VESSELS

Fig. 45-15

### HOW TO KNOW LABOUR HAS BEGUN

'There are three signs that labour has started, but don't wait for all three before sending for the midwife or coming to the hospital. We want to be with you from the beginning of labour, to help you as much as we can.

' **"Show"** we have already mentioned.

'**Breaking of the bag of waters.** The bag of waters usually breaks some hours after labour has begun, but it may do so earlier. There is no pain when this happens, and perhaps only a slight trickle of water will come away.

'**Hardening of the uterus** you can feel by placing your hand on your abdomen, and is accompanied by a feeling of abdominal discomfort. These contractions begin so gently that you won't realise you are in labour until you notice that they are coming regularly, probably every 15 minutes. Often there is backache as well, but not always. The contractions stretch and open up the neck of the uterus until it is large enough to allow the baby's head to pass through it. This stretching or dilating period is known as the first stage, and occupies the whole of labour, except for the last hour or two. If the contractions are weak, labour will be slow, and you would, of course, expect a big baby to take longer to be born than a small one.'

### False Labour

'You may be wondering about false labour, which is fairly common during the last weeks. In that case you won't have any "show"; the contractions are irregular and longer than true labour contractions which seldom last more than one minute. False pains may be due to colic, so make sure that you have a daily bowel movement during the later weeks of pregnancy, even if it means taking a mild laxative. If you are in doubt or think you have started labour, come to the hospital, especially if it is not your first baby. Certainly come if the contractions are strong, or if they are returning every 10 minutes or more often. And don't forget that you may start labour before your expected date. If you go beyond your date the doctor may give you a "drip" to start labour.'

'When labour starts, your external parts are washed and shaved or clipped. Then you will be given a suppository or a small enema and a shower or bath. You may be given a "drip" during labour and one of the various modern appliances may be attached to baby's scalp or to your abdomen. The "drip" stimulates your uterus to function well and the monitors keep a check on baby and you. All is well—no need to worry. You are getting the benefit of modern science for the safety of baby and yourself. You will be given something to ease the discomfort as soon as you really feel the need of it. If you attend the "preparation for childbirth" classes you will probably require fewer sedative drugs.

'Tell your husband or any near relative that they may come and sit with you, if you wish, during the first part of labour; bring a magazine to pass the time or you can listen to the radio or watch T.V. if you feel like it.

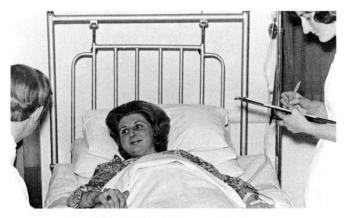

Fig. 45-16   Husband giving emotional support.
*Maternity Unit, Central Hospital, Irvine, Ayrshire.*

'One thing you should not do is to "bear down" until we have told you to do so. If you look at this diagram (Fig. 45-15) you will see that baby cannot get through the neck of the uterus until it is opened up sufficiently to allow him to pass. If you push too soon, the neck of the uterus hardens and won't stretch, causing you unnecessary pain and a longer labour. It is bad for baby, too. Towards the end of the second stage we shall ask you to hold your breath and push down, but only while the uterus is contracting. The muscles below (the pelvic floor) should be relaxed to make it easier for baby to be born, and you will be shown how to do this at the preparation for labour classes. Strangely enough, mothers usually complain less at this stage, and some prefer not to use the analgesia machine. But when you are drowsy from inhaling the analgesic gas you will experience very little discomfort and will certainly hear baby's first cry.

'Baby usually announces his arrival by a lusty yell, and you will experience a feeling of relief and great joy. He no longer needs oxygen and food through the umbilical cord; so it is tied and cut; now he will breathe and suck. Baby is wrapped in a warm bath towel and laid in a heated cot to rest after his intense participation in the experience of labour.

**Bonding.** You may want baby to be laid on your abdomen because some recommend this as a means of facilitating the bonding process. Remember that baby is wet and can readily be chilled: he has had a strenuous journey and needs warmth, quietness and gentle handling. You will love your baby very soon, if you haven't already created the bond during pregnancy.

'The after-birth comes away in about 5 minutes, then you are tidied up and given some food. You may feel tired but elated, so to make sure that you will have a sound sleep we usually give you a sedative. Baby's birthday is over: the little bundle is sleeping in his cot, and the majority of mothers say "it was well worth it" and "wasn't nearly as bad as I expected".'

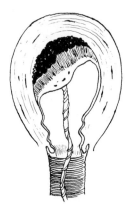

Fig. 45-17    Afterbirth separating from wall of uterus.

## REHEARSAL OF USE OF ANALGESIA MACHINES

*These are now used less frequently.*

### ENTONOX, TRILENE, PENTHRANE

#### The demonstration should be preceded by:

A talk on 'What happens during labour'. A course on tranquil labour. A tour round the labour and postnatal wards, and a glimpse of the babies.

#### THE PURPOSE OF THIS REHEARSAL IS:

To give the necessary tuition at a time when the woman is not distracted with pain or stupefied by drugs.

To reassure her regarding the safety and simplicity of the machine.

To make her familiar with the use of the mask.

To practise the various types of inhalation.

To gain her confidence and arouse enthusiasm for the analgesic gas.

Only the practical aspect of the subject should be taught and the mother's part in administration of the analgesic stressed. Much repetition will be necessary. Questions ought to be encouraged, but the midwife should tactfully keep them to the subject being taught. Teaching aids should be used, e.g. suitable illustrations of the birth canal. A machine similar to the one to be used during labour; extra masks for practice. Attractive pictures of babies and posters on health.

### The Demonstration as given

'You all want your labour to be as comfortable as possible, and we are eager to do what we can to help you. Today I am going to show you how you will use the apparatus during labour to relieve the sensation that some of you will call discomfort and others pain. This machine is perfectly safe for you and for baby. Not only is it simple to use, it is foolproof. The midwife is responsible for the working of the machine; all you have to do is to breathe in the analgesic gas.'

## ANALGESIC GAS AND ITS EFFECT

'The gas is easy and pleasant to take; it will make you feel calm and rather drowsy. It is not an anaesthetic, which is a substance that puts people to sleep and makes them unconscious. This gas is an analgesic, a substance that relieves pain without producing unconsciousness. If you decide that you don't want the gas, no one will force you to take it; it is there for your benefit, and doctors and midwives are only too willing that you should have it. Some mothers are very keen to be awake in order to hear their baby's first cry. I can assure you that under this gas you will certainly hear it, a sound that will fill your heart with joy. You won't miss anything at all; you will hear the midwife telling you when to inhale and when to stop, you will feel baby slipping out into the world, but it will be almost painless, so you can look forward to baby's birthday with pleasure.

'Here is the cylinder that contains the gas and oxygen; this piece of corrugated rubber tubing conveys the gas to the mask from which you will inhale. (During labour take care that you don't rest your arm on this tubing when you are inhaling gas or you won't get enough to be of any help.) We turn on the gas with this key, and it flows into the mask but it doesn't stream out as it does in your kitchen stove when you turn the gas on. You only get this gas when you actually inhale it (breathe it in).'

### THE USE OF THE MASK

'The mask you are holding is similar to the one you will use during labour; it has a broad and a narrow end. Place the mask on your face like this; the broad end is resting on my chin, the narrow end is on the bridge of my nose. Press the mask on firmly so that the rubber is in close contact with your face. Unless you do that, some of the gas will escape and you won't get the full benefit of it.

'As far as you are concerned all you have to do is to breathe in and out with the mask on your face. The midwife will know when a contraction is coming and she will tell you to inhale from the mask as soon as the uterus contracts, and that will be before you feel any pain. The contractions will not last longer than one minute, but it takes about 20 seconds, or eight deep breaths of gas before you get relief; that is why you must start inhaling before you feel the pain. Stop inhaling when the pain goes. You may be wondering what would happen if you kept on inhaling after the contraction had ceased, or for longer than one minute. You would become sleepy and drop the mask, so, you see, you cannot take too much gas.

'During the first stage of labour you can inhale the gas lying on your side or your back, whichever is the more comfortable. During the second stage, the midwife will tell you which of the two positions she prefers for baby's birth. Between contractions you will relax, but keep your mask beside you so that you can apply it again without delay.'

### *Practice*

'Will you lie down comfortably now, and practise using the mask without gas? One inhalation includes breathing out as well as breathing in. Breathe through your nose and mouth, and use your abdominal as well as your chest muscles. Take full, regular breaths. (The midwife sets the pace at 18 to 22 breaths per minute.)

'Put on your masks now, and when I say "Begin", start inhaling; keep time with me as I say, "In . . . out . . . in . . . out". When I say "Stop", remove your mask and relax.'

### SECOND STAGE (PUSHING) INHALATIONS

'When baby's head is just showing, the time has come when you can assist by pushing. You will know then that it won't be long until your baby is born. The neck of the uterus will have opened sufficiently to have permitted baby's head to pass through it, and the second stage will be well established. It is most important that you do not start pushing until the doctor or midwife tells you to do so. Pushing too soon will hinder rather than hasten baby's arrival, cause unnecessary pain, and may, later on, lead to prolapse of the uterus.

'The contractions will be coming every two or three minutes now. The midwife will "time" them and tell you to start inhaling about 20 seconds before the next contraction is due, in order that you will have enough gas in your body to relieve the pain while you are holding your breath and pushing baby downwards.'

### *Practice*

'When I say, "Begin", put on your masks quickly and start inhaling; keep this up until I say "Now". You will then take a quick breath, hold it, with lips tightly closed. Don't push here and now, you must only push when you are actually in the second stage of labour. At that time you will keep pushing without taking a breath for as long as you can, then you will take another quick breath of gas, and again push for as long as you can.

'When I say "Stop", remove your masks. During labour you may repeat the push twice; it all depends on how long you can hold your breath, but a long sustained push is more effective than a number of short ones. It may be necessary for you to push with each succeeding contraction for a period extending to half an hour with your first baby; then when baby's head is just about to be born the midwife will ask you to stop pushing and to breathe very deliberately.'

### DELIBERATE INHALATIONS FOR BIRTH OF BABY'S HEAD

'This type of breathing is only used for a matter of minutes, immediately before and during the birth of baby's head; the purpose being to prevent you from pushing, so that baby's head will emerge slowly and gently. If you pushed at this time, as you will feel very much like doing, the skin at the opening of the birth passage would tear, and stitches would be necessary. So, to avoid this, stop pushing and breathe deliberately with your mouth and throat open concentrating on breathing 'in' rather than breathing 'out' immediately your midwife tells you to do so. At the same time try to relax your pelvic floor muscles to allow baby to be born easily. There must be no lull between in and out or out and in, because if you breathe steadily without hesitating for one instant you will not push, and that is what we want. This is the time when you need the greatest amount of gas, and as you may be inhaling constantly, you will get the maximal relief. Another midwife usually helps you to hold the mask in position to make sure you are getting as much gas as possible. As soon as baby's head is born the mask is removed, but you will be deliciously drowsy. You will feel the baby's body slipping out quite painlessly. Very soon he will announce his arrival lustily, and you will be asking, "Is it a boy or a girl?" This for you is a very precious moment; your husband and you can admire him together.'

# A DATE WITH THE STORK

In preparing this talk, the instructions given should coincide with the requirements of the local maternity home or hospital. Suitable teaching aids are posters of attractive babies, fruit and vegetables, bottle of milk, iron tablets, nightdress for breast feeding.

### *The Talk as given*

'**As baby's birthday draws near** you may be surprised to find that you are eagerly looking forward to the big day that lies ahead. Do try to keep your thoughts on baby rather than on yourself. If you begin to think about your own labour, switch off immediately and dwell on the fact that thousands of babies are born, simply and easily, every day, and that having a baby is a natural event in a woman's life. Picture yourself tucking baby into his cot or wheeling the pram; happier thoughts. You will, of course, have been busy knitting, making or buying tiny garments for baby's arrival, and no doubt your husband and you have built many castles in the air regarding baby's future. But of all the preparations an expectant mother can make, none is more important than those for her own abundant good health.'

#### THE LAST FEW WEEKS

'**When your burden grows heavier** you will feel cumbersome and become more tired towards the end of the day; so do take things easily, get off your feet as much as you can, and go to bed early. You don't need to coddle yourself, for the woman who carries on with her housework has an easier and shorter labour than the pampered type of woman who treats herself as an invalid. During the last weeks the slight abdominal discomfort you may feel, cramp in your leg or a desire to pass water frequently, may be a bit tiresome, but they will soon pass. Keep your heart light, for it won't be long until baby is here; you will regain your slim lines and enjoy wearing your favourite frocks once again. You have, I hope, been taking the diet we recommended, one which includes 1,200 ml (2 pints) of milk, meat, fish, fruit and vegetables every day. Be sure to take your iron tablets, too, for baby and you both need a lot of iron during the last months.

'Do make sure that your bowels move every day, even if it means taking a mild aperient. We will, of course, give you a suppository or a small enema when labour starts, but it is better for you to have a regular motion every day until then.

'**Go out every day even if it is wet or cold,** so long as you are suitably clad. You need a change of scene as well as fresh air; the sight of other women wheeling their prams will remind you that very soon you will be doing the same.'

#### MAKE PLANS EARLY

'Make an effort to have all your arrangements completed before the end of the seventh month, for, as you know, babies do sometimes come too soon. Pack a small suitcase with the things you will need in hospital, or make out a list, for it isn't easy to think of what to take with you when labour starts at 02.00 hours. Your own dressing-gown, night dresses and slippers are always nicer than those the hospital can provide. Have two face cloths, so that one can be used for your face and breasts. By all means take cosmetics with you for afterwards, but for your own sake you should not apply lipstick, or nail-paint until labour is over. Your natural colour is a guide to the doctor or midwife as to how you are faring during labour. Take your purse and a little money with you for newspapers, telephone calls, or some item you may have forgotten to bring. Writing-paper and stamps you will almost certainly need.

Pack the case before you leave so that your husband won't have to search for them on that thrilling day when you are allowed to take your baby home.'

### STORK LATE IN ARRIVING

'Mothers often worry when the expected date arrives and the stork fails to appear. Don't let that disturb you, for babies rarely come on the exact date on which they are expected, in fact, half of the babies are a week late in arriving. It is, of course, possible that you have made a mistake in your dates. If you were taking the pill predicting the date of delivery is often difficult. Attend the clinic or your own doctor or midwife every week as usual; they will keep a watchful eye on your progress.

'**Let this, your first date with the stork, be a happy one.** Look forward to it calmly with a glow of anticipation in your heart, and when baby's birthday is over and he lies cuddled in your arms it will be one of your most treasured memories.'

## REHEARSAL OF LABOUR

This class should be a very practical one and not merely a recapitulation of all that has previously been taught on the physiology of labour. As far as is possible the woman's part in the procedure of labour should be rehearsed or explained; an effort being made by vivid word pictures—positions and practise-breathing to set the scene. The rehearsal should be patient-centred not procedure-centred. Likely happenings during the pre-labour days can be narrated, lightening and passing urine frequently being mentioned as a sign that baby is settling down into the pelvis in readiness for his outward journey. Advice can be given regarding the need for additional rest and how to avoid constipation.

Signs of false and true labour should be related to the woman as a person and what she ought to do; 'show' and breaking of the waters being described once more. They could be told about women inadvisedly waiting for the waters to break before leaving home, with resultant anxiety, or even birth in the ambulance. A reminder to have a case packed with toilet articles, etc., for hospital ready to avoid fluster should the call come suddenly during the night. What to do and when to come to hospital should be clearly explained, and time allowed for questions. Assurance should be given about the stork sometimes being late in arriving and the need to continue attending the clinic.

They are advised not to start rhythmic breathing at home: women become parched and tired when this is carried on too long. A brief résumé of what happens on arrival at the hospital is given: when husbands are to be present their helpful activities are discussed. A reminder is given about the need for sleep, and that the alleviation of discomfort by sedative drugs is all that is usually necessary during the first half of labour. All the labour positions, controlled breathing and holding the mask should be rehearsed. Relaxing the pelvic floor and the special breathing to counteract pushing during the perineal phase is practised. The gas and oxygen cylinder is put on view and a mask rehearsal given.

The midwife rounds out the lesson with additional comments and advice particularly concerning the actual birth. The third stage needs little description. To enlarge on the moment of joyous relief when baby is born and the thankfulness experienced when baby lies asleep in his cot is a happy note on which to end.

## CLASSES FOR HUSBANDS

**Too often the expectant father is made to play a minor or supporting rôle.** His feelings deserve greater consideration: he may be dubious as to how he will respond to the duties and responsibilities of fatherhood. He needs advice and encouragement. The average husband has little idea of what is required of him as an expectant father, but it is only reasonable that he should take an active interest in the subject of childbearing and have some knowledge of the physical and emotional demands it makes on his wife. During this century, men have been taking an increasing interest in the subject of childbearing and rearing. Mothers in the past may have been too possessive, but they should be advised to allow the father to participate in baby care from the very first weeks.

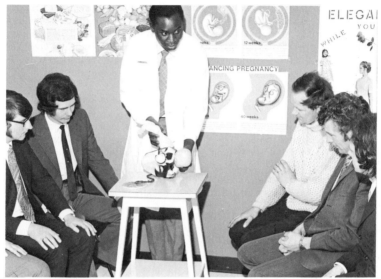

Fig. 45-18   Doctor giving talk on labour to expectant fathers.
*Maternity Hospital, Stirling.*

Midwives should arrange evening classes to which husbands are invited with their wives, teaching subjects such as:
**Keeping fit during pregnancy. The development of the baby before birth. What happens during labour. Family centred paternal care.**
They should not be encouraged to think of themselves as a small unique group but as modern sensible men. Some hospitals have classes for husbands after the evening visiting hour in pre- and postnatal wards.

## A WORD TO THE EXPECTANT FATHER

### The Talk as given

'The fact that you are attending these classes shows that you have an up-to-date outlook and are willing to share with your wife some of the responsibilities as well as the joys of parenthood. Women should not be expected to bear the whole burden of childbearing and rearing alone; your wife needs your help, encouragement and understanding.

**'If your wife is healthy and properly nourished she will feel well and enjoy her pregnancy;** a good diet is most important and it is quality rather than quantity that matters. During pregnancy the baby deprives a woman's body of vital substances, for a baby grows at the mother's expense. Unless your wife replaces these substances by having nourising food her body will suffer. Mothers are apt to neglect themselves, and to take what food is left after father and the children have been served, so you must see that she gets her fair share of body-building foods such as meat, fish, eggs and liver.

'**A well nourished woman stands up better to the stress of labour** and has more energy to look after baby and the home afterwards. Baby also benefits; he will be more vigorous when born, and will have fewer illnesses during the first year of life.

'Both baby and mother-to-be will profit from a daily outing; the change of scene will keep your wife more cheerful, she will enjoy her food, and sleep better. Of course she must have maternity garments in which she will feel less conspicuous; they are a necessity so do not grudge the money spent on them, for an expectant mother ought to enjoy a normal social life up to the last month.'

### Help as much as you can

'As the months wear on, your wife will be less able for the more strenuous household tasks. Assist her in turning heavy mattresses. If you already have an infant under 18 months old he will be heavy for your wife to lift, so do take care of him for a spell occasionally. See that your wife gets sufficient rest by lending a hand with the housework if extra domestic help is not available; otherwise you should not expect all the comforts and luxuries you usually enjoy at home.'

#### IRON IS VERY NECESSARY

'Baby, before birth, takes a great deal of iron from his mother's blood and unless your wife has a diet that is rich in iron she will become anaemic, feel breathless and tired; and pregnancy will be blamed for what is really due to anaemia. Liver is an excellent blood-forming food; encourage your wife to have it at least once a week. No doubt the doctor has prescribed tablets containing some form of iron, remind her to take them regularly every day.'

#### THE EMOTIONAL ASPECT

'There is no doubt that the nervous system is more sensitive during pregnancy, and especially with the first baby. Moods of depression may overwhelm your wife for no reason; she doesn't know why she is depressed, and on these occasions tears flow on the slightest provocation. There is no need to be dismayed at the prospect of such episodes, for they only arise very occasionally. It is simply futile to tell her to "snap out of it", and to ignore these moods is a subtle form of cruelty.

'The pregnant woman may seem unreasonable, and won't appreciate logical argument; she will more likely respond to tenderness and understanding. Help her to look on the bright side; planning some small treat or an outing will direct her thoughts into happier channels. The man who willingly and pleasantly gives his wife a cup of tea in bed during the miserable time of morning sickness is providing the best medical and psychological treatment for that condition. Every pregnant woman has vague fears—fear of pain, fear of the process of birth, fear of the unknown. Many of these fears are groundless, but to her they are none the less real. Her judgment is all tangled up in the web of her emotions, and she needs the stabilising influence of her husband's sound, well-balanced outlook.'

### CO-OPERATE WITH THE DOCTOR

'**See that your wife attends the clinic or her doctor regularly** and always uphold the advice she has been given; never suggest that it is unnecessary or that you do not approve. If, for example, your wife has been told to take extra rest, this may mean that her blood pressure is higher than it ought to be; it is most important that she carries out the doctor's instructions and I'm sure you will help her to do so. Your encouragement and sympathetic understanding at this time mean a great deal to her and will help to weld, even more securely, the marriage bond. Take an interest in the various activities arranged for expectant mothers at the clinic and encourage your wife to participate in them. The "Preparation for Childbirth" classes will help her to have an easier labour; at the course on baby-care she will be given advice on how to look after baby, and as you would expect, there is much to learn on that subject.'

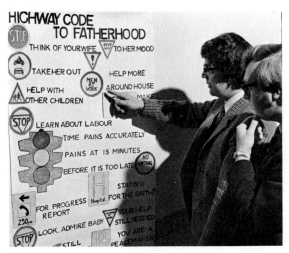

Fig. 45-19   Poster for expectant fathers.
*Maternity Unit, Central Hospital, Irvine, Ayrshire.*

### Learn about babies

**'It isn't fair to learn about babies by experience.** When studying baby care for the welfare of your own infant you will find this interesting subject absolutely fascinating. The information so gained will help to keep your child healthy and happy and the confidence such knowledge gives will enable your wife and you to enjoy your baby instead of worrying over your lack of experience. Learn about why babies cry and what to do in case you ever give in to the temptation to shake or spank your baby.

'A little knowledge and a lot of common sense will solve most of the simple baby problems, and a man is not as liable to panic over minor ailments as is the over-anxious mother. Take an interest in the preparations for the coming baby. Study catalogues of various makes of prams and learn about the good points to look for. It doesn't take much skill or ingenuity to make or remodel a few pieces of furniture and paint them in pastel shades. That is the sort of thing women appreciate.'

#### WHEN LABOUR STARTS

**'Don't expect your wife to go into labour on the exact day;** baby may arrive, one week, before or after the date given. There may be a few false alarms so I'll tell you the signs of true labour so that you can help to reassure your wife if she is in doubt. (These signs are well known to midwives and need not be repeated here.)

'Keep calm and help your wife to carry out the instructions she has been given at the clinic or by her doctor or midwife. As a rule there is no immediate urgency with first babies, but don't delay with subsequent ones as they sometimes arrive very quickly.'

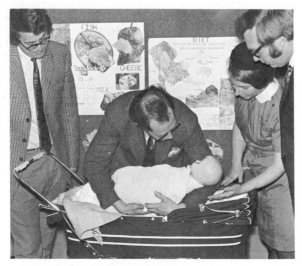

Fig. 45-20   Expectant fathers learning the correct 'hold' to support head and spine. *Maternity Unit, Central Maternity Hospital, Irvine, Ayrshire.*

### Should the husband be present at the birth?

'There is no valid objection if he can be of any assistance to his wife; his rôle is mainly a supportive one giving encouragement and emotional sustenance. In many hospitals in Great Britain, husbands are permitted to be in the labour ward while the baby is being born. They should not be made to feel that they ought to be present if this is contrary to their wishes.

'Watching the birth of a baby is an experience which may emotionally upset those who are closely related to the mother. The midwife's attention is concentrated on the two lives under her care at this critical moment and should not be diverted. The husband who intends to be present should attend classes so that he knows what to expect.

'It is, however, a matter of tradition as well as of personal opinion, but, the immediate safety of mother and baby should be considered. The parents should be permitted to decide and their wishes respected.'

---

## QUESTIONS FOR REVISION

**C.M.B.(Eng.) 30-min. question.** Outline a talk to expectant mothers on the importance of nutrition in pregnancy.

**C.M.B.(Eng.) 30-min. question.** What is the value of classes for preparation for childbirth and mothercraft? What subjects should be included in a series of such classes?

**C.M.B.(Scot.) 30-min. question.** Outline a plan for parenthood teaching.

**C.M.B.(Eng.) 30-min. question.** Outline a talk to expectant mothers and fathers on the effect of a first baby in a household.

**C.M.B.(Eng.) 30-min. question.** What is the value of classes in preparation for childbirth and parentcraft? What subjects should be included in a series of such classes?

**C.M.B.(Scot.).** How would you teach a woman and her husband to understand the processes of pregnancy and labour and the important things about the care of their newborn baby.

(N.Ire). Discuss the value of parentcraft education. Outline how you would plan a series of parentcraft classes for a small group of expectant mothers.

C.M.B.(Eng.). What is the value of a course of parentcraft instruction for expectant parents? What subjects should be included in such a course?

C.M.B.(Scot.). Outline a parentcraft talk in which you deal with the subject of the crying baby. Include the sources from which the parents may obtain help.

C.M.B.(Eng.). Discuss the scope and value of classes for expectant parents.

C.M.B.(Scot.). Describe a programme of health education in preparation for parenthood.

# 46
# Early Parenthood

*Budgeting for baby. A word to the new father. The layette. Napkins new and old. Handling, dressing, bathing baby. Health education: Advice to the ambulant woman, exercises and posture for the new mother. Preparing modified dried milk feeds. Planning baby's day. The crying baby. Sleep. Sore buttocks. Let father help. Sun baths. Standing and walking. Spoon and cup feeding, weaning, teething, potting. The toddler and the new baby. Prevention of accidents in the home*

### BUDGETING FOR BABY

The midwife ought to have some comprehension of housekeeping and budgeting and know the cost of equipment, such as prams, cots, baths, as well as the advantages and disadvantages of the various types, so that she is in a position to recommend articles at a suitable price to meet the needs of the different groups.

Expectant mothers may have been told what is required by neighbours or friends and be familiar with certain garments or articles; the teacher should not underestimate their knowledge and common sense. The intelligence and social background of groups may differ widely and the advice given must suit their mode of life. Some mothers may have difficulty in budgeting their weekly domestic allowance and on receiving the Maternity Grant may spend it unwisely. The midwife who is teaching expectant mothers needs understanding of such problems.

The market is flooded with a profusion of articles that attract the mother-to-be: but some are neither essential, serviceable nor commendable. The midwife must of course make allowance for the mother's youth, inexperience and desire to buy attractive items for her baby. It is always worth while visiting the baby equipment shops, or sending for catalogues to keep in touch with modern trends.

### The pram

Not all mothers can afford the well-sprung coach-built type of pram nor can these be negotiated in lifts or stored in multi-storied flats; the chrome chassis with folding body is reasonable in price. Good brakes are essential and the pram should not be easily tipped. The hood lining has less glare if it is grey or green. A thick mattress and extra blankets are necessary in winter when the carry-cot transporter is used, foam-padded sides are needed. Mothers should be advised not to use a push chair for babies during the first year of life; their spines need the support of a firm mattress.

### A WORD TO THE NEW FATHER

'Around the fourth day after confinement and on occasions, later, your wife may feel slightly depressed and dissolve into tears for no apparent reason. Be encouraging, because she may feel overwhelmed with her new responsibilities. Assure her of your assistance in the home, see that she gets good nourishing meals and sufficient sleep. This phase will pass when the glands in her body adjust to the postnatal state that follows childbirth.

'After baby is born your wife may feel weak and be unable to cope with her daily housework, so don't grumble if meals are late and the standard of housekeeping is not up to the usual level. A baby creates about three hours extra work daily and an inexperienced mother may take longer than that; lend a hand, this is only a temporary phase which will soon pass. Above all, try not to feel neglected and resentful; the maternal instinct is very strong at this time and the mother's whole attention is centred on her baby almost to the exclusion of everything else. Be unselfish, remember that your wife has endured all the discomforts of pregnancy and labour, allow her to enjoy the pleasant task of looking after your baby.'

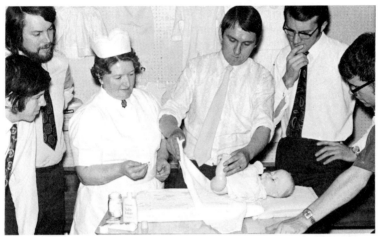

Fig. 46-1 Expectant fathers learning how to apply the napkin.
*Bellshill Maternity Hospital, Lanarkshire.*

### When Baby Cries at Night

When baby cries at night, as he may well do during the first week after going home from hospital, until he settles into a regular sleeping and feeding routine, be patient. A crying baby upsets the mother far more than the father, for the maternal instinct makes her unduly protective and overanxious. If you become irritable this only adds to the nervous tension your wife is experiencing. Your wife should seek medical advice if crying persists night after night.

#### LEARN TO ATTEND TO BABY

'Why not help with some of the little jobs for baby, many fathers enjoy doing them. If there are other children take over the care of the youngest one, toddlers are very liable to feel jealous and should be handled with patience, given a new toy and extra affection until they accept the new baby. Very soon baby will recognise you and give you a beaming smile of welcome, then you will appreciate the real joy of fatherhood.

**The new father has a very important part to play** at this time, and will reap great satisfaction by sharing the load of parenthood. Babies are a source of constant delight, and it is worth while studying how to handle them physically and psychologically, in order that they may develop into healthy happy persons.'

## BABY'S LAYETTE

The mother-to-be gets great pleasure in buying or making baby's layette, for this provides an outlet for her urge to prepare for her coming infant. It is understandable that her thoughts should turn to appearance, for she anticipates the joy of seeing her infant clothed in lovely garments. Without damping her enthusiasm, for we want to encourage her to take pride in her baby's clothes, she should be persuaded that baby's health and comfort depend to a great extent on how he is clothed; the question of cost, wearing and washing qualities must be considered, but there is no reason why suitable garments cannot also be attractive.

### WHAT THE MIDWIFE SHOULD KNOW ABOUT BABY CLOTHES

The midwife should be conversant with the requirements of baby clothes, the cost, advantages and disadvantages of various fabrics including those that are flame-proof, i.e. Proban. Brushed nylon does not catch alight but it may melt and burn the skin. Regulations banning the sale of inflammable night wear do not apply to garments for babies under one year. The teacher ought to know the good points of the various styles and be able to recommend the newer designs. Such information can be drawn on when necessary to strengthen the argument for, or against, some particular material or pattern. When fortified with such knowledge, the midwife can talk with greater confidence and conviction.

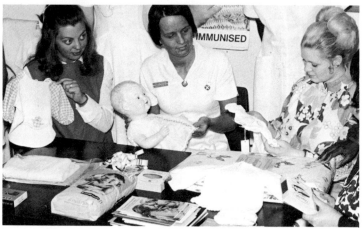

Fig. 46-2    Discussing the layette with prenatal clinic sister.
*Maternity Hospital, Stirling.*

### WARMTH AND COMFORT

Baby must be kept warm without causing undue perspiration, irritating his skin or inhibiting movement. Babies are usually grossly overclad in summer, and sun and air, with their health-giving properties, never reach their skins. Excessive heat causes baby to lose his appetite, and constant profuse perspiration is weakening; the moist skin being prone to chafing and infection. Baby catches one cold after another. The garments worn should vary, just as with adults, according to the temperature of the room or, if out of doors, the weather.

**Comfort is essential for sound sleep,** and to avoid the irritation that leads to persistent crying, fabrics ought to be soft, light in weight, and smooth in texture. Designs should be roomy with no tight bands or other restrictions. Clothing should not interfere with baby's natural desire to wriggle and kick. Movement stimulates the circulation of blood and the absorption of food, as well as developing the muscles in readiness for sitting, standing and walking.

Wool is expensive, irritating to some skins, and when badly washed the garment shrinks, becoming hard, tight and short. Pure wool in vests is irritating to some babies' skins; in pilches and stockings it shrinks with the constant wetting. A mixture of silk or cotton and wool is better for these garments, or wool and cotton mixtures, such as Osmalane. Orlon shawls and other garments should not be washed in very hot water; the fibres twist and the garment loses shape which cannot be rectified. Acrilan double knitting fibre is suitable for shawls and pram suits, it is soft and doesn't shrink.

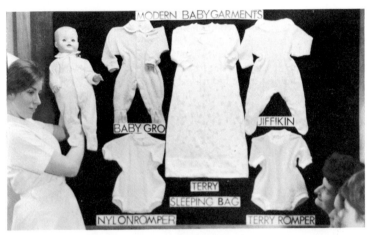

Fig. 46-3   Some baby garments.
*Mothercraft Department, Royal Maternity Hospital, Rottenrow, Glasgow.*

### How to give the Talk-Demonstration

Showing a layette to a group of women is comparatively easy, but the educational value of such a demonstration is extremely limited unless each garment is used as a pivot round which much good advice is concentrated. The garments should be immaculate, either freshly laundered or pressed for the occasion; a few of the more attractive items could be displayed on hangers, but it is probably better to exhibit each garment when describing it.

**Have an intriguing opening sentence,** such as: 'One of the joys of the lady-in-waiting is planning her baby's wardrobe'. 'Nothing gives the mother-to-be greater pleasure than sewing and knitting for the coming baby'. 'Who would think that fashions would change in the tiny garments babies wear; let me show you some of the latest models'.

**Arrange the clothes in the order in which you will show them,** e.g. begin at the skin and work outwards. It is advisable to have a plain, dark surface behind you, such as a blackboard, against which you hold the garments to show up the detail. Introduce the various articles in a different way to avoid monotony.

**Exhibit each garment sufficiently long** for the group to study the detail; a glimpse is not sufficient. You, the teacher, must only glance at the garment, your eyes should be on the audience. It is better not to pass the garments round until the end of the demonstration, or the attention of the audience will be distracted from the garment you are describing.

**Be prepared to answer questions** as to the approximate cost, and have a general idea regarding the amount of material and wool required. Hand out a typed list to those who wish to have it.

*N.B.*—No two people would agree on the number of garments they consider to be essential; mothers and midwives both have their personal preferences. Climate and financial status must be taken into account.

### *The Talk as given*

'I know you all want your babies to look adorable, for every mother pictures her beautifully dressed infant lying asleep in his cot. There is no reason why baby clothes can't be lovely, but we must consider other things besides appearance, for baby must be kept warm and comfortable, sweet and clean. The modern lady-in-waiting considers health and comfort before appearance when planning baby's wardrobe. Comfort is the important thing in baby's life, and as far as clothes are concerned it means freedom to wriggle and kick in garments made, in a roomy style, of fabrics that are smooth and soft. A comfortable baby is more likely to be contented during the day and to sleep soundly at night. Baby will be sleeping most of the time during the first three months so a touch of embroidery on the nightgown and a dainty matinée jacket will make him quite presentable for visitors.

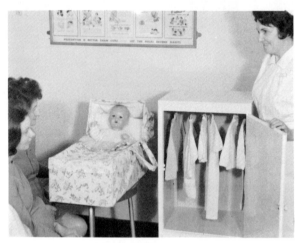

Fig. 46-4  Baby's wardrobe.
*Mothercraft Department, Royal Maternity Hospital, Rottenrow, Glasgow.*

'Baby must be kept warm in the cold winter months; there is a danger of chilling him at night so get a wall thermometer and keep the bedroom temperature at about 18·3°C. Don't keep him too warm in summer; if you keep him bundled in layers of wool he will become like a hothouse plant. It is weakening for baby to perspire all the time, and whenever a breath of cool air reaches him, he catches cold.'

## BABY GARMENTS

*'I will now show you the baby clothes.'*

### 'Vests (3 or 4)

'Bought vests are beautifully soft and kind to baby's skin. A wool and cotton or vincel and cotton mixture is also suitable. Do remember how quickly baby grows; your infant may weigh as much as 5·4 kg at three months, so select a roomy make of vest. The modern envelope neck slips easily over baby's head, yet it fits cosily round the neck with no draw-string for baby to pull tight. Sew on a tab like this to pin baby's napkin to.

### 'Gowns or Babygro suits (4)

'Some mothers prefer gowns of Osmalane or Clydella: a drawstring at the bottom makes it into a cosy sleeping bag. Do not have a waistband, they only hamper baby's breathing and the bow is uncomfortable to lie on. They are very old-fashioned.

'The modern mother prefers the Babygro or Baby Stretch sleeping suit with feet: it stretches and will fit baby from birth to 12 months. The press stud fastenings down the inside of the legs are convenient for nappy changing.

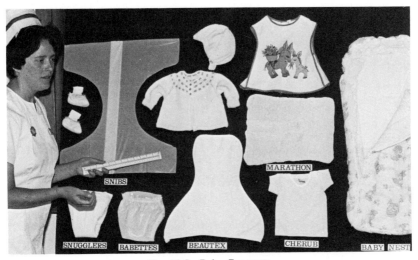

Fig. 46-5 Baby Garments.
*Royal Maternity Hospital, Rottenrow, Glasgow.*

### 'Shawls (2)

'The best pattern in shawls has a plain centre and a closely knitted border. The Shetland or lacy patterns are not now recommended as they aren't really warm, and baby's fingers get entangled in the meshes. Brushed cotton and 100 per cent acrylic shawls are on the market. I would like to recommend a snuggling blanket which is made from 0·9 metres of fine flannel. You can bind it with 4 cm ribbon like this. It is useful for everyday wear, is cosy at night, less expensive, and does not require to be stretched, when being dried, like a shawl.

**Quilted cotton and nylon sleeping bags are cosy,** some have a waterproof inner sheet.

### 'Dresses

'Dresses are not really necessary during the first three months. After the four-month milestone is passed the dainty polyester and cotton dresses that are so easy to launder may be worn when showing baby at her adorable best. The ready-made ones are extremely attractive; ask to see some of the dainty gingham dresses. Two piece angel top and pant sets are attractive for the active crawler.

### 'Matinée jackets (3)

'Baby need only wear these on cold days. They are a favourite gift to the new baby and are often knitted too loosely to have any warmth; but the cardigan-style buttons up to the neck and is really cosy. Don't you agree that this lemon-yellow one of baby nylon yarn is dainty, beautifully warm and a welcome change from pink or blue.

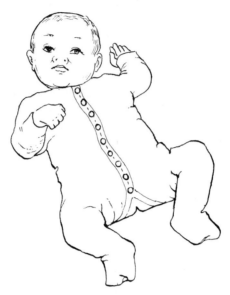

Fig. 46-6   Baby Stretch sleeping suit with Poppers.
*Royal Maternity Hospital, Rottenrow, Glasgow.*

### 'Leggings

'Along with the cardigan the leggings make a useful outfit to keep baby as warm as toast in the pram. Some mothers like them instead of dresses, but wool leggings shrink with constant wetting and washing. Tights in red, blue or white Bri-nylon, with matching Toppers make an attractive ultra-modern outfit. Two piece pram suits in acrylic are available.

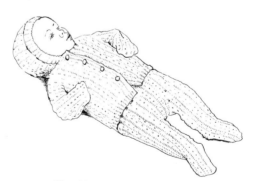

Fig. 46-7   Two-piece pram suit.

### Knitted hoods (2); Mitts (2 pairs)

'On fine days baby's head should be bare, but on cold windy days his ears should be kept warm, especially at teething time. This one is lined for additional warmth.

Some mothers find little use for hoods and gloves, but they are a necessity during winter in the northern counties of England and in Scotland. These are useful if baby scratches his face or sucks his fingers, as well as for keeping tiny fingers warm in wintry weather. Wool ones can be dangerous if baby sucks them and chews the knots that form. Sea island cotton mitts are excellent. Mothers should be warned that loose threads from the inside seam may wind around and severely damage tiny fingers. Seams should be oversewn securely.

### 'Bibs (6)

'Any soft material will do: some are made of four-fold butter muslin. If worn at feeding time they keep baby's gown sweet and clean; later on they are necessary when baby starts dribbling. **Beware of the plastic ones.** They have been known to blow over baby's face, and he can't breathe through plastic; he will suffocate.

'There is a bewildering range of fabrics and styles in baby clothes, but if you remember that baby must be kept warm, clean and comfortable, and that the garments should wash and wear well, the layette you select is almost certain to be a good one.'

## NEW AND OLD WAYS WITH NAPKINS

The 'terry' napkins are popular in Britain and the 0·6 metre square ones, folded in a triangular shape, soak up more urine than the narrow shaped ones. When two napkins are worn, one should be laid under or wrapped round the buttocks. Baby will need 8 or more napkins every day so at least two dozen will be needed to allow for washing and drying. Terry napkins involve more work than disposables but are much cheaper: an electric washing machine and tumble drier reduce the workload.

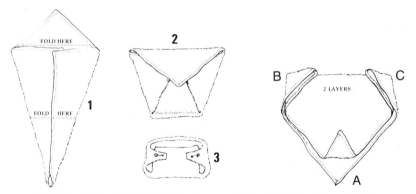

Fig. 46-8   1-2-3. The Pilch Method.        Fig. 46-9   The Triangular Fold.

*Bellshill Maternity Hospital, Lanarkshire.*

#### THE TRIANGULAR FOLD

Lay a medium-sized napkin folded cornerwise under the buttocks; bring the corner A, single fold, well up between baby's legs before wrapping the corners B around the inside of the thighs: this prevents soiling of B corners with stool. In this way all the ends are utilised to soak up urine.

A large napkin may be folded twice cornerwise, giving four layers; the three corners are pinned in front.

### THE PILCH METHOD

'Fold the napkin like this. Lay the broad end below the buttocks, and bring the narrower end up betweeen the legs: the fold from behind lapping over the one in front, and the safety pins being inserted horizontally and nearer the front so that baby won't have to lie on them. Try these methods and use the one you like best; experience will help you to decide.

'Turkish towelling ones should be 0·6 metres (24 inches) square. If two napkins are worn one should be laid under or wrapped round the buttocks: two being too bulky to bring between the legs during the first two months. They absorb the quantities of urine baby passes as he grows older. Maws disposable nappy liner is placed in the centre of the terry napkin.

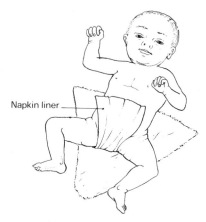

Napkin liner

Fig. 46-10   Napkin liner.

**One way napkin liners.** 'Marathon' or 'Johnson's' one way liner or 'Harrington's' disposable nappy roll liner all permit urine to pass through to the outer terry napkin while keeping the buttocks dry.

**Disposable napkins are convenient** but have to be changed more frequently than terry ones as baby grows older.

**Plastic pants should be washed when they get wet** and at least daily to avoid an unpleasant odour. They should not be too tight around the thighs.

## HOW TO HANDLE AND DRESS BABY

Many mothers would benefit from instruction on how to handle and dress their babies. It is evident that they do not realise how weak baby's spine is, for we see them unfastening the back of the dress of a three-weeks-old baby while they hold him in a sitting posture. They also carry very young infants in an upright position and sometimes neglect to support the head and spine properly.

### *The Talk as given*

'Have you noticed how a crying baby is soothed and quietened in the arms of an experienced person: this is because of the smooth firm way he is handled. A baby likes to feel supported and secure when he is lifted from his cot, so you must handle your baby deliberately yet gently, for quick jerking movements jolt and irritate him. Always support the head of a baby until he is over three months old, because his neck muscles are so weak. Watch while I show you how he should be lifted out of his cot. Slip your left hand under his shoulders and support his head on your arm like this. Slide your arm along his back to support the whole length of the spine; his head is now nestled in the crook of your elbow. At the same time put your right arm

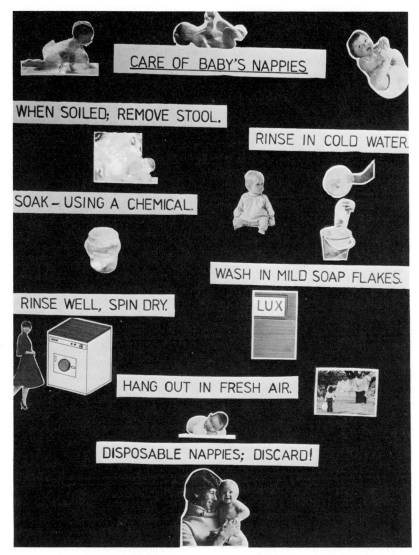

Fig. 46-11  Care of napkins.
*Bellshill Maternity Hospital, Lanarkshire.*

over and under the baby's buttocks. To lay him down continue to support his head and spine, then slip your hand out. I'll do that again. The bones in a baby's spine are not properly hardened; the muscles of the back are weak, so you should carry him like this. Don't sit him up when you are unfastening his clothes at the back. Turn him over and lay him face down on your knee. If you want your baby to have a nice straight back, let him lie flat in his cot or pram. Not until the fourth month should baby be propped up on pillows.

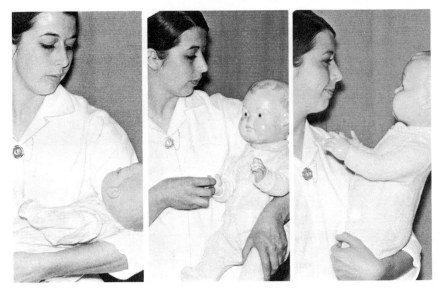

Fig. 46-12          Fig. 46-13          Fig. 46-14

Student midwife demonstrating how to hold a baby.

46-12 First three months; 46-13 second three months; 46-14 third three months.

*Simpson Memorial Maternity Pavilion, Edinburgh.*

'**Let me show you how to handle baby on your lap.** Sit on a low chair and separate your knees slightly to make a lap. To turn baby, grasp him by the body; lift and roll him towards you, on to his face. To turn him back, roll him in the same direction—towards you.

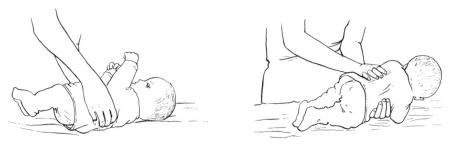

Fig. 46-15    Always roll baby towards you.

## DRESSING BABY

'Try to undress him without turning him oftener than is necessary. Undo all the available fastenings first, and you can slip loose garments off without moving baby very much. Babies don't like clothes being pulled over their heads, so put them off and on from below if you can. Remember, too, that babies don't like being bundled up tightly; they love freedom to wriggle and kick even during the very first weeks, so wrap his shawl loosely round his arms.

'This is the method of putting on a vest fastening at the front. The far-away arm goes in first. Slip your fingers into the wrist-end of the sleeve and draw his hand through the armhole to prevent tiny fingers or nails catching in the sleeve. Slip the vest behind his shoulders without raising him. Draw the arm nearest you into the sleeve in the same way, like this.'

'Now, I shall let you see the different positions we use when bathing a baby and in the next class you will see them again when I show you how to bath baby.'

## BATHING BABY

This is the most popular of all the talk-demonstrations, but one which demands greater teaching skill than the midwife might realise. The procedure embraces more than the woman can comprehend in one session, and demands the repetition which is so essential for good teaching. A lesson on handling, dressing and undressing baby should have been given at the preceding class, to allow more time for the actual bathing procedure and to avoid blurring the demonstration with too much detail.

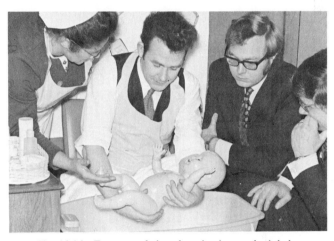

Fig. 46-16   Expectant fathers learning how to bath baby.
*Maternity Section, Central Hospital, Irvine, Ayrshire.*

*The following are eight ways in which repetition is employed in demonstrating how to bath a baby:*

1. The positions in which the baby is held are taught at the previous class.
(a) While washing the hair.  (b) Lowering the baby into the water.
(c) Turning baby over to wash the back. (d) Lifting baby out of the bath.
2. Each piece of equipment is discussed, before actually starting to bath the doll, stating why it has been selected and how it is used.
3. The complete bathing procedure is demonstrated on a doll.
4. Any difficult manoeuvre, such as in (1) and the grip used while holding the baby in the water, should be repeated.

5. One of the expectant mothers (*less than six months pregnant*) should be asked to bath the doll under the midwife's guidance. The audience are so intrigued watching her performance that they do not realise the process has been repeated.

6. A printed copy of the demonstration may be distributed, so that the woman can study the procedure at her leisure and refresh her memory if necessary.

7. Later, she will be shown how to bath her own baby, whether born at home or in hospital.

8. She is given the opportunity to do it herself under supervision.

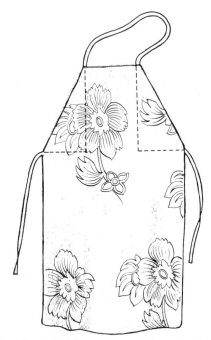

Fig. 46-17    Bathing apron made from a bath towel.

### The Bathing Demonstration as given

#### 'Introduction

'Bathing time should be one of the happiest hours of the day. Baby loves stretching and splashing in the nice warm water, and what is more adorable than a newly bathed baby? Bathing isn't just a job of work to be done as quickly as possible; it is one of the mothering times, an occasion when baby and mother get to know each other better. By the gentle way she handles her baby and the caressing tone of her voice a mother expresses her love. It is a bonding procedure.

#### 'Morning or evening

'Although many babies are bathed in the morning, there is no special reason why this should be so. Choose the time that suits you best; baby won't mind. Before the 18.00 hours feed is a good time; baby usually sleeps well after his bath, and night is the best time for sound sleep. The house is warmer in the evening, and when baby comes to the crawling stage he will need a bath at bedtime. We mustn't forget father, he may like to watch or to help. Allow yourself an hour at first, including preparation and clearing up; speed comes with experience.'

**On table or knee**

In hospital babies are usually bathed in their cots or on a table for convenience and speed. The table in many homes is in front of a window. In the home the knee is often preferred, the mother sitting near the fire or radiator; baby feels loved and secure being in such close contact with his mother.

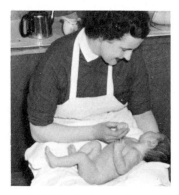

Fig. 46-18 Mothering. Prior to bath allowing baby to kick while undressed.

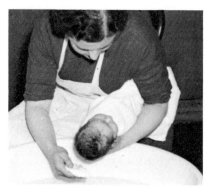

Fig. 46-19 Washing baby's hair. *Note*—Edge of bath at knee level. Body held securely with elbow. Head supported.

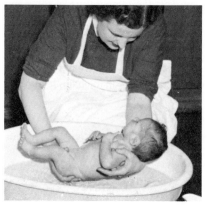

Fig. 46-20 Lowering baby into bath. *Note*—Head supported on wrist. Baby's left arm (*the far away one*) grasped securely. Left thigh being held and buttocks supported.
**Use the same grip when lifting baby out.**

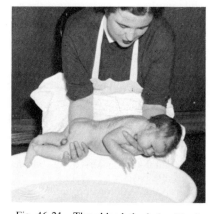

Fig. 46-21 The older baby being lifted out face downwards.
Baby's right arm and right thigh (*the far away ones*) are grasped securely.

Figs. 46-18–46-21 Demonstration of bathing baby as in the home.

## DISCUSSION OF EQUIPMENT

'Here we have everything set out that you are likely to need. This plastic baby bath is light in weight and does not get hot. (An oval washing-up bowl would do for the first three months.) Notice that the bath is placed on a strong stool to bring the edge of it to knee-level and so prevent backache from bending. This low chair without arms is similar to the one you will use when feeding baby.

'A tray is handy to hold baby's toilet articles which are few and simple. On this one there is a soap dish and cake of good face soap. Note the two wash cloths, a butter muslin one for the face and body; the Turkish one for the buttocks is washed with the napkins (some prefer disposable tissues). These cotton-wool balls in the glass jar are needed to clean baby's nose, but only to remove the smudges that can be seen. Here is a jar of cream for his buttocks, and a hairbrush. Talcum powder should be used sparingly if at all.

'His night-clothes, as you see, are warming on a screen by the fire, arranged, vest on top, in the order in which they will be put on. Baby's own soft face-towel and bath-towel are warming too.

'Have a pail like this beside you, to soak baby's napkins in until you are ready to wash them. Get a tiny chamber, if you like, to "catch what comes", but don't be too hopeful. We do not now recommend starting to train a baby until he is over eight months old; you only upset him by your over-anxiety, and he will gain control sooner if you begin training when he understands what you mean (see p. 803). This big jug is used to fill the bath. You will all want to have a bathing-apron like this one which is made from a bath towel and you would be wise to wear a plastic one underneath it to keep your lap dry, in case baby wets when his napkin is off.'

**PREPARATION**

'Have the room warm, windows and doors closed and everything ready before you start.

'**Always put the cold water into the bath first;** toddlers have been known to fall in while mother was away getting the cold water. Test the temperature of the water with a bath thermometer; it should be 37·7°C. If you haven't a thermometer, use your elbow; the water should feel gently warm, not hot. Don't use your hand, which could tolerate water that would burn baby's skin. Never add hot water while baby is in the bath, because of the risk of scalding him.

'Notice that the chair you will sit on is at the right-hand side of the fire, so that baby's head is cool, his feet warm. Wash your hands and put on the bathing apron.'

### The Actual Bath

'Baby is already undressed, all but his vest and napkin. Remove these and let him kick for a moment; he loves the freedom and it is good to let his skin become accustomed to the air. If his buttocks are dirty use the Turkish face cloth or disposable tissues.

'Wrap the bath towel round his arms and chest and wash his face with the butter muslin cloth, without soap. Do one side at a time so that you don't cover his nose and mouth with the face cloth. Dry his face gently and very thoroughly.

'**Watch how his body is being held with my left elbow,** while his head, grasped in my left hand, is brought to the edge of the bath. Wet and soap the hair properly, don't be afraid of the soft spot on the top of the head, if you don't keep it clean, scurf will form. Dry his hair thoroughly, and be sure to dry the creases behind the ears or they will become sore.

'Wet his body and legs with the face cloth, then soap both your hands and wash him like this; first neck, arms and hands, roll him towards you and soap his back, then do his body and legs and be sure to go into all the creases.

'**He is very slippery, so he must be held securely.** Place your left hand under his shoulders and grasp the left upper arm; his head will rest on your wrist. Put your right hand under his buttocks and grasp the left thigh. Lower him into the bath, keeping his head well out of the water. Rinse off the soap. When a baby is a month old, turn him over and wash his back like this.

'To lift him out of the bath grasp him in the same way, holding the "far away" arm and leg. Lay him face down on your lap and dry him carefully. Use a gentle mopping movement, don't rub briskly, his skin is very delicate; dry all the folds of skin thoroughly and be careful with his finger-nails, they are easily torn.

'**Shake a little talcum on your hand,** and rub it into the dry creases, smear some cream on his buttocks. Put on his vest, and remember to put your fingers into the sleeve and draw his hand through it as I showed you last week. Put on his napkin.'

The midwife should either dress the doll in night clothes or wrap the snuggling blanket over vest and napkin, and brush the hair. *She then stands up to face the audience with an appropriate closing sentence, such as,* 'Baby is now ready for his feed, then he will be drowsy, and when tucked into his cot will soon be fast asleep. Father and mother will enjoy a quiet evening.'

# HEALTH EDUCATION

### POSTNATAL EXERCISES; GOOD POSTURE

#### The Talk as given

'I'm sure you are all eager to look and feel as well as you did a year ago and, of course you want to reduce your waistline and slim your hips. It takes six to eight weeks, or even longer, for your overstretched muscles to return to normal and we will show you how to assist nature in doing this so that you can regain your trim figure. We hope that your childbearing organs and tissues have healed and are going back to their normal state. But we also want you to be full of energy—not tired and listless—and within the next few weeks ready and eager to resume your household duties.'

### GOOD WHOLESOME FOOD

'In order to be fit and well you must have nourishing meals with plenty of bodybuilding foods such as meat, fish, eggs, milk and cheese, as well as fruit and green vegetables that contain valuable minerals and vitamins. You need three cooked meals every day to build up your strength, foods rich in iron such as meat, liver, blood sausage, wholewheat bread and green vegetables will help to replace the blood you have recently lost. Good food helps to provide the energy you need in looking after your family and your home.'

### REST AND RECREATION

'Do ensure that you get sufficient sleep and rest after you go home. Go to bed at a reasonable hour so that you have at least nine hours' sleep; lie down during the afternoon if only for an hour. Get your husband to help you with any heavy work; it is very bad for you to lift heavy weights for at least six weeks, until your uterus and birth passage are back to their normal state. If you have to move something heavy, such as a big armchair, push, don't lift it. We will show you how to avoid straining your back if in the course of your daily housework you must lift something fairly heavy.

'Try to continue with some of your hobbies or social activities outside the home in order that you will be a cheerful companion for your husband and a good-natured mother to your children.'

### MAINTAINING GOOD POSTURE

'You will all admit that since baby was born you are tending to stand in a slovenly fashion and to walk in an ungainly manner; shoulders slumped forwards, abdomen bulging. This is because your muscles have lost the power to hold you erect and to enable you to walk gracefully. Try to be very figure conscious and cultivate the habit of good posture until your muscles and ligaments are restored to their natural strength again. We will help you, and we hope you will continue with good posture after you leave hospital.

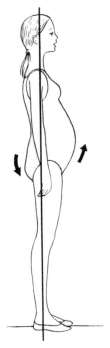

Fig. 46-22   Vertical line indicates centre of gravity. Shoulders should not be held back beyond this line or lordosis occurs.

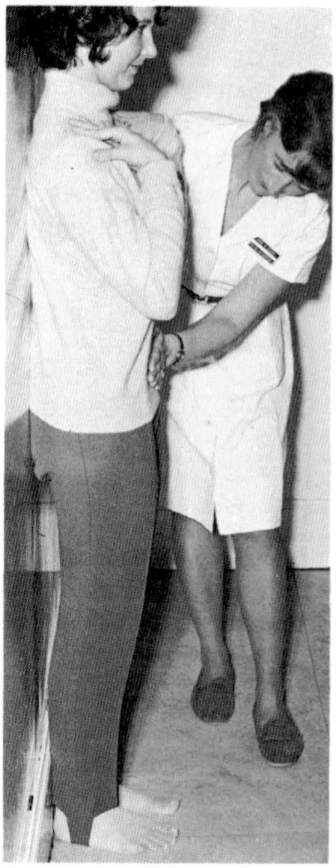

Fig. 46-23   Physiotherapist giving instruction *re* good posture in postnatal period.

'You must get rid of the backward-leaning stance you adopted during pregnancy or it will become an established habit. During the last months of pregnancy you had to lean backwards to counterbalance the size and weight of baby in your uterus. Make a conscious effort to stand erect and walk with a graceful carriage. Bad posture gives rise to low backache: it also induces a despondent outlook on life. If you hold yourself in a trim and confident manner your feelings and actions are more likely to be confident. A woman should maintain pride in her appearance even if she is a busy mother, and although she may have an excellent figure her appearance can be ruined by faulty posture. The abdominal wall muscles were grossly overstretched during the last three months of pregnancy. These muscles also worked hard during labour pushing baby out into the world; they are therefore lax or flabby and do not hold your abdominal organs snug in place as they ought to. We will teach you exercises that will tone up these muscles and help to flatten the bulging waistline.'

### WEAK PELVIC FLOOR MUSCLES

'While baby was actually being born the outlet of the birth passage was dilated or opened to a very great extent; the muscles of the pelvic floor were greatly overstretched and bruised: in fact, some of you required stitches. These pelvic floor muscles are meant to support and maintain the bladder and uterus in their natural places, but if they remain lax you will have difficulty in holding urine in your bladder for as long as you did previously. You may have heard of "falling of the womb"; this also is due to lax or slack pelvic floor muscles. We will teach you exercises that will strengthen the pelvic floor muscles.'

### POSTNATAL EXERCISE
*(Low chairs with reasonably firm seats, straight backs and no arms are provided)*

The women are seated throughout the lesson.
Outdoor shoes are worn not soft bedroom slippers.
The women wear tights into which their nightdresses are tucked.

## Good sitting posture

The mothers are asked to sit well back in the chairs.
Feet are placed on floor directly under the knees.
Hips and shoulders are pressed against the back of the chair.
The hollow of the back is flattened out.
The head is held erect.

*Hold position and count five slowly–Relax. Repeat six times*

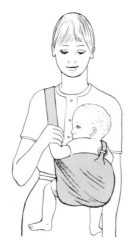

Figs. 46-24 Sling carrier leaves hands free.
*Royal Maternity Hospital, Rottenrow, Glasgow.*

## Strengthening the abdominal muscles

Draw the lower abdominal muscles inwards and upwards. Pull your 'tummy' in.

*Count five slowly–Relax. Repeat six times*

## Exercising pelvic floor muscles

Contract (*tighten*) the buttocks close together.
Contract (*draw up*) the pelvic floor muscles as you would do when urgently requiring to pass urine at a time when it is not convenient to do so.

*Count five slowly–Relax. Repeat six times*

# PREPARING MODIFIED DRIED MILK FEEDS

*Talk-Demonstration to Mothers*

The need for cleanliness should be stressed, reasons given and the danger of infection by germs explained.

## Hand washing

*This should be emphasised and carried out as part of the demonstration.*

'Hands that look clean may be covered with germs which are so small they cannot be seen. Your hand must go into the carton to scoop up the powder and, if not clean, will infect the milk. Wash your hands before preparing the feed, also before feeding baby (*and always after changing the napkin, which is usually done just before feeding*).'

## Clean utensils

'Everything used for making baby's food should be thoroughly washed and kept covered with a clean towel, in a cupboard free from dust and flies. A badly washed jug or dirty bottle brush will be a breeding ground for germs. Flies may infect the milk powder. Keep it in a glass jar with a screw top lid. The sugar jar should have a lid.'

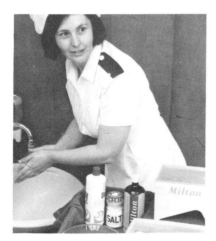
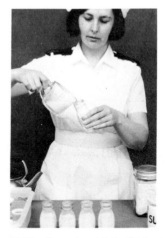

Fig. 46-25   Always wash your hands before making feeds.     Fig. 46-26   Preparing dried milk feeds.

*Aberdeen Maternity Hospital.*

## Accuracy in preparing feeds is most important

'Powdered milk, sugar and water must be measured carefully. If given too much sugar, baby will become fat and flabby; too little will prevent adequate weight gain.' Most dried milks have had sugar added to them. Baby will get too much salt if the milk powder added exceeds the required amount. Excess salt harms the brain cells.

*(Demonstration)*

## Requirements

Carton of modified Dried Milk with scoop, jar of sugar if not in milk powder.
Kettle of water.
Glass (*heat resisting*) measuring jug, 240 ml.
Casserole containing pyrex wide-mouth feeding bottle and teat in Milton 2, made from Milton crystals.
Knife, 4 g measure (teaspoon), bowl, bottle brush, soapless detergent.

## Preparation

Wash hands; scald jug, bowl and bottle brush with boiling water.
Allow kettle to cool for 10 minutes prior to making feed. (*Boiling water separates out the fat in the milk.*)

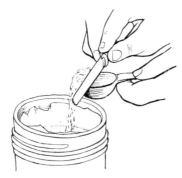

Fig. 46-27  Milk powder levelled with edge of knife. Powder must not be packed down.

### *Method*

Open pack or jar, remove lids from casserole and sugar jar.
Wash hands thoroughly. Remove bottle and teat from Milton solution, rinse them.
Measure 90 ml boiled water, pour into feeding bottle.
Measure 3 scoops powder (level with edge of knife), do not pack or heap the scoop, put into jug.

### *(Replace lids or close pack to avoid contamination by flies)*

Add a little of the measured warm water in the bottle to powder in jug and mix to a smooth cream. Add the remainder of the water, stirring constantly to remove any lumps. Pour into bottle and apply teat. Some do not use a jug: the milk powder is put into the bottle with a little water to mix it smoothly then the remainder of the water is added.

### HOW TO GIVE THE FEED

The napkin should be changed, mother's hands washed before feeding baby.
The bottle is placed in a jug of hot water until the milk is about 37·2° to 37·7°C. Many give feeds at living room temperature. Vacuum flasks should not be used to keep milk warm: organisms multiply in warm milk. Test the heat of the milk by allowing it to drip on the sensitive inner aspect of the wrist; milk should be at blood heat (gently warm). Mothers must be told never to put the teats in their mouths to

test the heat of the milk: and only to touch the neck of the teat when putting it on to the bottle.

Test the rate of flow by holding the bottle upside down. The milk should drip at approximately 2 ml (30 drops) per minute. If the hole is too small baby will take 15 or more minutes to get his feed and will swallow too much air and get colic. If the hole is too big baby will gulp his feed in less than five minutes.

*(Demonstrate how to enlarge a small hole with a darning needle heated by holding it in the flame of a match.)*

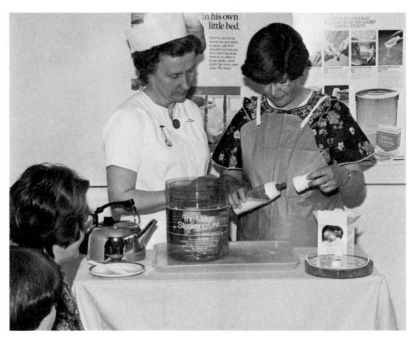

Fig. 46-28   Mother participating in demonstration: preparing a bottle feed.
*Queen Mother's Hospital, Glasgow.*

**Feeding position**
***Mothers should be warned against feeding baby in cot or pram with the bottle propped.***
The mother sits in a low chair with one foot raised on a footstool, cuddling baby as in the breast-feeding position.

A jug of hot water is within reach.

To keep baby's dress dry and sweet-smelling a bib (*not plastic*) should be worn or Kleenex tissue tucked under the chin.

It is advisable to hold the bottle like a pencil with the rim of the teat between the thumb and first finger. When the teat collapses, as it will when baby sucks the air out of the bottle, the fingers pinch the rim of the teat and allow air to enter. If the teat is removed from baby's mouth to do this he becomes annoyed. The bottle should be tilted at an angle to keep the neck of the bottle full of milk, thus avoiding undue sucking of air. Wind should be broken half-way through the feed. If the stomach is distended with air baby may not want to finish his feed. Wind is brought up again at the end of the feed, baby's bib being laid on mother's shoulder.

Rinse bottle and teat in cold water; turn teat inside out and rub between finger and thumb, rinse; clean bottle with brush and detergent, rinse and submerge in Milton 2, made up fresh daily from Milton crystals. The bottle and teat must remain submerged in Milton 2 between feeds.

*N.B.—Mothers should be given the opportunity to test the heat of the milk on their wrists, count the drops, apply teats and hold the bottles in the manner recommended.*

# PLANNING THE DAY FOR MOTHER AND BABY

This talk is only a guide, for each midwife knows best what will suit the women in her own area. It is probably better to discuss the subject in general, as an hour-by-hour plan would not suit every woman, nor would it be remembered unless a typed copy was given to each mother. Enjoy your baby is the perfect motif.

### The Talk as given

'Before you go home I would advise you to plan how you are going to manage your housework and at the same time give baby the care he will need. Some mothers make a lot of unnecessary work and tire themselves out; others make no plan at all and get into a hopeless muddle. Looking after baby will mean about three hours daily extra work, especially if it is your first baby, because you will be slow until you become more expert in handling him. The main thing is that you start off by getting baby to fit in with your usual routine. Babies are most accommodating; they don't mind whether they are bathed in the morning or the evening, so long as you keep to one or the other. Feeding times can be put back or forwards half an hour, or even an hour, if they clash with family meals. Baby can be fed at 05.00; 09.00; 13.00; 17.00 hours instead of the usual 06.00; 10.00; 14.00; 18.00 hours. It is unnecessary and unwise to disorganise the household for baby.'

### Take things easily

'During the first month, you will tire readily and will require some extra help with the heavy work, so do accept any offer of assistance you may get from relatives or friends. It is, however, better that you yourself should bath baby, a pleasant task at which you can sit down. Encourage your husband to help with the heavier jobs, not for six to eight weeks should you lift heavy weights. Don't attempt to keep your house like a new pin if it means being on your feet from early morning until late at night. A home that is reasonably clean and tidy, well-cooked meals and a happy mother are better for everyone concerned than an immaculate house with a tired irritable mother.'

### Have a flexible plan

'I am not going to set out a plan, hour by hour, from 06.00 hours until 22.00 hours at night. A hundred and one unexpected things may crop up in the course of the day, and some require your immediate attention; if life is a frantic race with the clock, you will soon be a nervous wreck. No rigid scheme will suit every household. Mothers vary in their ability as housewives, and some are stronger than others; babies differ in the amount of attention they demand. By all means have a plan, but for baby's sake let it be a flexible one. Don't be too strict at first regarding feeding times, for some babies object to being regimented by the clock. The restless wiry baby seems to need more food than the placid sleepy one, and often likes to have it every three rather than every four hours. Let baby have some say regarding feeding times if he is the type who objects to the usual schedule. The doctor or health visitor at the child health clinic will advise you if any difficulty arises.

'**Baby usually starts the day bright and early,** around 06.00 hours, but after you have fed him you can have another short sleep until it is time to prepare breakfast. When baby wakes up again, about 09.30 hours, face, hands and buttocks are washed and clean clothes put on; give the 10.00 hours feed and settle him for sleep in the pram out of doors.

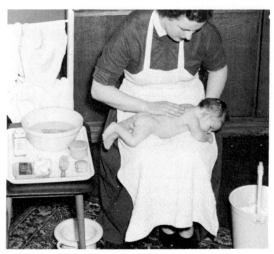

Fig. 46-29   Baby's morning toilet.
*Bath given during evening.*

'When you have finished baby's daily washing have a rest with your feet up while you take a nourishing drink. Housework and cooking usually occupy the remainder of the morning. If your husband and children do not come home at midday, be sure to have a proper meal yourself, as it is important that you keep up your strength and your supply of milk. Before the 14.00 hour feed allow baby to have at least five minutes on your lap kicking with his napkin off; chat to him, and he will learn to know the sound of your voice. These mothering times are essential for baby's happiness, and he enjoys the exercise, too. Finish your household jobs, and then have another rest with your feet up while you drink a cup of tea before you take baby out. The air in the parks or the suburbs does baby and you more good than the air in the crowded shopping centres, which is laden with dust and petrol fumes, so do get away from the traffic.'

## TAKE FATHER INTO CONSIDERATION

'Between 17.00 and 18.00 hours, depending on when father comes home, is a good time for baby's bath. You will find out, of course, whether father prefers to see baby being bathed or whether this should be done before he comes home. When fed and tucked into his warm cot baby will probably sleep until the 22.00 hour feed. Plan to have a quiet evening by the fire, reading, viewing television, or talking to your husband; bathing baby in the evening is one way of ensuring this. You should go to bed immediately after baby's last feed, and your husband will give you a beaker of cocoa, milk or Ovaltine to help to keep up your supply of breast milk. Relax and read if it is too early for you to go to sleep. Do try to arrange an outing with your husband at least once a week; it is good for you to get away from baby for a short time occasionally, and although you may be satisfied to stay at home, your husband will no doubt appreciate an outing with you. See that baby and father get their fair share of your love and attention, but try to have a little leisure for yourself, or you will only become overtired and disgruntled. Remember, it is mainly the mother who makes the home a happy place. If baby, father and you are all thriving and contented, your plan is a success; you are a good wife and mother.'

## WHEN BABY CRIES

*Because some parents 'batter' young babies when annoyed due to their crying, midwives should keep that fact in mind. Parents need advice on this subject.*

### The Talk as given

'Many mistakes in baby care are made when trying to pacify a crying infant, so it is necessary that you should know some of the reasons why babies cry and how to deal with them. In moderation crying is good for babies; it expands their lungs, and the vigorous waving of arms and legs that accompanies crying is a splendid form of exercise. Crying is baby's language, and his only way of letting us know that something is annoying him. He may be uncomfortable, too hot, thirsty, hungry, or in pain, but even an experienced midwife cannot tell which of these is the cause during the first week of life. It doesn't take much to make tiny babies cry, so don't decide he is hungry or ill until you have investigated the other causes.

'A new baby may scream furiously as though in agony yet he may only be tired of lying on one side. Turn him over and give him a friendly pat and a word of comfort; he will very likely settle down and go to sleep again. You may expect your baby to have at least half a dozen spells of crying throughout the day, and occasionally at night. Always think of the simple things first before you conclude that he is in pain or ill. To a mother the cry of her infant makes such a tremendous appeal that she is apt to worry unnecessarily. Keep calm and investigate the situation.

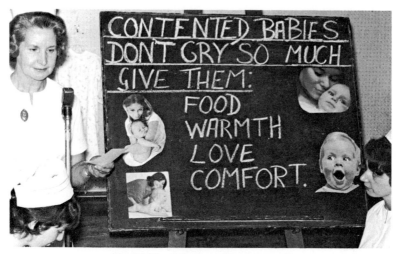

Fig. 46-30   Talk also relayed to wards.
*Bellshill Maternity Hospital, Lanarkshire.*

### 'Is his napkin wet?

'It may be that his napkin is wet, but in my opinion babies are not disturbed by wet napkins if the cot is warm. Cold, wet napkins are uncomfortable, and if baby's buttocks are sore, they will hurt when he passes water or a motion.

### 'Is he too warm?

'Is his face red, and does his head look or feel moist? Is the bedroom stuffy? Babies, like adults, sleep best in a well-ventilated room. Mothers often make the mistake of overclothing their babies, especially in summer. I saw a baby protesting bitterly about the heat one hot August afternoon; he was swaddled in four layers of wool, yet his mother was wearing a cool cotton frock. By all means keep baby warm in winter, but allow the air to reach his skin in summer.

### 'Is he uncomfortable?

'Have you wrapped him up too tightly? Babies love to squirm and move their arms and legs when they want to, and it infuriates even tiny babies when they can't. It may be that the pure wool vest you knitted for him is driving him frantic; many babies cannot tolerate wool next to their skins. If baby continues to scream, you had better lift him. Straighten his clothes, and make him comfortable; cuddle and soothe him before you lay him down again. During the night, if he refuses to settle, give him a few ml of boiled water; he will be thirsty with crying and more so if he is hot.

### 'Is he thirsty?

'It is now being realised that babies do cry bitterly because they are thirsty; mouthing their fists as though hungry. This may be due to the increased amount (4 times) of salt in cow's milk. When the mother heaps or packs powdered milk the baby may get 6 times as much salt as he requires. The mother thinks crying is due to hunger and gives more milk which increases thirst because of the high salt content.

### 'Is he hungry?

'Water will not pacify a hungry baby, so you had better feed him. With a first baby, the mother's milk supply may not be plentiful until the third or fourth week, so take nourishing drinks as well as three good meals a day. You will never teach a baby to sleep all night by letting him cry for an hour or more, and you have your husband to think of too; he, as well as you, needs a good night's sleep. We used to condemn night feeds, but not now. When baby gets enough food during the day he usually sleeps all night.

'If you have disturbed nights go to the child health clinic or consult the health visitor, who will be pleased to advise you. Persistent crying is more often due to some fault in the feeding routine rather than that the breast milk does not agree with baby. He may be getting too much or too little food, take him to the child health clinic and this will be investigated. No two babies are exactly alike in the amount of food they require; the thin restless infant often needs more food and more cuddling than the placid baby, so seek and take the advice of an expert.

'Newborn babies do not cry because of bad temper. Be patient, and don't expect too much of an infant who is only ten days old. Give him time to settle into a satisfactory sleeping and feeding routine.'

### Pain or illness

'Wind may give rise to pain, but you will avoid this by letting baby break wind after each feed. Colic, is rare in breast-fed babies. With each piercing shriek baby will draw up his legs and will continue to cry even after you have picked him up. Lay him face downwards on your knee over a hot-water bottle with a little warm (not hot) water in it. Give him some warm water to drink. A baby who is ill may whimper rather than cry but you would notice that there was something wrong, such as cough, cold, vomiting, diarrhoea, or feverishness.'

### 3 Months' colic

Evening colic occurring between the 18.00 and 22.00 hours feeds is seen in breast- and bottle-fed babies. It is thought to be due to gaseous distension of the bowel due to slow feeding with concomitant air swallowing. This may be rectified by 'breaking wind' and enlarging the hole in the teat if necessary. A too high sugar content may cause excessive formation of gas.

Midwives are aware that the hyperactive baby may need a sedative such as phenobarbitone 7·5 mg, thirty minutes before feeds. The antispasmodic dicyclomine syrup (Merbentyl), 2·5 to 5 ml, before the 18.00 hour feed gives relief in most cases.

#### GENERAL ADVICE ON CRYING

'**Try not to let crying become a habit;** baby should not have to scream for the normal care all babies need.

'It is the placid, good-natured woman who makes the best mother; so make up your mind to keep calm. Mothers who are always in a state of anxiety about their babies seem to produce the same anxious state in their infants. Don't get worked up over every whimper: on the other hand don't lose control of yourself and handle your baby roughly when his crying exasperates you: seek medical advice.

'Babies may look very fragile, but they are not weaklings. This is when a patient, level-headed husband can be a tower of strength to a worried young mother, for sound commonsense can be applied to baby care as well as to other things. Baby's needs are simple—food, warmth, comfort and love, and when these are given satisfactorily baby will be as good as gold and brighten your home like a ray of sunshine.'

*Midwives must take some responsibility in preventing the 'battered baby' syndrome by teaching mothers how to cope with the crying baby. (See also p. 697.)*

# SLEEP

Use as teaching aids a cot and bedding; a doll; sleeping garments. Give demonstration of dressing baby for sleep; putting baby to bed.

### The Talk as given

'It is easy to see what a soothing effect sleep has on babies, for no matter how cross they are when they fall asleep, they wake up good-natured and ready to smile again.

'**At first baby will sleep 20 out of the 24 hours;** he only stays awake long enough for napkin changing, feeding and bathing. Gradually he sleeps for shorter periods during the day, and at six months sleeps 17 out of the 24 hours.

'Baby feels drowsy after a feed, so you should settle him comfortably into the cot or pram then, and he will soon be fast asleep. The most important and the longest sleep is at night, and when baby is properly fed during the day, he is more likely to sleep all night.'

#### A BED TO HIMSELF

'Baby should have a little bed of his own. If he sleeps with mother he breathes warm stale air, and there is always the danger that the heavy blankets or mother's arm might lie over his face. A basket may be suitable for the first three months, but baby very soon grows out of it and might topple it over in his attempts to sit up to see what is going on.

'The mattress should be firm and enveloped in a rubber cover. Pillows are not necessary: in fact, they are dangerous for young babies. If baby rolls over, and babies whose arms are wrapped in tightly are more likely to do this, he may burrow his face into a soft pillow with serious results. The Divine pillow and the Visavent mattress have air spaces that lessen the danger of suffocation. Two light, wool, cotton, or Acrilan cellular blankets will be needed, and if a top sheet is not provided, the washable top cover may be folded in over the top of the blankets. The cot should always be clean and sweet-smelling. Air it at feeding times; once a day you can strip and air it in the sunshine or fresh air.

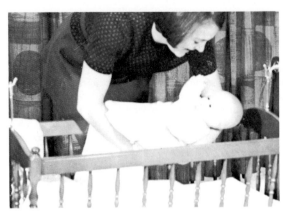

Fig. 46-31   Spine and head supported while laying baby in cot.
*Aberdeen Maternity Hospital.*

'A carry-cot with adjustable straps is useful for travel during the first four months. In winter an extra lining blanket and mattress are needed for warmth if the carry-cot is used as a bassinet.'

### PUTTING BABY TO SLEEP

**'Always lay baby on his side in case he should be sick:** if lying on his back he might inhale into his lungs the milk he vomits and choke. A number of babies die each year because of this. Lay him on his right and left sides alternately so that both lungs will expand well. Have baby's cot in your own bedroom during the first nine months at least, so that you can hear what is going on. For a number of years a separate room for baby was recommended, but in case he should vomit and choke,

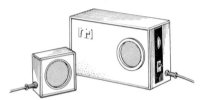

Fig. 46-32   Alarm to relay baby's cries.
*Courtesy Mothercare.*

it is now considered safer to have baby near his mother. Don't worry about this, it is only a wise precaution. A baby alarm should be obtained if baby is not within hearing distance. As baby grows older he should go to sleep by himself, so lay him down awake from the very beginning. This will save you time and trouble later on, and after a nursery rhyme or a story your child will go happily to sleep.

'When baby is sleeping out of doors see that the back of the pram-hood faces into the wind, and that in summer he is shaded from the rays of the mid-day sun. Choose a quiet spot, if you can. A cat net may be necessary.

'If babies are overtired they are very fretful, and sometimes they scream, refuse food and cannot be pacified. When this happens you may think baby is ill, try cuddling and soothing him to sleep with a lullaby he knows.'

# THE CARE OF BABY'S SKIN

### *The Talk as given*

'Baby's skin should be pink and smooth like the petal of a rose, and as soft as silk. Because the texture is so fine, baby's skin is very easily irritated, therefore you should take every care to avoid this. The time to begin is when you are planning baby's layette. Choose vests with a mixture of silk or cotton and wool; they are much less irritating.

'The red blotches of a wool rash are so itchy and irritating that baby and you will have a few disturbed nights. Should you bath him? Yes! but let the water be slightly cooler than usual; pat him dry, gently, with a soft towel. A sweat rash is often troublesome, especially in summer when baby is likely to be kept too hot. Tiny pin-point blisters that are hard, and make the skin feel rough, appear on the forehead and body. No wonder baby is cross. Bath him as usual to remove the perspiration, and dab on a very little baby talcum powder; keep him less warm and give extra water to drink.'

## SORE BUTTOCKS

'Sore buttocks generally begin as a reddened area, but with a little care this can usually be prevented. They are due to various causes, such as:

'Not washing baby's buttocks properly when they are soiled.

'Leaving wet napkins on too long, especially under plastic pants; the skin becoming soggy and then breaking.

'Using napkins that are too rough; this happens when Turkish towelling is dried quickly, for example, near the fire. Napkins should, where possible, be dried out of doors.

'Washing the napkins with a strong soap, washing soda, bleaching powder or "blue" and not rinsing them properly. Napkins should be rinsed in three waters.

'Sore buttocks sometimes occur during the first ten days of life, when baby has loose stools because he is taking too much milk or is not digesting it properly. Copious oily applications combined with wearing plastic pants will make the skin soggy and encourage infection.

'Prevention is the best treatment, and that means the avoidance of the causes already mentioned.' (The midwife should refer to page 492 for curative treatment.)

### Scurf

'I'm sure you have all seen a baby with a dark greasy patch on the front of his head. The scales from it fall on to the face, and the next thing you see is a red, sore area on baby's cheek. This may be the beginning of extensive skin trouble, so don't allow the scurf to form. Wash the soft spot on baby's head every day, rinse off the soap thoroughly, and rub the hair briskly with a Turkish towel.'

### Sensitive skins

'Some babies have extremely sensitive skins. I've seen little cheeks red and sore with rubbing on a harsh blanket or shawl. To avoid this, fold the cot sheet over the top of the blanket. Tiny chins get sore, too, when dribbling or slavering. Dry the chin gently, use a soothing face cream, change his bibs frequently, and tie a silk scarf around his neck. Do dry baby's face thoroughly; he objects, I know, but you must insist, or rough red patches will form on his cheeks and cold winds will make them raw and sore.

'Crops of spots commonly appear during the first year which mothers often say are due to teething, but are more likely to be the result of some new food baby isn't yet accustomed to. Always give new foods, such as eggs or fruit, in small quantities until you see what happens. The treatment is to dab on some cooling lotion and give him a few ml of milk of magnesia.

'Of course you mustn't expect all these skin conditions to affect your baby, but it is wise to prevent them if you can. Aim at having the bloom of the fresh air and the tan of the sun on your baby's skin, and he won't have many skin blemishes. What is more, he is likely to be a healthy little lad.'

## THE NEW FATHER

This talk should be given to the mothers of first babies. So often the father's point of view is overlooked, and this leads to domestic disharmony.

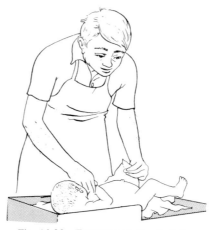

Fig. 46-33     Encourage father to help.

### *The Talk as given*

'Now that you are going home, have you given any thought as to how you are going to deal with the very important person: No, not His Majesty the baby—the new father. The average man has very little idea of what is expected of him, and it isn't easy being a father for the first time, so help him as much as you can. Don't make the mistake of being too possessive with your baby. True enough, you provide most of the care baby needs, but try to make your husband feel that he also is of importance. A baby should bind and not separate his parents. You have the advantage of having learned how to look after baby, but let your husband feel that baby is his as well as yours; consult him, ask his opinion, bring him into the picture.'

### LET FATHER HANDLE BABY

'Allow your husband to share some of the pleasant little jobs for baby, but do try to let the first occasion be a happy one. Of course he is going to feel awkward and embarrassed too; ignore this, and don't forget to give a word of encouragement. Use a little psychology. Do not hand a screaming infant to your hungry husband while you finish some item of housework; it would be more tactful to get him to tuck baby into his cot, when drowsy after a feed, while you put the final touch to the evening meal. Be lavish in your praise, for success will encourage him to attempt the more complicated tasks. There is no denying this is one of the dangerous corners in married life, and for your own happiness as well as your husband's you should try to negotiate it successfully. I wouldn't say a father would be actually jealous of his own child, but until now your husband has received all your love and attention; meals were ready on time, and a smiling wife greeted him at the end of the day. Now, the home is noisy and untidy, meals hastily prepared and often late, his wife harassed and irritable. The new father offers to help or maintains a friendly silence behind the newspaper, astonished that such a tiny scrap of humanity can have such a devastating effect on his home-life. Not until baby is old enough to give him a welcoming smile will he experience the real joy of fatherhood.

'That is a gloomy picture, and I have purposely painted it like that as a warning, so that you will realise what can happen; but you aren't going to let it be like that.'

### READJUST THE DAILY ROUTINE

'You may well be thinking, "What about me, the mother, don't I get any consideration?": Of course you do. I know you need extra rest; you may not be an experienced housewife, and the thought of the extra work you will have to do fills you with dismay. Fortunately, relatives and friends are often willing to lend a hand, and your husband should be encouraged to do so if extra domestic help is not available.

'It will be necessary to readjust your daily routine to allow for at least three hours' extra work. You will recall that I explained "How to plan your day" in a previous talk. You may have to lower temporarily your standards of housekeeping and do the essentials only until you feel stronger. Admittedly baby needs a lot of your attention, but he won't need as much as you are likely to lavish on him. Your second baby will get far less handling and will be a healthier, happier baby because of it. Make up your mind to make a success of motherhood by doing your best to keep your husband and children healthy and happy. Let your husband experience the joys as well as the responsibilities of fatherhood; help him to adjust to this new home situation: encourage him. Give him a fair share of your love and attention if you want him to be a home-loving, devoted husband and father. It is well worth making an effort to achieve this.'

## THE INFANT AFTER THE FIRST MONTH

### SUN AND AIR-BATHS

#### *The Talk as given*

'You all know that baby must have fresh air; that is why you buy a pram in which to take him to the park. Babies, like flowers, grow and flourish in fresh air and sunshine, so while the summer days are here catch every sunbeam. But there is little value in taking baby to the park for a short airing if he spends the remainder of the time in a room with closed windows. I have seen a pram out of doors in which it was impossible to see the baby. The hood was up and the front opening closed half-way by a waterproof protector. No fresh air could reach the baby at the bottom of that pram.

### Air-baths

'Besides having fresh air to breathe, baby will thrive better if you give him air-baths. This is one way of hardening baby so that he will not catch colds so readily. The baby who is always bundled up perspires so much that whenever the slightest breath of a cool breeze reaches him he gets another cold. Start air-baths when baby is 4 weeks old. Before his water-bath allow him to lie naked on your lap for five minutes. Don't chill him in a cold room or by having the window wide open. As time goes on take every opportunity to expose his arms and legs, and you will find he will develop a healthy tan even if there is no sunshine.'

### Sun-bathing

'You may start sun-baths when baby is 3 months old. Go easily at first, for sun-tanning must be done slowly. Expose the legs only, for three minutes the first day. Increase the time by one minute each day, and expose a little more every day, until the whole body is getting the sun for 20 minutes. Then, when he is tanned all over he can remain in the sun for longer periods. Be sure to protect his head and the back of his neck with a suitable sun hat, especially from the hot mid-day sun. Whatever you do, don't attempt to tan your baby all in one day, especially at the seaside where the air is so much stronger. If you do, you will have a sick, sunburned child.

'You will soon see the results of sun- and air-baths; rosy cheeks will glow under a golden tan; abundant energy, and a splendid appetite are signs of a healthy, thriving baby.'

### *Treatment of Sunburn*

'Sunburn is very painful, so baby will be as cross as can be; he will be feverish—off his food—and he may vomit. Give him plenty of water to drink, but don't bath him. With the tips of your fingers, and using a feather-light touch, smear on plenty of cooling-cream, and keep him out of the sun for a few days until he is better.'

## FROM KICKING TO WALKING

Use teaching aids such as a play-pen with a blanket covered by a plastic or a rubber and a cotton sheet; examples of simple, safe playthings to be found in the home, such as—

### A wooden spoon: plastic napkin ring: reels on tape.

Stress the danger of toys with lead paint, sharp edges, and loose parts that may be swallowed.

### *The Talk as given*

'Your baby at the moment is a helpless mite, yet at the end of a year he will be a sturdy little fellow, standing on his own two feet, and ready for walking. But before he can stand and walk, his bones must be strong and his muscles firm.

'A mother is apt to think that if her baby is properly fed and she gives him vitamin drops and puts him out in the fresh air, she is doing all that is necessary. But that isn't enough, baby must get plenty of exercise. I have seen babies of 10 months whose legs were too weak and flabby to support the weight of their bodies. These babies had been bundled up in their prams for long periods, and their leg muscles were not developed because of lack of exercise.

'During the long summer days babies get a glorious opportunity to exercise. If you look into a pram and see a pair of active bare brown legs you will also see bright eyes and a beaming smile, for the baby who is given the chance to kick with perfect abandon amuses himself happily. In the winter, baby must, of course, be wrapped up to keep him warm, so he ought to get his exercise indoors. Stretching and squirming strengthen baby's back in readiness for sitting up. Kicking with freedom and vigour not only develops good leg muscles, it helps the formation of straight bones and enables baby to strengthen those eager limbs of his in readiness for standing and walking.'

## EXERCISE DURING THE FIRST MONTHS

'Begin exercising baby as early as you like. At two weeks give him five minutes to kick when you change his napkin at feeding times. He will be hungry, so arms and legs will wave furiously. Then when you undress baby in the morning, and at bath-time in the evening, let him kick naked on your lap; turn him over and stroke his back to encourage him to stretch. If you haven't got a play-pen lay baby on a clean napkin over a rubber and cotton sheet, on the floor, the settee, or your own bed. (Don't leave him for a second, for it is surprising how a tiny baby can roll or wriggle to the edge of a wide bed in a matter of minutes.) Turn him over on his tummy, he will raise his head and arch his back. Let him roll about for 10 minutes. About the fourth month baby will start pushing his feet on your knee. Hold him around the body, taking the weight off his legs, and let him get the feel of his feet. His legs will grow stronger each week, and he will learn to control them. Encourage him to walk up your body, and he will gurgle with delight at this new game.

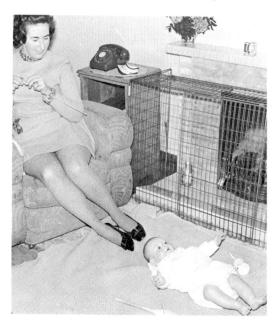

Fig. 46-34   Baby having exercise on the floor. Note efficient fire guard.
*Maternity Section, Central Hospital, Irvine, Ayrshire.*

'Let baby have a few simple toys; in the play-pen, a ball that he has to stretch to reach, four empty reels threaded on a tape, a red plastic napkin ring will please him as much as the expensive toys will. Rubber or woolly animals are more suitable for the pram. Playing with toys gives practice in muscle control and co-ordination. Out of doors there are so many things he loves to watch, and if you give him an occasional smile and a cheery word of greeting, baby will be perfectly content. Busy, active babies are healthy and happy.'

'A play-pen is a good investment for baby's health and happiness; in it he gets more exercise than is possible in the pram. With safety he can roll about and get all the exercise he needs from about the fourth month. Play-pen babies rarely crawl; their legs are so well developed that they stand and walk. During the ninth month, and sometimes before then, baby will pull himself on to his feet in his pen, and what fun it is; he bumps down for the sheer delight of pulling himself up again.

'You needn't worry about early standing being the cause of bow-legs. It is the pale, fat flabby baby who has had neither vitamin drops nor exercise who gets bow-legs. You can depend on it that a baby will not attempt to stand until his legs are strong enough to bear his weight, but don't urge him to do so until he himself wants to. He may try to stand up in his pram, and I need hardly remind you how easily baby can fall out of it; so do use a set of safety harness after the seventh month, especially if his legs are strong.

'From the time the baby stands it will be about two months before he walks by himself. To maintain his balance he keeps his feet wide apart, but very little will topple him over. Help him by removing bulky napkins. Clumsy, hard shoes are difficult to negotiate on polished floors, and after one or two nasty bumps baby loses confidence. A few babies walk before they are a year old, the majority are fifteen months.'

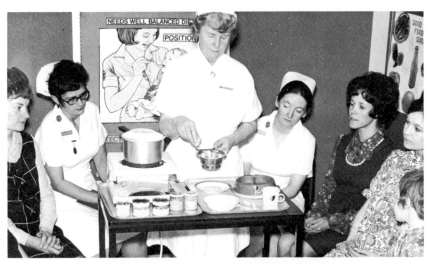

Fig. 46-35   Using the Mouli grinder. Liver being cooked.
*Maternity Hospital, Stirling.*

## SPOON AND CUP FEEDING

Much experience of baby feeding is necessary before the midwife is qualified to advise on this subject. The talk on weaning should probably be omitted until the need arises, when it could with greater advantage be given to individual mothers.

*The Scottish report on infant feeding 1970 states that there is no need to give solids prior to 4 months and no fresh cow's milk during the first year.*

Use teaching aids such as colourful baby-china: spoon and pusher: vitamin drops: tin of cereal baby food.

### The Talk as given

'The first thing baby gets from a spoon is vitamin drops; usually when he is three weeks old. It is given for sturdy growth. Spoon-feeding should not be begun until baby is over 16 weeks old, but baby experts have different opinions.

'Take the advice of the doctor who knows your baby; he will tell you which foods baby should have; I am just offering a few hints as to how you should prepare and give them.'

## Cereals and egg yolk

'Cereals are not now introduced until the fourth month, when baby can have 4 ml of cereal baby food. After cooking mix it to a creamy consistency with whatever milk he is having. He will try to suck it at first and will spill most of it but he will soon learn. Gradually increase by 4 ml every two weeks until he is getting 30 ml daily.

'**Egg yolk is excellent for babies because it contains iron** and other invaluable substances. Start with 4 ml of lightly boiled egg—no more or you may upset him. Offer it as a great treat, let him see the yellow colour, and don't force it on him like medicine. Give egg every other day before the 10.00 hours feed if you like. Baby should be 8 months old before he gets half an egg, and 15 months before he has a whole egg. Baby has to get accustomed to many different kinds of food, to the flavour and texture of more solid things such as milk pudding and sieved vegetables. But if we are too late in introducing them baby may have become so attached to sucking milk that he refuses anything else. Tinned baby foods are convenient.

'Some infants get very annoyed when offered solid food before having the breast or bottle; this is probably because they are thirsty and want a drink first. Others resent solid food either before or after. A baby may object to any change in the routine he knows and enjoys, so humour him a little. Putting a little egg yolk on the tip of the spoon with the vegetable might help, for it is quite a good plan to introduce a new food along with one he already knows.

'At 4 months you could give sieved vegetable. Begin with cooked lettuce, as it is so easily digested, but you can use any fresh green vegetable that has been boiled until tender and rubbed through a fine sieve. 4 g (one teaspoonful) will be enough to begin with. If he refuses it, try again in a week or two.

'The Mouli grinder and sieve is useful for fruit, vegetables, fish and meat.'

## Liver is good for babies

'One very special food for babies is calf's or lamb's liver which helps baby to form rich red blood. Cut a small slice, 0·8 cm (one-third of an inch) thick, put it between two saucers with 4 ml (one teaspoonful) of warm water, and steam it for 20 minutes over a saucepan that is boiling briskly. Liver should be thoroughly cooked. Rub it through a fine sieve, and give 4 g (one teaspoonful) with the sieved vegetable. Increase the amount until at 6 months he is having 15 g (one tablespoonful).'

## WEANING

'Don't hurry over weaning: it should take about four weeks. Baby is now accustomed to so many different foods that it is just a question of getting him to give up sucking and to use a cup and spoon. Continue with modified dried milk.

'**The first week.** He will have one meal without sucking, usually the midday meal. Serve minced chicken, fish, liver or meat with 15 g (one tablespoonful) of vegetable and potato. Give a small helping of pudding or stewed fruit and a drink of milk from his cup.

**'The second week.** He will have two meals with no bottle, i.e. breakfast in addition to the midday meal: porridge; or cereal; or half an egg; wholewheat bread and butter, milk 200 ml.

| On waking 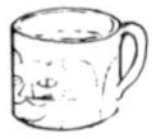 | Juice of half an orange diluted. 60ml |
| --- | --- |
| 8·0am 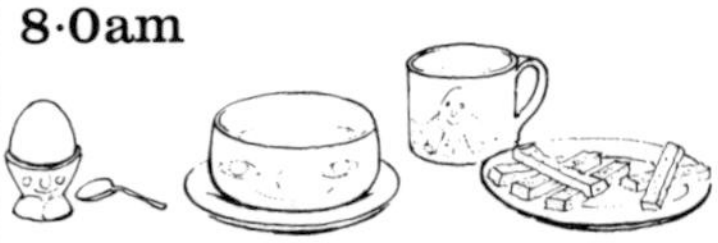 | Oat flour or Farex or baby cereal 2 tablespoons. or ½ egg or 1 rasher lean bacon chopped. Toast and butter. Milk 200 ml |
| 12·0 noon 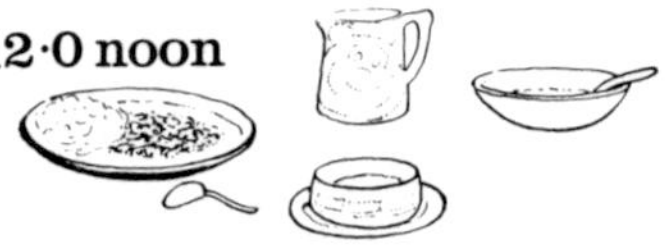 | Vegetable soup 4 tablespoons or mashed veg. 2 tablespoons. Meat, chicken or liver minced, 2 tablespoons minced. Grated apple or milk pudding, 2 tablespoons. Milk 100 ml |
| 4·0pm 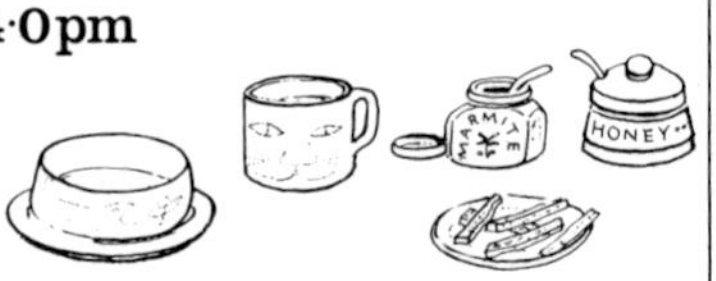 | Fish or other milk soup or custard or cheese or egg sandwich. Banana or stewed apple —sponge finger, Liga rusk or bread and butter. Milk 100 ml |
| 10·0pm 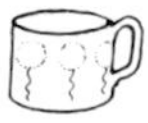 | Milk 200 ml |

Protein, vitamins and minerals are essential. Egg once daily morning or evening.
Fresh milk 600ml. Avoid too many starchy, rich or greasy foods.

Fig. 46-36   Suggested foods at one year.

**'The third week.** He will have three meals with no bottle, i.e. supper at about 17.00 hours, as well as the other two meals: cereal; baby food. He will probably wish to have a drink of milk at 22.00 hours until he is about a year old.

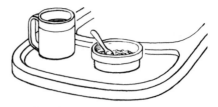

Fig. 46-37   Meals on high chair.

**'At one year.** Baby should have 600 ml of milk every day. Always remember it is the body-building foods as well as fruit and vegetables with their minerals and vitamins that baby needs. Starchy foods make fat, flabby babies, but a baby with strong straight bones and firm muscles is far healthier in every way.

'Don't worry if your baby is slow in drinking from a cup, giving up the bottle or in feeding himself; some babies develop at a slower rate without being actually backward. Allow him to feed himself as soon as he wants to even if he makes a mess. Some feed themselves at 10 or 12 months, others later. If he refuses to eat the foods you serve, don't fuss or show any anxiety or you will have more and more trouble. The mother who can keep calm at meal times will usually manage to get her infant to eat the foods that build bonny babies.'

## TRAINING BABY TO KEEP DRY

### *The Talk as given*

'The most successful method is to start potting at the ninth month. Babies take longer to gain control when potting is started early; an investigation carried out on a large number of babies proved this quite conclusively. You may hold baby out from the second week, if you like, so long as you realise that you are not training him. Catch what comes, and be satisfied, but if you think you are teaching him to wait until you pot him again, you are going to be bitterly disappointed. Baby is too young to know what you are trying to teach him. After all, the sensation of water in the bladder is a very delicate one, and if after seven months he is no further ahead, you are going to get discouraged, and slack off in your efforts at the very time when you should be starting to train him.

'We all know the type of mother who is determined to have the perfectly trained baby, dry at all costs. She is thinking more of her own reputation as a good manager than of what is best for baby. Poor lamb, he is potted before and after feeds, before he goes out and when he comes in, before he goes to sleep and when he wakes up. No wonder he hates the pot and rebelliously refuses to use it on many occasions as soon as he is old enough to register his objection. He is shamed and blamed, scolded and spanked, and all this fuss gets him so worked up that he can't relax and do what is wanted. The happy baby becomes stubborn and bad tempered, and later develops into a defiant or sulky toddler.

'Baby has to learn to control bowel and bladder but he also has to learn self-control which for him is difficult. Constant reprimanding and thwarting only makes the process harder. Try to appreciate how much he has to learn when he does not understand "why".'

#### START TRAINING BABY AT NINE MONTHS

'Study his habits; note when he usually passes water and make your efforts coincide with "his times", which will most likely be every two or three hours.

'Always hold him out in the same place, so that he will learn where you want him to do it.

'Use a special word and he will soon know what it means.

'Show him the water when he has passed it, and again use the special word. It is at this point that baby is really beginning to learn bladder control. Don't hold him out for longer than three or four minutes. Praise his success with a word or two; ignore failure. Be careful not to overpraise, or his feelings will be hurt on the days when he gets no praise. Keep steadily on, week after week, with persistent regularity, cheerful and hopeful. There will be periods of success and many setbacks; eventually, at about 15 months, he will tell you when he has passed water, and, not until about 18 months, will he tell you he wants to do it. Baby learns first that he has done it, later he learns that he is going to do it. Leave off the napkin when he can go for two hours. When busy playing, he may ignore the need until it is too late;

remind him, for the memory of a child is short. Overlook occasional lapses. Active or highly strung children take longer than the placid type, and boys are rather slower than girls. It does, however, take longer to gain bladder control at night. Few children are dry all night at two years, and most are nearly three before they can do without napkins. Bowel training starts at the same time as bladder training, although baby may have had success with the pot prior to that time. He is quite well trained at 12 or 15 months.

'It is the patient mother who plods steadily on, never expecting too much of a mere infant, who has the greatest success; the strict disciplinarian who makes such a "to do" about a perfectly natural function takes far longer to train her baby and may make him feel unloved. It is most important for a child to feel that he himself is loved although his behaviour may not be approved of.

'If at $3\frac{1}{2}$ years he is still wetting, much encouragement is required; he needs all the help you can give him. Patience and perseverance are indeed excellent qualities in a mother.'

# TEETHING

### *The Talk as given*

'There is always great rejoicing in the home when baby cuts his first tooth. The event is often anticipated for weeks and sometimes months, because from about the fourth month baby has been dribbling or slavering. But there is no connection at all between teething and dribbling, except that they occur at the same time. To digest starchy foods such as oat-flour or Farex, baby is now producing saliva, and it dribbles down his chin until he learns to swallow it. Day after day mother looks at his gums, and although it always seems as if a tooth is just ready to come through, nothing happens. Then without warning two tiny teeth are seen peeping through the lower gum; baby has cut his first teeth and never even made a whimper. That is what usually happens; it is the double ones that are apt to upset baby and cause disturbed nights; they come through during the second year.'

#### TIMES OF CUTTING TEETH

'The first two teeth may appear during the sixth month, but don't worry if your baby has no teeth even at 9 months as long as he is a sturdy infant; babies grow and develop at different rates. You will be attending your doctor or the child health clinic, and they will advise you what to do if teething is slow.

'If you would like to know when baby gets his teeth, I'll tell you an easy way to remember.

'He should have six teeth less than his age in months.

**At 12 months baby has  6 teeth.**
**At 18 months baby has 12 teeth.**
**At 24 months baby has 18 teeth.**

'By the time he is $2\frac{1}{2}$ years old the 20 baby teeth will be cut.'

### Care during teething

'In cold weather see that baby has a cosy vest that fastens well up in front, for when his dress is sopping wet with saliva he is more likely to catch cold. Soft muslin bibs (four layers) are very satisfactory, but **do not use a plastic bib:** they have been known to blow over baby's nose and mouth with disastrous results. If baby is at the crawling stage his hands will get dirty, and as he is sucking his fingers a great deal at this time, wash them often. There is nothing to beat soap and water to prevent infection; have clean floors, clean clothes, clean toys. Baby's resistance to germs is lowered when he is upset with teething, and a cold may develop into bronchitis. Cotton play trousers with shoulder straps worn over a knitted dress or suit can be easily washed. They keep baby clean and warm. Use a plastic spoon with a rounded edge when feeding him, the sharp edge of a metal spoon will hurt his gums and make him cry.

'Give him something to bite on. It must be clean and unbreakable, not sharp. Bone teething rings are usually recommended, but as a rule baby prefers something a little softer, a rubber toy or his own fingers.'

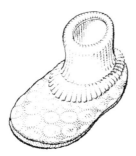

Fig. 46-38 Warm pram shoes.
*Courtesy Mothercare.*

### TEETHING TROUBLES

'It is true some babies are upset, but we must not blame teething for every illness that occurs during the two years of teething time. If his gums are hot and painful he will be restless and cross. Give him frequent sips of cool water; it soothes his gums, and, if feverish, he needs the extra fluid. If he isn't hungry don't coax him to eat. Baby needs less food when he is feverish, and don't give any new foods or he may be upset.

'Some babies seem to have skin spots at teething time, but doctors think they are probably due to some food that baby hasn't become accustomed to. Moisten some bicarbonate of soda and dab it on to soothe the itching. See that his bowels move every day; the extra water should help, but use a mild laxative such as milk of magnesia, if necessary. If his urine is dark in colour or has a strong smell, you will know he isn't getting enough to drink.

'Out of doors let him wear a helmet or hood, or tie a scarf round his ears if there is a cold blustering wind, for teething babies do get pain in their jaws.

'A teething baby has a very sensitive nervous system, so if he is having a bad day keep him quiet, give extra mothering and prevent the other children from trying to amuse him; excitement only makes things worse. A warm bath and early to bed is good treatment.

'All these things are not going to happen to any one infant, and the majority of babies cut their teeth with no trouble whatsoever, so don't let the teething bogey worry you unduly.'

## THE TODDLER AND THE NEW BABY

Some toddlers resent the intrusion of a new baby and may suffer intense jealousy if the parents do not show understanding. An endeavour should be made to avoid the psychological trauma which may ensue. Jealousy can be exhibited in various ways, such as temper tantrums, whining, bed-wetting and reversion to baby habits; these may not be manifest until months later.

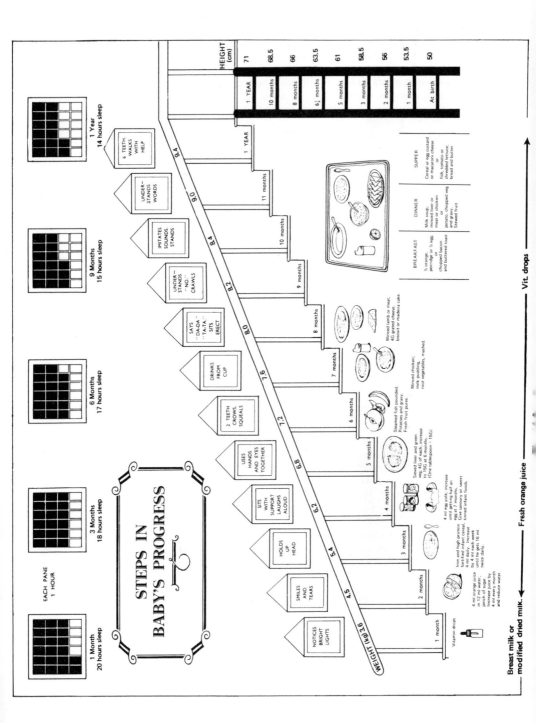

It would be considerate if the toddler saw the new baby for the first time in a cot rather than in the mother's arms. Should domestic assistance be given by a relative or home-help, it might be discreet to allow her, rather than the mother, to attend to the new baby in the toddler's presence. Nor would it be advisable for the baby to be fed by the mother in the same room as the toddler. Allowing him to help with the bath and other matters will tend to make him feel that the baby belongs to him.

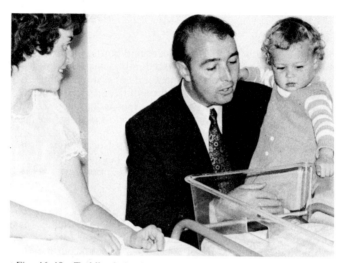

Fig. 46-40  Toddler being introduced to the new baby in hospital.
*Simpson Memorial Maternity Pavilion, Edinburgh.*

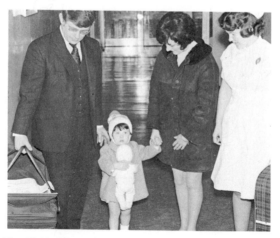

Fig. 46-41  The toddler is given a doll from the new baby.
*Maternity Section, Central Hospital, Irvine, Ayrshire.*

During this period the father usually devotes more time to the toddler who will revel in this. He should also be given a particularly coveted toy but should be spared hearing excessive adulation of the baby by visitors and ought not to see the gifts they bring. If parents give the toddler extra attention and assure him of their love by a more than usual display of affection he will more readily accept and enjoy the new baby.

## PREVENTION OF ACCIDENTS IN THE HOME DURING THE FIRST YEAR

**Young mothers should be warned about potential dangers.**

### Choking and suffocating

Baby should be laid on his side after feeds and bottles should never be propped otherwise the infant may inhale regurgitated milk.

**Babies are nose breathers** and if due to nasal congestion the nose is blocked the infant does not know to breathe through his mouth and may suffocate. The doctor will prescribe drops to clear the nose. For this reason the baby should sleep in his mother's bedroom. Overlaying is uncommon today as most babies have their own cots.

**Plastic bibs** can blow over baby's face and suffocate him. Soft pillows are dangerous. Toddlers should not play with plastic bags.

**Cats** have been known to lie over a baby's face in pram or cot: a cat net provides protection from stray cats.

### Burning

Dangers to be avoided are leaking hot water bottles; putting hot water into the bath before the cold water: heating an enamel potty in front of the fire: baby pulling on the table cloth and upsetting hot tea or soup: pot handles protruding over the edge of the stove.

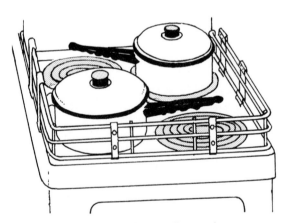

Fig. 46-42   Safety rail on cooker.

A fire guard is essential when the crawling stage is reached and flame-proof fabrics should be used. Bri-nylon melts when set alight and burns the skin.

### Miscellaneous dangers

Prams and cots may be tipped over by an active baby or an older child: harness is essential. All electrical appliances are potential dangers and little fingers are sometimes poked into electric sockets, ingenuity is needed to prevent opening doors and falling downstairs. Drawstrings around the neck may be pulled tight. Chewing toys with lead paint. Cheap toys with pins to fix the eyes in position, and those with sharp edges. Medicines not in locked cupboards or not out of reach.

Babies should not be left alone with a slice of apple or a rusk. They may choke on a crumb, peanuts being light may be inhaled and cause a serious lung disturbance.

---

### QUESTIONS FOR REVISION

What advice would you give in response to the mother's questions: What will I do if baby screams during the night? How soon can I take baby out in the pram? How will I know if baby is too hot? How many hours should a baby sleep during 24 hours? How will I know baby is crying too much? If baby chokes when I am giving him his bottle what will I do? Why should I not use a pillow? Why are plastic bibs condemned? My husband wants the baby to be circumcised. My mother says the baby is tongue-tied and thinks this should be cut. Are green motions serious? How do I clean baby's nose and mouth? Should baby sleep in a separate room?

**C.M.B.(Scot.) 30-min. question.** Outline a programme for the education of the patient in preparation for labour and parenthood.

**Short C.M.B. questions.**

**Eng.** Education of expectant fathers.

**Eng.** Preparation of infant milk feeds in the home.

**Scot.** What would you teach mothers about bottle feeding?

**Scot.** Outline a talk to expectant fathers. Explain why the following are not recommended (a) propping feeding bottles, (b) using plastic bibs, (c) having drawstrings in garments around the neck.

# 47
# Principles and Psychology of Education
## APPLIED TO THE INSTRUCTION OF EXPECTANT MOTHERS

*The learning process; arousing interest; promoting understanding: psychology of education; motivation, attention, making contact, repetition. Methods of learning, methods of teaching, teaching aids. Demonstration. Discussion. Drawing. TV Broadcasts.*

This subject can only be dealt with at a very rudimentary level in the few pages available within the limits of a textbook for midwives. An endeavour has been made to elucidate some of the principles and the psychology of education to enable midwives to teach expectant mothers the processess of childbearing and child-rearing.

**Midwives are well equipped to teach parentcraft:** they have knowledge and experience of the obstetric and paediatric aspects but they may not know how people learn or how to help them to learn.

### THE EXPECTANT MOTHER'S POINT OF VIEW

**The teacher should be sensitive to the emotional state of the pregnant woman and** endeavour to imagine her thoughts and feelings at this time. She is going through one of life's enriching experiences; sentiment runs high so the teacher should not be too mundane and matter of fact in her approach. Notes of lectures given to student midwives on pregnancy or babies are not suitable; they frequently contain bald statements of a scientific nature that have no appeal for the mother-to-be. A more personal, even sentimental approach is needed and facts ought to be clothed in words that reflect the mother's joy in creation.

Acceptance of advice will be influenced by the expectant mother's knowledge and experience: traditional and cultural beliefs may have to be overcome. Some will accept advice when the benefits are stated others respond to logical argument.

### THE LEARNING PROCESS

**Learning is a complex, slow process** whereby new knowledge is linked to what is already known. It involves thinking which is a process of exercising the mind and using mental imagery. By seeking clues from already known matter, a conclusion is arrived at by logical reasoning: the conclusion is then tested by critical analysis.

**The process of learning involves remembering and recall;** the person being taught should be able to apply the new knowledge to a different procedure or situation. To assist the learning process every statement made should be crystal clear: each sentence should carry the lesson a stage further on. This may necessitate making definite, even dogmatic, pronouncements, a measure usually advisable when teaching the novice. Having given what you consider is the best method, don't confuse the issue by making alternative suggestions. Do not clutter the talk with unnecessary words.

**Most people have to be told or shown what to do at least three times before they really learn:** repetition is therefore very necessary, but it should not be too obvious. Explanations should be made wherever possible, for unless people understand, they do not learn; they may look without seeing, and hear without comprehending. The 'reason why' should be stated in order to be convincing, particularly when something contrary to common practice is being recommended. The reasons given may so impress the mother that she remembers what she is told, e.g. why cold water ought to be put into baby's bath before the hot water.

**Only when the pupil learns has she been taught.** Teaching is not merely 'telling' or pouring information into the mind. It consists in causing people to learn and involves using methods and providing circumstances in which learning can take place.

## THE PRINCIPLES OF EDUCATION

**The principles of education are founded on the laws of learning** which incorporate the reasons that motivate and govern the teaching and learning processes. Methods of teaching are grounded on the principles and psychology of education. If an educational principle is violated or ignored the teaching method is unlikely to be successful.

### Finding the growing point

It is essential to have some idea of what the class know already, so that new knowledge can be linked and added to what is already known. The multipara has had experience of pregnancy, labour and baby care. The well educated woman will have read widely on associated subjects. It is a sound principle to teach the simple before the complex: the normal before the abnormal, to go from known to unknown.

## AROUSING INTEREST

**This is one of the essentials in teaching.** There are many and varied reasons why people are interested in a particular subject or problem. Interest may have to be aroused as when teaching arithmetic to a schoolboy so his teacher links the subject to something he will be interested in such as cars or aeroplanes. When learning 'meets a need' interest is high. Teaching the expectant mother is comparatively easy because her need is great: she is aware that her knowledge of childbearing and childrearing is scant; she is eager to learn.

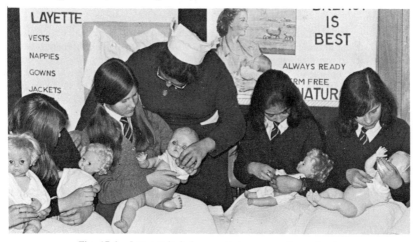

Fig. 47-1   Interest in baby care being aroused at school.

**To maintain interest her need must be met and satisfied.** She should be given the sort of information she requires; shown what she wants to see, e.g. how to bath baby, a model layette. We will of course teach her what we think she ought to know and this may entail giving two different subjects in one lesson in order that her interest in mothercraft is maintained.

**Interest can be stifled** if the subject matter is too difficult, the language too technical, as could happen if information suitable for student midwives is given to mothers-to-be. Conversely, if the subject matter is too elementary, boredom ensues. When delivered too rapidly brain fag occurs and interest wanes.

**The teacher, by her personality, enthusiasm, choice of words,** ability to paint vivid word pictures, can hold interest. Skilful use of the voice gives meaning to what is being said and amplifies the learning process. Awareness of platform deportment and voice production enables the teacher to give an interesting performance.

PROMOTING UNDERSTANDING

The woman does not learn unless she understands and knows the reasons why she should accept and practise what she is being taught. Explanation is essential and teaching-aids can be used to elucidate the problem.

**Explanation is given** by the teacher but the pupil draws her own conclusions. She sees 'the light' when the new facts become meaningful: cohesion between existing knowledge, previous experience, and the subject being taught having occurred. Expectant mothers are usually mature adults, many having well established ideas, accomplishments and attitudes that have to be taken into consideration.

## THE PSYCHOLOGY OF EDUCATION

Psychology is concerned with how the mind works. Individual behaviour is influenced by emotional stimuli that give rise to responses or feelings; learning is an emotional as well as an intellectual pursuit. The teacher applies her knowledge of psychology which has given her insight regarding how people learn and this enables her to further the learning process. Psychologically the pupil will get emotional satisfaction and find joy in achievement from the learning process, when (a) the subject matter meets her need, (b) the method of teaching increases her understanding of the subject, (c) the experience is pleasurable.

### PSYCHOLOGICAL PROCEDURES THAT FURTHER LEARNING

**Motivation**

**Learning is more effective when imbued with a sense of purpose.** The expectant mother's need is urgent; she is interested and willing to learn. The maternal instinct motivates her to prepare for and learn how to look after her baby. The fact that she will experience labour intensifies her curiosity in the process and she wants to know how she can be helped to cope with the stress that may occur. The midwife has a receptive pupil to teach; she must endeavour to meet her needs and to foster her acquiescent attitude.

**Attracting and holding attention**

**Attention is the outward expression of interest;** i.e. being mentally alert, looking, listening and thinking. When attention is diligently applied the state of concentration is reached.

**To hold the attention of a group,** the mind of each one must be kept active. The vitality of the teacher and her ability to paint vivid word pictures, the interest of the subject, the setting up of an attractive display, handing out typed recipes or instructions, passing round samples of fabrics and patterns, allowing the members of the group to participate in demonstration or discussion all help to maintain attention.

Every available teaching device should be utilised to hold attention, including the teacher's personality, expressed in her bearing, deportment, voice production and choice of words.

### Remembering

Having understood and accepted the suggested idea remembering is the next stage in the learning process. Most people have to be told or shown three times before the new knowledge is firmly entrenched and can be recalled.

### Repetition

**Repetition is utilised to compensate for the inevitable forgetting that** occurs. To avoid boring the pupils, repetition should be subtle and varied. Facts can be presented in a different context, linking them to the basic principle, the form of presentation can be varied, visual or auditory.

**Bathing baby is often taught inadequately** for lack of repetition; this procedure provides a good example of how repetition can be employed with subtlety and variety.

### Eight examples of repetition used when teaching how to bath baby

(1) Midwife gives demonstration of bathing baby, using a doll.
(2) Description and use of equipment.
(3) Demonstration by mothers of the bathing positions with repetition of difficult manoeuvres.
(4) Detailed demonstration of complete bath using doll.
(5) Demonstration of bathing by a mother under direction of teacher.
(6) Given printed copy of procedure.
(7) Shown how to bath her own baby.
(8) Baths her baby under close supervision.

### Recapitulation

This is a form of repetition but is usually a rapid revision or summing up of the main points at the end of the talk. It ought to take place throughout the lesson as the need and opportunity arises, in order to be useful and meaningful. Mere reiteration suggests that learning is a mechanical process depending on memory when it is a state of growth involving understanding and reasoning.

## METHODS OF LEARNING

**Learning by rote** is merely memorising words without understanding their meaning and having no appreciation of the significance of the idea being conveyed.

**Trial and error.** Learning by making mistakes is slow, extravagant in material, time and effort as well as being dangerous when health is concerned. Wise persons benefit from other people's mistakes and are guided by a teacher who shares with them her knowledge and experience.

**Trial and success.** This mental process, similar to trial and error, should be practised by those who plan for the future. The procedure or situation is visualised mentally, applied to the principles of education, thinking and reasoning, identifying the problem in the light of existing knowledge and past experience: then accepting or rejecting the proposition.

**Problem solving** is the method currently much in vogue. It is a form of mental 'trial and success.' It involves

(a) appreciation of and understanding the problem;
(b) consideration of benefits, advantages and disadvantages;
(c) thinking—reasoning and critical analysis of the situation;
(d) arrival at a conclusion;
(e) solution of the problem.

# METHODS OF TEACHING

Method is concerned with how the subject matter is presented and involves learner, teacher and subject matter. The teacher must have an aim clearly defined as to what she is trying to accomplish and this entails planning the programme so that the subject unfolds in logical sequence toward the desired goal.

### Preparing the Talk

Start preparing the talk in ample time; read all the books available to you on the subject: draw on your own knowledge and experience. Jot down suitable facts under headings, check and re-check them, for all statements made must be correct and up to date, as well as practical. If in doubt consult an expert. Never underestimate the intelligence of your audience and be prepared to answer their questions.

**A clear plan should be made out** and the subject-matter arranged systematically rather than giving it as a jumble of unrelated facts. Search your brain for an exciting opening sentence. Set the matter aside for a few days and go back to it with a fresh outlook; new ideas may come while the subject is simmering in your mind. Write up the talk as fully as you wish, choosing words which depict what you mean to convey with vividness and exactitude. Again set the material aside, then read it over with a critical eye and select only the best of it, prune ruthlessly; the improvement will be marked. Polish it until the style is fluent yet lucid. Set it aside once more, then read it aloud and listen to the sound of the words, remembering that they are to be heard and not read. If you get someone to read it to you the faults in construction will be even more evident. Continue polishing and rearranging until it cannot be improved any further. By this time you are saturated with the subject-matter although you have not actually memorised it. 'Time' it to the required length.

**Choose intriguing non-medical titles,** e.g. Pregnant and pretty. The latest fashions for ladies-in-waiting. What every expectant father should know. Cries in the night.

Arrange headings on filing cards, using red and blue ink to catch the eye. Think of these headings as islands between which you must swim; you won't founder for you are buoyed up with a very comprehensive knowledge of the subject, without such notes, the teacher tends to ramble and may omit some very important points.

**Practise the delivery of one heading** until it is mastered: do the second one, then both together and continue until the whole is ready for delivery. This apparently simple talk will, when given with effortless ease, belie all the hard work that has gone into its preparation.

**Parentcraft should be presented in** such a way that baby-care is depicted as a happy experience. An effort can be made to create a bright friendly atmosphere: a little kindly humour will help to make the talk sparkle. In order that those of less than average intelligence will understand what is being taught, the language used should be within their range of comprehension: the lay equivalent of medical terms given.

## MAKING CONTACT

This term is used to designate the mental and psychological link that a good teacher creates between the learners and herself and is one of the most vital factors in teaching. Contact is made by the teacher when she looks at and talks to the audience as individuals in whom she is interested and to whom she is eager to pass on her ideas. Her gaze is directed towards the whole group yet every member feels that she is being looked at; the spoken word is heard by each individual as though meant for her personally.

**Examples of how to make contact**

**When demonstrating 'baby's layette'** the midwife's eyes ought to be on the audience so that her personality is projected towards them; she should only glance at the garment she is displaying.

**When demonstrating 'baby's bath'** she must frequently look at and address the group if only to say 'watch carefully what I'm going to do now' or 'I'll do that over again' or to explain a point. If the midwife's whole attention is concentrated on what she is doing with her hands no contact is made, and only an intense interest in the subject will hold the attention of the group.

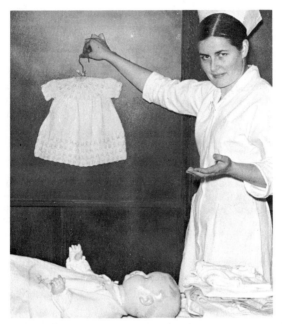

Fig. 47-2   Education in mothercraft teaching. Student midwife making contact. Talking to the audience, not to the garment. Clear background.

*Simpson Memorial Maternity Pavilion, Edinburgh.*

**When using teaching aids** such as posters, blackboard or baby clothes they ought to be given only a fleeting glance. **Teach the audience not the blackboard.**

**Failing to make contact**

No contact is made when a lecturer is so engrossed in her subject or indifferent to the educational needs of her audience that she appears to be quite oblivious of their presence. Under no circumstances should a talk on a simple subject like baby-care be read. Listening to any lecture being read is dull and boring in the extreme because this breaks the vital contact so necessary between speaker and audience. When the eyes are glued to the reading desk there is no opportunity for the personality to bring the spoken word to life.

Notes should be held in the hand or placed on a lectern, if on a table this entails looking down and away from the audience which creates a break in contact.

A good teacher needs some of the attributes of the actor; physical mental and emotional faculties must all be utilised.

## TEACHING AIDS

These should be set out in readiness to start without delay in order that the rhythm of the talk will not be interrupted. Introducing a visual teaching aid at the precise moment when required, adds to the vitality of the lesson.

**Teaching aids are utilised to amplify verbal teaching,** but it should be realised that no matter how unique these are in conception or artistic in execution they are only of value if they simplify the lesson or make it more interesting and enjoyable. They are not substitutes for teaching.

### Baby clothes and equipment

These are absolutely essential for teaching baby-care and can be displayed for their attractive, decorative value, and to create the atmosphere that appeals to mothers even although not utilised in the lesson being taught. Some manufacturers will supply garments and equipment, patterns of materials and catalogues on request. Baby equipment is discussed under the appropriate demonstrations.

## POSTERS

They should be arresting in colour and design, conveying the message at a glance. Posters ought to be designed with racial customs in mind: being appropriate to the country and people. Advice given ought to be positive, good rather than bad methods being depicted. Printing should be legible at a distance, captions short and pithy. Many commercial posters are so colourful and pleasing that they introduce an aesthetic quality as well as having educational worth.

Flannelgraphs supply a variation of poster and blackboard, but being somewhat limited in their usefulness are not so popular. Printed headings can be presented quickly; gaily coloured felt cut-outs are excellent to depict the generative organs and fetus *in utero*: cut-outs from glossy magazines make a colourful display of fruits and vegetables. The peg board and the magnetic board lend variety for display purposes.

**The portoscope or overhead projector is** suitable when teaching small groups. Coloured diagrams should be carefully planned and labelled to emphasise salient points. Notes are set out 6–8 words per line. There is scope for ingenuity in the use of colour and intriguing design.

## THE BLACKBOARD (Chalk Board)

This well-tried device is a most valuable teaching aid, too often used only to jot down words or on which to scribble a poorly conceived diagram. It is worth while going to the trouble of achieving proficiency in its use.

### Start with an empty blackboard

There is great educational value in teaching step by step while building up a drawing or setting out headings. The necessary action breaks the monotony of talk. Coloured dust-free chalk should be used with vigour and gay abandon to give emphasis, variety and beauty. Study from a distance the colours that show up well in close proximity to each other, such as red and yellow, green and white. Blue can rarely be seen beyond the front row. Do not hold the chalk like a pencil. Use half a stick, one end in the palm, the point projecting 1.25 cm beyond the tips of the thumb and first two fingers. Apply sufficient pressure to make a bold decisive line.

White boards are difficult to clean when large-scale eradication is necessary during the lesson.

### How to draw

As an aid to drawing look at the object for six times as long as it will take to draw it, noting the proportions of length to breadth, the ratio of the size of one part to another, e.g. cervix to corpus, the convexity of curves and other details. Thus the visual image is transmitted to the brain which then guides the hand.

Practise drawing heavy bold lines, vertical, horizontal and semi-circular, right across the blackboard with a wide sweep of the arm, using shoulder and elbow rather than wrist. Continue until convincing lines can be executed under perfect control. Wavy thin lines are not readily visible and convey the impression that the teacher is lacking in resolution.

Printing is legible, but round writing is done more quickly. Practise writing rows of words 10, 5, 2·5, 1·25 cm in size. From the back of the room it will be evident that medium size is the most legible.

### A clear plan

Decide how to arrange blackboard headings and sub-headings for each lesson. Avoid too much detail. The outline should be intelligible, because of its orderly arrangement to anyone who was not present at the lesson. It also provides an excellent means for recapitulation. Duplicate the foundation drawing rather than cluttering it with detail to such an extent that the structure or idea depicted is neither comprehensible nor recognisable.

### Learning from the blackboard

The blackboard is a valuable aid to learning; a means whereby understanding of the subject is enhanced, not merely a vehicle for the statement of facts.

The teacher is the link between audience and blackboard and the vital contact with the audience must be constantly maintained. While writing, turn towards the audience as far as is possible.

Long silences while writing are wasteful and create an intangible barrier. Explain what you are drawing; spell a difficult or new word, stop to explain a point.

Using the blackboard as an effective aid to learning requires teaching skill of a high order.

### BULLETIN BOARD FOR EXPECTANT MOTHERS

A bulletin board is ideal for exhibiting printed matter or illustrations that will educate or interest expectant mothers. The layout must be attractive to catch the eye. Bright, gaily coloured cut-outs from the cookery section of women's magazines. Booklets from baby food manufacturers are a source of attractive baby photographs; pages from catalogues of baby equipment showing the latest in prams, baths, etc., are always appreciated.

**Educational exhibits.** Maternity benefits, immunisation. Family planning.

**Health education.** Foods that build bonny babies. Foods that prevent anaemia. Keeping food clean, covered, cool. Good posture.

Mottoes and pictures relating to home and motherhood.

*Illustrations from midwifery textbooks are not suitable.*

## FILMS AND FILM STRIPS

These are admirable to depict situations that are beyond the scope of classroom presentation by the teacher, e.g. the birth of a baby. The teacher will make her own comments as the method shown may be at variance with those approved of by the teacher or her employing authority. Films can be used to show the childbearing process as a whole and give expectant mothers insight into the facilities available for their welfare.

Their great disadvantage is that the viewers are passive observers rather than active participants and do not benefit from the personal relationship that should exist between the teacher and her audience. They do not suit the people of all countries: they allow no opportunity for repetition or consolidation and may be too quick for those with lower intelligence or language difficulty.

Discretion should be used in showing films of the actual birth: many parents leave the room because the procedure disturbs them. After all, the mother does not witness the actual birth naturally. This film if used should be the culmination of a series of lessons leading up to the moment of birth.

### Showing slides

This educational technique for illustrating lesions and exhibiting statistical and other graphs is being over-used by the indifferent teacher as a vehicle for stating facts rather than elucidating ideas; 'telling' rather than 'teaching'. Unless enhanced by the teacher's personality, vivid word pictures and the full range of vocal performance the monotony of presentation and the darkened room become soporific.

### RADIO BROADCASTS

These are of value in presenting another point of view to those who have basic knowledge and experience of the subject. They are apt to be talks or demonstrations given by experts on the subject rather than well-planned lessons by experienced teachers. Audio-visual cassettes (in individual booths) are useful to give information and advice for immigrant mothers who do not understand English.

## TELEVISION BROADCAST

Giving a polished visual presentation of any one aspect of obstetrics requires many hours of preparation. No matter how experienced, proficient and confident the midwife may be, regarding her professional ability, she ought to ensure that the ideas she promulgates are sound and up-to-date, her methods and equipment modern. Planning the procedure in detail and adequate rehearsal are absolutely essential.

### Pictorial representation

The midwife as a personality will be subjected to critical appraisal so she ought to try to present a favourable image of a knowledgeable and efficient midwife; a member of the obstetric team rather than an independent practitioner. Her appearance, demeanour and speech will portray the presence or absence of her caring concern for mother and baby. Her attitude to the father and to the establishment of the bonding process will be obvious so she must consider the effect of what she is and does, as well as of what she says.

**Her approach should exude kindly competence;** a domineering exhibition of superiority being abhorrent. When giving necessary commands her voice ought to be well modulated: strident dictatorial speech precluded. To avoid using repetitive, boring, phraseology the midwife could select beforehand a variety of sentences to encourage the woman in labour. In a recent broadcast the words 'Good girl' were repeated 18 times in about 20 minutes. The midwife should rehearse the procedure in detail and decide what she will say at any given moment: this being essential for the production of a first class performance.

### The environment

Selecting and arranging a suitable photographic environment enhances the artistic quality of the visual display. A plain uncluttered background is desirable without windows, radiators etc: the bed can be moverd from its usual position to a more expedient one. The whiteness of walls and linen can be contrasted by using green gown and towels. Electronic monitors add interest but should not dominate the situation.

**Educational expertise**

Brief explanations shuld be given, when possible, to promote understanding. If time permits the midwife should state what she is doing and why.

The audience is likely to consist of three main categories and an attempt should be made to meet some of their needs.

(1) **Expectant mothers** will glean information: they will also gain assurance by noting the kindly way in which patients are treated.

(2) **The public** should be told, if the occasion arises, of the benefits of certain procedures that some object to, i.e., induction of labour, electronic monitoring, episiotomy.

(3) **Practising midwives** will note the manual dexterity and teaching ability of the broadcasting midwife. They will expect ideas and information to be up-to-date and methods of treatment to be modern: a caring attitude exhibited.

## THE DEMONSTRATION

This method of teaching is enhanced if the members of the class can participate in the procedure.

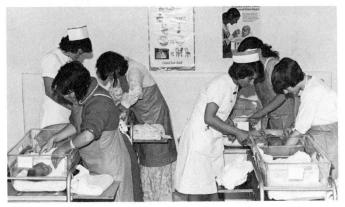

Fig. 47-3   Mothers participating in bathing demonstration.
*The Queen Mother's Hospital, Glasgow.*

Set up an attractive display; hang model baby garments on the walls; buy or borrow the type of articles used in the home (not hospital equipment); see that everything is in perfect condition. You need hardly ask a busy mother to prepare things nicely for her baby if you don't do so when demonstrating. Towels and baby's layette ought to be freshly laundered or pressed and arranged in the order in which they are to be used. Check each item so that nothing is missing. Use each garment as a pivot round which to give information. Introduce each item in a different way. Hold it long enough for the audience to grasp the details. Have a plain dark background. Talk to the expectant mothers not to the garment.

**Rehearse the procedure** and know exactly what you will say when you are doing a certain thing. When undertaking a comprehensive demonstration such as bathing baby, it is a good idea to have an assistant to carry out the procedure while the teacher explains what is being done. In that case a complete rehearsal must be arranged beforehand. Analyse each movement made before demonstrating such manoeuvres as turning baby on the knee, e.g. show how to grasp baby's body and in which direction to turn him. These details are appreciated by the learner.

**It is advisable to use a doll for bathing and** dressing, because then you can be as slow as you wish without any danger of chilling: a crying baby distracts the audience. When bathing a doll without the use of water, it is absolutely imperative that the face cloth be dipped into imaginary water and wrung out realistically, the non-existent soap rinsed off and the doll dried properly, otherwise the illusion is broken and the demonstration ruined.

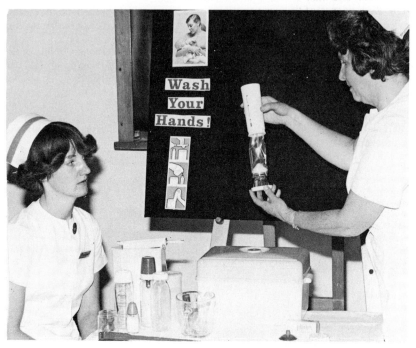

Fig. 47-4    Disposable bottle shows up well against a plain dark background.
*Royal Maternity Hospital, Rottenrow, Glasgow.*

### Select the Opening Statement with Discernment

While standing make a few remarks on the purpose or some other aspect of the demonstration. It may be worth while discussing the equipment, giving advantages and prices.

**Speak slowly and deliberately,** letting each sentence convey some particular point. Repeat any important part of the procedure. Explain why you do a certain thing in a particular way, or the audience may think it is only a whim of yours. Draw attention to apparently trivial points, for they have neither the knowledge nor the experience of the teacher, e.g. the gentle drying of baby's fingers to avoid injury to the nail folds. Look at the audience as often as you can to maintain contact.

**Omit unnecessary detail,** and do not make the mistake of the inexperienced teacher who tries to tell her students all that she knows on the subject; teach a little at a time but teach it well. Short silent periods are invaluable to allow the mothers to concentrate on what you are doing; if you chatter the whole time, they become so confused and cannot mentally absorb all that you are saying, nor differentiate between the significant and the insignificant. Emphasise what they should, rather than what they should not, do. Use the words 'don't' and 'never' sparingly.

**To bring the lesson to a close,** rise, if seated, and face the audience. Do not waver and then stop in an indecisive manner; work up to a climax by slowing the rate of speech and increasing intensity of feeling. Have the final sentence memorised, make it arresting or appealing. Any remarks about leaflets or equipment can be made afterwards.

*A woman less than 24 weeks pregnant may demonstrate again, any procedure, under the guidance of the teacher.*

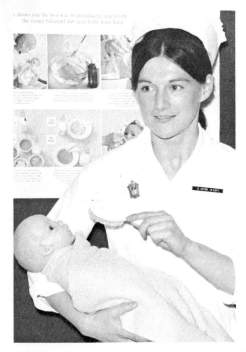

Fig. 47-5 Climax of bathing demonstration. Baby wrapped in shawl. Midwife brushes hair and says 'after his feed baby will sleep soundly. Father and mother will enjoy a quiet evening together'.

*Simpson Memorial Maternity Pavilion, Edinburgh.*

### THE GROUP DISCUSSION

Sitting around a table chatting may give satisfaction and pleasure to the vocal members of the group but unless they have valid opinions to express that the novice can benefit from, the discussion may be a sterile educational project. Discussion is not a fertile method of imparting new knowledge but can be utilised (*a*) to clarify misunderstood ideas or procedures, (*b*) to create desirable attitudes and (*c*) to gain assurance from the experience of those who have knowledge or have been in similar circumstances.

**The first essential is good leadership,** i.e. (*a*) knowing how to exercise persuasive authority, (*b*) guiding rather than directing, (*c*) promoting the interaction of opinions, (*d*) drawing out the reticent members by phrasing questions in such a way that their response is more than 'yes' or 'no'. e.g. it is better to ask, following a visit to the labour ward or nursery: 'What did you see that interested you?' rather than

'Was it interesting?'. Initiative is required to fill in awkward pauses, redirecting the course when necessary in order to keep the subject moving onward.

**Planning is absolutely imperative;** a rambling discussion leads nowhere. A tentative flexible plan should be formulated so that the subject unfolds in logical sequence.

**Knowledge of the subject in all the wider aspects** that concern parents is essential. Topics such as family planning have cultural, racial, intellectual, religious and emotional overtones that may dominate logical reasoning. Mothers should be encouraged to bring up problems or partly understood facts but questions of opinion are more suitable for a mixed discussion group.

### QUESTIONING

It is no longer considered advisable to attempt to teach by questioning. Unless the answer can be deduced from (*a*) their previous knowledge and experience or (*b*) what the teacher has already taught them, questioning is a time wasting pursuit. An occasional question can be asked during a lesson, and planned revision by questioning is an admirable device (more appropriate when teaching student midwives).

---

### QUESTIONS FOR REVISION

**How would you motivate** expectant mothers to attend parentcraft classes?

**Describe how** the woman's cultural and traditional beliefs influence her attitude to baby care?

**Why should** the 'reason why' be given?

**Give 3 ways** in which the teacher can maintain interest by her personal qualities. Give instances in which repetition can be utilised without causing boredom?

**What do** you mean by (*a*) making contact: (*b*) the growing point: (*c*) problem solving as a method of learning: (*d*) learning by rote: (*e*) recapitulation: (*f*) trial and error: (*g*) vivid word pictures?

**Why is it** a good working rule (*a*) to teach the normal prior to the abnormal: (*b*) to meet the needs of the learners: (*c*) to encourage participation by the class.

The blackboard is a valuable teaching aid when used intelligently:- enlarge on this statement.

How would you conduct a discussion group?

Why is questioning not a fruitful method of teaching?

# 48
# Platform Deportment and Public Speaking

*Overcoming nervousness. Stance, Appearance Gestures. Breath Control. Tone. Articulation. Rate. Faults.*

*Although the teaching of parenthood is usually given to small groups informally the midwife feels more confident when she is aware of the procedure on a more formal basis as outlined below.*

## OVERCOMING NERVOUSNESS

Even although the midwife knows her subject and is well rehearsed, the prospect of the ordeal will no doubt make her nervous. All good speakers experience some degree of stage-fright which is a state of nervous tension rather than fear; a necessary stimulus to effective public speaking.

**Tension is usually evident** in the hands and face, so relax both: slow deep breathing helps to induce calmness.—Think of the audience instead of yourself: it is almost certain that they know much less about the subject than you do. They are eager to learn: you should be eager to teach them.

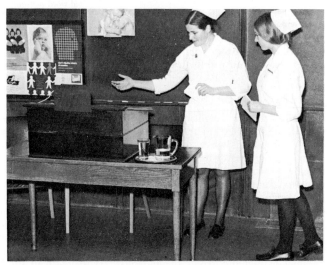

Fig. 48-1   Student midwives being taught platform deportment. Speaker being shown to her seat on the right of 'the chair'.

*Simpson Memorial Maternity Pavilion, Edinburgh.*

## An attractive appearance

It is the duty of a speaker to look her best as a compliment to the audience, and clothes with simple lines and clear contrasting colours show up well from a distance. A midwife ought to wear uniform if possible as a symbol of her competence to speak on the subject. An immaculate uniform appeals to the audience.

**Entering the room.** Have a smile in your heart if not on your lips when you enter

823

the room and maintain a degree of poise and composure. A chairman will not be necessary for an informal talk to a group of mothers who know you, but if being introduced by a chairman she will precede you when entering the room and show you to the seat on the right of 'the chair'.

**Seated on the platform all eyes will be on you** and the slightest sign of nervousness will be noted, so resist the impulse to fiddle with your hair or uniform. Let your hands lie idly on your lap though you may feel tempted to clutch your notes. Look over the audience with a friendly eye but give no visible sign of recognising anyone you know.


## OPENING THE TALK

**When called on by the chairman rise gracefully and** on no account must you speak until you are on your feet and facing the audience. With your gaze embrace the group, wait for silence and begin, turning slightly towards the chairman as you address her as 'Madam Chairman'.

Do not fix your eyes on any one individual, neither should you stare straight ahead into space as you concentrate intently on what you are saying. Looking at the floor gives the speaker a most pathetic demeanour and riveting the eyes on the ceiling, as though imploring help, will only rouse pity in the minds of the audience. If you gaze out of the window the group will do likewise and you will no longer hold their attention.

**Avoid the trivial subterfuge of telling an amusing anecdote to** get on good terms with the audience; a friendly manner, a talk well prepared and delivered will do all that is necessary. The telling of stories to stress a point is an excellent teaching device but stories, humorous or otherwise, should arise out of and not be superimposed upon the subject matter.

**Use a confident tone** to bolster your own morale a thin tremulous voice will make you even more nervous and will distress the audience on your behalf.


### GRACEFUL STANCE AND APPROPRIATE GESTURES

Stand gracefully with the weight of the body poised lightly on the balls of the feet; heels should be about 20 cm apart, toes of the right foot being 10 cm in front of the left to give a solid stance that allows free movement of knee, hip and shoulder joints without loss of balance, for your whole body is brought into play when speaking expressively. Hands ought to be cupped together lightly at waist level and shoulders held well back to give ample breathing capacity. On no account lean on chair or table, an ungraceful even ugly attitude; stand well away from both in case you are tempted to lean on either of them.

Make appropriate gestures, only when the urge to do so is spontaneous, in order to emphasise a point; they should appear to be so natural that the audience is not aware that gestures are being made. Arms should be curved, wrists relaxed. Avoid mannerisms: they distract and irritate the audience. Try to create an atmosphere of tranquillity by maintaining poise and making only the movements that are absolutely necessary.

**Do not pace the platform, fiddle with buttons, toy with the chalk,** trifle with the duster, jingle coins or keys. These mannerisms are intensely annoying to an attentive audience; they also develop into habits that are very difficult to eradicate.


### ENDING THE TALK

**Plan how to end your talk:** prepare a special plea or message. Work up to a climax, don't 'just stop'.

# HINTS ON PUBLIC SPEAKING

Speech is concerned with breath control, voice production and diction. Beautiful audible speech can be acquired with training and practice. Voice is part of the personality and the mode of delivery must be in harmony with this.

## BREATH CONTROL

The passage of a steady stream of air through the larynx is essential for the production of vocal sound. Fairly deep breaths should be taken in, through the nose and mouth, with no apparent effort; the shoulders not being raised during the process. The expiration of air is controlled by the diaphragm and not by a tightening of the muscles of the throat, the vocalised breath being allowed to flow evenly and directed forwards on to the lips and tip of the tongue.

**To be audible** the voice must have carrying power and this requires sufficient breath. If the audience have to make an effort to hear they cannot absorb what is being said. To amplify the volume of sound, breathe more deeply but under control. If not regulated properly the extravagantly used breath gives a gasping toneless quality to the spoken word and necessitates frequent inhalations: the sound produced lacks carrying power.

### Practice

Inhale a full breath and let it flow out steadily while you say 'one, two . . . one, two . . .' for 20 to 30 seconds. Do not continue speaking after the breath is finished or the sound will be toneless. Increase the time taken to expel the breath as an exercise only; no attempt is made while speaking in public to breathe excessively deeply, but expiration must be steady and under control.

## THE PRODUCTION OF TONE

**Tone is produced in the larynx,** but it emanates from the mind. the tone of voice expresses what is felt emotionally, or can be made to simulate this as is done in acting. Facial expression also influences tone, e.g. it is not possible to speak in a pleasant tone of voice while frowning, or conversely to speak crossly with a smile on the face.

**Variations in tone give interest and liveliness to the performance.** The voice has all the possibilities of an orchestra: by varying tone, pitch and volume this can be achieved. Mental boredom will be evident in the tone of voice and it may be necessary to 'pep-up' oneself in order to speak convincingly. To produce a round musical tone the oral cavity must be resonant, and this is achieved by depressing the lower jaw as in yawning. The back of the tongue should be relaxed and must not block the passage of vocalised breath which should be directed forwards and on to the hard palate. No tightening or squeezing of the throat muscles should take place, and the lips and mouth ought not to be forced beyond their normal limits in shaping words.

Much of the beauty and musical tone of the spoken word is dependent on the proper enunciation of the vowel sounds. In shaping these the cavity of the mouth may have to be round, ovoid or flattened, and many of the most exquisite words in the English language have the 'oh' or 'ah' vowel sounds, which permit maximal resonance in the oral cavity. Tones are also modified and beautified by the emotion of the speaker and her ability to interpret this in sound. An artistic quality can be given to words and conveyed by the tone of voice.

**The volume of tone should be regulated according to the size of the room.** The conversational tone suited to an informal small group would not project the voice to a large audience in a lecture theatre.

*Practise saying*

**'Lovely lilacs bloom in the valley.'** Allow the mind to dwell on the mental image conjured up by these words, and try to interpret and convey it in colourful sound. Suffuse the vowel sounds with a warm glow; allow the tongue to linger for a second on the consonant 'L.' Concentrate on tone and smooth flowing breath.

*For comparison repeat the following lines*

**'Dirty British coaster with a salt-caked smoke stack.'** Speak the words briskly, no beauty of tone is required; accentuate the consonants and use a jerky rhythm to denote the chugging of a ship.

**Modulation** is the passing from one tone to another in order to clothe the words with meaning and beauty and to give interest, variety and expression to speech. Speaking in a monotone, no matter how lovely the tone may be, is liable to act as a soporific.

**Pitch** is the level at which sound is produced on the vocal register, and may be high, middle or low. It is regulated by tightening or loosening the vocal cords. For a high note they are tightened; for a low note the vocal cords are relaxed and a pleasing musical sound with good carrying power is produced. The middle pitch is most commonly used. When a high pitch is used the tone is thin and squeaky as in depicting excitement or agitation and is not pleasant to listen to. A change of pitch is used to indicate a new idea or subject.

Speakers sometimes make the mistake of raising pitch and shouting in response to complaints from members of the audience at the back of the hall that they cannot hear. This is quite wrong; the speaker ought to lower pitch, articulate more precisely, relax the lower jaw, breathe deeply and increase the volume of air expelled. Shouting tightens the throat muscles and interferes with voice production in the larynx.

**Inflection** is the gliding up and down of pitch on a syllable or individual word as an aid to clarifying the idea being expressed, e.g. when asking a question a rising inflection is used. Speaking on one pitch is most monotonous to listen to.

## ARTICULATION

Articulation is concerned with the clear enunciation of vowel sounds and the precision with which consonants are delivered. Slovenly articulation of the consonants 'T', 'B' and 'P' is a common cause of mumbling, and the consequent inaudibility of speech.

Words should be articulated by the lips, the teeth, the tip of the tongue, and when doing so, the voice is brought well forwards to facilitate its carrying power. Avoid shaping the mouth beyond its normal range.

*Practise the following*

'Bat-pat'; 'Tip-top'; 'Pip-pop'; 'Bab-tab'; also the sentences, 'The lips, the teeth, the tip of the tongue'. 'The cat sat on the mat'. Exaggerate chipping off the consonants neatly like coins from the mint.

**Avoid the hissing sibilants**

This may occur when a word ends and the next one begins with the letter 'S'.

*Practise the following*

'Luscious strawberries'; 'Sing a song of sixpence'; 'English roses'; 'Irish shamrocks'; 'Scottish thistles'. 'The hissing of sibilants is especially unpleasing.'

Use the point of the tongue and speak well forward in the mouth, permitting the tongue to sound the letter 'S' for the minimal length of time.

## RATE

It is imperative when speaking in public, that the words are spoken slowly enough to be heard and understood. If a stream of words, indistinguishable one from another, is poured out, the audience will grasp only a minute part of their meaning. Even if the words are clearly articulated the rate at which new ideas are being presented may be more rapid than the rate at which they can be absorbed. The necessary mental effort is so great that members of the audience allow their attention to wander. Emphasis on some special point may be made by slowing the rate to an impressive degree, as in giving warning of impending danger or in working up to a climax. Unimportant points can be described more rapidly but enunciation must be crisp to ensure clarity.

**The pause** is one of the most telling devices in public speaking; being not only effective, but almost dramatic in intensity. The audience listens more intently to hear what follows the pause or concentrates on what has just been said. Multiple pauses are the refuge of the badly prepared speaker; dull and boring. As an aid to speaking more slowly, think in words, and not in sentences as is usually done during conversation. Give each word its full value, articulating the first and last letters meticulously (if they should be sounded) as well as the body of the word. Speak deliberately and make an effort to enunciate the words distinctly without actually disjointing them.

### The choice and use of words

Words are used to convey meaning and portray ideas, but they also express feeling: they should, therefore, be selected with care and discrimination. Vivid word-pictures may be used to recreate a scene or give vitality to an incident. Words may sound beautiful in themselves, or they may be loved by the hearer because of their association, e.g. 'home' is more attractive than 'hostel'; 'a field of golden corn' than 'a street littered with rubbish'. These facts should be kept in mind when choosing words.

The meaning of the words can be enhanced by the manner in which they are spoken, and the midwife can increase the effectiveness of her talk or demonstration in this way. *When saying*, 'Rub the hair briskly with a Turkish towel', speak tersely to suggest the action; use a fairly high pitch and sound consonants crisply. *When saying*, 'Cuddle your baby', linger on the vowels, use a round musical tone, low pitch, slow rate; above all 'feel' in your mind what you are trying to express with your voice.

The fluent speaker has a deep and wide knowledge of her subject on which she can draw and a large and varied vocabulary from which she can select the appropriate word without hesitation. The reading of good prose is of inestimable value, experience in public speaking is, of course, beneficial, but adequate preparation of the talk is absolutely essential. Sheer garrulousness should not be emulated.

### Some Common Faults in Public Speaking

**Inadequate emotional power** is often due to inhibition in expressing emotion. Forget yourself and think of the audience. Try to visualise the situation and to feel more acutely, use facial expression to suit the emotion.

**Lack of emphasis** may be due to insecurity regarding the subject-matter or in facing an audience. Volume should be amplified; thorough preparation of both is essential.

**Shrill or unmusical tone** may be due to tightening the throat muscles or rigid lower jaw and lack of resonance.

**Absence of variety** occurs when the full range of volume, tone, pitch and rate are not utilised.

**Indistinct speech** is due to rigidity of the lower jaw and immobility of the lips. Slurred speech is due to flabbiness of the tip of the tongue, which should be used with precision.

**Inaudibility** may be due to insufficient volume or to dropping of the voice at the end of a sentence; the flow of breath must be sustained to the last letter of the final word in the sentence. Deeper inspiration and more frequent breaths are needed.

The persistent use of a word such as 'now' prior to stating a new idea or saying quickly 'Is that clear': or 'Do you see': without waiting for a reply becomes a habit. This was said over forty times in one talk. (There is no need to ask, except in rare instances. The good teacher anticipates the perplexities of her students and explains difficult points in various ways in order that all will understand.)

# 49
# Questions for Revision and Assessment of Knowledge

*Student midwives can use these tests individually to assess their knowledge. Tutors may care to utilise them for planned pre-final revision classes. Midwives returning to practise can update their knowledge.*

## QUIZ NO. 1

### CLINICAL TESTS THAT MIDWIVES MAY BE INVOLVED WITH

| Test | Purpose | see Page |
|------|---------|----------|
| Silverman's | | 530 |
| Coomb's | | 570 |
| Guthrie's | | 542 |
| Moro's | | 488 |
| Barlow's | | 593 |
| Bishop's | | 601 |
| Apgar's | | 320 |
| Ortolani's | | 593 |
| Huhner's | | 675 |
| Papanicolaou | | 678 |
| Saling's | | 302 |
| Singer's | | 51 |
| Kleihauer's | | 567 |
| Dextrostix | | 539 |
| Alpha fetoprotein | | 109 |
| B.C.G. | | 210 |
| Oxytocin stress test | | 108 |
| Lecithin sphingomyelin | | 110 |
| Oestriol assay | | 108 |
| Baxter F1 | | 235 |
| Prepuerex | | 80 |
| H.A.I. | | 215 |
| Multistix | | 669 |
| Haemoglobin | | 211 |
| Serum bilirubin | | 570 |
| Mammography | | 680 |
| Thermography | | 680 |
| V.D.R.L. | | 221 |
| Billings | | 459 |

## QUIZ NO. 2

### DIFFERENTIATE BETWEEN

**Prenatal:**

(*a*) hydatidiform and carneous mole; (*b*) static ultrasonography and a real-time scan; (*c*) missed and habitual abortion; (*d*) vasa praevia and placenta praevia;

(e) quickening and lightening; (f) threatened and therapeutic abortion; (g) placenta praevia and abruptio placentae; (h) an engaged and a non-engaged head; (i) gestational and menstrual age; (j) positive and probable signs of pregnancy; (k) chemical and overt diabetes; (l) unwed and unsupported mothers; (m) cephalic and vertex presentation; (n) multipara and multigravida; (o) homozygous and heterozygous; (p) multiple pregnancy and multiparity.

### Intranatal:

(a) analgesia and amnesia; (b) fetal hypoxia and anoxia; (c) metabolic and respiratory fetal acidosis; (d) hand and foot PV; (e) cervical and shoulder dystocia.

(a) Syntometrine and Syntocinon; (b) fetal heart rate early and late deceleration; (c) cleidotomy and craniotomy; (d) delayed and obstructed labour; (e) contraction and retraction of uterine muscle; (f) ergometrine and Syntometrine; (g) restitution and external rotation of the head; (h) the three degrees of cephalopelvic disproportion; (i) retraction, Bandl's and constriction ring; (j) podalic and bi-polar version. (k) Brandt Andrews manoeuvre and controlled cord traction; (l) upper and lower uterine segment; (m) Entonox and Trilene; (n) false and true labour; (o) pubiotomy and symphysiotomy.

### Neonatal:

(a) physiological jaundice and icterus gravis; (b) hypoglycaemia and hypocalcaemia; (c) encephalocele and anencephaly; (d) stool with melaena and meconium; (e) haemorrhagic and haemolytic disease of the newborn; (f) epispadias and hypospadias; (g) phototherapy and spectrophotometry; (h) preterm and previable baby; (i) microcephaly and micrognathia.

(a) Supplementary and complementary feeds (b) hydrops fetalis and hydrocephaly; (c) CPAP and CNAP; (d) light for date and preterm baby; (e) perinatal and neonatal death; (f) notification and registration of birth; (g) caput succedaneum and cephalhaematoma.

### Postnatal:

(a) laparotomy and laparoscopy; (b) vesico-vaginal and recto-vaginal fistula; (e) postpartum 'blues' and psychosis; (f) stress and paradoxical incontinence.

### Miscellaneous:

(a) nuclear and extended family; (b) dizygotic and monozygotic twins; (c) maternity allowance and maternity grant; (d) millimetre and centimetre; (e) symbol for microgram and kilogram; (f) the protected and the deprived child; (g) alimony and affiliation order; (h) mammography and thermography; (i) embryo and fetus; (j) android and anthropoid pelvis; (k) presentation and prolapse of cord; (l) placenta succenturiata and circumvallata; (m) true and false pelvis; (n) amelia and phocomelia; (o) pharmacological and pharmaceutical drug names; (p) elective and classical Caesarean section; (q) nullipara and primipara; (r) tubal and vas ligation; (s) social trends and social pressures.

# QUIZ NO. 3

## NOTABLE NAMES

*To evaluate the percentage, select 50 questions and allow 2 marks for each correct answer.*

# QUIZ NO. 4

## WHAT WOULD YOU DO IN HOSPITAL PENDING THE ARRIVAL OF THE DOCTOR?

**In the Prenatal Ward: a woman is admitted with** (*a*) a threatened abortion; (*b*) acute pyelonephritis in severe pain. (*c*) Prodromal signs of eclampsia are manifest in patient with pre-eclampsia. (*d*) Cardiac patient develops signs of acute heart failure.

**In the Labour Ward:**

 **Woman is admitted** (*a*) with history of contact with rubella; (*b*) bleeding freely with an inevitable abortion; (*c*) fetus in transverse lie in advanced labour; (*d*) in prolonged labour, dehydrated and with ketonuria; **during labour** (*a*) impending amniotic fluid embolism is suspected; (*b*) cord prolapsed during the first stage of labour.

 (*a*) **Fetus** of patient having Syntocinon drip induction shows signs of distress; (*b*) patient having an epidural block has signs of hypotension; (*c*) severe bleeding occurs in a patient who has had a hydatidiform mole evacuated; (*d*) shoulder dystocia occurs (baby large); (*e*) deep transverse arrest of the head is diagnosed PV.

 (*a*) **Patient** having a blood transfusion shows signs of reaction; (*b*) severe atonic third stage haemorrhage occurs; (*c*) the perineal phase is prolonged; (*d*) Apgar score is 2 at one minute.

## The Nursery:

(*a*) Baby with spina bifida and myelomeningocele; (*b*) umbilical haemorrhage occurs 2 hours after birth; (*c*) baby 2 days old is having a convulsion; (*d*) preterm baby has early signs of idiopathic respiratory distress syndrome; (*e*) baby with intracranial injury is still restless after sedation; (*f*) baby is having an apnoeic episode; (*g*) baby has congenital dislocation of hip.

## The postnatal ward

**The following occurs:** (*a*) pulmonary thrombo-embolism; (*b*) high temperature on the third day; (*c*) signs of psychosis; (*d*) 'flushed' breast; (*e*) brisk haemorrhage on the 7th day; (*f*) deep vein thrombosis.

### WHAT ARE THE DANGERS OF?

Buccal pitocin; a prolonged second stage of labour; shoulder presentation; contracted pelvis; teratogenic drugs; placental insufficiency; the grande multipara; postmaturity; eclampsia; apnoeic episodes in the neonate; prolapse of cord; icterus gravis; Mendelson's syndrome; deep vein thrombosis; bi-polar version; amniotic embolism; neonatal hypothermia; inversion of uterus; hypofibrinogenaemia; persistent mento-posterior; fetal hypoxia; hydatidiform mole; retrolental fibroplasia; plastic bibs; hypernatraemia.

# QUIZ NO. 5

## HOW COULD YOU

### Assess:

(*a*) **The measurement** of the diagonal conjugate; (*b*) **the capacity** of the pelvic outlet; (*c*) **the suitability** of the home for confinement; (*d*) **the estimated** date of delivery; (*e*) **the dilatability** of the cervix at 39 weeks; (*f*) **whether** the head is engaged.

### Treat:

(*a*) severe haemorrhage from an incomplete abortion; (*b*) the patient having an eclamptic convulsion; (*c*) acute heart failure in pregnancy; (*d*) postpartum haemorrhage; (*e*) inversion of uterus.

The baby (*a*) of a diabetic mother; (*b*) having an apnoeic episode; (*c*) having a convulsion; (*d*) with sore buttocks; (*e*) with an inflamed umbilicus.

The woman with (*a*) afterpains; (*b*) cracked nipples; (*c*) painful haemorrhoids; (*d*) insomnia.

### Record on partogram

(*a*) uterine contractions; (*b*) dilatation of cervix; (*c*) descent of head; (*d*) rotation of head.

### Perform:

(*a*) intubation of asphyxiated baby; (*b*) injection of lignocaine for episiotomy; (*c*) manual expression of breast milk; (*d*) vaginal examination; (*e*) an episiotomy; (*f*) cricoid pressure.

### Teach the expectant mother

(*a*) how to protect her unborn child, (*b*) how to relax, (*c*) the benefits of breast feeding; (*d*) how to bath her baby; (*e*) how to deal with a crying baby; (*f*) the need for bonding; (g) to cope with the stress of labour; (h) the benefits of electronic monitoring equipment; (i) to record fetal movement; (j) the content of a suitable diet in pregnancy.

### Prepare

A talk on (a) the expectant father; (b) the role of the husband during labour; (c) the role of the new father.

### Deal with

(a) an unsupported mother-to-be, 14 years old; (b) an immigrant expectant mother; (c) obtaining blood for the Guthrie test; (d) topping up an epidural analgesic; (e) inhibiting lactation.

### Cope with

The woman who has (a) serious signs of pre-eclampsia; (b) antepartum haemorrhage type undiagnosed; (c) glycosuria; (d) apprehension regarding labour; (e) postpartum 'blues'.

## QUIZ NO. 6

### WHY SHOULD?

### The midwife:

(a) have knowledge of pelvic anatomy; (b) recognise signs of previous childbirth; (c) be a competent practitioner; (d) know how to teach; (e) know the hazards of adding drugs to i.v. infusion fluids; (f) accept the aid of electronic monitors; (g) understand the mechanism of labour.

### The expectant mother:

(a) attend the prenatal clinic early in pregnancy; (b) be weighed at each prenatal visit; (c) the blood be examined for alpha fetoproteins? (d) the blood group be determined during pregnancy? (e) amniocentesis by carried out on pregnant women over 40 years of age? (f) pregnant women be told not to take drugs unless prescribed by the doctor? (g) take alcohol sparingly if at all; (h) the pregnant woman's breasts be examined? (i) the lecithin/sphinogomyelin ratio sometimes be carried out at 34 weeks? (j) be screened during pregnancy.

### During labour:

(a) The suture inserted for an incompetent cervix be removed prior to the onset of labour; (b) a partogram be an advantageous way of recording the progress of labour; (c) the woman have the constant companionship and supervision of a midwife; (d) no vaginal examination be made outwith the theatre in cases of antepartum haemorrhage; (e) the woman with multiple pregnancy be delivered in hospital; (f) the husband be encouraged to remain with his wife during labour; (g) the bladder be emptied every 2 hours; (h) fetal heart monitors be used; (i) foam rubber wedges be used to produce a lateral tilt during Caesarean section?

### The baby:

The mother (a) see and touch her baby soon after birth; (b) visit her baby in the intensive care nursery two or three times every day; (c) give her baby tender loving care; (d) take her baby to the child health clinic? (e) the baby be breast fed; (f) have a Dextrostix test; (g) be given neurological tests; (h) be screened; (i) have continuous positive airway pressure; (j) be admitted to the neonatal intensive care unit; (k) be given phototherapy; (l) have the Guthrie test done.

# QUIZ NO. 7

## HOW WOULD YOU DETERMINE

**During pregnancy**

(*a*) a multiple pregnancy from polyhydramnios; (*b*) that the woman had pre-eclampsia; (*c*) hyperemesis from morning sickness; (*d*) the positive signs of pregnancy; (*e*) that the woman had a justo minor pelvis; (*f*) the expected date of delivery; (*g*) whether an abortion was complete or incomplete; (*h*) that eclampsia was imminent; (*i*) that the woman was anaemic; (*j*) that medical aid was urgently needed; (*k*) that fetal growth was retarded; (*l*) the period of gestation; (*m*) cephalo-pelvic disproportion.

**During labour:**

(*a*) that labour was 'true' rather than false; (*b*) the latent from the active phase; (*c*) that labour was progressing normally; (*d*) that the fetal condition was satisfactory; (*e*) that the membranes were intact; (*f*) that the second stage was in progress; (*g*) that third stage haemorrhage was atonic and not traumatic; (*h*) that the placenta had separated and descended; (*i*) that the placenta was complete; (*j*) that the second twin was in the transverse lie; (*k*) when to 'top up' an epidural analgesic; (*l*) that rupture of uterus was impending; (*m*) that the uterus was hypotonic; (*n*) maternal distress; (*o*) fetal distress; (*p*) the station of the head PV; (*q*) the presence of a third degree perineal laceration.

**The baby:**

(*a*) was light for date rather than preterm; (*b*) that intubation was necessary.

**The presence of** (*a*) congenital dislocation of hip; (*b*) imperforate anus; (*c*) oesophageal atresia; (*d*) Down's syndrome.

(*a*) That vomiting was serious; (*b*) oral thrush from a milky tongue; (*c*) that the baby was getting insufficient breast milk; (*d*) the i.v. needle in a scalp vein was displaced.

**During the puerperium:**

**Whether** (*a*) involution was progressing normally; (*b*) the postpartum 'blues' were minor or suggestive of psychosis; (*c*) medical aid was necessary; (*d*) the woman needed additional supervision by the Health Visitor; (*e*) the presence of (1) puerperal sepsis; (2) mastitis; (3) venous thrombosis.

# QUIZ NO. 8

## REARRANGE THE CONDITION FOR WHICH THE DRUG MAY BE PRESCRIBED

| Drug | Wrong condition | State correct condition |
| --- | --- | --- |
| Jectofer | hookworm | |
| methyldopa | tuberculosis | |
| methotrexate | anaemia | |
| mannitol | hypertension | |
| Apresoline | massive oedema | |
| diazepam | cerebral oedema in newborn | |
| Nupercaine | pre-eclampsia | |
| isoniazid | induction of labour | |
| fibrinogen | acute heart failure | |
| aminophylline | trichomoniasis | |

| Drug | Wrong condition | State correct condition |
|------|-----------------|-------------------------|
| chlormethiazole | psychosis | |
| naloxone | abruptio placentae | |
| frusemide | labour pain | |
| Lanoxin | blood coagulation disorder | |
| prostaglandin | renal failure | |
| Alcopar | heart failure in newborn | |
| Flagyl | choriocarcinoma | |
| Nardil | analgesia for episiotomy | |
| lignocaine | asphyxia neonatorum | |
| Phenergan | Staph. infection | |
| promazine | neonatal haemorrhagic states . | |
| Vasogen | epidural analgesia | |
| clomiphene | venous thrombosis | |
| Buscopan | anti-spasmodic | |
| phenindione | tranquilliser | |
| bupivacaine | to induce ovulation | |
| Konakion | sore buttocks | |
| Kanamycin | improve blood supply | |
| Lomodex | anti-histamine | |

# QUIZ NO. 9

## ENLARGE ON THE FOLLOWING STATEMENTS IN DETAIL

**The prenatal clinic:**

It should be (a) a school for expectant mothers; (b) have a friendly welcoming atmosphere; (c) expectant mothers should feel at ease with the obstetric staff; (d) understanding of obstetric advice given should be ensured; (e) helpful advice re minor disorders should be offered.

**The expectant mother:**

(a) **Her emotional welfare is important;** she responds to kindly understanding counsel rather than logical argument; (b) her sensitivity is heightened: this includes apprehension as well as joy in creation; (c) she should be motivated to provide in her body a health-giving environment for the fetus; (d) she is receptive to advice on 'preparation for motherhood'.

**The husband:**

(a) **Can support his pregnant wife** by consideration and patient, kindly care; (b) should be encouraged to participate in the duties and responsibilities of child bearing and rearing; (c) can be a tower of strength to the apprehensive mother of a young baby.

**The fetus:**

(a) **The fetus is a potential parent;** (b) although the baby may be unwanted at the time of conception the majority are welcomed at birth; (c) the quality of fetal life is being improved; (d) the fetus needs a daily 'fresh air outing' before birth as well as afterwards.

**Labour:**

(a) **Labour is now safer and easier** than at any previous time; (b) the sun should not set twice on the woman in labour; (c) the uterine muscle fibres act as 'living ligatures' to prevent third stage bleeding; (d) 'baby's birthday' should be a happy memory; (e) the labour ward should have a relaxing home-like atmosphere: the staff create this.

### The postnatal ward:

(a) **Mothers should be able to relax and enjoy their babies;** (b) rigid routine, rush and bustle are detrimental to the necessary calm atmosphere needed; (c) advice should be given without dictating or dominating and include 'reasons why'.

### The baby:

(a) **Babies do not thrive without 'mothering';** (b) giving the baby too much love is safer than giving too little; (c) breast milk has not been excelled as a food for newborn babies; (d) crying is his only language; (e) he has to learn a tremendous amount during the first year of life.

### The midwife:

(a) **Is a teacher and supervisor of expectant mothers,** a competent practitioner, a counsellor during the postnatal period; (b) deals proficiently with urgent complications in the doctor's absence; (c) performs a sentinel role during pregnancy and labour, (d) eliminates fear in her patients by instilling confidence and serenity based on elementary understanding of the process of labour.

(a) Electronic monitors extend her powers of observation; (b) should endeavour to prevent stillbirths and neonatal deaths, thereby reducing the perinatal mortality rate; (c) reverting to the basic role of 'delivery woman' would be a retrograde step; (d) should teach schoolgirls in preparation for their reproductive role.

**Demonstrates her interest** in and concern for the pregnant woman as an individual as well as an obstetric patient.

Should explain to expectant mothers the advantages of modern methods and electronic equipment.

## QUIZ NO. 10

### WHAT ADVICE OR INFORMATION WOULD YOU GIVE IN THE FOLLOWING CIRCUMSTANCES? (Explain in detail.)

### Prenatal:

To (a) the unsupported expectant mother who is considering adoption; (b) the mother-to-be who is reluctant to give up smoking; (c) the older primigravida who is apprehensive about labour; (d) the woman who is contemplating transfer home 48 hours after delivery; (e) the married woman who plans to work full time until the 28th week; (f) the primigravida who is eager to have her baby at home.

### To the sophisticated mothers-to-be who ask questions on:

(1) **Choosing** (a) a modern layette; (b) equipment for bottle feeding; (c) the ideal pram; (d) the best type of napkin.

(2) **Subjects such as** (a) ultrasonography; (b) electronic monitoring equipment; (c) vasectomy; (d) amniocentesis; (e) multiple pregnancy; (f) induction of labour; (g) episiotomy; (h) forceps; (i) restoration of her figure.

### Intranatal:

The woman who is having (a) epidural analgesia; (b) Entonox; (c) **who refuses** (i) pethidine; (ii) episiotomy; (d) **How to** relax, breathe rhythmically, push effectively.

### Re the baby:

**To mother** (a) feeding of baby with cleft palate; (b) baby with splint for dislocated hip; (c) whose baby is mongoloid; (d) not gaining weight.

**How to deal with** (*a*) persistent crying at night; (*b*) sore buttocks; (*c*) skin rash; (*d*) possetting; (*e*) constipation.

## Postnatal:

**(1) to the woman who objects to hospital routine,** e.g. self demand feeding, restrictions on visitors: **(2) at counselling discussions on** (*a*) the crying baby; (*b*) attending the Child Health Clinic; (*c*) planning baby's day; (*d*) the new father; (*e*) family relationships; (*f*) 'post partum blues'; (*g*) handling the toddler; (*h*) attending the postnatal clinic; (*i*) 'fertility control'; (*j*) stillbirth; (*k*) to the mother of a handicapped baby.

# QUIZ NO. 11
## GIVE REASONS WHY

### Prenatal:

(*a*) the date of quickening should be recorded: (*b*) fetal growth should be assessed during pregnancy; (*c*) fresh blood is transfused in cases of abruptio placentae; (*d*) pregnant women should refrain from taking alcohol other than very sparingly; (*e*) the pregnant woman is asked to keep a kick-count chart.

(*a*) bi-parietal cephalometry is carried out; (*b*) a real time ultrasonic scan is made; (*c*) serial urinary oestriol excretion assays are made.

### Intranatal:

(*a*) the Bishop cervical score is used: (*b*) prostaglandin is sometimes preferred to induce labour: (*c*) the fetal scalp electrode is used: (*d*) gauze swabs for Caesarean section should be in bundles of five: (*e*) the perineal phase of the second stage should not exceed 30–45 minutes.

(*a*) The i.v. drip may have to be stopped when inducing labour: (*b*) buccal pitocin is now disapproved of: (*c*) the intravaginal route of administering prostaglandins is preferred to the oral and intravenous routes.

(*a*) The fetal heart rate pattern should always be checked when the membranes rupture; (*b*) late fetal heart deceleration (Dip 2) is more serious than early (Dip 1); (*c*) intermittent auscultation of the fetal heart rate during labour is inadequate.

### Neonatal:

(*a*) continuous positive airway pressure (CPAP) is applied to the newborn; (*b*) babies are admitted to special or intensive neonatal care units; (*c*) intermittent positive pressure ventilation (IPPV) is employed; (*d*) babies are screened at birth; (*e*) the Dextrostix test is used; (*f*) brown fat is important.

### *The following are used?*

Sellick's manoeuvre; Mauriceau Smellie Veit grip; assessing fundal height; estimating Hb in the puerperium; bi parietal cephalometry; Lovset manoeuvre; placental localisation; Burn's Marshall manoeuvre; measuring the diagonal conjugate; insertion of cervical suture; measuring abdominal girth; diagnosing the type of APH; adopting the dorsal position in labour; fetal blood sampling; assessing the central venous pressure; giving naso-jejunal feeds; giving cytotoxic chemotherapy; phototherapy; intubation; testing the Moro reflex; a mechanical ventilator; mammography; cervical cytology; thermography; prenatal screening; fetal kick-count chart; oxytocin stress challenge test; notification of births; an episiotomy; induction of labour; health education; Guthrie test; genetic counselling; external version; accurate record keeping; giving magnesium trisilicate; bonding; urinary oestriol assay; the obstetric flying squad.

# QUIZ NO. 12

## WHAT COULD BE DONE TO

### During pregnancy:

**Motivate expectant mothers** to attend parentcraft and health education classes.
**Prevent** (a) anaemia; (b) rubella; (c) preterm labour; (d) eclampsia.
**Assist** (a) the unsupported expectant mother; (b) the subfertile woman; (c) the woman with language problems; (d) the bonding process.
**Detect** (a) rubella; (b) fetal growth retardation; (c) spina bifida; (d) fetal death; (e) cephalo pelvic disproportion; (f) the amount of bilirubin in amniotic fluid.
**Treat** (1) heartburn; (2) morning sickness; (3) constipation; (4) mild varicose veins; (5) pruritus; (6) haemorrhoids.

### During labour:

**Relieve** (a) pain; (b) emotional distress; (c) fear; (d) backache; (e) cramp in the leg.
**Prevent** (a) fetal hypoxia; (b) postpartum haemorrhage; (c) perineal laceration; (d) injury to the bladder; (e) sepsis; (f) Mendelson's syndrome; (g) vena-caval compression; (h) ketoacidosis.
**Detect** (a) hypertonic uterine action; (b) occult prolapse of cord; (c) fetal heart base line irregularity; (d) fetal distress; (e) ketoacidosis; (f) maternal distress.
**Record** (a) strength and frequency of uterine contractions; (b) the FH rate; (c) the blood pressure; (d) the latent and active stages; (e) descent of the head; (f) condition of baby prior to transfer to postnatal ward.
**Treat** (a) hypotonic uterine action; (b) a retained placenta; (c) neglected shoulder presentation; (d) hypovolaemic shock; (e) umbilical cord three times around the neck; (f) cervical dystocia: (g) prolapse of cord; (h) fetal distress; (i) shoulder dystocia.

### The baby:

**Ensure** (a) correct identification; (b) giving correct information re the sex of the baby over the telephone; (c) recognition of hypoglycaemia.
**Prevent** (a) hypothermia; (b) ophthalmia; (c) infection in the nursery; (d) omphalorrhagia; (e) retrolental fibroplasia; (f) sore buttocks; (g) kernicterus.
**Treat:** (a) the asphyxiated baby; (b) physiological jaundice; (c) baby with; (1) cleft palate; (2) spina bifida; (3) oesophageal atresia; (4) club foot; (5) intracranial injury; (6) thrush.

### During the puerperium:

(a) arrange for rooming-in; (b) meet the woman's psychological needs; (c) deal with the mother who feels incompetent re baby care; (d) complains of pain in the perineum; (e) stimulate the supply of breast milk?
**Comfort the mother of** (a) a stillborn baby; (b) handicapped baby; (c) baby with severe cleft palate.

### Miscellaneous:

(a) prepare the room for a home confinement; (b) use the neonatal Ambu bag; (c) decide whether the home was suitable for 24 hour transfer from hospital; (d) keep informed re the financial allowances mothers are entitled to; (e) prepare a talk on (i) fashionable baby garments; (ii) cries in the night; (iii) cuddle your baby?

# QUIZ NO. 13

## WHAT ARE THE ADVANTAGES *(if any)?*

**Prenatal:**

**Advocating additional rest** for (a) multiple pregnancy; (b) pre-eclampsia.

(a) **Giving** pelvic floor exercises; (b) **assessing** pelvic capacity PV; (c) **screening** for high risk pregnant women; (d) applying face cream to prevent striae; (e) **determining** whether the woman is primigravid or multigravid.

**Diagnosing** (a) asymptomatic bacteriuria; (b) diabetes; (c) contracted pelvis; (d) inevitable abortion; (e) multiple pregnancy; (f) pre-eclampsia; (g) anaemia; (h) cardiac disease; (i) cephalopelvic disproportion; (j) malpresentation; (k) lecithin/sphingomyelin ratio.

**Treating** (a) asymptomatic bacteriuria; (b) varicose veins; (c) morning sickness; (d) inverted nipples; (e) candidiasis; (f) gonorrhoea.

**Giving** (a) an iron preparation to all pregnant women; (b) instruction on parentcraft to adoptive parents; (d) advice re fertility control.

**Counselling expectant mothers** re (a) drugs; (b) rubella; (c) anaemia; (d) smoking; (e) overeating; (f) recording the date of quickening; (g) bonding; (h) avoiding an excessive or moderate alcohol intake.

**Intranatal:**

**Admitting** (a) the preterm baby in utero; (b) the woman early in labour; (c) woman with multiple pregnancy, breech presentation.

**Withholding food during labour:** giving magnesium trisilicate.

Shaving the pubic area.

**Relief of pain** using (a) epidural block; (b) pethidine; (c) Entonox; (d) rhythmic breathing.

**Using** (a) foam rubber wedges; (b) Apgar score; (c) controlled cord traction; (d) rubber bands for umbilical cord; (e) the partogram.

**Differentiating between** (a) hypotonic and hypertonic uterine action; (b) dip 1 and dip 2 FH decelerations; (c) restitution and external rotation of the fetal head; (d) atonic and traumatic PPH; (e) first and second stages of labour.

**Neonatal:**

(a) clearing the airway prior to baby's first breath; (b) nursing baby in the prone position; (c) mask wearing in the nursery; (d) operating on the baby with spina bifida within hours of birth; (e) Barlow's test; (f) developmental assessment.

**Using** (a) overhead heat when resuscitating the baby; (b) Vitamin K for newborn babies (c) napkin liners; (d) disposable napkins; (e) phototherapy; (f) Dextrostix test.

**Postnatal:**

(a) self perineal care; (b) giving shower 6 hours after delivery; (c) allowing children to visit; (d) measuring and recording the fundal height; (e) 24 hour transfer home.

**Miscellaneous**

**Knowing how:** (a) to teach expectant parents; (b) to comfort the grieving mother; (c) to speak and demonstrate in public; (d) to act as counsellor; (e) to be a helpful member of the obstetric team.

## QUIZ NO. 14

### A SELECTION OF DRUGS THAT MIDWIVES MAY HAVE TO ADMINISTER

| Drug | Prescribed for | Page | Drug | Prescribed for | Page |
|------|----------------|------|------|----------------|------|
| nitrazepam | | 206 | methotrexate | | 174 |
| Aludrox | | 291 | promazine | | 261 |
| rifampicin | | 210 | Konakion | | 574 |
| Sodium Amytal | | 160 | nupercainal | | 155 |
| mag. trisilicate | | 622 | Sabin vaccine | | 215 |
| Pergonal | | 677 | chlorpromazine | | 480 |
| polymyxin | | 561 | cloxacillin | | 473 |
| Alcopar | | 211 | methoxyflurane | | 266 |
| Kaomycin | | 564 | trichloroethylene | | 265 |
| protoveratrine | | 190 | cephalexin | | 218 |
| chloramphenicol | | 561 | Fersamal | | 212 |
| mannitol | | 196 | papaveretum | | 263 |
| Lomodex | | 474 | ethambutal | | 210 |
| Stemetil | | 186 | Vasogen | | 493 |
| Macrodex | | 474 | Nardil | | 481 |
| heparin | | 475 | clomiphene | | 677 |
| diazepam | | 191 | Bromocriptine | | 506 |
| chlorothiazide | | 191 | chlormethiazole | | 190 |
| diamorphine | | 477 | bupivacaine | | 623 |
| Kannasyn | | 223 | digoxin | | 206 |
| fibrinogen | | 235 | cephradine | | 472 |
| Triplopen | | 222 | cyclizine | | 186 |
| nystatin | | 220 | Parentrovite | | 219 |
| meclozine | | 186 | Cendevax | | 215 |
| Pregfol | | 212 | frusemide | | 191 |
| metronidazole | | 219 | minovular | | 460 |
| dequalinium | | 563 | Loestrin | | 460 |
| prostaglandin | | 601 | erythromycin | | 562 |
| chlordiazepoxide | | 190 | phytomenadione | | 476 |
| promethazine | | 263 | amitriptyline | | 481 |
| gentamicin | | 565 | Marevan | | 475 |
| carbenicillin | | 563 | betamethazone | | 529 |
| methyldopa | | 202 | Lanoxin | | 571 |
| Hydrallazine | | 190 | aminophylline | | 205 |

## QUIZ NO. 15

### WHAT TREATMENT MAY BE GIVEN WHEN?

**In pregnancy:**

(a) profuse bleeding from an inevitable abortion occurs; (b) woman is admitted with hyperemesis; (c) proteinuria and hypertension are diagnosed at 28 weeks; (d) patient with pre-eclampsia develops serious signs; (e) major cephalo-pelvic disproportion is diagnosed at 36 weeks; (f) hookworm disease is diagnosed; (g) woman's Hb is 8 g/dl at 36 weeks' gestation; (h) the membranes rupture at 38 weeks; (i) for heartburn, varicose veins, asymptomatic bacteriuria, cervical incompetence, missed abortion, hydatidiform mole.

**During labour:**

(a) cord prolapses during first stage; (b) signs of vena caval compression are manifest; (c) woman with a cervical suture goes into labour; (d) hypotension occurs during epidural analgesia; (*e*) delay in birth of second twin; (*f*) woman develops ketoacidosis; (*g*) delay due to deep transverse arrest occurs; (*h*) signs of amniotic embolism are manifest; (*i*) third degree perineal laceration occurs; (*j*) fetal distress during first stage; (*k*) acute polyhydramnois is present. (*l*) transverse lie in early labour, membranes intact; (*m*) delay due to extended legs in breech presentation; (*n*) late fetal heart-rate deceleration occurs; (*o*) post partum haemorrhage occurs.

## To the baby:

(*a*) Apgar score is 3 at 5 minutes; (*b*) club feet are present; (*c*) pronounced physiological jaundice is manifest; (*d*) baby develops epidemic gastro-enteritis; (*e*) signs of idiopathic respiratory distress syndrome are evident; (*f*) congenital dislocation of hip is diagnosed; (*g*) grass green vomiting occurs; (*h*) blood glucose is 1.6 mmol/l; (*i*) baby is admitted with hypothermia; (*j*) Erb's paralysis is present; (*k*) a convulsion occurs; (*l*) omphalorrhagia occurs.

## During the puerperium:

(*a*) a sutured episiotomy breaks down; (*b*) deep vein thrombosis is diagnosed; (*c*) lactation must be inhibited; (*d*) puerperal sepsis is diagnosed on the third day; (*e*) painful engorged haemorrhoids are present; (*f*) Hb is 7.5 g/dl on the third day; (*g*) a flushed breast; (*h*) vesico-vaginal fistula; (*i*) pulmonary thrombo-embolism.

# QUIZ NO. 16

## WHAT DO YOU UNDERSTAND BY?

### The midwife:

(*a*) her supportive role; (*b*) a competent practitioner; (*c*) her intention to practise; (*d*) a counsellor; (*e*) a teacher of expectant parents; (*f*) an obstetric team member.

### Pregnancy:

(*a*) amniocentesis; (*b*) asymptomatic bacteriuria; (*c*) the older primigravida; (*d*) real-time ultrasonic scanning; (*e*) nicotine dependence; (*f*) an abdominal pregnancy: (*g*) kick count chart; (*h*) lecithin/sphingomyelin ratio.

### The Fetus:

(*a*) improving the quality of fetal life; (*b*) genetic anomalies; (*c*) fetal wellbeing; (*d*) gestational age; (*e*) growth retardation; (*f*) crown rump length; (*g*) an open neural tube defect.

### Labour:

(*a*) cervical effacement; (*b*) the active management of labour; (*c*) precipitate labour; (*d*) the fourth stage of labour; (*e*) inhalational analgesia; (*f*) 'breathing the head out'; (*g*) the vacuum extractor; (*h*) the mechanism of labour; (*i*) axis traction.

### The Baby:

(*a*) notification of births; (*b*) child health clinic; (*c*) a sibling; (*d*) plantar creases; (*e*) hypernatraemia; (*f*) surfactant; (*g*) brown fat; (*h*) the weaning process; (*i*) fetal alcohol syndrome; (*j*) a test feed; (*k*) rooming in; (*l*) intravenous alimentation.

### Contraception:

(*e*) Billing's mucus test; (*b*) Depo-Provero; (*c*) post pill amenorrhoea; (*d*) the rhythm method; (*e*) intrauterine device; (*f*) withdrawal bleeding; (*g*) the Dutch cap.

**Social problems:**

(*a*) unsupported child; (*b*) Marriage Guidance Council; (*c*) registered child minder; (*d*) socio-economic factors; (*e*) marital relationship; (*f*) immigrant group of pregnant women; (*g*) high perinatal mortality rate; (*h*) permissive attitude to sexual relations; (*i*) putative father; (*j*) legal aid; (*k*) adoption order; (*l*) delinquent child.

**Miscellaneous:**

(*a*) oncology; (*b*) TLC; (*c*) environmental health; (*d*) health education; (*e*) vital statistics; (*f*) cervical cytology; (*g*) emotional support; (*h*) handicapped child; (*i*) cot deaths; (*j*) the pain threshold; (*k*) thermography; (*l*) nuclear family; (*m*) artificial insemination; (*n*) ethical problems; (*o*) Home Help service; (*p*) genetic counselling.

# QUIZ NO. 17

## WHY ARE THE FOLLOWING PROCEDURES OR APPLIANCES USED

**Prenatal:**

**Tests** (*a*) blood group; (*b*) haemoglobin; (*c*) alpha feto-protein; (*d*) rubella antibodies. **Weight assessment;** amniocentesis; urine analysis.

**History taking** (*a*) family; (*b*) medical; (*c*) obstetrical; (*d*) present pregnancy.

**Ultrasonography** (*a*) placental localisation; (*b*) biparietal cephalometry; (*c*) crown rump measurement; (*d*) fetal movement and breathing.

**Means for detection** of (*a*) fetal growth retardation; (*b*) fetal abnormality; (*c*) malpresentation; (*d*) twins; (*e*) size of fetus; (*f*) cephalo-pelvic disproportion.

**Intranatal:**

**Using the** (*a*) fetal scalp electrode; (*b*) electronic fetal heart monitor; (*c*) electrocardiograph; (*d*) partogram; (*e*) foam rubber wedges.

**Delivering the baby** (*a*) in the dorsal position; (*b*) by the Burn's Marshall method; (*c*) by the Lovset method.

**Assessing** (*a*) descent of the head in fifths abdominally; (*b*) uterine tonus by abdominal palpation; (*c*) differentiating between early and late fetal heart deceleration.

**Emptying the bladder** every 2 hours. Taking blood pressure every 4 hours.

**Neonatal:**

**Giving** (*a*) naso-jejunal feeds; (*b*) intravenous alimentation; (*c*) self demand feeding; (*d*) low solute feeds.

**Using** (*a*) apnoea monitor alarm; (*b*) continuous positive airway pressure (CPAP); (*c*) blood gas analyser; (*d*) radiant heat shield; (*e*) replacement blood transfusion.

**Appliances in use** (*a*) Denis Browne splint; (*b*) Ambu bag; (*c*) laryngoscope; (*d*) dental plate; (*e*) Barlow splint; (*f*) apnoea alarm mattress; (*g*) radiant heat shield; (*h*) humidifier; (*j*) phototherapy unit.

**Tests** (*a*) Dextrostix; (*b*) Moro reflex; (*c*) Guthrie; (*d*) Ortolani; (*e*) Coombs; (*f*) test feeds; (*g*) gastric aspirate.

**Postnatal:**

(*a*) giving Rh anti-D immunoglobulin; (*b*) doing the haemoglobin test; (*c*) **Using** the rooming in plan; (*d*) planned 48 hour transfer home; (*e*) early ambulation.

**Miscellaneous**

(a) real-time scan; (b) kick count chart; (c) Cardiff infusion system; (d) electrocardiograph; (e) urinary oestriol assay.

# QUIZ NO. 18

## HOW WOULD YOU

**During pregnancy:**

**Give** health education, **take** the history of the present pregnancy, **deal** with the older primigravida, **obtain** evidence of fetal wellbeing; **treat** morning sickness; **teach** the expectant mother how to (a) relax; (b) **cope** with labour; **persuade** expectant fathers to share in childrearing; **try to prevent** congenital abnormalities; **try to foster** good mother, baby and family relationships; **monitor** fetal wellbeing; **treat** a patient with pre-eclampsia; **cope with** haemorrhage from an incomplete abortion; **do Pawlik's manoeuvre; prepare** for amniocentesis: **suspect** fetal death.

**During labour:**

**Deliver a baby** face to pubes; **deal with** shoulder dystocia; **record** labour on a partogram; **perform** an episiotomy; **deal with** prolapse of cord in second stage; **do mouth to mouth** ventilation; **deal with** transverse lie of second twin; **supervise** a woman having an i.v. infusion induction and epidural block; **deliver a baby** presenting by the face; **try to prevent** a perineal tear; **transport** a preterm baby from home to hospital; from the labour ward to the nursery; **deal with fetal distress; meet the woman's emotional needs;** top up an epidural block: use the Mauriceau Smellie Veit grip?

**Care of the baby:**

**Perform** intubation; **nurse** the baby of a diabetic mother; **give** intermittent positive airway pressure; **give** phototherapy; **give a** nasogastric feed; **take** blood for the Guthrie test; **observe** baby during replacement transfusion, **treat** sore buttocks, oral thrush, omphalitis, paronychia.

**The puerperium:**

**Teach a woman** (a) to express her breast milk; (b) to strengthen her pelvic floor muscles; (c) how to cope with her baby when excessive crying occurs?

**Comfort the mother** of (a) a handicapped baby; (b) a stillborn baby.

**Treat:** (a) a 'broken down' perineum; (b) a sutured third degree tear; (c) engorged breasts; (d) cracked nipples; (e) 'the blues'; (f) after-pains; (g) haemorrhoids.

**Give:** (a) Rh anti-D immunoglobulin; (b) psychological support.

**Deal with:** (a) a flushed breast; (b) pulmonary thrombo-embolism; (c) retention of urine?

**Miscellaneous:**

**Inculcate the woman's confidence** in the maternity hospital staff. Convince her that a team of experienced experts is an advantage?

**Promote bonding** of mother and baby? **Motivate the mother** to give 'tender, loving care' to her baby? **Try to prevent** non-accidental injury? **Conduct a discussion group** with postnatal mothers?

## QUIZ NO. 19

**Give the time** *(approx)* **in minutes, hours, days or weeks.**
*Verify by the page number.*

| See page | Subject | State | Min | Hours | Days | Weeks |
|---|---|---|---|---|---|---|
| 158 | When fetus is viable ............... | | | | | |
| 187 | When pre-eclampsia occurs ............. | | | | | |
| 54 | When fetus weighs 700 G ............... | | | | | |
| 78 | When quickening occurs ............. | | | | | |
| 36 | That the sperm is capable of fertilisation ............. | | | | | |
| 83 | Days in pregnancy ............. | | | | | |
| 59 | When the post. fontanelle closes ............. | | | | | |
| 67 | When fundus reaches umbilicus in pregnancy ............. | | | | | |
| 67 | When pregnant uterus is at the summit of symphysis ............. | | | | | |
| 69 | When prickling occurs in the breasts ............. | | | | | |
| 237 | When lightening occurs ............. | | | | | |
| 664 | When the biparietal diameter can be measured by sonar ............. | | | | | |
| 109 | When amniocentesis is done for Down's syndrome ............. | | | | | |
| 110 | When amniocentesis is done for lecithin/sphing omyelin ratio ............. | | | | | |
| 122 | When the pregnant woman is seen up to 20 weeks ............. | | | | | |
| 122 | When the pregnant woman is seen 20–36 weeks ............. | | | | | |
| 122 | When the pregnant woman is seen 36–40 weeks ............. | | | | | |
| 241 | That the first stage of labour lasts ............. | | | | | |
| 241 | That the second stage of labour lasts ............. | | | | | |
| 241 | That the third stage of labour lasts ............. | | | | | |
| 402 | Prolonged labour lasts over ............. | | | | | |
| 138 | When the fetal head engages ............. | | | | | |
| 150 | Hours of sleep pregnant woman should have ............. | | | | | |
| 121 | First visit of pregnant woman to clinic ............. | | | | | |
| 567 | When Rh anti-D immunoglobin is given postnatally ............. | | | | | |
| 143 | When cephalo-pelvic disproportion is diagnosed ............. | | | | | |
| 515 | Of gestation for the preterm baby ............. | | | | | |
| 439 | The length of the puerperium ............. | | | | | |
| 335 | Syntocinon takes to act ............. | | | | | |
| 335 | Ergometrine takes to act ............. | | | | | |
| 335 | Syntometrine takes to act ............. | | | | | |
| 610 | The optimal time for external version ............. | | | | | |
| 681 | When a birth is registered in England ............. | | | | | |
| 681 | When a birth is registered in Scotland ............. | | | | | |
| 681 | When a birth is notified ............. | | | | | |
| 450 | When a shower can be given after delivery ............. | | | | | |
| 173 | That hydatidiform mole is diagnosed ............. | | | | | |
| 153 | That morning sickness begins ............. | | | | | |
| 449 | After delivery when Hb is estimated ............. | | | | | |
| 493 | When physiological jaundice occurs ............. | | | | | |
| 460 | That post-pill amenorrhoea lasts ............. | | | | | |
| 502 | When the healthy newborn baby is fed after delivery ............. | | | | | |
| 488 | That newborn babies sleep in 24 hours ............. | | | | | |
| 491 | That the umbilical cord comes off ............. | | | | | |
| 520 | When is first feed given to preterm baby ............. | | | | | |
| 563 | Oral thrush occurs ............. | | | | | |
| 320 | That the Apgar score is made ............. | | | | | |
| 534 | Iron is unnecessary for newborn until ............. | | | | | |
| 539 | When the Dextrostix test is made after birth if necessary ............. | | | | | |
| 542 | The Guthrie test is made ............. | | | | | |

## QUIZ NO. 20

### WHICH METHOD DO YOU PREFER? GIVE REASONS WHY

**Pregnancy:**

(a) Rail or air travel (b) foods rich in iron or tablets; (c) to determine cephalo-pelvic disproportion; (d) to prepare the nipples for lactation; (e) to motivate expectant mothers to give up smoking; (f) to prevent constipation; (g) to diagnose multiple pregnancy from polyhydramnios: (h) to obtain a mid-stream specimen of urine.

**Labour:**

(a) home or hospital for delivery; (b) an admission tub bath or shower with mobile hand spray; (c) vulval shaving, clipping, a mini prep or neither; (d) ligatures, rubber bands or plastic clamps for the umbilical cord; waiting for the cord vessels to cease pulsating or not prior to ligating the umbilical cord; (e) delivery in the dorsal or left lateral position; (f) using foam rubber wedges to prop up the woman in labour or not; (g) using pudendal nerve block or epidural; (h) using beads, wrist bands or foot prints for baby identification; (i) controlled cord traction or the Brandt Andrew manoeuvre; (j) continuous fetal monitoring or using Pinard's stethoscope intermittently.

**Baby:**

(a) breast or bottle feeding: fresh or dried milk: self demand or four hourly feeds: milk warm or at room temperature; (b) washable or disposable napkins; (c) baby with Down's syndrome to be kept at home or in an institution: parents of mongoloid baby to be told sooner or later; (d) in treatment of sore buttocks; (e) bathing on knee or table, morning or evening.

**Puerperium:**

Transfer home at 24, 48 hours or 7th day: treatment of (a) cracked nipples; (b) engorged breasts; (c) to suppress lactation; (d) afterpains: (e) using the contraceptive pill, condom, intrauterine device.

**Miscellaneous:**

(a) group or individual parentcraft teaching; (b) adoption or fostering for the baby of the unwed mother? (c) an electric breast pump, hand pump, or manual expression; (d) teaching 'fertility control' during pregnancy or puerperium.

## QUIZ NO. 21

### GIVE THE CORRECT PHARMACOLOGICAL NAME

| Pharmaceutical | Pharmacological name arranged in wrong order | Place correct pharmacological name below |
|---|---|---|
| Sparine | chlordiazepoxide | |
| Narcan | bupivacaine | |
| Pentothal | nitrazepam | |
| Largactil | diazepam | |
| Marcain | promethazine | |
| Phenergan | phenelzine | |
| Nardil | chloropromazine | |
| Flagyl | phenindione | |
| Kannasyn | thiopentone | |
| Heminevrin | promazine | |
| Valium | kanamycin | |
| Syntometrine | pentazocine | |
| Fortral | oxytocin | |
| Librium | naloxone | |
| Lanoxin | frusemide | |
| Syntocinon | ergometrine maleate | |
| Dindevan | metronidazole | |
| Mogadon | chlormethiazole | |
| Lasix | lignocaine | |
| Xylocaine | digoxin | |
| Ceporex | methicillin | |
| Apresoline | methyldopa | |
| Celbenin | cephalexin | |
| Aldomet | hydrallazine | |

## QUIZ NO. 22

### HOW WOULD THE MIDWIFE IN HOSPITAL

#### Decide

When to administer: (a) pethidine prescribed by the doctor: (b) Entonox; (c) naloxone; (d) Syntometrine; (e) lignocaine; (f) promazine (Eng.); (g) magnesium trisilicate; (h) bupivacaine for topping up epidural; (i) oxygen to the preterm baby.

#### Proceed regarding

(a) the second twin; (b) prolapse of the cord; (c) fetal distress; (d) convulsion in the neonate; (e) haemorrhage from an incomplete abortion; (f) traumatic postpartum haemorrhage; (g) a pulmonary thrombo-embolism; (h) the Dextrostix test; (i) making an episiotomy.

#### Screen for high risk patients

(a) pregnant woman; (b) fetus; (c) neonate.

#### Deal with

(a) severe asphyxia neonatorum; (b) baby with epidemic gastroenteritis; (c) an apnoeic episode; (d) the bereaved mother; (e) accelerated labour; (f) inverted uterus.

**Help to avoid**

(*a*) hypernatraemia; (*b*) eclampsia; (*c*) ophthalmia neonatorum; (*d*) anaemia in the pregnant woman ; (*e*) neonatal hypothermia; (*f*) post partum haemorrhage.

**Treat the woman in labour**

(*a*) who is having epidural analgesia;
(*b*) with incipient signs of fetal distress;
(*c*) who is receiving prostaglandin E₂ vaginally;
(*d*) who is a diabetic;
(*e*) when there is fetal growth retardation;
(*f*) who had a previous Caesarean section;
(*g*) when pre-eclampsia is present.

## QUIZ NO. 23

### INSTRUMENTS AND APPLIANCES

*For what reasons might the following instruments or appliances be used in obstetric practice?*

| Page | | Page | |
|---|---|---|---|
| 555 | Rubber nasal prongs | 618 | Wrigley's forceps |
| 323 | Hollister clamps | 570 | bilirubinometer |
| 654 | Gregory box (modified) | 625 | Tuohy's needle |
| 229 | Fenwell pressure apparatus | 590 | Holter valve |
| 168 | Karman catheter | 522 | Slow syringe pump |
| 547 | Ambu bag | 517 | silver swaddler |
| 557 | Negative pressure chamber | 594 | Denis Browne splint |
| 433 | Iris scissors | 476 | Hanley pump |
| 554 | humidifier | 553 | Draeger unit |
| 603 | Palmer pump | 549 | laryngoscope |
| 463 | laparascope | 594 | Barlow's splint |
| 678 | Ayres spatula | 483 | electronic thermometer |
| 115 | real-time scanner | 436 | central venous pressure manometer |
| 604 | Tekmar apparatus | 540 | oxygen analyser |
| 644 | Malmstrom extractor | 165 | braided mersilk cervical suture |
| 532 | contactless alarm mattress | 297 | fetal scalp electrode |
| 400 | cardiotocograph | 618 | Kielland's forceps |
| 554 | positive pressure chamber | 260 | foam rubber wedge |
| 544 | radiant heat shield | 654 | Blease Samson resuscitator |
| 625 | millipore filter | 586 | neonatal dental plate |
| 198 | oral rubber wedge | 461 | Saf T Coil |
| 288 | Studd's stencil | 657 | Blond Heidler wire saw |
| 603 | Cardiff infusion unit | 601 | Nelaton Catheter |
| 201 | ultrasound BP monitor | 557 | Penlon resuscitator |
| 483 | electronic thermometer | 11 | Ohio intensive care centre |

## QUIZ NO. 24

### GIVE AN ALTERNATIVE TERM FOR:

Sonar; antenatal; chloasma; dizygotic twins; platypelloid pelvis; calorie; abortion; battered baby; placenta; accidental APH; ectopic gestation; strabismus; umbilicus; teratogen; proteinuria; fetus papyraceous; hypovolaemia; Bandl's ring; exchange transfusion; bregma. Siamese twins; amniotic fluid; frank breech; omphalitis; vas ligation; unavoidable APH: funic presentation: the growth hormone; effacement of cervix; loss of FH beat to beat variation; Sellick's manoeuvre; Down's syndrome; cephalic presentation; carneous mole; umbilical cord; hour glass contraction.

Vesicular mole; ventouse; flying squad; gynaecoid pelvis; Mendelson's syndrome; palmar crease; malacosteon pelvis; secondary postpartum haemorrhage; fertility control; torticollis; candidiasis; Trilene; high blood pressure; climacteric; gravid; domiciliary; caput; nicotine dependence; assay; glycosuria; centigrade; Entonox; conception; bicornuate uterus; lactation; mentum; parturition; sinciput; abruptio placentae; venereal disease; habitual abortion; the abused baby; amniotomy; brachial palsy; transverse cervical uterine ligaments; puerperal haemorrhage; intranatal; haemorrhoids; identical twins; parenteral alimentation; normal saline; nuchal; pelvic measurement; pertussis; trimester; molar pregnancy; platypelloid pelvis; pseudocyesis; neonatology; transverse lie; wire saw decapitator.

# QUIZ NO. 25

## WHAT IS MEANT BY?

(a) hermaphroditism; (b) an affiliation order; (c) incompetent cervix; (d) weaning; (e) SI units; (f) cervical cytology; (g) localisation of the placenta; (h) genetic anomalies; (i) persistent occipito-posterior position; (j) i.v. alimentation; (k) blighted ovum; (l) endometrial biopsy; (m) neutral thermal range; (n) fetoscopy; (o) nuclear family; (p) primary health care team; (q) the show; (r) obstructed labour; (s) electronic monitor; (t) Community Physician; (u) neonatal developmental assessment; (v) non-accidental injury; (w) local supervising authority; (x) Health visitor; (y) trimester; (z) central venous pressure.

(a) anti-D immunoglobulin; (b) Erb's paralysis; (c) ano-rectal atresia; (d) hypoglycaemia; (e) intraventricular haemorrhage; (f) IPPV; (g) CPAP; (h) nasal rubber prongs; (i) apnoea; (j) 'feto-maternal bleed'; (k) emotional support; (l) rim of cervix; (m) cervicograph; (n) established labour; (o) electrolyte replacement; (p) base line FH rate; (q) type 1 Dip; (r) hypoxia; (s) pH of blood; (t) pudendal nerve block; (u) ketoacidosis; (v) haemolysis; (w) crowning; (x) bonding; (y) the social history; (z) grande multipara.

(a) Low solute infant feeds; (b) acceleration of labour; (c) elective Caesarean section; (d) intrauterine growth retardation; (e) small for date baby; (f) the expanding role of the midwife; (g) a real time scan; (h) prescription only medicines (POM) (i) artificial insemination; (j) ovulation induction clinic; (k) brown fat; (l) a dyad; (m) oncology; (n) abbreviated birth certificate; (o) nullipara; (p) social classes 1 to 5; (q) environmental health; (r) fertility control; (s) uterine tonus; (t) vena caval occlusion; (u) sternal recession; (v) gravity drip feed; (w) precipitate labour; (x) ultrasonography; (y) nutritional anaemia; (z) the extra amniotic route for prostaglandin.

# QUIZ NO. 26

## ELABORATE ON THE FOLLOWING

### (1) The aims of

(a) prenatal care; (b) notification of births; (c) health education; (d) neonatal intensive care; (e) family planning; (f) therapeutic abortion; (g) parentcraft teaching; (h) sex education in schools; (i) screening pregnant women; (j) neonatal paediatric follow up clinics.

**(2) The facilities available**

For parents caring for their child with (*a*) spina bifida; (*b*) Down's syndrome; (*c*) cleft palate; (*d*) dislocated hip; (*e*) birth palsy.

**(3) The conditions that cause**

(*a*) fetal anoxia; (*b*) prolapse of cord; (*c*) bleeding in early pregnancy; (*d*) intracranial injury; (*e*) transverse lie; (*f*) mental retardation; (*g*) fetal growth retardation; (*h*) preterm labour.

**(4) Why schoolgirls should be**

(*a*) given anti-rubella vaccine; (*b*) taught about pregnancy, labour and baby care; (*c*) encouraged to adopt a wholesome attitude regarding breast feeding; (*d*) given sex education before puberty.

**(5) Investigations made**

(*a*) the pH of the blood; (*b*) surfactant in the fetal lungs; (*c*) quantity of chorionic gonadotrophin in urine; (*d*) amount of protein in urine; (*e*) rubella antibodies; (*f*) blood glucose level; (*g*) amount of breast milk taken at one feed; (*h*) bilirubin in amniotic fluid.

**(6) Diagnosis of**

(*a*) Rh antibodies; (*b*) hypofibrinogenaemia; (*c*) phenylketonuria; (*d*) melaena; (*e*) blighted ovum; (*f*) vasa praevia; (*g*) fetal death; (*h*) hookworm infection; (*i*) cervical cancer; (*j*) vulval haematoma; (*k*) brow presentation; (*l*) overdistended bladder in the postnatal woman.

**(7) Why expectant mothers should be given a simple explanation of subjects such as**

(*a*) induction of labour; (*b*) postpartum blues; (*c*) epidural block; (*d*) forceps delivery; (*e*) electronic monitoring; (*f*) ultrasonic scanning; (*g*) episiotomy.

# QUIZ NO. 27

## NEWER TERMINOLOGY *(definitions)*

| Old | Newer | State Definitions |
|---|---|---|
| moniliasis | candidiasis | |
| premature baby | preterm baby | |
| calorie | Joule | |
| hypotensive drugs | anti-hypertensive | |
| hare lip | cleft lip | |
| accidental haemorrhage | abruptio placentae | |
| toxaemia of pregnancy | pre-eclampsia | |
| $\mu$g | microgram | |
| hydramnios | polyhydramnios | |
| venereal disease | sexually-transmitted disease | |
| normal saline | isotonic saline | |
| antenatal | prenatal | |
| Secondary PPH | puerperal haemorrhage | |
| twins, triplets | multiple pregnancy | |
| the mongol | Down's syndrome | |
| elderly primipara | older primipara | |
| Sanitary Inspector | Environmental Health Officer | |
| nephritis | renal disease | |
| liquor amnii | amniotic fluid | |

| Old | Newer | State Definitions |
|---|---|---|
| child welfare clinic | child health clinic | |
| Family allowance | child benefit | |
| polyhydramnios | acute polyhydramnious | |
| sacro-cotyloid diameter | sacro-cotyloid dimension | |
| battered baby | non-accidental injury | |
| uniovular twins | monozygotic twins | |
| binovular twins | dizygotic twins | |
| pyelitis | pyelonephritis | |
| centigrade | Celsius | |
| asphyxia livida | mild asphyxia | |
| asphyxia pallida | severe asphyxia | |
| albuminuria | proteinuria | |
| supine hypotensive syndrome | vena caval compression | |
| defaulters | non-attenders | |

# GLOSSARY

## OF TERMS AND OBSTETRICAL CONDITIONS

**Acid-base balance.** The degree of acidity or alkalinity of the blood is governed by the amount of acid or bicarbonate present in the blood. This is reflected in the pH which rises in alkalaemia and falls in acidaemia. Changes in the acid-base balance of fetal and neonatal blood are measured by the Astrup Micro-Equipment, e.g. when fetal distress or respiratory distress syndrome is present. This is essential prior to undertaking chemical correction by the administration of glucose and sodium bicarbonate.

**Amnesic.** A drug that causes loss of memory (of pain). Scopolamine is a good example, also being hypnotic. Diazepam (Valium) and promethazine (Phenergan) have some amnesic action.

**Anaesthetic.** A central nervous system depressant given by inhalation or i.v. injection characterised by loss of consciousness and pain.

**Analgesic (local).** A substance that interrupts nerve impulses by blocking nerve endings, as in pudendal nerve block and epidural analgesia.

**Ante-.** Prefix meaning 'before' or 'in front of', e.g. antenatal, before birth; anteflexion of uterus, a uterus which bends forwards.

**Antibody.** A serum protein which is formed in response to an antigenic stimulus and reacts specifically with the antigen.

**Atresia.** Closure or absence of a usual opening or canal; e.g. oesophageal atresia.

**Autosome.** The chromosomes not concerned with sex determination are known as autosomes. The human cell has 22 pairs of autosomes and one pair of sex chromosomes.

**Axis-traction.** Used when pulling on the fetal head in the direction of the axis of the pelvic canal. For this purpose midwifery forceps are used, with a special axis-traction handle which permits alteration in the direction of pull, according to whether the head is in low or mid-cavity.

**Baptism of infants.** This religious rite signifies entry into the Church and is generally accompanied by name-giving. The ritual consists in the 'pouring on' (*the baby's head*) of water at the same time saying: 'I baptise thee in the name of the Father and of the Son and of the Holy Ghost'.

**Bi-** or **Bis-.** Prefix meaning 'two'; e.g. bi-manual, two hands, as in bi-manual examination of the pelvic organs, bi-manual compression of uterus; bi-polar, two poles or extremities, as in bi-polar version; bis-acromial diameter, the measurement between the two acromion processes.

**Bifid.** Cleft, divided into two; e.g. spina-bifida.

**Bilirubin.** The orange pigment of bile. This gives the yellow tint to the skin and conjunctiva in cases of jaundice. The serum bilirubin test is carried out on the blood of babies suffering from icterus neonatorum.

**Biology.** The science of life and of living things.

**Biopsy.** Examination of tissue from the living body; e.g. from the cervix in cases of suspected carcinoma; from the endometrium in cases of infertility.

**Bohn's nodules.** Small white nodules, having no significance, seen on the centre of the palate of the newborn. They may be present during the first few days of life and disappear spontaneously. Sometimes they are mistaken for thrush, which does not appear till after the fourth day.

**Breast-pump.** An appliance with glass funnel and rubber bulb, used to extract milk from the lactating breast by suction; it is worked either by hand or electricity.

**Brown fat.** A source of heat for the newborn infant, is deposited as pads of adipose tissue between the scapulae, around the neck and the blood vessels that leave the heart and kidneys. The blood going to the brain and other vital organs is warmed by brown fat. When the baby is cold the temperature receptors in the skin send impulses to the brain which via the sympathetic nervous system relays impulses to the brown fat. The nerve endings in the brown fat release noradrenaline that activates the heat producing cycle; glucose and oxygen are essential. Preterm babies have a small amount of brown fat so chilling must be avoided and heat supplied.

**Cardinal ligaments.** The transverse cervical ligaments of the uterus (Mackenrodt's ligaments).

**Caul.** A cap. This is the part of the amnion which covers the child's face when it is born with the amnion intact.

**-cele.** Suffix, meaning a 'tumour', usually one containing fluid; e.g. cystocele, a protrusion of the bladder into the vagina; meningocele, a tumour containing cerebrospinal fluid.

**Chromosomes.** Thread-like bodies situated within the nucleus of the cell which carry genetic information. Sex chromosomes determine the sex of the individual; XX in women, XY in men. Chromosomes not responsible for sex determination are known as autosomes.

**Circumcision.** Excision of part of the penile prepuce or foreskin, to allow it to be drawn back over the glans for the purpose of adequate cleansing of the part. This procedure is no longer recommended as a routine measure. Circumcision is a religious rite among Jewish people, being performed by the Mohel on the eighth day, if the health of the child permits.

**Climacteric.** The change of life or menopause.

**Colpos.** The vagina; e.g. colporrhaphy, suturing of the vagina; haematocolpos, collection of blood in the vagina due to imperforate hymen or atresia of the vagina.

**Community.** All the people living within a defined geographical area. The hospital is part of the community.

**Community medicine.** This is concerned with the health status of population groups rather than individuals and with conditions that affect health, pure food, milk, water.

**Community nurse or midwife.** One who gives attention to patients in their own homes. She may be based in the hospital.

**Craniotabes.** A condition characterised by thinning of the bones of the vault of the skull, due to the failure of ossification. This is most common in preterm babies: it is also an early sign of rickets. On applying pressure along the suture lines, the thin bone can be dented.

**Cyesis.** Pregnancy; e.g. pseudocyesis, a phantom or false pregnancy.

**Cytology.** The study of tissue cells. From desquamated fetal cells found in amniotic fluid, obtained by abdominal amniocentesis, the sex and maturity of the fetus can be determined. Chromosomal abnormalities, e.g. trisomy 21, as in Down's syndrome, can be detected. Cervical epithelial cells obtained by Papanicolaou smear are examined for the recognition of early cancer of the cervix.

**Decidual cast.** The decidua, triangular in shape, when it is shed intact from the uterus, as occurs in some cases of tubal pregnancy. The decidua is, however, usually passed in shreds.

**Dolichocephaly.** A head which is long from front to back. This is believed by some authorities to be a cause of face presentation; others consider dolichocephaly to be due to the moulding resultant from the extended head.

**Duhressen's incisions.** Incisions of the cervix, rarely made in cases of extremely slow dilatation of the os, to facilitate delivery of the child. Three incisions are usually made when the os is 6–7 cm dilated at 10-2-6 'on the clock'.

**Dyad.** A couple, e.g. mother and father, mother and baby.

**Dystocia.** Difficult labour.

**-ectomy.** Suffix meaning 'cutting out', e.g. hysterectomy, removal of uterus.

**Electrolyte.** A substance which in solution is capable of conducting an electric current and is decomposed by it, e.g. sodium, chloride, potassium, bicarbonate.

**Endo-.** Prefix, meaning 'within' or 'lining'; e.g. endometrium, membrane lining the uterus.

**Epidemiology.** The study of general health and disease in the community.

**Erythroblastosis fetalis.** A condition in which there are immature erythrocytes in the blood-stream of the newborn. This is the body's response to excessive destruction of red cells by haemolysis, e.g. due to Rh incompatibility.

**Ex-.** Prefix, meaning 'out of'; e.g. exogenous source of puerperal sepsis, organisms introduced from 'without' into the vagina; exomphalos, protrusion of the intestines out of the umbilicus (or omphalos).

**Extra-uterine pregnancy.** A pregnancy occurring outside the uterus; e.g. tubal, abdominal. (*See also* Ectopic gestation, p. 172.)

**Fecundation.** Impregnation or conception. (*See also* Superfecundation.)

**Fetation.** Impregnation or conception. (*See also* Superfetation.)

**Fetoscopy.** Fetoscopy is a technique, carried out at the 16th to 18th week of pregnancy, whereby the external surface of the fetus in utero can be inspected and abnormal conditions such as spina bifida and anencephaly detected. Fetal blood sampling and skin biopsy can also be carried out when indicated. Under local analgesia a cannula with a needlescope 1.7 mm and a fine glass fibre light source is introduced via the abdominal and uterine walls. To avoid the placenta it is located by using a real-time ultrasonic scanner immediately prior to the fetoscopy.

**Fontanelle.** A little fountain. The membranous space at the junction of two or more sutures in the fetal skull. It was so named because, in days prior to the discovery of the circulation of blood, the pulsation felt suggested the bubbling of a small fountain.

**Funis.** A cord. A term sometimes applied to the umbilical cord. Funic souffle.

**Gamma globulin.** Plasma proteins are divided into 4 main groups: albumin and the alpha, beta and gamma globulins. It is in the gamma globulin fraction that man carries his antibodies.

**Ganglion.** A semi-independent nervous centre from which nerves radiate; e.g. the paracervical ganglion, a sheath of nerves, situated behind and on either side of the cervix, also known as Frankenhäuser's plexus.

**Gene.** The genetic molecule or unit present in the chromosomes of the ovum and spermatozoon, which transmits the inherited factors or characteristics of the parents.

**Genitalia.** The organs of generation; the external and internal genital organs.

**Genotype.** The genetic constitution of an individual. This term is used when investigating paternal blood in cases of Rh incompatability when the father's genotype may be Rh positive homozygous or Rh positive heterozygous.

**Gestation.** Pregnancy; e.g. ectopic gestation.

**Gonad.** A reproductive gland, e.g. the ovary in the female, the testis in the male.

**Gonadotrophic.** The term used to describe a substance which stimulates the gonads; e.g. the follicle-stimulating hormone and the luteinising hormone of the anterior pituitary gland.

**Gram-negative.** The term applied to bacteria which do not retain the stain when acted upon by Gram's iodine solution. The gonococcus is Gram-negative.

**Gravid.** Pregnant; e.g. retroverted gravid uterus.

**Gravidarum.** Meaning 'of pregnant women'; e.g. hyperemesis gravidarum.

**Haem-.** Prefix, meaning 'blood'; e.g. haematuria, blood in the urine; haemolysis, breaking-down of red blood cells.

**Haematocrit.** Expresses the percentage volume of red corpuscles in uncoagulated whole blood. It is used as a screening test for anaemia and in following the course of water and electrolyte disorders. Normal 50 to 60 per cent.

**Hermaphroditism.** A condition in which the generative organs of both sexes are present. True hermaphroditism is exceedingly rare in human beings and pseudo-hermaphroditism is more commonly of the male type. The penis is small, the testes are present but undescended, and the scrotum being divided into two halves resembles the labia majora.

In the female type the clitoris is enlarged and resembles the penis, the labia may be adherent and contain the ovaries, thereby giving the appearance of male genitalia. The midwife must always examine the external genital organs carefully, prior to stating the sex, and in cases of doubt must obtain medical advice before making any pronouncement or filling up forms.

**Herpes gestationis.** A skin disease affecting 1–4,000 pregnant women and characterised by the appearance of papules, vesicles and pustules which may extend over the whole body. The patient suffers from itching and burning which may cause insomnia. This rare condition is considered to be toxic in origin and may recur in subsequent pregnancies. Treatment is by systematic steroids and as the condition occurs in the mid-trimester teratogenic effects are unlikely. Soothing local applications may help.

**Heterozygous.** Having an inherited characteristic in which the zygotes are composed of diverse elements. The term is applied in cases of Rh incompatability, to describe the genotype of an Rh positive father. The positive heterozygous man has inherited an Rh negative gene from one of his parents and an Rh positive gene from the other. The genes in his spermatozoa may therefore be either negative or positive. If negative, the fetus will also be negative, and consequently there will be no incompatability with the Rh negative mother. If positive, the fetus will also be positive, and there may be incompatability with the Rh negative mother.

**Heyn's apparatus for abdominal decompression.** This apparatus, a fibreglass dome, is placed over the abdomen, in an effort to reduce pain of labour. It is not widely used in Britain.

**Hirsutes.** An abnormal growth of hair, the term usually being applied to a female with the male distribution of hair.

**Homozygous.** Having an inherited characteristic in which the zygotes are composed of the same type of elements. The term is applied in cases of Rh incompatability to describe the genotype of an Rh positive father. The positive homozygous man has inherited an Rh positive gene from each of his parents. The genes in his spermatozoa will all be positive, the fetus will also be positive and there may be incompatability with the Rh negative mother.

**Human placental lactogen.** (HPL) is secreted by the syncytiotrophoblast into the maternal circulation. The term somatotrophin was previously applied. Growth hormone-like changes in pregnancy, may be due to H.P.L. The amount in maternal blood and urine indicates feto-placental-unit functioning. Low levels after 30 weeks suggest high fetal risk.

**Hydro-.**   Prefix meaning 'water'; e.g. hydrocephaly, water in the ventricles of the brain; hydraemia, a watery condition of the blood such as occurs normally during pregnancy.

**Hydrorrhoea gravidarum.**   A condition in which, during the later months of pregnancy, there is a discharge from the uterus of clear fluid which may persist intermittently. This may be amniotic fluid which escapes, owing to the rupture of the amniotic sac, at a high level. It may also be due to inflammation of the decidual glands, and in such cases there is pain in the lower abdomen.

**Hypo-.**   Prefix, meaning 'under'; e.g. hypotonic uterus, one which has poor tone.

**Hypovolaemia.**   Low or decreased blood volume as occurs in haemorrhage.

**Ichthyosis (congenital).**   A skin disease in which scales or plaques of smooth, dry, horny skin peel off: the whole body being involved. Numerous fissures run between the plaques. The normal skin folds are obliterated and ectropion (eversion) of the eyelids is present. Such severe cases are fatal. Recovery may take place in mild forms of the disease which sometimes occur after birth.

**Immunoglobulin.**   A serum protein that is produced in response to an antigen and reacts specifically to it.

**Impaction.**   Tight wedging; jamming of one object inside another; e.g. impaction of breech, face or shoulder (*presentation*) in the pelvic canal.

**Impetigo herpetiformis gravidarum.**   A dangerous form of impetigo, affecting pregnant women. Pustules appear on the trunk and thighs; the temperature is raised; vomiting, delirium and grave prostration ensue. Injections of blood-serum from a normal pregnant woman have been given with varying degrees of success. The mortality rate is high, but, fortunately, the disease is rare.

**Indicating point.**   The denominator or part of the presentation that indicates the position of the fetus in relation to the six areas of the mother's pelvis.

**Iniencephaly.**   A fetus with a protrusion of the brain in the occipital region.

**Inter-.**   Prefix, meaning 'between'; e.g. intertuberischial diameter, the distance between the inner borders of the ischial tuberosities.

**Intra-.**   Prefix, meaning 'within'; e.g. intracranial haemorrhage, bleeding within the skull; intrapartum eclampsia when the condition occurs during labour.

**Intra-ligamentous pregnancy.**   This occurs when the Fallopian tube ruptures and the fetus continues to develop within the folds of the broad ligament.

**Iso-immunisation.**   The prefix 'allo' is preferred by some authorities as being more accurate. This has been defined as the process whereby antibodies are formed in an individual in response to the injection of an antigen from another individual of the same species, e.g. Rh negative mother immunised by the antigens in the red cells of her Rh positive fetus or by the antigens in the red cells in a transfusion of Rh positive blood (inadvertently) given to her.

**Joule (J).**   The term used in nutritional science for the calorie. The large or kilocalorie equals 4·184 kilojoules (approximately 4). 1,000 kilojoules equals one megajoule.

**Kelvin (K).**   The unit of thermodynamic temperature. It is an absolute scale of temperature which has its zero at minus 273°C.

**Kluge's sign of pregnancy.**   Varicosities of the veins in the region of the vaginal orifice.

**Klumpke's paralysis.**   The forearm and hand are affected, due to injury of the lower part of the brachial plexus. It is less common than Erb's paralysis in which the upper part of the brachial plexus is injured and the upper arm affected.

**Kyphotic pelvis.** When there is kyphosis (*angular curvature of the spine*) in the lumbar region, the misdirected body-weight causes a narrowing of the pelvis from side to side, particularly at the outlet. The deformity of hump-back is obvious in such a case.

**Legal aid.** This is provided by solicitors on the legal aid panel to persons whose income is below set limits.

**Lysis.** A breaking down; e.g. haemolysis, breaking down of red blood cells. This may occur in the fetal blood, due to Rh incompatability.

**Mal.** Prefix, meaning 'bad'; e.g. malpresentation, such as breech, face, brow, shoulder; malposition, such as right and left occipito-posterior, right and left mento-posterior; malformation, such as cleft lip.

**Menarche.** The initial onset of menstruation.

**Micro-.** Prefix, meaning 'small'; e.g. microcephaly, a very small head; microcytic hypochromic anaemia, in which the red blood cells are small.

**Micrognathia.** Because the mandible is poorly developed the lower jaw and chin recede. The baby should not lie on his back as the tongue may fall backwards and block the larynx.

**Miscarriage.** The word is synonymous with the word 'abortion'. Patients prefer the term miscarriage' and use it to describe a spontaneous abortion: they associate the word 'abortion' with criminal induction.

**Mole (mol).** The term used to record the concentrations or amounts of substances whose molecular weights are known, e.g. concentrations in blood plasma as millimoles per litre (mmol/l). Urinary output in 24 hours will be reported in moles (mol) or millimoles (mmol). For drugs, grams, milligrams and millilitres will continue to be used for safety reasons.

**Multigravida.** Multi, meaning 'more than one'; gravida, meaning 'pregnant'. A woman who has been pregnant more than once is a multigravida.

**Multipara.** Multi, meaning 'more than one'; parere, meaning 'to bear'. A woman who has borne more than one child is a multipara. A primigravida, having borne no child, is designated as para 0, a woman pregnant for the second time as para 1.

**Nates.** The buttocks. The natal cleft, the furrow between the buttocks.

**Neo-.** Prefix, meaning 'new'; e.g. neonatal, the newborn; neoplasm, a new growth, a term usually applied to one that is malignant.

**Nuclear family.** A home based social structure: parents and their offspring living permanently together.

**Nullipara.** A woman who has not given birth to a child.

**-oma.** Suffix, meaning 'tumour'; e.g. carcinoma, tumour of malignant origin; fibroma, tumour of fibrous and muscle tissue.

**Oncology.** The term is derived from the Greek word 'oncos' meaning a mass. It is at present applied to the study of tumours and in practice its clinical application is total patient care in cancer.

**-orrhaphy.** Suffix, meaning 'suturing of'; e.g. perineorrhaphy, suturing of perineum; trachelorrhaphy, suturing of cervix.

**Osmolality.** This is the total concentration of non-permeating particles (solute) in a solvent. Water molecules pass through the wall of the cell and keep the osmolality of the intracellular and the extracellular fluids equalised. Osmolality is measured in milliosmoles per litre: 280–300 m Osm/kg $H_2O$.

Electrolyte disturbances will upset plasma osmolality, therefore in low birth weight babies receiving parenteral nutriment this is monitored. Babies suspected of having sustained brain damage at birth will have their plasma osmolality monitored so that steps can be taken to avoid further cerebral oedema.

**-otomy.** Suffix, meaning 'incision of' or 'cutting into'; e.g. hysterotomy, cutting into the uterus.

**Para-.** Prefix, meaning 'alongside of' or 'near'; e.g. parametrium, the connective tissue surrounding the uterus; parametritis, inflammation of the parametrium.

**Paracervical nerve block.** To relieve pain when the cervix is 5 or more cm dilated 10 ml lignocaine one per cent is injected via the lateral vaginal fornices into the base of the broad ligaments. The effect only lasts for 1 to $1\frac{1}{2}$ hours. Fetal bradycardia may occur so the method is losing favour.

**Pascal (Pa).** A unit of pressure, the term used to express pressures. Partial pressure of blood gases currently reported in mmHg will be measured in kilopascals (kPa). 1 mmHg equals 133 Pa. The international practice of using mmHg for blood pressure will be continued for a few years.

**Paternity Tests.** If a blood group gene is present in the child and absent in the mother it must have come from the father. Lack of this gene in the alleged father absolves him from paternity. Presence of the gene does not denote that he is the father of the child.

**Pathic.** Meaning 'pertaining to disease'; e.g. pathogenic or disease-producing organisms; neonatal pathology, science of disease of the newborn.

**$P_{CO_2}$.** This symbol denotes the partial pressure or tension of carbon dioxide in the blood; normal being approx. 40 mm Hg. In cases of respiratory acidosis the $P_{CO_2}$ is raised.

**$P_{O_2}$** is the symbol for the pressure of oxygen in the blood, normal being approx. 100 mm Hg in arterial blood. Levels below 70 mm Hg denote serious oxygen lack.

**pH.** This is the symbol for expressing acidity or alkalinity. The normal pH of the blood is 7·35 to 7·4. When the fetus is hypoxic the increased acid produced raises the acidity of the blood and the pH falls. When below 7·3 the fetus is at high risk and its condition vigilantly monitored: if 7·2 or below, immediate delivery is essential; 6·9 could be fatal.

**Phenylketonuria.** Sign of a hereditary disease characterised by increase of phenylalanine in the blood. The Guthrie test for phenylalanine in the blood is the most efficient method available, 1–10,000 cases are positive; one drop of blood obtained by heel prick is dripped on to the filter paper and dried, the test being done not before the 8th and prior to the 14th day of life. Early dietary therapy prevents mental retardation.

**Placenta membranacea.** A thin layer of placental tissue, covering the whole of the amniotic sac instead of being confined to one area. The condition is very rare.

**Poly-.** Prefix, meaning 'much' or 'many'; the prefix poly is now used (polyhydramnios) when describing the amount of amniotic fluid formerly known as hydramnios. Polydactyly, having supernumerary fingers or toes.

**Pre-.** Prefix, meaning 'before'; e.g. prenatal, before birth; premonitory sign, a forewarning.

**Previable baby.** One of less than 28 weeks' gestation.

**Primigravida.** Gravida, meaning 'pregnant'. A woman pregnant for the first time.

**Primipara.** Parere, meaning 'to bear'. A woman giving birth to a child for the first time. During pregnancy she is para 0. The author saw a patient, pregnant for the thirteenth time (*a case of habitual abortion*) give birth to her first baby. She was a primipara although a multigravida.

**Prone position.** Lying face downwards; e.g. semi-prone position as used in eclampsia.

**Prostaglandins.** They are a group of at least 14 naturally occurring long chain fatty acids found in most mammalian tissues and in high concentration in seminal fluid. They are concerned with processes such as intestinal motility, mediation of inflammation, fertility and parturition. Prostaglandin is liberated from the endometrium in the menstrual fluid and appears in amniotic fluid and maternal blood in increasing amounts when labour is established. It may be responsible for the release of oxytocin and the maintenance of smooth muscle tone and uterine contractions. The six prostaglandins of the E and F series are $E_1$, $E_2$, $E_3$, $F_1$, $F_2$, $F_3$. In obstetric practice $E_2$ is most widely used.

**Ptyalism.** Excessive salivation. A slight increase in salivation may occur during pregnancy, and in rare cases the excessive flow amounts to 1,000 ml per day. The woman does not swallow the saliva, because of nausea, and with loss of appetite, impaired digestion and dehydration her nutrition suffers. Sleep is interfered with. The treatment is to give fluids, intravenously if necessary, also sedatives and astringent mouthwashes. The condition is rare.

**Pubiotomy.** An operation previously performed in cases of contracted pelvis, now superseded by Caesarean section. One transverse ramus of the os pubis is divided with a Gigli saw to enlarge the pelvic brim. The baby is then born *per vaginam*.

**Pyo-.** Prefix, meaning 'pus'; e.g. pyosalpinx, pus in the Fallopian tube; pyonephrosis, pus in the kidney.

**Rectocele.** Prolapse of the rectum into the vagina.

**Recto-vaginal fistula.** This is an artificial opening between the rectum and vagina which occurs most commonly when a sutured third degree perineal tear does not heal properly. It may be suspected by the midwife when faeces are seen on the perineal pad, usually on the third or fourth day postpartum.

**Retro-.** Prefix, meaning 'behind'; e.g. retroplacental clot, a clot lying behind the placenta, occurring in severe abruptio placentae; retroversion, backward displacement (*of uterus*).

**Ringer's lactate solution.** Sodium lactate, 1·2 ml; sodium chloride, 3·0 g; potassium chloride, 0·2 g; calcium chloride, 0·1 g; water to 500 ml administered i.v. in prolonged labour and in haemorrhage until blood is available. Some add dextrose anhydrous, 25 g.

**Sex determination.** Fetal sex is being determined by measuring the concentration of testosterone in amniotic fluid. When the fetus is male, testosterone is higher during the second trimester.

**Sibling.** One of a group of children of the same parents.

**Spontaneous evolution.** A process by which the fetus may be expelled in cases of shoulder presentation. This can only occur with a large pelvis and a small fetus, and mainly when it is preterm or macerated. One arm and shoulder are forced down on to the pelvic floor and are stemmed under the pubic arch. The body, breech and limbs, in that order, are driven past the shoulder. The head is born last.

**Spontaneous expulsion.** This process begins in a manner similar to spontaneous evolution, but is even more rare. The shoulder presents and the body becomes doubled up and driven through the pelvis in that attitude until the breech and legs escape; the shoulders and head are born last.

**Spurious pregnancy.** An imaginary or phantom pregnancy. (*See under* Pseudocyesis, p. 83).

**Stridor (congenital).** This is characterised by a crowing inspiration. In the absence of cyanosis or other pathological sign, the condition may be due to a poorly developed larynx, small glottis or large epiglottis. The paediatrician will diagnose the cause.

**Superfecundation.** The fertilisation of two ova during one intermenstrual period, at different acts of coitus, will result in dizygotic twins. There is no way of proving that superfecundation has occurred.

**Superfetation.** The fertilisation of two ova during different intermenstrual periods (*the first three months of pregnancy*). This a very rare occurrence. The fact that one twin weighs 1300 to 1800 g more than the other is not diagnostic of superfetation. A fetus papyraceous is sometimes wrongly attributed to super-fetation.

**Syndrome.** A group of signs and symptoms which, when considered together characterise a disease or condition, e.g. Respiratory distress syndrome.

**Teratogen.** An agent, i.e. drug, organism, believed to cause congenital abnor-malities, e.g. Thalidomide, rubella.

**Thermo-neutral environment** is the temperature in which the baby uses the least amount of energy to keep warm, as in a heated incubator in a warm nursery.

**Trimester.** A period of three months. The nine months of pregnancy can be divided into three trimesters (*a*) The first, (*b*) second or mid, and (*c*) the third.

**Trisomy.** A chromosome additional to the normal complement = 47 instead of 46. In Down's syndrome the extra chromosome is commonly Trisomy 21.

**Vagitus uterinus.** The crying of the fetus *in utero*. If air is introduced into the fetal sac, or if gases develop and the fetus inspires these, it may emit sound during their expiration. Cases have been reported by reliable observers, in which the baby has been born alive a number of hours after 'cries' had been heard. It is a rare phenomenon.

# Index